AF806480

Reconstructive Transplantation

Raffi Gurunian • Antonio Rampazzo
Frank Papay • Bahar Bassiri Gharb
Editors

Reconstructive Transplantation

Springer

Editors
Raffi Gurunian
Department of Plastic Surgery
Cleveland Clinic
Cleveland, OH, USA

Antonio Rampazzo
Department of Plastic Surgery
Cleveland Clinic
Cleveland, OH, USA

Frank Papay
Department of Plastic Surgery
Cleveland Clinic
Cleveland, OH, USA

Bahar Bassiri Gharb
Department of Plastic Surgery
Cleveland Clinic
Cleveland, OH, USA

ISBN 978-3-031-21519-3 ISBN 978-3-031-21520-9 (eBook)
https://doi.org/10.1007/978-3-031-21520-9

© Springer Nature Switzerland AG 2023, corrected publication 2023
This work is subject to copyright. All rights are reserved by the Publisher, whether the whole or part of the material is concerned, specifically the rights of translation, reprinting, reuse of illustrations, recitation, broadcasting, reproduction on microfilms or in any other physical way, and transmission or information storage and retrieval, electronic adaptation, computer software, or by similar or dissimilar methodology now known or hereafter developed.
The use of general descriptive names, registered names, trademarks, service marks, etc. in this publication does not imply, even in the absence of a specific statement, that such names are exempt from the relevant protective laws and regulations and therefore free for general use.
The publisher, the authors, and the editors are safe to assume that the advice and information in this book are believed to be true and accurate at the date of publication. Neither the publisher nor the authors or the editors give a warranty, expressed or implied, with respect to the material contained herein or for any errors or omissions that may have been made. The publisher remains neutral with regard to jurisdictional claims in published maps and institutional affiliations.

This Springer imprint is published by the registered company Springer Nature Switzerland AG
The registered company address is: Gewerbestrasse 11, 6330 Cham, Switzerland

Preface

In 1869, the first successful skin transplant was performed by renowned Swiss surgeon Jacques-Louis Reverdin. Along with the advent of transplantation immunology, the beginning of the twentieth century witnessed the emergence of vascularized composite allograft transplantation (VCA), which has become the highest level of reconstruction in human history. Since then numerous VCAs have been reported globally. VCAs have made replacement of complex tissues possible in a 3-dimensional form providing both function and aesthetic, particularly in case of upper extremity and face transplantations.

I am humbled to have the opportunity to participate in one of the most challenging and complex microsurgical reconstructions as part of the face transplantation team at Cleveland Clinic, performing the second and the third transplants in 2014 and 2017, respectively. These unforgettable transplantation experiences inspired me to compile the book *Reconstructive Transplantation* whose idea was born in 2019 with an aim to gather global knowledge that has been gained in various VCAs performed in humans.

The book was tremendously set back by the Covid pandemic, and its production was certainly delayed due to unforeseen factors. Despite all the hardships, it gives me great pleasure to see that the book is finally published.

Chapters of this book have been contributed by eminent surgeons and physicians both nationally and internationally in the field of VCA. They made history by having performed technically and immunologically challenging VCAs with exceptional outcomes. Also, failures and lessons learned have been reported with honesty. I am sincerely thankful to all the contributing authors, and my co-editors Antonio Rampazzo, MD, Frank Papay, MD, and Bahar Bassiri Gharb, MD, for their unrelenting hard work they put in for the creation of this book.

The book begins with a chapter "History of VCA" contributed by Dr. Maria Siemionow who relentlessly paved the road for VCA beginning with landmark animal studies in the 1990s and finally accomplishing the first US face transplant in 2008 at Cleveland Clinic Foundation.

There are 34 chapters in the book, 19 of which have been allocated to face and upper extremity transplantations as these have been the most frequently performed VCAs across the world. One exceptionally well-written chapter is dedicated to immunosuppressive protocols in VCA. In addition, abdominal wall, lower extremity, knee and penile transplantation chapters are included. All these chapters reflect global VCA practices, immunosuppressive protocols used, and outcomes from countries such as the Unites States, Canada, Germany, Austria, France, Spain, Poland, Finland, Italy, India, and Turkey. While chapters on the same subject show similarities in technique and immunosuppressive regimens, the reader will be able to appreciate unique variances and nuances among chapters contributed by different authors. Also included are special chapters on laryngeal transplantation, and uterus transplantation that shed light on their current state. Successful uterus transplantations have made live births possible, which was once unimaginable and unthinkable.

Reconstructive Transplantation provides a historical snapshot of VCA across the world at this point in time, which is an accumulation of decades of hard work and research globally. I hope this book will be considered as a paramount resource in this regard.

The chapters of this book are testament that technical challenges in VCA have been largely overcome so far. As it stands today, rejection remains a significant challenge, and maintenance requires life-long use of immunosuppressive treatment which carries significant risk of malignancy and infection. The future of VCA will depend on de-sensitization and advances in immunomodulating protocols with a hope that one day immunological tolerance can be achieved for better outcomes.

Cleveland, OH, USA Raffi Gurunian

Contents

Contributors

Andrew Atia Division of Plastic, Maxillofacial, and Oral Surgery, Department of Surgery, Duke University Medical Center, Durham, NC, USA

Mario A. Aycart Division of Plastic Surgery, Brigham and Women's Hospital, Boston, MA, USA

Juan P. Barret Department of Plastic Surgery and Burns, Vall d'Hebron Barcelona Hospital Campus, Universitat Autònoma de Barcelona, Barcelona, Spain

Maureen Beederman Section of Plastic and Reconstructive Surgery, The University of Chicago Medicine, Chicago, IL, USA

Massimo Del Bene Plastic Surgery, Monza, Italy

Steven L. Bernard Department of Plastic Surgery, Cleveland Clinic, Cleveland, OH, USA

Laxminarayan Bhandari CM Kleinert Institute for Hand and Microsurgery, Louisville, KY, USA

Kleinert Kutz Hand Care Center, Louisville, KY, USA

Department of Surgery, University of Louisville, Louisville, KY, USA

Daniel E. Borsuk Maisonneuve Rosemont Hospital, Montreal, QC, Canada

Sainte-Justine University Healthcare Centre, Montreal, QC, Canada

Division of Plastic and Reconstructive Surgery, University of Montreal, Montreal, QC, Canada

Daniel Bula Oncologic and Reconstructive Surgery, Maria Sklodowska-Curie, National Research Institute of Oncology, Gliwice Branch, Gliwice, Poland

Antonio Peri di Caprio Ospedale San Gerardo—Monza, Monza, Italy

Matteo Cescon General Surgery and Transplantation Unit, IRCCS Azienda Ospedaliero-Universitaria di Bologna, Bologna, Italy

Curtis L. Cetrulo Jr Division of Plastic Surgery, Massachusetts General Hospital, Boston, MA, USA

Harvard Medical School, Boston, MA, USA

Riccardo Cipriani Plastic Surgery, IRCCS Azienda Ospedaliero-Universitaria di Bologna, Bologna, Italy

Federico Contedini Plastic Surgery, IRCCS Azienda Ospedaliero-Universitaria di Bologna, Bologna, Italy

Jennifer Cooley USAISR - The United States Army Institute of Surgical Research, San Antonio, TX, USA

Demetrius M. Coombs Department of Plastic Surgery, Cleveland Clinic, Cleveland, OH, USA

Giuseppe D'Amico Department of General Surgery, Transplantation Center, Digestive Disease and Surgery Institute, Cleveland Clinic, Cleveland, OH, USA

Stephanie Dapke UR-7516 CHIMERE, Amiens, France

Bernard Devauchelle Department of Maxillofacial Surgery, CHU Amiens-Picardie, Facing Faces Institute, Amiens, France

Michael Diefenbeck Scientific Consulting in Orthopedic Surgery, Hamburg, Germany

Risal Djohan Department of Plastic Surgery, Cleveland Clinic, Cleveland, OH, USA

Nasuh Utku Dogan Department of Gynecology, Faculty of Medicine, Akdeniz University, Antalya, Turkey

Jean Michel Dubernard Department of Transplantation, Hôpital Edouard Herriot, HCL, Lyon, France

Bijan Eghtesad Transplantation Center, Cleveland Clinic, Cleveland, OH, USA

Detlev Erdmann Division of Plastic, Maxillofacial, and Oral Surgery, Department of Surgery, Duke University Medical Center, Durham, NC, USA

Mustafa Gökhan Ertosun Department of Plastic, Reconstructive, and Aesthetic Surgery, Akdeniz University School of Medicine, Antalya, Turkey

Tommaso Falcone Obstetrics and Gynecology and Women's Health Institute, Cleveland Clinic, Cleveland, OH, USA

D. Gregory Farwell Department of Otolaryngology Head and Neck Surgery, University of California-Davis Medical Center, Sacramento, CA, USA

Department of Otolaryngology-Head and Neck Surgery, University of Pennsylvania Health System, Philadelphia, PA, USA

Brian Gastman Department of Plastic Surgery, Cleveland Clinic, Cleveland, OH, USA

Aram Gazarian Chirurgie de la Main et du Membre Supérieur, Hôpital Edouard Herriot, HCL, Lyon, France

Chiara Gelati Plastic Surgery, IRCCS Azienda Ospedaliero-Universitaria di Bologna, Bologna, Italy

Bahar Bassiri Gharb Department of Plastic Surgery, Cleveland Clinic, Cleveland, OH, USA

Jordan Gornitsky Maisonneuve Rosemont Hospital, Montreal, QC, Canada

Lawrence J. Gottlieb Section of Plastic and Reconstructive Surgery, The University of Chicago Medicine, Chicago, IL, USA

Marion Goutard Division of Plastic Surgery, Massachusetts General Hospital, Boston, MA, USA

Harvard Medical School, Boston, MA, USA

Devajyoti Guin Department of Plastic and Reconstructive Surgery, Amrita Hospital, Faridabad, Haryana, India

Raffi Gurunian Department of Plastic Surgery, Cleveland Clinic, Cleveland, OH, USA

John E. Hanks Department of Otolaryngology Head and Neck Surgery, Boston University School of Medicine, VA Boston Healthcare System, Jamaica Plain, MA, USA

Alexander de Heinrich Department of Plastic, Reconstructive, Hand and Burn Surgery, Munich Clinic Bogenhausen, Academic Teaching Hospital Technical University Munich, Munich, Germany

Department of Surgery, University Hospital for Visceral, Transplant and Thoracic Surgery, Medical University of Innsbruck, Innsbruck, Austria

Office of Plastic and Reconstructive Surgery, Munich, Germany

Jorge Andres Hernandez Division of Plastic, Maxillofacial, and Oral Surgery, Department of Surgery, Duke University Medical Center, Durham, NC, USA

Gunther O. Hofmann Klinik für Unfall-, Hand- und Wiederherstellungschirurgie, Universitätsklinikum Jena, Jena, Germany

Klinik für Unfall- und Wiederherstellungschirurgie, Berufsgenossenschaftliches Klinikum Bergmannstrost, Halle (Saale), Germany

Andrew Hollins Division of Plastic, Maxillofacial, and Oral Surgery, Department of Surgery, Duke University Medical Center, Durham, NC, USA

Liza Johannesson Annette C. and Harold C. Simmons Transplant Institute, Baylor University Medical Center, Dallas, TX, USA

Jean Kanitakis Department of Dermatology, Hôpital Edouard Herriot, HCL, Lyon, France

Hülya Kapucu Wake Forest University Health Sciences, Wake Forest Institute for Regenerative Medicine, Winston Salem, NC, USA

Nima Khavanin Department of Plastic and Reconstructive Surgery, Johns Hopkins University School of Medicine, Baltimore, MD, USA

Sarah E. Kinsley Division of Plastic Surgery, Brigham and Women's Hospital, Boston, MA, USA

Martin H. Kirschner Ludwig-Maximilians-University of Munich Klinikum Großhadern, Munich, Germany

Łukasz Krakowczyk Oncologic and Reconstructive Surgery, Maria Sklodowska-Curie, National Research Institute of Oncology, Gliwice Branch, Gliwice, Poland

Arda Küçükgüven Plastic, Reconstructive and Aesthetic Surgery Clinic, University of Health Sciences, Ankara Training and Research Hospital, Ankara, Turkey

Patrik Lassus Department of Plastic Surgery, Helsinki University Hospital, University of Helsinki, Helsinki, Finland

Alexandre G. Lellouch Division of Plastic Surgery, Massachusetts General Hospital, Boston, MA, USA

Harvard Medical School, Boston, MA, USA

L. Scott Levin Department of Surgery, Division of Plastic Surgery, Hospital of the University of Pennsylvania, Philadelphia, PA, USA

Benedetto Longo Division of Plastic and Reconstructive Surgery – Breast Unit, Tor Vergata University Hospital, Department of Surgical Sciences, School of Medicine and Surgery, Tor Vergata University of Rome, Rome, Italy

Robert R. Lorenz The Head and Neck Institute, Cleveland Clinic, Cleveland, OH, USA

David G. Lott Division of Laryngology; Otolaryngology-Head and Neck Surgery, Mayo Clinic Arizona, Phoenix, AZ, USA

Head and Neck Regenerative Medicine and Transplantation Program, Mayo Clinic Arizona, Phoenix, AZ, USA

Elise Lupon Division of Plastic Surgery, Massachusetts General Hospital, Boston, MA, USA

Harvard Medical School, Boston, MA, USA

Adam Maciejewski Oncologic and Reconstructive Surgery, Maria Sklodowska-Curie, National Research Institute of Oncology, Gliwice Branch, Gliwice, Poland

Christine McAndrew Department of Surgery, Division of Plastic Surgery, Hospital of the University of Pennsylvania, Philadelphia, PA, USA

Pratik Mehta Annette C. and Harold C. Simmons Transplant Institute, Baylor University Medical Center, Dallas, TX, USA

Zvjezdana Milacak Department of Plastic, Reconstructive, Hand and Burn Surgery, Munich Clinic Bogenhausen, Academic Teaching Hospital Technical University Munich, Munich, Germany

Department of Surgery, University Hospital for Visceral, Transplant and Thoracic Surgery, Medical University of Innsbruck, Innsbruck, Austria

Maria Elisa Lozano Miralles Plastic Surgery, IRCCS Azienda Ospedaliero-Universitaria di Bologna, Bologna, Italy

Plastic Surgery, Policlinico di Modena, University of Modena and Reggio Emilia, Modena, Italy

Emmanuel Morelon Department of Transplantation, Hôpital Edouard Herriot, HCL, Lyon, France

Claude Bernard Lyon I University, Lyon, France

Gaetano Musumarra Ospedale San Gerardo—Monza, Monza, Italy

Amit Nair Division of Transplantation/Hepatobiliary Surgery, University of Rochester, Rochester, NY, USA

Serdar Nazif Nasir Department of Plastic, Reconstructive and Aesthetic Surgery, Hacettepe University Faculty of Medicine, Ankara, Turkey

Marina Ninkovic Department of Plastic, Reconstructive, Hand and Burn Surgery, Munich Clinic Bogenhausen, Academic Teaching Hospital Technical University Munich, Munich, Germany

Department of Surgery, University Hospital for Visceral, Transplant and Thoracic Surgery, Medical University of Innsbruck, Innsbruck, Austria

Milomir Ninkovic Department of Plastic, Reconstructive, Hand and Burn Surgery, Munich Clinic Bogenhausen, Academic Teaching Hospital Technical University Munich, Munich, Germany

Department of Surgery, University Hospital for Visceral, Transplant and Thoracic Surgery, Medical University of Innsbruck, Innsbruck, Austria

Office of Plastic and Reconstructive Surgery, Munich, Germany

Jakub Opyrchał Oncologic and Reconstructive Surgery, Maria Sklodowska-Curie, National Research Institute of Oncology, Gliwice Branch, Gliwice, Poland

Ömer Özkan Department of Plastic, Reconstructive, and Aesthetic Surgery, Akdeniz University School of Medicine, Antalya, Turkey

Department of Plastic, Reconstructive, and Aesthetic Surgery, Akdeniz University School of Medicine, Antalya, Turkey

Özlenen Özkan Department of Plastic Surgery, Faculty of Medicine, Akdeniz University, Antalya, Turkey

Department of Plastic, Reconstructive, and Aesthetic Surgery, Akdeniz University School of Medicine, Antalya, Turkey

Tuna Özyürekoglu CM Kleinert Institute for Hand and Microsurgery, Louisville, KY, USA

Kleinert Kutz Hand Care Center, Louisville, KY, USA

Department of Surgery, University of Louisville, Louisville, KY, USA

Department of Orthopedics, University of Louisville, Louisville, KY, USA

Frank Papay Department of Plastic Surgery, Cleveland Clinic, Cleveland, OH, USA

Palmina Petruzzo Department of Transplantation, Hôpital Edouard Herriot, HCL, Lyon, France

Department of Surgery, University of Cagliari, Cagliari, Italy

Antonio Daniele Pinna Abdominal Transplant Center, Weston, FL, USA

Valentina Pinto Plastic Surgery, IRCCS Azienda Ospedaliero-Universitaria di Bologna, Bologna, Italy

Fabio Santanelli di Pompeo Division of Plastic Surgery, Sant'Andrea Hospital, NESMOS Department, School of Medicine and Psychology, "Sapienza" University of Rome, Rome, Italy

Luca Del Prete Department of General Surgery, Transplantation Center, Digestive Disease and Surgery Institute, Cleveland Clinic, Cleveland, OH, USA

Cristiano Quintini Department of General Surgery, Transplantation Center, Digestive Disease and Surgery Institute, Cleveland Clinic, Cleveland, OH, USA

Antonio Rampazzo Department of Plastic Surgery, Cleveland Clinic, Cleveland, OH, USA

G. Srilekha Reddy Department of Plastic and Reconstructive Surgery, Amrita Institute of Medical Sciences, Kochi, Kerala, India

Richard J. Redett Department of Plastic and Reconstructive Surgery, Johns Hopkins University School of Medicine, Baltimore, MD, USA

Stephanie Ricci Obstetrics and Gynecology and Women's Health Institute, Cleveland Clinic, Cleveland, OH, USA

Elliott Richards Obstetrics and Gynecology and Women's Health Institute, Cleveland Clinic, Cleveland, OH, USA

Leonardo V. Riella Department of Medicine, Massachusetts General Hospital, Boston, MA, USA

Eli Saleh Maisonneuve Rosemont Hospital, Montreal, QC, Canada

Graham S. Schwarz Department of Plastic Surgery, Cleveland Clinic, Cleveland, OH, USA

Viviana M. Serra López Department of Surgery, Division of Plastic Surgery, Hospital of the University of Pennsylvania, Philadelphia, PA, USA

Mohit Sharma Department of Plastic and Reconstructive Surgery, Amrita Hospital, Faridabad, Haryana, India

Maria Z. Siemionow Department of Orthopaedics, University of Illinois at Chicago, College of Medicine, Chicago, IL, USA

Nicholas R. Sinclair Department of Plastic Surgery, Cleveland Clinic, Cleveland, OH, USA

Andrea Sisti Department of Surgery, University of Texas Medical Branch (UTMB), Galveston, TX, USA

Zvi Steinberger Department of Surgery, Division of Plastic Surgery, Hospital of the University of Pennsylvania, Philadelphia, PA, USA

Simon G. Talbot Upper Extremity Transplantation, Brigham and Women's Hospital, Boston, MA, USA

Harvard Medical School, Boston, MA, USA

Pierre Tawa Division of Plastic Surgery, Massachusetts General Hospital, Boston, MA, USA

Harvard Medical School, Boston, MA, USA

Giuliano Testa Annette C. and Harold C. Simmons Transplant Institute, Baylor University Medical Center, Dallas, TX, USA

Sylvie Testelin Department of Maxillofacial Surgery, CHU Amiens-Picardie, Facing Faces Institute, Amiens, France

Chad M. Teven Northwestern University Feinberg School of Medicine, Chicago, IL, USA

Philipp Tratnig-Frankl Division of Plastic Surgery, Massachusetts General Hospital, Boston, MA, USA

Harvard Medical School, Boston, MA, USA

Dmitry Tuder Alamo Orthopedics, San Antonio, TX, USA

Fatma B. Tuncer Division of Plastic Surgery, University of Utah School of Medicine, Salt Lake City, UT, USA

Andreas Tzakis Department of General Surgery, Transplantation Center, Digestive Disease and Surgery Institute, Cleveland Clinic, Cleveland, OH, USA

Anil Vaidya Department of General Surgery, Transplantation Center, Digestive Disease and Surgery Institute, Cleveland Clinic, Cleveland, OH, USA

Frithjof Wagner Berufsgenossenschaftliche Unfallklinik Murnau, Murnau am Staffelsee, Germany

Abhijeet Wakure Department of Plastic and Reconstructive Surgery, VPS Lakeshore Hospital and Research Center, Kochi, Kerala, India

Erin L. Weber Department of Surgery, Division of Plastic Surgery, Hospital of the University of Pennsylvania, Philadelphia, PA, USA

Chiara Zanfi General Surgery and Transplantation Unit, IRCCS Azienda Ospedaliero-Universitaria di Bologna, Bologna, Italy

Fatih Zor Department of Surgery, Wake Forest University Health Sciences, Wake Forest Institute for Regenerative Medicine, Winston Salem, NC, USA

Part I
Introduction

History of Vascularized Composite Allotransplantation

1

Maria Z. Siemionow, Hülya Kapucu, and Fatih Zor

1.1 Introduction

The longer you look back, the farther you can look forward
Winston Churchill

Reconstruction of severe tissue loss such as complex facial defects and limb amputations is one of the most challenging procedures of reconstructive surgery. In a survey, members of American Council of Academic Plastic Surgeons (ACAPS) and the Southeastern Society of Plastic and Reconstructive Surgeons (SESPRS) agreed that microsurgery is one of the most important plastic surgery innovation of the past decades. The advancement of microsurgery during the last century opened new reconstructive options for defects which were not previously reconstructible [1]. Vascularized composite allotransplantation (VCA), which was formerly known as the Composite Tissue Allotransplantation (CTA) has emerged as a new application of microsurgery. This new field of reconstructive surgery has gained significant interest in a short period of time. Compared to innovations of the past, ACAPS and SESPRS members agreed that VCA (which includes hand and face transplantation) is considered one of the five most important innovations of the modern era [2]. Currently, VCA represents the highest level of the reconstruction pyramid, and thus the outcomes are expected to outweigh what the "classical" reconstructive surgery can offer even with the application of the most advanced microsurgical techniques. Another worldwide survey among plastic surgeons confirmed that major changes in hand surgery and craniomaxillofacial surgery will be related to the VCA transplantation in the future [3].

The history of VCA revealed that clinical applications of solid organ transplantation (SOT) proceeded for many decades the first applications of VCA. The main reason for this late introduction of VCA relies on many differences between SOT and VCA [4]. VCA is still considered as primarily a non-lifesaving procedure and consists of a number of tissues, including skin, subcutaneous tissue, muscles, nerves, tendons, bones and cartilage, and arteries and veins, with each tissue representing a different immunogenic response [5, 6]. The heterogeneous tissue composition of VCA transplants introduces potentially more significant immunogenic response compared to solid organ transplants [7]. These unique features of VCA are responsible for a slower pace of progress in the field of VCA. In this chapter, we will present the history of VCA transplantation from the first anecdotal reports in the ancient times to the current applications of VCA in reconstructive surgery.

1.2 VCA Records in the Ancient History

1.2.1 Transplantation in the Antient Times

The idea of transplanting tissues or organs is almost as old as the human history. Greek mythology and religious texts presented many examples such as Icarus and his father Daedalus who tried to fly with the support of the bird wings, and the Chimera which represented the coexistence of three different organisms: the goat, the lion, and the dragon [8, 9]. The concept of transplantation was reported in the Egyptian, Chinese, Indian, and early Christian mythology as early as 2000 BC. Lord Ganesha, in a myth from the twelfth century BC, is one of the best-known and most-worshipped deities in Hinduism. After being beheaded, an elephant's head was attached to Ganesha's body by his father, thus bringing him back to life with the divine attributes [10, 11]. This myth is

M. Z. Siemionow (✉)
Department of Orthopaedics, University of Illinois at Chicago, College of Medicine, Chicago, IL, USA
e-mail: siemiom@uic.edu

H. Kapucu · F. Zor
Department of Surgery, Wake Forest University Health Sciences, Wake Forest Institute for Regenerative Medicine, Winston Salem, NC, USA
e-mail: fzor@wakehealth.edu

© Springer Nature Switzerland AG 2023
R. Gurunian et al. (eds.), *Reconstructive Transplantation*, https://doi.org/10.1007/978-3-031-21520-9_1

the first documented and successful example of the brain and head transplantation, which still inspires both the transplant and the neurosurgical community [12, 13].

In ancient Chinese texts, doctor Pien Ch'iao exchanged the hearts of two warriors to equally balance the good spirits in both the individuals. This document not only described the surgery but also mentioned the use of potent drugs to aid in the healing process, thus emphasizing the importance of the posttransplant period which is still the main challenge in transplantation [14]. In the Old Testament, Ezekiel, referring to the heart transplant, said, 'I will also give you a new heart ... I will remove the stony heart from its flesh and give you a flesh heart,' and was perhaps the one of the oldest reference to a heart allograft transplant [15]. Despite many ancient reports on transplantation concept from Chinese and Eastern literature, perhaps the most famous myth about transplantation in the antiquity is the event known as the "black leg miracle" reported by Saint Cosmas and Saint Damian in the third century AD. These twin brothers successfully transplanted the leg of a recently deceased Ethiopian Moor by replacing the malignant and gangrenous foot of an elderly Roman soldier in church. This myth has created the new concept of cadaver transplantation. Although these myths are not derived from the historical facts, they show that the fascination with human transplantation has been around for many centuries [16, 17].

During post-classical period, there are only few reports on transplantation, such as Chinese doctor Hua Tuo who was known to replace the diseased organs with the healthy ones. Unfortunately, all of Tuo's medical texts were destroyed and his surgical procedures were prohibited [18].

1.2.2 Transplantation During Modern History

The field of transplantation during the modern history was mainly focused on autotransplantation.

In the second century BC, Indian surgeon Sushruta, who pioneered skin grafting and rotational pedicle flaps for nasal reconstruction, laid the foundations of plastic surgery by describing more than a dozen ways of how to reconstruct the ears and the lips [19]. Advances in skin grafting techniques continued throughout the fifteenth century AD, leading to optimization of these surgical techniques. In the sixteenth century, Gaspare Tagliacozzi, a specialist in the rhinoplasty, successfully performed a nasal reconstruction on a patient who lost his nose, using a flap from the patient's upper arm [20].

Allografts were widely used during this period; however, success was not achieved when compared with the autografts. Since the allografts were always failing, Tagliacozzi and other surgeon-scientists discovered that this was probably due to "*the force and power of individuality*" [21]. This can be accepted as the first report on the human as well as tissues individuality and could be referred to the transplant immunology, emphasizing the importance of the origin of the transplanted tissues. Resurrected in London in the early 1800s, plastic surgery and transplantation became popular again after successes with the free skin grafts. During the second half of the 1800s, other methods of organ transplantation such as parabiosis were investigated. This was the physical union of two living animals of the same species. Although, never successful, these studies concluded that the higher is the animal in the phylogenetic scale, there was the greater difficulty in achieving successful transplantation [22]. Around the same time, the public noticed the activities of the tooth transplant recipients, and the experimental transplant studies in France were the subject of protests by some groups [23].

1.2.3 History of Transplant Biology

Early 1900s focused on investigating the unsuccessful outcomes of the allotransplantations and transplant biology. The studies during this period concluded that there are individual differences or complex protein substances within each cell that cause rejection of the transplanted tissue. These studies also led to a belief that transplantation between individuals is impossible due to the inherent differences between individuals at the cellular level [24]. In addition to the donor-related differences, Holman showed increased immunity to the second grafting, concluding that "*each group of grafts develops its own antibody*" [25]. Experience gained by skin grafting between identical twins and successful transplantation outcomes provided information and courage necessary to proceed with kidney transplantation two decades later [26].

During the Second World War, Medewar conducted several studies on skin grafting and rejection. He succeeded for the first time to take microscopic pictures showing the transplant rejection in great detail and called the process as actively acquired immune reaction [21]. Owen performed studies in cattle twins which shared circulatory system due to union of the placentas. He was granted to be the first to prove that two genetic types can live together in the same organism without any rejection signs [27]. Owen postulated that seeding of the each other's bone marrow before birth caused cross-colonization and permitted the two different blood types to live together resulting in tolerance. In 1953, Brent and Medawar succeeded to experimentally overcome the allogeneic barrier which was reported for the first time in the literature [28]. Their experiment was based on the recapitulation of Owen's observation in mice. Briefly, they injected spleen cells from the skin-donor strain into the embryo of the recipient strain and showed that these mice tolerated allogeneic skin from the donor mice. During the same time, studies from Simonson and Mitchison demonstrated that acute allograft rejection was not mediated by the antibodies but by the direct attack of the lymphocytes [29, 30]. These studies became the cornerstone of the current concept of the tolerogenic immunomodulation and conditioning studies.

1.2.4 Brief History of Immunosuppression

The first greatest contribution to experimental and clinical transplantation was the establishment and progress of microsurgical techniques and free tissue transfers [31]. Following Murphy, who successfully anastomosed femoral artery of a wounded soldier in 1897, Alexis Carrel described reproducible technique for vascular anastomosis as well as methods for transplantation of whole organs and was awarded the Nobel Prize for pioneering vascular anastomosis techniques and as recognition of his work on organ transplantation [32]. The second groundbreaking progress was the innovation of the induced immunosuppression which was first provided by the total body irradiation (TBI) in rodents to prevent skin graft rejection, and this concept was later used in humans [33]. The side effects of the TBI limited its use and caused emergence of novel immunosuppressive drugs. Antimetabolite 6-mercaptopurine was the first potent immunosuppressive drug used in experimental and clinical transplantation [34, 35]. The first immunosuppressive combination protocol including azathioprine and corticosteroid was later developed by Starzl et al. and became the standard immunosuppressive therapy [36]. The advent of cyclosporine (CsA) made a major contribution to the organ transplantation by dramatically improving allograft survival and making widespread clinical application of the extrarenal transplantation possible [37].

1.3 History of Experimental VCA

The success of clinical VCA depends on experimental studies as well as experience with the solid organ transplantation studies, and both can be considered as the "pathfinders" for the development field of VCA. Experimental animal models constitute the workhorse of the VCA as they help to determine the technical feasibility and evaluate the effects of various immunosuppressive protocols and novel tolerance inducing strategies. Following Carrel's introduction of vascular anastomosis, Ullmann performed the first experimental kidney transplantation, Carrel and Guthrie performed the first heart transplant in animals, which was followed by other investigators. However, all the attempts undertaken have failed invariably.

After the proven efficacy of various immunosuppressives protocols, numerous research teams began investigating limb allograft transplant models in the rats, dogs, and rabbits. Over the past 20 years, many VCA models have been developed to test transplantation of different body parts and to assess effects of various immunosuppressive protocols. Experimental models can be divided into two main categories, small and large animal models, which can further be classified according to the transplanted organ and/or tissue as presented in Table 1.1 [38]:

Table 1.1 Experimental models of the VCA and their specific features

	Experimental model	Tissues included and specific features
Skin containing VCA models	Groin flap/extended groin flap	Skin, fat, and lymphoid tissue. Simple, used in immunologic studies, small skin component
	Semimembranosus muscle and epigastric skin transplant model	Skin, fat, muscle, and lymphoid tissue. Used for microcirculatory, physiologic, and immunologic studies
	Total abdominal wall transplant model	Skin, fat muscle, and lymphoid tissue. Contains large skin component
Hindlimb models	Rat hindlimb transplant model[a]	Popular, technically challenging, contains all tissue components including vascularized bone marrow and nerve
	Groin-thigh osteomyocutaneous transplant model	Alternative model to hind limb transplant less challenging technique, low mortality
Immuno-modulatory VCA models	Unilateral or bilateral vascularized femur transplant model	Femoral bone, bone marrow, cartilage and muscle, applied for bone marrow-induced chimerism studies
	Composite vascularized skin/bone transplant model	Combination of groin flap with vascularized femur transplantation, enables follow-up of rejection
	Vascularized osteomyocutaneous iliac transplant model	Iliac bone, bone marrow, abdominal wall musculature, and wide skin island
	Vascularized sternum transplant model	Sternum, skin and muscles. Contains bone marrow
	Thymus transplant model	Used for evaluation of effect of thymus on tolerance induction
	Osteomyocutaneous sternum, ribs, thymus, pectoralis muscles, and skin transplant	Includes all three important immunologic tissues (bone marrow, thymus, and skin) for immunology and tolerance studies

(continued)

Table 1.1 (continued)

	Experimental model	Tissues included and specific features
Facial allograft models	Full face/scalp transplant model	Includes ear, neck, and facial skin without eyelids and nose, high mortality
	Hemiface/scalp transplant model	Unilateral ear, neck, and facial skin. Used for immunologic studies in facial transplantation
	Hemiface calvarium transplant model	Temporal muscle and parietal bone included to hemiface scalp model, contains bone marrow
	Hemiface mandible tongue allotransplantation model	Mandibular bone and tongue are included into hemiface model. Contains bone marrow
	Maxilla transplant model	Response of maxillary bone to transplantation
	Midface transplant model with sensory and motor units	First model to evaluate motor and sensory recovery after face transplantation
	Total osteocutaneous hemiface transplant model	Includes entire hemiface: vascularized nose, premaxilla, eyelids, upper and lower lips, external ear, and facial skin for immunological, histological, and biological evaluation of different facial tissues
	Composite face and eyeball transplant model	Evaluation of optic nerve regeneration and evaluation of orbit content
Other models	Penis transplant model	Penis including corpora cavernosa and spongiosum
	Uterus transplant model	Uterus
	Larynx transplant model	Larynx, trachea and thyroid gland

Yellow color—models already translated to clinical application, green color—models not translated to clinical application yet
[a] Clinically translated as upper extremity transplant

1.3.1 Rat Hindlimb Allotransplantation Model

The rat hindlimb transplantation model was described by Shapiro and Cerra in 1978 [39]. The orthotopic hind limb transplant model in the rat can be used for functional, immunological, and ischemia-reperfusion studies [40]. Hindlimb transplantation in the rat is a complex procedure involving bones, muscles, nerves, vessels, and skin. Based on the publications, the rat hindlimb transplantation model has been used successfully in many functional and immunological studies and therefore may be considered as the current gold standard animal model tested in the reconstructive transplantation research.

The access to standard VCA models allows for reliable and reproducible surgical procedure where robust and reproducible data can be collected for the statistical assessment and comparative analysis.

1.3.2 Rat Face Transplantation Models

There are several face transplantation models including full face, hemiface, and various facial subunits transplantation, which were developed to evaluate survival as well as immune response of various facial structures [41]. Siemionow et al. were the first to develop a full-face scalp allotransplantation model in rats, which was based on the bilateral common carotid artery and external jugular vein [42]. However, the surgical procedure of full-face transplantation was challenging with a high mortality rate which led to the development of combined hemi-face/scalp allotransplantation model. This technique was further modified to form the basis for the development of different facial allograft models by inclusion of various craniomaxillofacial subunits [43]. The first model that evaluated the motor and sensory recovery after facial allotransplantation was developed by Zor et al. [44]. This composite midface transplant model with the sensory and motor neuromuscular units included premaxilla, mystacial pad, and nose and included the infraorbital and facial nerves. A total osteocutaneous hemifacial allotransplantation model was developed in order to extend the application of the combined face/scalp transplantation in the rat model [45]. This new model, which included all hemifacial soft tissues as well as the premaxillary bone segment with nose components, enabled immunological, histological, and biological evaluation of different facial tissues and structures in the one complex composite allotransplantation scenario. The most recent advancement in facial allotransplantation models is the development of composite face and eyeball allotransplant model with the optic nerve [46]. This experimental model allows for the evaluation of optic nerve regeneration and the effect of allotransplantation on the composite facial tissues including periorbital contents.

1.3.3 Immunomodulatory VCA Models

With the advent of tolerance inducting strategies, immunomodulatory models have been described for better understanding of transplantation tolerance. These models include vascularized bone and bone marrow transplantation and immunologically privileged tissue transfers, such as thymus, in order to assess correlation between donor specific chimerism and immune tolerance. Vascularized bone marrow transplantation was described by Agaoglu [47], confirming efficient engraftment of donor cells into the recipient's bone marrow compartment, leading to the development and maintenance of chimerism. Another method of tolerance induction in the experimental studies was tested after thymus transplantation. The first thymus transplantation was described by Jiang et al. in 1999 and was tested thereafter in different research scenarios. One of the important and complex models to study VCA acceptance and rejection was the composite osseomusculocutaneous sternum, ribs, thymus, pectoralis muscles, and skin allotransplantation model [48, 49]. This model including three important immunological tissues (bone marrow, thymus, and skin) demonstrated the direct effects of thymus transplantation on the induction and maintenance of the donor-specific chimerism [48, 49].

1.3.4 Large Animal Models

Large VCA animal models are accepted as the preclinical translational models developed for the assessment of feasibility of different immunosuppressive protocols in preparation to the clinical VCA application. Several large animal models of VCA including dogs, rabbits, and swine have been described [50, 51].

Ustuner et al. reported the transplantation of a radial forelimb osteomyocutaneous flap transplants between size-matched, outbred pigs using a daily oral regimen of CsA, MMF, and prednisone [52, 53]. The same group also reported visual scoring of skin rejection in swine VCA model [54]. Swine hemi-facial composite tissue allotransplantation model was developed by Kuo et al. to investigate the new strategies for preclinical facial allotransplantation studies [55]. Later Villamaria et al. described gracilis myocutaneous flap allotransplantation model in swine. This model included a large quantity of muscle which enabled evaluation of the effects of ischemia reperfusion injury on the allograft survival [56]. Swine heterotopic hind limb transplant model included transplantation of partial limb of donor animal to the groin of the recipient. This model is used to study the role of different protocols and donor bone marrow infusion on VCA survival [57]. Finally, porcine orthotopic forelimb vascularized composite allotransplantation model was described by Fries et al. and represents the first load-bearing porcine limb transplant model. The authors reported on their technical, procedural, and logistic experiences [58]. The porcine model has also served to investigate techniques to induce tolerance to the VCA transplants [59, 60]. A preclinical swine model of whole eyeball transplantation was described by Pittsburgh group [61].

Non-human primate (NHP) models of VCA were studied primarily in Cynomolgus monkeys. The first successful model of facial VCA including facial subunits (skin, muscle, bone) have been described by Barth et al. This model provided a platform for further investigation of VCA tolerance and preclinical immunosuppressive protocols [62]. Later, the same group presented prolonged survival of facial VCA under tacrolimus treatment. However, a very high rate of posttransplant lymphoproliferative disorder (PTLD) was reported with this protocol [63]. In another study, Barth et al. investigated the effect of vascularized bone marrow (VBM) component on the allograft survival. They showed that VBM containing grafts demonstrated prolonged rejection-free survival when compared to VCA without VBM. This is the first study in large animal model confirming immunomodulatory role of VBM [64]. Later, Mundinger et al. developed a fibular VCA model in NHP to investigate the healing and the rejection patterns of bone component and associated tissues [65]. In contrast to the literature reports and clinical evidence, they reported early skin loss, replacement of donor bone marrow, and chronic rejection. Limb transplantation model in NHPs was developed by Cendales et al. The model included the sensate osteomyocutaneous radial forearm flap without any functional impairment. The transplant was reported to be well tolerated by the recipient animal and allowed for systematic preclinical evaluation of therapeutic maneuvers to improve allograft survival [66].

1.3.5 Other VCA Models

Several research groups have focused on other types of rat and large animal VCA, such as larynx, penile, and vascularized knee joint transplants. Several mouse VCA models have also been described in the literature. These models included hindlimb, forelimb, and facial subunits transplantation. However, these models have not been popularized due to either technical problems or lack of clinical relevance of the model.

Uterus transplantation became a new VCA organ studied in different animal models to lay the groundwork for preparation as the alternative treatment for infertility [67–70]. However, uterus transplantation differs from hand and face transplantation since it does not require lifelong immunosuppression.

Laryngeal and penis allotransplantation models are the examples of other VCA transplants tested and reported in the literature. However, these models are not clinically translational models [71].

1.4 History of Clinical VCA

Clinical applications of VCA have progressed rapidly due to the discovery of immunosuppressive therapies in the 1980s. Although the most successful outcomes have been achieved following hand transplantation and face transplantation, other clinical VCA transplants have been reported including the trachea, peripheral nerve, flexor tendon apparatus, vascularized knee, larynx, abdominal wall, penis, and uterus transplantation as outlined in Table 1.2. The experience gained from solid organ transplantation motivated surgeons to try the world's first-hand transplantation in Ecuador in 1964. However, the transplanted hand had been lost from acute allograft rejection within 2 weeks due to the inadequate immunosuppressive treatment [72]. In November 1997, a conference was held in Louisville, Kentucky, known as the *First International Symposium on Composite Tissue Allotransplantation*.

The first short-term successful hand transplant was performed on September 23, 1998, in Lyon, France by a team led by Dubernard [73]. Although, early postoperative period was uneventful with the evidence of functional recovery, the transplanted hand was amputated in 2001 at 29 months posttransplant after several rejection episodes due to the patient noncompliance with the immunosuppressive regimen [74]. Since the first successful hand transplantation in Lyon, over 100 hand transplantation procedures have been performed all over the world [73, 75]. In 1998, a few months after the first hand transplant was performed in Lyon France, team led by Breidenbach performed the first US hand transplantation, which still represents the longest over 20 years survival of hand allograft [76]. Following first reported cases of hand transplantation, surgeons and transplant immunologists from around the world met to discuss a number of ethical, clinical, and research issues related to hand transplantation [77].

On November 15, 2004, Cleveland Clinic received the world's first IRB approval for human face transplantation. About a year later, on November 27, 2005, the first successful partial face transplant took place in Amiens, France [78]. The patient received lower and central facial subunits, including the tip of the nose, lips, and chin. Although the functional outcomes and patient quality of life were satisfactory, the patient developed multiple rejections of face allograft and died in 2016 due to the development of cancer secondary to chronic immunosuppressive therapy. In 2008, the world's first near-total face transplantation was performed in the US by team lead by Siemionow. During the

Table 1.2 Clinical applications of VCA

VCA type	First application	Specific features
Total knee joint	1996—Hofmann	• Encouraging short-term results, including ambulation • High graft failure rates in long term follow up
Larynx	1998—Strome	• Provides breathing without tracheostoma, normal swallowing, and voice production • Not popularized despite encouraging results • Almost all candidates have advanced larynx cancer which limits use of immunosuppression
Unilateral/bilateral upper extremity	1998—Dubernard	• Can be considered the gold standard orthoplastic reconstruction for devastating upper limb injuries in selected patients • Patient survival and graft survival in Western countries are above 90% • Long term follow-up showed that chronic rejection is a major problem for graft/functional loss
Uterus	2000—Fageeh	• Temporary transplantation eliminates lifelong immunosuppression • Satisfactory pregnancy and childbirth rates make it a popular technique for female infertility treatment
Abdominal wall	2003—Levi	• Includes skin, rectus sheath with rectus muscles, internal and external oblique muscles, transversus abdominis, and peritoneum • Facilitates closure of the abdominal domain following multivisceral or isolated small bowel transplant and serves as sentinel flap
Ovary	2005—Mhatre	• Alternative treatment of primary ovarian insufficiency (e.g., Turner syndrome) • Good take-up and follicular development on USG. Hormonal rise has indicated functioning graft
Face/ craniomaxillofacial	2005—partial, Dubernard 2008—near total, Siemionow 2008—full, Lantieri	• Different units/subunits of craniomaxillofacial region can be transplanted with or without bony tissue involvement • Provides optimal functional and aesthetics results with high patient satisfaction • Chronic rejection represents currently the major problem leading to the graft loss
Unilateral/bilateral lower limb	2006—Zuker 2011—Cavadas	• Technically comparable to upper extremity transplantation • High perioperative complications due to reperfusion injury and hemodynamic instability • Unpredictable functional outcomes due to poor nerve regeneration and weight bearing function
Genitourinary penis	2014—van der Merwe	• New evolving application of VCA with insufficient long-term outcomes • Functional effect achieved in clinical applications is surprisingly good, and clears the path for future procedures
En bloc neck organs	2015—Grajek	• Neck organs including larynx, trachea, pharynx, and esophagus, functioning thyroid, and parathyroid glands • Early outcomes indicate normal endocrine homeostasis and independent speech, swallowing, and breathing

22-hours procedure, transplanted facial allograft included cheeks, the nose, lower eyelids, upper lip, alveolus, soft palate, and underlying bony structures and maxilla supporting the replaced facial subunits. Since 2005, there have been over 40 reports of facial allotransplantation around the world [79]. Finally, in 2015, a group led by Grajek from Poland, performed the first en bloc neck organs including larynx, trachea, pharynx, and esophagus, functioning thyroid and parathyroid glands [80].

1.4.1 Other Clinical VCA Applications

Besides hand and face transplantation, there are other clinical applications of VCA including larynx, trachea, knee, femur, abdominal wall, peripheral nerves, tongue, scalp/external ear, penis, uterus, flexor tendon apparatus, lower extremity, and muscles [81].

Following the first attempt by Kluyskens in 1969 [82], the first successful laryngotracheal allotransplantation was performed at the Cleveland Clinic in 1988 [83]. The patient was able to generate voice at 3 days after transplant. The patient reported improved quality of life (including senses like smell and taste), adequate daily communication and emotional expression.

In 1908, the first pioneering clinical whole-joint transplantation was performed by Lexer [84]. There were other attempts of knee joint transplantations; however, they either did not include vascular supply or were not supported by immunosuppressive treatment. The first successful allogeneic vascularized knee joint transplantation was performed by Hoffman team in 1996 [85]. Although the early postoperative results were encouraging, late results were disappointing due to the high rate of chronic rejection and graft failure [86]. Additionally, since the knee joint transplant was denervated, this led to the development of neuropathic arthropathy, loss of proprioception of the transplanted allograft causing microtrauma and subsequent transplant fractures.

Flexor tendon apparatus allotransplantation has an important place in the history of clinical VCA. Although many authors attempted tendon allograft transplantation, the first successful clinical VCA including flexor tendon mechanism was performed by Peacock from the cadaver sources [87]. Peacock tried to differentiate these structurally complex grafts including multiple tissues from the solid organ grafts and proposed the term "composite tissue allografts," which is the former terminology for VCA [88]. His results were also encouraging with "successful" active movement of tendons in 7/10 patients. In 1988, Guimberteau successfully transplanted the vascularized flexor tendon apparatus attached to the ulnar vascular pedicle and provided short term immunosuppression [89].

Abdominal wall transplantation was first described by a group led by Levi in 2003 in order to solve the problems associated with difficult closure of the abdomen [90]. The allograft included both rectus abdominis muscles, overlying fascia, subcutaneous tissues, and skin and was harvested based on the bilateral inferior epigastric vessels. Despite different outcomes, current clinical experience demonstrates that abdominal wall transplantation is surgically feasible providing the tension-free closure of the abdomen and is also immunologically justified.

The first peripheral nerve VCA was reported by Mackinnon and co-workers in St. Louis. They reported seven clinical cases of nerve allotransplantation supported with 12–26-month period of immunosuppression. This procedure is unique since it does not require lifelong immunosuppression. In addition, the use of tacrolimus in the immunosuppressive protocol supports nerve regeneration [91].

In 2003, a total tongue VCA was performed in a patient who underwent total tongue resection after tongue cancer [92]. The early postoperative period was uneventful with limited swallowing function of the tongue and improved patient satisfaction. However, the patient died from recurrence of the carcinoma, which emphasizes the importance of careful case by case assessment and patient selection when considering reconstruction with VCA after cancer resections that require immunosuppression. Same problem occurred in the world's first bilateral ear and scalp transplantation, performed by Hui in 2004. The patient received the transplantation after resection of advanced melanoma; however, the reports on initial technical success were followed by reports on the recipient's death [93].

Penis is unique in terms of histology and morphology of the skin, corpora urethra, and glans. Thus, VCA provides a good option for penile reconstruction. The first penile transplantation was performed in China by Hu in 2006 [94]. The patient was able to void spontaneously at postoperative day 10; however, the transplanted penis was amputated at day 14 due to psychological distress and request of the patient and his wife. The first successful penile transplantation was performed 8 years later, in South Africa [95], which was followed by the first US penis transplantation in 2016 [96]. Despite these encouraging results, penile transplantation is yet far from a routine clinical applications, due to multiple challenges that have to be still overcome [97].

The first uterus transplantation was performed by Fageeh et al. in Saudi Arabia in 2006 [98]. Despite early success, the graft was lost at 3 months posttransplant, secondary to vascular problems resulting from the pedicle torsion or kinking. In 2014, Brännström performed the first successful uterus transplant confirming that a live birth is possible after uterus transplantation. One of the key advantages of the uterus transplant is that the immunosuppression is given temporary since the organ can be removed after successful pregnancy.

Deceased donor uterus transplantation with the delivery of the live birth was also reported [99]. However, similar to the concerns observed after penis transplantation, uterus transplantation has raised many ethical and philosophical questions due to the religious and cultural concerns [100]. As a part of reproductive transplantation Mhatre performed the first vascularized ovary transplantation in 2005, but it did not gain popularity [101].

Lower extremity transplantation (LET) is another controversial topic in the field of VCA. Up to date only few cases of LET have been reported [71]. First successful complete LET has been performed between ischiopagus twins by Zuker et al. in 2006 [102]. World's first bilateral transfemoral allotransplantation was performed by Cavadas in 2011. This patient developed primary central nervous system posttransplant lymphoproliferative disease (PTLD). Although the transplanted limbs were removed and immunosuppressive treatment was discontinued, the patient died. Other efforts of LET have also resulted in extremity loss and patient's death.

1.5 History to Be Made in the Field of VCA

There are three major research areas related to the field of VCA, where a groundbreaking advancements are expected in next decade. These topics include a new approaches to *bypass the immunological barrier, to solve the problem of chronic rejection, and to overcome organ shortage.*

Bypassing the Immunological Barrier The first one is solving the immunologic barrier against allotransplantation. Currently, VCA is accepted as a viable option for patients suffering from severe and complex tissues defects which are not amenable to the currently available reconstructive techniques. Improving "only" quality of life at the expense of lifelong systemic immunosuppression carrying severe side effects is currently the major concern limiting the routine clinical application of VCA. Thus, development of the new tolerance inducing strategies is considered at the holy grail for VCA. Several methods have been tested to solve the immunologic barrier against VCA. Cellular therapies have confirmed immunomodulatory and tolerogenic properties when tested in the context of VCA transplantation [103]. However, these approaches are still far from routine clinical applications. Siemionow et al. created donor–recipient chimeric cells both in vivo and in vitro for therapeutic applications in VCA and solid organ transplantation [104, 105]. Supportive therapy with chimeric cells resulted in improved graft survival (up to 100 days) when combined with short-term 7-day course of immunosuppression.

Another method for bypassing the immunological barrier is the application of gene editing technologies for evading immunosurveillance. To date, few important studies have been conducted in transplantation models and confirmed the option to modify the immune response and prolong survival of solid organs and VCA transplants [106, 107]. Gene editing in the transplantation field focuses primarily on the modification of antigenicity of the allograft or the immune response against alloantigens [108, 109]. The first techniques of genetic engineering of the allograft was performed by transfection of cells with the antisense oligodeoxynucleotides (ODN), which prevents translation of different proteins by specifically binding to mRNA. Other mechanisms such as splicing inhibition and translational arrest were also reported [110–113]. The advance of CRISPR-Cas9 technique provided simple, versatile, highly specific, and efficient gene editing with potential applications in VCA [114]. However, despite the tremendous advances in gene editing technologies in recent years, its application in the vascularized tissues is still developing due to many unknowns such as vector efficiency, vector toxicity, control of gene expression, and biosecurity. Current advances in the novel, more specific and sensitive methods of genomic editing may open a new era in bypassing the immunological barrier in the field of VCA transplantation.

1.5.1 Solving the Chronic Rejection

Although current immunosuppressive medications are effective in preventing acute allograft rejection, they are still not able to prevent chronic rejection (CR) in VCA [115]. There are reports on the hand and face transplant outcomes where recipients have lost their grafts secondary to chronic rejection [116–119]. Thus, CR is emerging as a major threat to the field of VCA and the long-term outcomes. There are currently no reliable serum/blood markers for CR. Thus, in addition to the development of new strategies minimizing side effects and toxicity of immunosuppression, it is equally important to identify diagnostic tools and novel therapies allowing to prevent development of vasculopathy and treat CR in VCA [120–122].

1.5.2 Overcoming Organ Shortage

The organ shortage represents a complex problem which cannot be easily solved by administrative or organizational measures undertaken by organ sharing organizations. Current research related to the problem of organ shortage is mainly focusing either on tissue regeneration or on xenotransplantation. There are examples of engineered tissues and organs such as skin substitutes and bladder that have been already introduced to the clinic, and new tissue engineering approaches and designs are currently tested [123, 124].

However, these are not vascularized tissues, which will develop vascularization following implantation into the body. At the moment, there are no reports on successful vascularization of the laboratory generated organs or tissues. Moreover, VCA is different from the solid organs and regeneration of VCA tissues is much more complex, and in addition to the restoration of vascularization, there is the need for tissues innervation specific for the multiple tissue types [125]. Xenotransplantation has the potential to solve the organ shortage problem [126, 127]. However, immunologic barrier against xenotransplantation is much more complex and difficult to overcome [128, 129]. Moreover, there are many other challenges, such as the risk of xenogenic infection, ethical, legal, religious, and social concerns that need to be resolved before clinical application of organs of xenogenic origin [130–132].

Finally, there is still a "wish-list" of potential VCA transplants such as allografts composed of different functional units or new VCA composed of complex structures such as the whole eye transplantation. Experimental studies of the whole eye transplantation including optic nerve have already been performed, as well as the first cadaver studies testing technical feasibility of the composite periorbital–eyeball transplantation. These pioneering studies may allow for clinical application of these new VCA transplants in the near future [46, 133, 134].

In conclusion, despite the advances in basic and translational research and expansion of clinical applications, VCA is still considered as the experimental procedure and depends on many disciplines for the ultimate success. The current research and clinical studies and innovative developments in the VCA filed will make contribution to the future history of VCA transplantation.

References

1. Siemionow M. The miracle of face transplantation after 10 years. Br Med Bull. 2016;120(1):5–14.
2. Hultman CS, Friedstat JS. The ACAPS and SESPRS surveys to identify the most influential innovators and innovations in plastic surgery: no line on the horizon. Ann Plast Surg. 2014;72(6):202–7.
3. Ozturk S, Karagoz H, Zor F. The future of plastic surgery: surgeon's perspective. J Craniofac Surg. 2015;26(8):e708–13.
4. Weissenbacher A, Hautz T, Pratschke J, Schneeberger S. Vascularized composite allografts and solid organ transplants: similarities and differences. Curr Opin Organ Transplant. 2013;18(6):640–4.
5. Oda H, Ikeguchi R, Aoyama T, Ohta S, Noguchi T, Kaizawa Y, et al. Relative antigenicity of components in vascularized composite allotransplants: an experimental study of microRNAs expression in rat hind limb transplantation model. Microsurgery. 2019;39(4):340–8.
6. Lee WP, Yaremchuk MJ, Pan YC, Randolph MA, Tan CM, Weiland AJ. Relative antigenicity of components of a vascularized limb allograft. Plast Reconstr Surg. 1991;87(3):401–11.
7. Siemionow MZ, Zor F. Experimental studies in face transplantation: rodent model. In: Siemionow MZ, editor. The know-how of face transplantation. London: Springer; 2011. p. 41–53.
8. Rubin CT. Daedalus and icarus revisited. New Atlantis. 2005;8:73–91.
9. Wu S, Xu H, Ravindra K, Ildstad ST. Composite tissue allotransplantation: past, present and future-the history and expanding applications of CTA as a new frontier in transplantation. Transplant Proc. 2009;41(2):463–5.
10. Marino IR, Cirillo C. An abridged photographic history of organ transplantation. Exp Clin Transplant. 2014;12(Suppl 1):11–6.
11. Kumar R, Kalra SK, Mahapatra AK. Lord Ganesha: the idol neurosurgeon. Childs Nerv Syst. 2008;24(3):287–8.
12. Lamba N, Holsgrove D, Broekman ML. The history of head transplantation: a review. Acta Neurochir. 2016;158(12):2239–47.
13. Ren XP, Ye YJ, Li PW, Shen ZL, Han KC, Song Y. Head transplantation in mouse model. CNS Neurosci Ther. 2015;21(8):615–8.
14. Kahan BD. Pien Ch'iao, the legendary exchange of hearts, traditional Chinese medicine, and the modern era of cyclosporine. Transplant Proc. 1988;20(2 Suppl 2):2–12.
15. Boadt L. Review: a new heart and a new soul: Ezekiel, the exile and the Torah. J Semit Stud. 2005;50(1):217–8.
16. Brandacher G, Khalifian S, Lee WPA. Reconstructive transplantation: from scientific dream to clinical reality. In: Brandacher G, editor. The science of reconstructive transplantation. New York: Springer; 2015. p. 3–11.
17. Gordon CR, Serletti JM, Black KS, Hewitt CW. The evolution of composite tissue allotransplantation: the twentieth century realization of "Cosmas and Damian". In: Hewitt CW, Lee WPA, Gordon CR, editors. Transplantation of composite tissue allografts. Boston: Springer; 2008. p. 13–25.
18. Tubbs RS, Riech S, Verma K, Chern J, Mortazavi M, Cohen-Gadol AA. China's first surgeon: Hua Tuo (c. 108-208 AD). Childs Nerv Syst. 2011;27(9):1357–60.
19. Bath K, Aggarwal S, Sharma V. Sushruta: father of plastic surgery in Benares. J Med Biogr. 2019;27(1):2–3.
20. Gurunluoglu R, Gurunluoglu A, Arton J. Great teachers of Gaspare Tagliacozzi (1546-1599). J Med Biogr. 2017;25(3):161–9.
21. Murray JE. Organ transplants: a type of reconstructive surgery. Can J Surg. 1965;8(4):340–50.
22. Finerty JC. Parabiosis in physiological studies. Physiol Rev. 1952;32(3):277–302.
23. The natural history of human teeth - John Hunter. Available from: https://library.uthscsa.edu/2015/03/the-natural-history-of-human-teeth-john-hunter/?word=james.
24. Loeb L. Transplantation and individuality. Physiol Rev. 1930;10(4):547–616.
25. Holman E. Protein sensitization in isoskingrafting. Is the latter of practical value. Surg Gynecol Obstet. 1924;38:100–6.
26. Starzl TE. Peter Brian Medawar: father of transplantation. J Am Coll Surg. 1995;180(3):332–6.
27. Owen RD. Immunogenetic consequences of vascular anastomoses between bovine twins. Science. 1945;102(2651):400–1.
28. Billingham RE, Brent L, Medawar PB. Actively acquired tolerance' of foreign cells. Nature. 1953;172:603–6.
29. Simonsen M, Buemann J, Gammeltoft A, Jensen F, Jorgensen K. Biological incompatibility in kidney transplantation in dogs. I. Experimental and morphological investigations. Acta Pathol Microbiol Scand. 1953;32(1):1–35.
30. Starzl TE. History of clinical transplantation. World J Surg. 2000;24(7):759–82.
31. Wing-Yee CW. Evolution and clinical application of microsurgery. BMC Proc. 2015;9(Suppl 3):53.
32. Aida L. Alexis Carrel (1873-1944): visionary vascular surgeon and pioneer in organ transplantation. J Med Biogr. 2014;22(3):172–5.

33. Murray JE, Merrill JP, Dammin GJ, Dealy JB Jr, Walter CW, Brooke MS, et al. Study on transplantation immunity after total body irradiation: clinical and experimental investigation. Surgery. 1960;48:272–84.
34. Calne RY. The rejection of renal homografts. Inhibition in dogs by 6-mercaptopurine. Lancet. 1960;1(7121):417–8.
35. Schwartz R, Dameshek W. The effects of 6-mercaptopurine on homograft reactions. J Clin Invest. 1960;39:952–8.
36. Starzl TE, Marchioro TL, Waddell WR. The reversal of rejection in human renal homografts with subsequent development of homograft tolerance. Surg Gynecol Obstet. 1963;117:385–95.
37. Halloran PF. Immunosuppressive drugs for kidney transplantation. N Engl J Med. 2004;351(26):2715–29.
38. Zor F, Siemionow M. Vascularized composite allotransplantation models. 2015. p. 151-9.
39. Shapiro RI, Cerra FB. A model for reimplantation and transplantation of a complex organ: the rat hind limb. J Surg Res. 1978;24(6):501–6.
40. Kern B, Sucher R. Small animal models for reconstructive transplantation. In: Brandacher G, editor. The science of reconstructive transplantation. New York: Springer; 2015. p. 53–61.
41. Zor F. Facial vascularized composite tissue allotransplantation. Gulhane Med J. 2013;55(2):156.
42. Ulusal BG, Ulusal AE, Ozmen S, Zins JE, Siemionow MZ. A new composite facial and scalp transplantation model in rats. Plast Reconstr Surg. 2003;112(5):1302–11.
43. Siemionow M, Zor F. Experimental studies in face transplantation: rodent model. New York: Springer; 2011. p. 41–53.
44. Zor F, Bozkurt M, Nair D, Siemionow M. A new composite midface allotransplantation model with sensory and motor reinnervation. Transpl Int. 2009;23(6):649–56.
45. Kulahci Y, Altuntas SH, Karagoz H, Cwykiel JM, Zor F, Siemionow M. A new total hemiface allotransplantation model in rats. Microsurgery. 2016;36(3):230–8.
46. Zor F, Polat M, Kulahci Y, Sahin H, Aral AM, Erbas VE, et al. Demonstration of technical feasibility and viability of whole eye transplantation in a rodent model. J Plast Reconstr Aesthet Surg. 2019;72(10):1640–50.
47. Agaoglu G, Unal S, Siemionow M. Transplantation of the vascularized bone allograft into the inguinal region. Plast Reconstr Surg. 2005;115(6):1794–5.
48. Bozkurt M, Klimczak A, Nasir S, Zor F, Krokowicz L, Siemionow M. Composite osseomusculocutaneous sternum, ribs, thymus, pectoralis muscles, and skin allotransplantation model of bone marrow transplantation. Microsurgery. 2012;33(1):43–50.
49. Zor F, Bozkurt M, Cwykiel J, Karagoz H, Kulahci Y, Uygur S, et al. The effect of thymus transplantation on donor-specific chimerism in the rat model of composite osseomusculocutaneous sternum, ribs, thymus, pectoralis muscles, and skin allotransplantation. Microsurgery. 2020;40(5):576–84.
50. Kulahci Y, Bayram Y, Karagoz H, Sever C, Sahin C. Experimental craniofacial composite tissue allotransplantation (CCTA) models in rats. Arch Clin Exp Surg. 2012;1(3):181.
51. Hong SH, Eun SC. Experimental forelimb allotransplantation in canine model. Biomed Res Int. 2016;2016:1495710.
52. Ustuner ET, Zdichavsky M, Ren X, Edelstein J, Maldonado C, Ray M, et al. Long-term composite tissue allograft survival in a porcine model with cyclosporine/mycophenolate mofetil therapy. Transplantation. 1998;66(12):1581–7.
53. Ustuner ET, Majzoub RK, Ren X, Edelstein J, Maldonado C, Perez-Abadia G, et al. Swine composite tissue allotransplant model for preclinical hand transplant studies. Microsurgery. 2000;20(8):400–6.
54. Zdichavsky M, Jones JW, Ustuner ET, Ren X, Edelstein J, Maldonado C, et al. Scoring of skin rejection in a swine composite tissue allograft model. J Surg Res. 1999;85(1):1–8.
55. Kuo YR, Shih HS, Lin CC, Huang CC, Yang JC, Wu WS, et al. Swine hemi-facial composite tissue allotransplantation: a model to study immune rejection. J Surg Res. 2009;153(2):268–73.
56. Villamaria CY, Rasmussen TE, Spencer JR, Patel S, Davis MR. Microvascular porcine model for the optimization of vascularized composite tissue transplantation. J Surg Res. 2012;178(1):452–9.
57. Wachtman GS, Wimmers EG, Gorantla VS, Lin CH, Schneeberger S, Unadkat JV, et al. Biologics and donor bone marrow cells for targeted immunomodulation in vascularized composite allotransplantation: a translational trial in swine. Transplant Proc. 2011;43(9):3541–4.
58. Fries CA, Villamaria CY, Spencer JR, Rickard RF, Gorantla VS, Davis MR. A porcine orthotopic forelimb vascularized composite allotransplantation model: technical considerations and translational implications. Plast Reconstr Surg. 2016;138(3):461.
59. Swearingen B, Chang J, Mathes DW. Use of large-animal and nonhuman primate models for reconstructive transplantation. In: Brandacher G, editor. The science of reconstructive transplantation. New York: Springer; 2015. p. 63–76.
60. Horner BM, Randolph MA, Duran-Struuck R, Hirsh EL, Ferguson KK, Teague AG, et al. Induction of tolerance to an allogeneic skin flap transplant in a preclinical large animal model. Transplant Proc. 2009;41(2):539–41.
61. Erbas VESH, Oksuz S, Dong L, Miller MR, Shojaati G, Wollstein G, Chan KC, Sigal I, Kostereva N, Raval S, Ibrahim T, Goldberg JL, Benowitz L, Schuman JS, Zor F, Solari M, Washington KM, Gorantla VS. Abstract 16: a preclinical swine model for whole eyeball transplantation: planning and procedural aspects. Plast Reconstr Surg. 2016;4(4S):42.
62. Barth RN, Bluebond-Langner R, Nam A, Stanwix M, Shipley S, Bartlett ST, et al. Facial subunit composite tissue allografts in nonhuman primates: I. Technical and immunosuppressive requirements for prolonged graft survival. Plast Reconstr Surg. 2009;123(2):493–501.
63. Barth RN, Nam AJ, Stanwix MG, Kukuruga D, Drachenberg CI, Bluebond-Langner R, et al. Prolonged survival of composite facial allografts in non-human primates associated with posttransplant lymphoproliferative disorder. Transplantation. 2009;88(11):1242–50.
64. Barth RN, Rodriguez ED, Mundinger GS, Nam AJ, Ha JS, Hui-Chou H, et al. Vascularized bone marrow-based immunosuppression inhibits rejection of vascularized composite allografts in nonhuman primates. Am J Transplant. 2011;11(7):1407–16.
65. Mundinger GS, Nam AJ, Hui-Chou HG, Stanwix MG, Jones LS, Drachenberg CB, et al. Nonhuman primate model of fibula vascularized composite tissue allotransplantation demonstrates donor-recipient bony union. Plast Reconstr Surg. 2011;128(6):1193–204.
66. Cendales LC, Xu H, Bacher J, Eckhaus MA, Kleiner DE, Kirk AD. Composite tissue allotransplantation: development of a preclinical model in nonhuman primates. Transplantation. 2005;80(10):1447–54.
67. Yu B, Liu Z, Zhang C, Wu Y, Han J, Li H, et al. Allogeneic uterus transplantation in a rhesus model: a short-term graft viability study. PLoS One. 2020;15(12):e0243140.
68. Zhang X, Liu J, Wu Q, Liu Z, Yan Z. Uterus allo-transplantation in a swine model: long-term graft survival and reproductive function. Med Sci Monit. 2018;24:8422–9.
69. Kengelbach-Weigand A, Lotz L, Schmid R, Lang W, Beckmann MW, Hoffmann I, et al. Intra- and postoperative blood flow monitoring in a sheep model of uterus transplantation. In Vivo. 2019;33(2):325–36.
70. Johannesson L, Enskog A. Experimental uterus transplantation. Best Pract Res Clin Obstet Gynaecol. 2014;28(8):1198–210.
71. Kulahci Y, Karagoz H, Zor F. Experimental models of penile and lower limb transplantation: are they really translational? Curr Transpl Rep. 2018;5(4):344–8.

72. Park SH, Eun SC, Kwon ST. Hand transplantation: current status and immunologic obstacles. Exp Clin Transplant. 2019;17(1):97–104.
73. Dubernard JM, Owen E, Herzberg G, Lanzetta M, Martin X, Kapila H, et al. Human hand allograft: report on first 6 months. Lancet. 1999;353(9161):1315–20.
74. Kanitakis J, Jullien D, Petruzzo P, Hakim N, Claudy A, Revillard JP, et al. Clinicopathologic features of graft rejection of the first human hand allograft. Transplantation. 2003;76(4):688–93.
75. Siemionow MZ, Kulahci Y, Bozkurt M. Composite tissue allotransplantation. Plast Reconstr Surg. 2009;124:e327.
76. Breidenbach WC, Gonzales NR, Kaufman CL, Klapheke M, Tobin GR, Gorantla VS. Outcomes of the first 2 American hand transplants at 8 and 6 years posttransplant. J Hand Surg Am. 2008;33(7):1039–47.
77. Swearingen B, Ravindra K, Xu H, Wu S, Breidenbach WC, Ildstad ST. Science of composite tissue allotransplantation. Transplantation. 2008;86(5):627–35.
78. Devauchelle B, Badet L, Lengelé B, Morelon E, Testelin S, Michallet M, et al. First human face allograft: early report. Lancet. 2006;368(9531):203–9.
79. Siemionow M. The decade of face transplant outcomes. J Mater Sci Mater Med. 2017;28(5):64.
80. Grajek M, Maciejewski A, Giebel S, Krakowczyk Ł, Ulczok R, Szymczyk C, et al. First complex allotransplantation of neck organs: larynx, trachea, pharynx, esophagus, thyroid, parathyroid glands, and anterior cervical wall: a case report. Ann Surg. 2017;266(2):19–24.
81. Kollar B, Tasigiorgos S, Dorante MI, Carty MJ, Talbot SG, Pomahac B. Innovations in reconstructive microsurgery: reconstructive transplantation. J Surg Oncol. 2018;118(5):800–6.
82. Kluyskens P, Ringoir S. Follow-up of a human larynx transplantation. Laryngoscope. 1970;80(8):1244–50.
83. Strome M, Stein J, Esclamado R, Hicks D, Lorenz RR, Braun W, et al. Laryngeal transplantation and 40-month follow-up. N Engl J Med. 2001;344(22):1676–9.
84. Lexer E. Substitution of whole or half joints from freshly amputated extremities by free plastic operation. Surg Gynecol Obstet. 1908;6:601–7.
85. Hofmann G, Kirschner M, Wagner F, Land W, Buehren K. First vascularized knee joint transplantation in man. Transplantation. 1996;8:46–7.
86. Diefenbeck M, Nerlich A, Schneeberger S, Wagner F, Hofmann GO. Allograft vasculopathy after allogeneic vascularized knee transplantation. Transpl Int. 2011;24(1):e1–5.
87. Peacock EE Jr. Homologous composite tissue grafts of the digital flexor mechanism in human beings. Plast Reconstr Surg. 1960;25(4):418–20.
88. Tobin GR, Breidenbach WC, Ildstad ST, Marvin MM, Buell JF, Ravindra KV. The history of human composite tissue allotransplantation. Transplant Proc. 2009;41(2):466–71.
89. Guimberteau J, Baudet J, Panconi B, Boileau R, Potaux L. Human allotransplant of a digital flexion system vascularized on the ulnar pedicle: a preliminary report and 1-year follow-up of two cases. Plast Reconstr Surg. 1992;89(6):1135–47.
90. Levi DM, Tzakis AG, Kato T, Madariaga J, Mittal NK, Nery J, et al. Transplantation of the abdominal wall. Lancet. 2003;361(9376):2173–6.
91. Mackinnon SE, Doolabh VB, Novak CB, Trulock EP. Clinical outcome following nerve allograft transplantation. Plast Reconstr Surg. 2001;107(6):1419–29.
92. Birchall M. Tongue transplantation. Lancet. 2004;363(9422):1663.
93. Jiang HQ, Wang Y, Hu XB, Li YS, Li JS. Composite tissue allograft transplantation of cephalocervical skin flap and two ears. Plast Reconstr Surg. 2005;115(3):31–5.
94. Hu W, Lu J, Zhang L, Wu W, Nie H, Zhu Y, et al. A preliminary report of penile transplantation. Eur Urol. 2006;50(4):851–3.
95. Bateman C. World's first successful penis transplant at Tygerberg Hospital. SAMJ. 2015;105(4):251–2.
96. Cetrulo CL Jr, Li K, Salinas HM, Treiser MD, Schol I, Barrisford GW, et al. Penis transplantation: first US experience. Ann Surg. 2018;267(5):983–8.
97. van der Merwe A, Moosa MR, Barsdorf N. Ethical and societal challenges in penis transplantation. Curr Opin Organ Transplant. 2020;25(6):594–600.
98. Fageeh W, Raffa H, Jabbad H, Marzouki A. Transplantation of the human uterus. Int J Gynecol Obstet. 2002;76(3):245–51.
99. Tardieu A, Dion L, Collinet P, Ayoubi JM, Garbin O, Agostini A, et al. Uterus transplantation: questions and future prospects. J Gynecol Obstet Hum Reprod. 2019;48(1):1–3.
100. Milliez J. Uterine transplantation: FIGO committee for the ethical aspects of human reproduction and women's health. Hoboken: Wiley Online Library; 2009.
101. Mhatre P, Mhatre J, Magotra R. Ovarian transplant: a new frontier. Transplant Proc. 2005;37(2):1396–8.
102. Zuker RM, Redett R, Alman B, Coles JG, Timoney N, Ein SH. First successful lower-extremity transplantation: technique and functional result. J Reconstr Microsurg. 2006;22(4):239–44.
103. Matar AJ, Crepeau RL, Duran-Struuck R. Cellular immunotherapies in pre-clinical large animal models of transplantation. Biol Blood Marrow Transpl. 2020. https://doi.org/10.1016/j.bbmt.2020.09.032.
104. Kwiecien GJ, Cwykiel J, Madajka M, Bobkiewicz A, Uygur S, Siemionow MZ. Donor-recipient chimeric cell transplantation as a novel rescue therapy for acute radiation syndrome: a preliminary report. Plast Reconstr Surg. 2014;133(4S):1013–4.
105. Cwykiel J, Zor F, Klimczak A, Siemionow M. Comparison of in-vivo created donor-recipient chimeric cell therapy and bone marrow cell therapy as a supportive treatment in face allograft model: 2293. Transplantation. 2010;90:47.
106. Isaka Y. Gene therapy targeting kidney diseases: routes and vehicles. Clin Exp Nephrol. 2006;10(4):229–35.
107. Yang Z, Rostami S, Koeberlein B, Barker CF, Naji A. Cardiac allograft tolerance induced by intraarterial infusion of recombinant adenoviral CTLA4Ig1. Transplantation. 1999;67(12):1517–23.
108. Itano H, Mora BN, Zhang W, Ritter JH, McCarthy TJ, Yew NS, et al. Lipid-mediated ex vivo gene transfer of viral interleukin 10 in rat lung allotransplantation. J Thorac Cardiovasc Surg. 2001;122(1):29–38.
109. Sato M, Keshavjee S. Gene therapy in lung transplantation. Curr Gene Ther. 2006;6(4):439–58.
110. Mathieu P, Chauveau C, Bouchet D, Guillot C, Tesson L, Anegon I. Genetic engineering in allotransplantation of vascularized organs. Curr Gene Ther. 2002;2(1):9–21.
111. Myers KJ, Dean NM. Sensible use of antisense: how to use oligonucleotides as research tools. Trends Pharmacol Sci. 2000;21(1):19–23.
112. Walder RY, Walder JA. Role of RNase H in hybrid-arrested translation by antisense oligonucleotides. Proc Natl Acad Sci U S A. 1988;85(14):5011–5.
113. Wood KJ. Gene therapy and allotransplantation. Curr Opin Immunol. 1997;9(5):662–8.
114. Das K, Eisel D, Lenkl C, Goyal A, Diederichs S, Dickes E, et al. Generation of murine tumor cell lines deficient in MHC molecule surface expression using the CRISPR/Cas9 system. PLoS One. 2017;12(3):e0174077.
115. Gorantla VS, Demetris AJ. Acute and chronic rejection in upper extremity transplantation: what have we learned? Hand Clin. 2011;27(4):481–93.

116. Krezdorn N, Lian CG, Wells M, Wo L, Tasigiorgos S, Xu S, et al. Chronic rejection of human face allografts. Am J Transplant. 2018;19(4):1168–77.
117. Morelon E, Petruzzo P, Kanitakis J, Dakpe S, Thaunat O, Dubois V, et al. Face transplantation: partial graft loss of the first case 10 years later. Am J Transplant. 2017;17(7):1935–40.
118. Kaufman CL, Breidenbach W. World experience after more than a decade of clinical hand transplantation: update from the Louisville hand transplant program. Hand Clin. 2011;27(4):417–21.
119. Kaufman CL, Ouseph R, Blair B, Kutz JE, Tsai TM, Scheker LR, et al. Graft vasculopathy in clinical hand transplantation. Am J Transplant. 2012;12(4):1004–16.
120. Hautz T, Zelger B, Brandacher G, Mueller H, Grahammer J, Zelger B, et al. Histopathologic characterization of mild rejection (grade I) in skin biopsies of human hand allografts. Transpl Int. 2012;25(1):56–63.
121. Kanitakis J, Badet L, Petruzzo P, Beziat JL, Morelon E, Lefrancois N, et al. Clinicopathologic monitoring of the skin and oral mucosa of the first human face allograft: Report on the first eight months. Transplantation. 2006;82(12):1610–5.
122. Womer KL, Vella JP, Sayegh MH. Chronic allograft dysfunction: mechanisms and new approaches to therapy. Semin Nephrol. 2000;20(2):126–47.
123. Atala A. Bioengineered tissues for urogenital repair in children. Pediatr Res. 2008;63(5):569–75.
124. Ojeh N, Pastar I, Tomic-Canic M, Stojadinovic O. Stem cells in skin regeneration, wound healing, and their clinical applications. Int J Mol Sci. 2015;16(10):25476–501.
125. Yang T-L, Yoo JJ, Siemionow MZ, Atala A. Tissue engineering for facial reconstruction. In: Siemionow MZ, editor. The know-how of face transplantation. London: Springer; 2011. p. 447–62.
126. Starzl TE, Fung J, Tzakis A, Todo S, Demetris AJ, Marino IR, et al. Baboon-to-human liver transplantation. Lancet. 1993;341(8837):65–71.
127. Taniguchi S, Cooper DK. Clinical xenotransplantation: past, present and future. Ann R Coll Surg Engl. 1997;79(1):13–9.
128. Auchincloss H Jr, Sachs DH. Xenogeneic transplantation. Annu Rev Immunol. 1998;16:433–70.
129. Galili U, Wang L, LaTemple DC, Radic MZ. The natural anti-Gal antibody. Sub-cellular. Biochemistry. 1999;32:79–106.
130. Tanabe YN, Randolph MA, Shimizu A, Lee WP. Xenotransplantation model for vascularized musculoskeletal tissues in rodents. Microsurgery. 2000;20(2):59–64.
131. Lu T, Yang B, Wang R, Qin C. Xenotransplantation: current status in preclinical research. Front Immunol. 2019;10:3060.
132. Sykes M, Sachs DH. Transplanting organs from pigs to humans. Sci Immunol. 2019;4(41):6298.
133. Zor F, Karagoz H, Kapucu H, Kulahci Y, Janjic JM, Gorantla VS. Immunological considerations and concerns as pertinent to whole eye transplantation. Curr Opin Organ Transplant. 2019;24(6):726–32.
134. Siemionow M, Bozkurt M, Zor F, Kulahci Y, Uygur S, Ozturk C, et al. A new composite eyeball-periorbital transplantation model in humans: an anatomical study in preparation for eyeball transplantation. Plast Reconstr Surg. 2018;141(4):1011–8.

2 Immunosuppression Protocols in VCA Transplantation

Amit Nair and Bijan Eghtesad

2.1 Introduction

Vascularized composite allografts (VCAs) comprise a heterogenous group of tissues that share both a common anatomical and functional framework as well as blood supply [1]. The advent, successes, and increasing applications of VCA transplantation owe much to the lessons learned from decades of experience with immunosuppressive protocols utilized in other solid organ transplantation (SOT) arenas such as the kidney, heart, and liver. Their composite nature aside, VCAs also distinguish themselves from other SOT paradigms based on the typical background circumstances of potential recipients, along with the unique immunological challenges these grafts inexorably pose.

VCAs often consist of tissues that include components of the integumentary system/skin and/or bone marrow, thus rendering these allografts quite immunogenic compared to their visceral counterparts. Additionally, there is often a substantial incidence of prior sensitization of potential recipients by transfusions of blood products, given the frequent rate of trauma-related index events that ultimately lead to indications for VCA transplantation [2]. It is therefore not surprising that the incidence of acute rejection after implantation of VCAs is rather high at around 80% in the first postoperative year, with the skin often being the prime target [3, 4]. Yet another consideration is the fact that most VCA recipients are younger, with many years of immunosuppression ahead of them toward maintaining a transplant that rather than being lifesaving, is essentially aiming to improve the quality of their lives. Indeed, the current Achilles heel of VCA transplantation is the lack of an optimal immunosuppressive regime that balances durable anti-rejection properties with minimal short- and long-term adverse effects.

2.2 Historical Perspectives

The strong immunogenicity of allografted skin, capable of eliciting a systemic response and immunization from the recipient, was demonstrated across several clinical experiments earlier on during the twentieth century. The ravages during the period of the Second World War accelerated investigations into this realm to help consolidate a treatment for wartime injuries, without success [5]. Concurrent with the advent of kidney transplantation into clinical practice in the 1950s, transplantation of composite tissues such as flexor tendons gained popularity, aided by the lack of requirement for anti-rejection medications for these particular tissues. The first attempt at VCA transplantation was made in 1964 with the technically successful implantation of a hand under Azathioprine and steroid coverage, which nonetheless unfortunately failed from acute rejection just a few weeks later [6]. Despite significant subsequent progress in the field of transplant immunosuppression further to the realization of the anti-rejection effects of Cyclosporin A (1976) and later, Tacrolimus (1990), clinical activity in VCA waned until the late 1990s, when the use of Tacrolimus along with mycophenolic acid became more mainstream in SOT [7]. One of the earliest and durable successes of VCA was reported from Louisville, KY, USA back in 2000 with the implantation of a cadaveric hand utilizing Basiliximab induction therapy and immunosuppression maintenance with Tacrolimus, Mycophenolate mofetil, and Prednisolone [8]. Twenty years later and concurrent with the exponential development in this field with the introduction of abdominal wall, penile, laryngeal, uterine, and facial transplantation in the interim, this particular graft continues to function well [9].

A. Nair
Division of Transplantation/Hepatobiliary Surgery, University of Rochester, Rochester, NY, USA
e-mail: amit_nair@urmc.rochester.edu

B. Eghtesad (✉)
Transplantation Center, Cleveland Clinic, Cleveland, OH, USA
e-mail: eghtesb@ccf.org

© Springer Nature Switzerland AG 2023
R. Gurunian et al. (eds.), *Reconstructive Transplantation*, https://doi.org/10.1007/978-3-031-21520-9_2

2.3 Immunosuppression in VCA

The drugs discussed further in the sections below are not part of an exhaustive list but are nonetheless most often used in the realm of VCA transplantation.

2.3.1 Induction Regimes

Anti-rejection treatments in VCA transplantation have mostly evolved from those used in kidney transplantation, and as such, there is no standardized "one size fits all" protocol. As mentioned above, an important consideration for VCAs relates to the increased risk of acute cellular rejection, especially in the first year after implantation, underscoring the frequent need for induction immunosuppression at the outset. Induction agents serve to help reduce the incidence and/or intensity of early acute rejection episodes through multiple mechanisms unique to the drug used. In the area of extremity VCA transplantation, the majority of patients receive recombinant Anti-thymocyte Globulin (rATG) as an induction agent, with Interleukin (IL)-2 and CD-52 inhibition (using the monoclonal antibodies Basiliximab and Alemtuzumab, respectively) following closely behind [10]. Notably some patients have been managed without any induction therapy at all [11]. In facial transplantation, rATG and Basiliximab have been utilized interchangeably [12], whereas in uterine transplantation the use of rATG is more consistent [13, 14]. Alemtuzumab and rATG have been the most commonly used induction agents in abdominal wall transplantation [15]. The implications of induction therapy in terms of infection and long-term risk of malignancy are not entirely clear, as the occurrence of these events are also related to the type and degree of maintenance immunosuppression. Their observed safety profile nonetheless instills continued confidence in their ongoing usage in VCA transplantation.

2.3.1.1 Recombinant Anti-thymocyte Globulin

The potent clinical immunosuppressive properties of anti-lymphocyte globulin were recognized in the late 1960s with promising results reported further to its first use in kidney transplantation [16]. These sera were obtained by equine immunization, a trend that continued with the first iterations of anti-thymocyte globulin which appeared in the 1980s. rATG was introduced into the realm of transplantation in 1984 and is now the predominant drug in its class. It is a polyclonal serum produced by immunization of rabbits or horses against human thymus tissue and has potent antilymphocyte properties, thought to be mediated primarily by T-cell depletion, although other mechanisms such as complement-dependent cell lysis, B-cell apoptosis, and anti-plasma cell effects are all believed to contribute to its action. The onset of its effects is prompt and broad, allowing upfront intense immunosuppression, with patients typically beginning to recover their lymphocyte counts within 3 months at standard dosing protocols [17].

For induction, rATG is usually administered at a cumulative dose of 3–5 mg/kg (usually at 1.5 mg/kg/day) as higher doses bring an increased risk of side effects. As the drug may exert cross-reactive depletive effects on circulating nonlymphoid cells, it must be administered under caution in patients with thrombocytopenia and leucopenia. Although safely tolerated in the majority of instances including patients with renal dysfunction, other reported adverse reactions include cytokine release syndrome, cardiorespiratory effects (mostly hypotension, but rarely as significant as pulmonary edema and myocardial infarction), and delayed serum sickness. Due to its broader immunosuppression, rATG is thought to confer an increased risk of viral infections (such as Cytomegalovirus) in the posttransplant period in comparison to IL-2 inhibitors, although this point remains contentious.

2.3.1.2 Basiliximab

Basiliximab is a chimeric (human/murine), monoclonal antibody directed against the alpha chain (CD25/Tac antigen) subunit of the IL-2 receptor, expressed in abundance on activated T-lymphocytes [18]. Following its initial FDA approval for use in 1998 toward prevention of acute rejection in kidney transplantation, this drug has gained much popularity across several SOT protocols, especially in comparison to its related predecessor Daclizumab, with which it shares a similar mechanism of action. A portion of its appeal over Daclizumab stemmed from a quicker dosing schedule (20 mg on Day-0 and Day-4) in addition to favorable costs, but the latter nonetheless is in the process of being phased out worldwide due to risks of hepatotoxicity and immune-mediated neurological reactions. In liver transplantation, Basiliximab usage has been relatively common in those patients with associated kidney injury (since clearance of the drug is nonrenal), where it permits the delayed introduction of maintenance therapy with innately nephrotoxic Calcineurin inhibitors (CNI) by a few days. Considered a T-cell nondepleting agent, Basiliximab's duration of action approximates 5 weeks. Its safety profile is considered more favorable than rATG, with less incidence of cytokine release syndrome.

2.3.1.3 Alemtuzumab

Alemtuzumab is anti-CD52 inhibitor was first reported in 1983 as a potent anti-T cell antibody that showed potential in reducing the incidence of graft versus host disease in bone marrow transplant patients through in vitro pretreatment [19]. In its present form, it is a chimeric IgG1 monoclonal antibody that within SOT has found most applicability in off-label induction protocols for kidney transplantation. CD52 is a cell surface glycoprotein that is found on circulating T- and B-cells and to some extent on natural killer cells and monocytes. Through complement and antibody-mediated cell lysis, Alemtuzumab induces rapid and significant upfront lymphopenia that has allowed for improved rates of acute rejection in the short term after kidney transplantation in low-risk recipients. Usual administration is via intravenous or subcutaneous routes, at a total dose of 30–60 mg over two doses. The drug is usually well tolerated but with intravenous administration can be associated with cytokine release syndrome. Replenishment of depleted lymphocytes can typically take from 6 months to a year, so appropriate infective prophylaxis must be undertaken [20].

2.3.2 Maintenance Regimes

Triple therapy with a CNI (Tacrolimus or Cyclosporin), steroids, and Mycophenolate Mofetil (MMF) is considered the standard for maintenance immunosuppression in VCA transplantation.

2.3.2.1 Tacrolimus

Following its acceptance into the compendium of anti-rejection medications in 1993 for liver transplantation, Tacrolimus (FK-506) has since become the mainstay of maintenance regimes for the majority of SOT immunosuppression protocols. This macrolide drug was initially isolated in 1984 from *Streptomyces tsukubaensis* and was shown to inhibit T-lymphocyte activation and IL-2 production through a process of calcineurin phosphatase inhibition via FK binding protein [21]. Initial data suggested an improved rate of acute rejection for Tacrolimus over Cyclosporin, with comparable graft survival in kidney and liver transplantation. However, accumulating evidence suggests that Tacrolimus provides a survival benefit too besides decreased hypertension, but with an increased incidence of diabetes [22, 23]. It is orally administered in the majority of instances, with variable bioavailability (an empty stomach ensures better absorption), subsequent hepatic metabolism and biliary excretion. It is typically commenced at 0.05 mg/kg daily in divided doses. Dosing adjustments are not often required except with significant hepatic impairment, and although the drug is associated with nephrotoxicity, no renal adjusted dosing is required. Other adverse effects include hypertension, tremors, headaches, dyslipidemia, and thrombotic microangiopathy among others. Possible drug interactions must be considered too, especially with those that affect the cytochrome P450 enzyme system which is utilized by the liver to metabolize Tacrolimus. Upfront target trough Tacrolimus levels are 8–12 ng/ml in most VCA programs although there is scope to gradually reduce this with time and graft stability.

2.3.2.2 Cyclosporin

This CNI peptide pre-dates Tacrolimus, having been first isolated in 1971 from the fungus *Tolypocladium inflatum*. Cyclosporin was the cornerstone of maintenance immunosuppression after its approval for use in SOT in 1983, up until the advent of Tacrolimus. At the time, the introduction of Cyclosporin conferred a significant improvement in graft survival after SOT which until then had relied on a largely ineffectual combination regime of Azathioprine and steroids. In present day, Cyclosporin still plays an important role in this SOT, especially in patients intolerant of Tacrolimus. The drug has a mechanism of action similar to the latter, although its calcineurin inhibition occurs via inhibition of cyclophilin rather than FK binding protein. Side effects include hypertension, gum hyperplasia, and hirsutism. The drug is less diabetogenic than Tacrolimus but shares with it a degree, albeit lesser, of nephrotoxicity. Pharmacokinetics shares many features with Tacrolimus in terms of bioavailability, hepatic metabolism and drug interactions. Target trough levels in the short-term after transplantation are 150–300 ng/ml [24].

2.3.2.3 Mycophenolate Mofetil

Mycophenolate Mofetil (MMF) is an anti-metabolite with depletory actions on T- and B-lymphocytes via its binding of the enzyme inosine monophosphate dehydrogenase and resultant inhibition of intracellular purine synthesis. It has been in clinical use for over 20 years for both kidney and liver transplantation and plays an important role in providing a CNI-sparing effect, due to its lack of nephrotoxicity. The drug has all but supplanted Azathioprine in the standard triple-therapy maintenance immunosuppression utilized in SOT patients due to its more favorable side effect profile. Oral bioavailability is excellent and the drug undergoes hepatic metabolism and significant enterohepatic circulation before being excreted in the urine. Adverse effects include cytopenias, gastrointestinal disturbances including diarrhea, and risk of opportunistic infections including CMV viremia [25]. It has teratogenic potential which therefore precludes its use during embryo transfer/implantation in uterine transplantation recipients. In most other VCA regimes, MMF plays an important role in maintenance immunosuppression as well as steroid minimization/cessation protocols.

2.3.2.4 mTOR Inhibitors

The two most commonly employed drugs in this class are Sirolimus (Rapamycin) and Everolimus. These macrolide derivates the mammalian target of Rapamycin (mTOR) complex, which is an intracellular kinase enzyme involved in cell proliferation with resultant effects on T/B-cell regulation. The main remit of these agents within transplantation is toward facilitating CNI minimization/avoidance due to their lower risks of nephrotoxicity, with added potential benefits in terms of reduced CMV viremia and reduced risk of posttransplant malignancy [26]. Notable adverse effects include dyslipidemia, bone marrow suppression, noninfectious pneumonitis, and increased risk of wound-related complications. Additionally, some data suggests that Sirolimus is associated with an increased risk of early postoperative vascular thrombosis such as within the hepatic artery after liver transplantation. These drugs are therefore typically commenced weeks to months after upfront CNI therapy, once the risk of wound/vascular complications has much reduced.

2.3.2.5 Steroids

Corticosteroids were the first medications used in the attempts to prolong organ survival in transplantation [27] and are certainly the most commonly used in current day as part of induction and maintenance therapy in both SOT and VCA recipients. Through the binding of cytosolic glucocorticoid receptors, steroids influence transcription of genes leading to reduction of pro-inflammatory cytokines along with lymphopenia/modulation of lymphocyte function. In more recent years, with the availability of better drugs to maintain viability of grafts, along with an increasing recognition of the long-term deleterious effects of chronic steroid use (such as diabetes, hypertension, muscle atrophy/myopathy, osteoporosis), transplant programs are increasingly exploring the feasibility of steroid withdrawal/sparing protocols. Despite this tendency, these drugs are still the most used first-line option in the treatment of rejection in transplantation.

2.3.2.6 Belatacept

This intravenous drug is a fusion protein of IgG and CTLA-4 (cytotoxic T-cell lymphocyte associated antigen-5) that acts toward T- and B-cell co-stimulation blockade. Belatacept has found most application in kidney transplantation within CNI replacement/minimization regimes. It has shown some efficacy in minimizing DSA formation, although similar benefits do not translate into the area of ACR. Its use is however limited to Epstein–Barr virus seropositive patients due to concerns about development of posttransplantation lymphoproliferative disorder (PTLD) in those with no immunity to the virus. The agent has only been used sporadically in VCA patients, with varying degrees of success [28].

2.3.2.7 Topical Immunosuppression

A novel aspect to extremity and facial VCA is the accessibility offered and therefore the ability to deliver topical immunosuppression as an alternative to oral therapy. This model has been explored in several preclinical VCA studies using topical Tacrolimus or Rapamycin with encouraging, albeit transient effects [29]. Sporadic clinical reports also note the efficacy of topical steroids and Tacrolimus for early rejection in extremity transplantation. Nonetheless their applicability still remains largely experimental [30].

2.3.2.8 Immunosuppression Minimization Protocols

Reduction of maintenance anti-rejection drugs in SOT has always been an attractive proposition toward lessening the risks of long-term immunosuppression and has not surprisingly been explored in VCAs too. There are infrequent reports of success with steroid withdrawal in carefully selected VCA recipients, but such efforts are usually met with increased rates of rejection and nephrotoxicity from the required compensatory increases in CNI therapy [3]. As with SOT, per-protocol reduction in immunosuppression is to be considered on an individual basis, and mostly for patients who have shown stability with initial maintenance regimens. The addition of mTOR inhibitors may permit the reduction in CNI dosing, and on occasion, complete conversion from CNI to the former may be possible. Belatacept can also help in this scenario, with its use being occasionally reported to this effect in VCA patients.

2.4 Rejection

2.4.1 Acute Rejection

Acute rejection (AR) remains a significant impediment to durable graft survival in VCA transplantation and can occur despite good compliance with immunosuppressive treatment regimes. As any cutaneous component of a VCA is often the primary target of the rejection process, their ease of accessibility (along with any associated sentinel flap) permits early clinical suspicion and tissue biopsy. In tissues with a mucosal component (such as with buccal mucosa of facial VCAs and endometrial lining of uterine allografts), biopsies of this layer may provide adjunctive value toward a diagnosis too [31].

T- and B-cell-derived pathways both play important roles in the pathogenesis of AR. Despite the high incidence of pretransplant sensitizing events in recipients of VCAs, episodes of B-cell-dependent antibody-mediated rejection (AMR) are less frequently observed than T-cell-facilitated acute cellular rejection (ACR). This is correlated with a low incidence of donor-specific antibodies (DSAs) in VCA recipients in comparison with that observed in SOT (or alternatively a higher presence of asymptomatic DSAs). The mechanisms for this observation remain largely unexplained, although the typically seen prolonged warm ischemic time, gradual/staged reperfusion, and resultant ischemic preconditioning with graft accommodation may play a role, at least in extremity VCA transplantation [32].

2.4.1.1 Diagnosis and Grading of Acute Rejection

In contrast to that seen with traditional SOT themes (such as kidney and liver) where acute rejection is frequently first suspected on the basis of biochemical alterations on blood tests, VCAs currently offer no such serum laboratory markers. This perhaps makes early suspicion/diagnosis more challenging in the latter. Invariably, tissue biopsy is required to refute/confirm a diagnosis.

The Banff working group convened in 2007 to formulate a skin-themed histological grading system for diagnosis of ACR in VCA transplantation. This essentially stratifies rejection from mild (grade 1) through severe (grade 3) based on increasing degree of perivascular allograft inflammation and epithelial changes, with grade 4 rejection denoting frank epidermal necrosis.

The diagnosis of AMR in VCAs is generally made following clinical suspicion in the absence of a classical cellular infiltrate on tissue biopsy, with detection of DSAs lending supportive evidence. Although positive graft endothelial immunostaining with C4d (a degradation product of the classic complement cascade) along with circulating DSAs are essentially diagnostic of AMR in SOT paradigms, this constellation of findings is rare in VCA transplantation, especially so in extremity VCAs [32]. Nonetheless, on account of their rarity and lack of diagnostic consensus, AMR is currently not included in the Banff grading system for classification of VCA rejection [31]. A pre-emptive strategy to offset having to treat full blown AMR, by periodic screening for threshold levels of DSAs in the circulation along with institution of appropriate treatment when required, is also an option.

2.4.1.2 Treatment

ACR

Cases of mild ACR can at times be managed by increasing maintenance immunosuppression intensity including a small tapering cycle of oral steroids. The mainstay of ACR treatment however, especially in moderate to severe cases, is high-dose intravenous steroids, usually methyl prednisolone. T-cell-depletive therapies such as rATG and Alemtuzumab can also play an important role in higher degree/steroid-resistant cases.

AMR

B-cell-depletive therapies form the foundation for treatment of AMR episodes. Modalities that have been utilized include high-dose intravenous steroids, therapeutic plasma exchange (TPE), intravenous immunoglobulin (IVIG), rATG, Bortezomib, and Rituximab [2], with TPE and IVIG becoming the de facto drugs against which newer therapies are assessed in trials involving kidney transplant recipients with AMR [33].

TPE

In AMR, TPE (plasma pheresis/plasma exchange [PLEX]) entails the removal of circulating antibodies through a process of ex vivo segregation of cellular components from blood, leaving behind an antibody-rich plasma component, which is then discarded. The latter is replaced/substituted by albumin, fresh frozen plasma (FFP) or other colloid solution, and the separated cells resuspended in this before being returned to the circulation. Manual separation of plasma from blood was first described in 1914 but its first clinical application dates back to 1952 in the use of hyperviscosity syndromes. Now with applications across a multitude of immunological indications, TPE is nonetheless always used in conjunction with other agents such as high-dose IVIG in managing AMR. TPE therapy usually amounts to 5–6 once-daily sessions, often followed by additional low-dose IVIG therapy (100 mg/kg) [34]. The drawbacks of TPE include its non-selectivity, which means that plasma proteins such as albumin and non-incriminatory immunoglobulins get removed during the process. Additionally, replenishment using FFP brings with is an infective risk. Further variations to TPE have thus emerged, including double-filtration plasma pheresis (DFPP) and immunoadsorption which in addition to improving the selectivity of antibody removal also reduce these aforementioned risks [35].

IVIG

IVIG is prepared from the pooled sera of a multitude of blood donors and has since its first use in the 1980s (as a stimulant for patients with immunodeficiency) has had its scope broaden considerably, concurrent with the recognition of its immunomodulatory properties. In AMR, IVIG is understood to have depletive actions on circulating antibodies, with the interval between doses allowing for further antibodies from the allograft to leach back into the circulation for targeting. Nonetheless, it is often employed (and recommended to be used) in tandem with TPE or other agents such as Rituximab for maximal efficacy [36, 37]. Typically utilized dosing is at 1–2 g/kg. Adverse effects reported include headaches, bronchospasm, and rarely aseptic meningitis, thrombotic events and acute renal failure.

Rituximab

This chimeric (human/murine) monoclonal antibody exerts its effects by binding to and blocking the cell surface protein CD20 found on B lymphocytes. It has durable lymphodepletive effects usually lasting 6–12 months, but notably does not affect plasma cells (which can continue to be a source of anti-HLA antibodies). Rituximab has been utilized often in treatment of refractory B-cell lymphomas and within SOT, as a pretransplant induction/desensitization protocols for high risk patients. Its value in AMR is debatable, with recent data in kidney transplantation indicating a possible benefit [38]. Usual dosing is 375 mg/m^2 body surface area, and the drug is usually well tolerated, despite concerns about risks of infections in the short to medium term. In AMR treatment, most protocols invariably combine Rituximab with TPE and IVIG, although it is often resorted to as second-line treatment/in instances of steroid-resistant AMR.

Bortezomib

Bortezomib is a proteasome inhibitor with potent activity against plasma cells, which it depletes through a process of apoptosis. It is established in the treatment of myeloma and in recent years has found increasing application as a second/third-line treatment for AMR in SOT. The evidence for it however in this context is at present weak, especially so as a sole agent, which is likely explained in part by evidence of a rebound increase in antibodies with time in preclinical studies [39]. In practice, it is as with most other non-first-line agents in AMR, used along with TPE and IVIG. The drug is usually well tolerated, but reported side effects include reductions in circulating counts of platelets or neutrophils, anemia, peripheral neuropathy, and gastrointestinal disturbances.

Eculizumab

Eculizumab, a C5 inhibitor that interferes with the complement activation cascade, has anecdotal efficacy in AMR in SOT recipients. As rejection is mediated through several pathways rather than complement activation alone, the drug's effects are therefore understandably limited. Its use is usually in conjunction with other anti-rejection agents (and not as monotherapy), that too in refractory cases of AMR. Additionally, there are suggestions that Eculizumab may be less efficacious in the absence of C4d positivity of rejected tissue [40].

2.4.2 Chronic Rejection

Chronic rejection (CR) has been reported more frequently in recent years with accumulating experience in extremity and craniofacial VCAs [4]. Repeated episodes of ACR or AMR can lead to a state of CR, as can long-term suboptimal immunosuppression. Histological diagnosis of CR in its early stages can often be challenging in VCAs since the hallmark features of allograft vasculopathy (as seen in SOT) are not often observed. The CR process here nonetheless focuses on the skin and vessels, with relative sparing of nerves. A recent proposal to streamline the diagnosis of CR in VCAs suggests the presence of features such as capillary thrombosis, vasculopathy with intimal proliferation, skin atrophy, adnexal loss, and fibrosis among others could indicate the early stages of this process [41].

As CR often leads to gradual loss of function and ultimately graft loss, efficient strategies to halt it are much needed but unfortunately lacking. As chronic AMR is the most often encountered type of rejection in SOT, medical management protocols using modalities employed for AMR such as TPE, IVIG, Rituximab, Bortezomib, and Eculizumab are often explored, with limited success. In extremity transplantation, advanced cases of CR may ultimately only be amenable to the radical but pragmatic option of amputation.

2.5 Desensitization and Tolerance Induction Protocols

The prevalence of DSAs in VCA transplant waitlisted patients makes upfront desensitization therapies an attractive proposition, thereby permitting better access to the donor pool, which is regardless stifled by the paucity of suitable donor allografts (as opposed to an actual dearth of deceased donors). This logistical hurdle and the resultant unpredictability of VCA transplantation timing nonetheless make opportune preoperative tackling of sensitization less feasible. Such treatments can alternatively also be instituted immediately after transplantation toward the same effect, i.e., reduction of DSAs that could otherwise hasten the occurrence of AMR. A notable exception is the use of living donation for uterine transplantation, where timings can be controlled. The approaches used in desensitization are again, similar to that employed in therapies for AMR, viz. TPE, IVIG, and various antibody treatments. Newer generation agents showing promise in early reports have encouragingly appeared, including Imlifidase (a *Streptococcus pyogenes*-derived IgG cleaving enzyme), Carfilzomib (proteasome inhibitor), and Tocilizumab (IL-6 inhibitor) among others [42]. Their impact in the area of VCA transplantation is yet to be established.

The induction of tolerance in VCA transplantation is also an area of on-going research, since the benefits of minimizing chronic immunosuppression are obvious. Explored avenues in preclinical models have included attempted priming of regulatory T cells to be permissive against donor antigen, regulatory T-cell augmentation, and induction of recipient chimerism through irradiation and injection of mesenchymal stromal cells [3].

2.6 Conclusions

The arena of VCA transplantation has expanded significantly in over two decades, evolving from a field primarily dealing with extremity and craniofacial allografts to its current scope which includes organs such as the abdominal wall, uterus, penis, and larynx. The immunobiology of VCA transplantation shares many features with that seen in SOT, and much of the current VCA immunosuppressive recommendations draw from the experience gained in SOT paradigms. Nonetheless VCAs are a distinct commodity and bring with them their own challenges. Further understanding of the rejection process in VCAs is required, as is a comprehensive grading system. Maintenance immunosuppression and rejection episodes are best managed at a multidisciplinary level to optimize outcomes. The establishment of a VCA transplantation waiting list by the Organ Procurement and Transplantation Network (OPTN) in the United States in 2014 has formalized the status of VCAs in the national transplant landscape and in conjunction with other national registries will hopefully help generate further data on immunosuppression trends and challenges in this field.

References

1. Wainright JL, Wholley CL, Cherikh WS, Musick JM, Klassen DK. OPTN vascularized composite allograft waiting list: current status and trends in the United States. Transplantation. 2018;102(11):1885–90.
2. Moris D, Cendales LC. Sensitization and desensitization in vascularized composite allotransplantation. Front Immunol. 2021;12:682180.
3. Iske J, Nian Y, Maenosono R, Maurer M, Sauer IM, Tullius SG. Composite tissue allotransplantation: opportunities and challenges. Cell Mol Immunol. 2019;16(4):343–9.
4. Geoghegan L, Al-Khalil M, Scarborough A, Murray A, Issa F. Pre-transplant management and sensitisation in vascularised composite allotransplantation: a systematic review. J Plast Reconstr Aes. 2020;73(9):1593–603.
5. Gibson T, Medawar PB. The fate of skin homografts in man. J Anat. 1943;77(Pt 4):299–310.
6. Gilbert Fernandez JJ, Febres-Cordero RG, Simpson RL. The untold story of the first hand transplant: dedicated to the memory of one of the great minds of the Ecuadorian medical community and the world. J Reconstr Microsurg. 2019;35(3):163–7.
7. Tobin GR, Breidenbach WC, Ildstad ST, Marvin MM, Buell JF, Ravindra KV. The history of human composite tissue allotransplantation. Transplant Proc. 2009;41(2):466–71.
8. Jones JW, Gruber SA, Barker JH, Breidenbach WC. Successful hand transplantation. One-year follow-up. Louisville Hand Transplant Team. N Engl J Med. 2000;343(7):468–73.
9. Benedict JL, Barth RN. How to help patients considering VCA. AMA J Ethics. 2019;21(11):E960–7.
10. Petruzzo P, Sardu C, Lanzetta M, Dubernard JM. Report (2017) of the international registry on hand and composite tissue allotransplantation (IRHCTT). Curr Transp Rep. 2017;4(4):294–303.
11. Petruzzo P, Lanzetta M, Dubernard JM, Landin L, Cavadas P, Margreiter R, et al. The international registry on hand and composite tissue transplantation. Transplantation. 2010;90(12):1590–4.
12. Rifkin WJ, David JA, Plana NM, Kantar RS, Diaz-Siso JR, Gelb BE, et al. Achievements and challenges in facial transplantation. Ann Surg. 2018;268(2):260–70.
13. Richards EG, Farrell RM, Ricci S, Perni U, Quintini C, Tzakis A, et al. Uterus transplantation: state of the art in 2021. J Assist Reprod Genet. 2021;38(9):2251–9.
14. Ricci S, Bennett C, Falcone T. Uterine transplantation: evolving data, success, and clinical importance. J Minim Invasive Gynecol. 2021;28(3):502–12.
15. Honeyman C, Dolan R, Stark H, Fries CA, Reddy S, Allan P, et al. Abdominal wall transplantation: indications and outcomes. Curr Transp Rep. 2020;7(4):279–90.
16. Starzl TE, Marchioro TL, Porter KA, Iwasaki Y, Cerilli GJ. The use of heterologous antilymphoid agents in canine renal and liver homotransplantation and in human renal homotransplantation. Surg Gynecol Obstet. 1967;124(2):301–8.
17. Thiyagarajan UM, Ponnuswamy A, Bagul A. Thymoglobulin and its use in renal transplantation: a review. Am J Nephrol. 2013;37(6):586–601.
18. Berard JL, Velez RL, Freeman RB, Tsunoda SM. A review of interleukin-2 receptor antagonists in solid organ transplantation. Pharmacotherapy. 1999;19(10):1127–37.
19. Hale G, Bright S, Chumbley G, Hoang T, Metcalf D, Munro AJ, et al. Removal of T cells from bone marrow for transplantation: a monoclonal antilymphocyte antibody that fixes human complement. Blood. 1983;62(4):873–82.
20. van der Zwan M, Baan CC, van Gelder T, Hesselink DA. Review of the clinical pharmacokinetics and pharmacodynamics of alemtuzumab and its use in kidney transplantation. Clin Pharmacokinet. 2018;57(2):191–207.
21. Fung JJ. Tacrolimus and transplantation: a decade in review. Transplantation. 2004;77(9 Suppl):S41–3.
22. Ong SC, Gaston RS. Thirty years of tacrolimus in clinical practice. Transplantation. 2021;105(3):484–95.
23. Muduma G, Saunders R, Odeyemi I, Pollock RF. Systematic review and meta-analysis of tacrolimus versus ciclosporin as primary immunosuppression after liver transplant. PLoS One. 2016;11(11):e0160421.
24. Tedesco D, Haragsim L. Cyclosporine: a review. J Transp Secur. 2012;2012:230386.
25. Kaltenborn A, Schrem H. Mycophenolate mofetil in liver transplantation: a review. Ann Transplant. 2013;18:685–96.
26. Waldner M, Fantus D, Solari M, Thomson AW. New perspectives on mTOR inhibitors (rapamycin, rapalogs and TORKinibs) in transplantation. Br J Clin Pharmacol. 2016;82(5):1158–70.
27. Starzl TE. History of clinical transplantation. World J Surg. 2000;24(7):759–82.
28. Giannis D, Moris D, Cendales LC. Costimulation blockade in vascularized composite allotransplantation. Front Immunol. 2020;11:544186.
29. Safi AF, Kauke M, Nelms L, Palmer WJ, Tchiloemba B, Kollar B, et al. Local immunosuppression in vascularized composite allotransplantation (VCA): a systematic review. J Plast Reconstr Aesthet Surg. 2021;74(2):327–35.
30. Schnider JT, Weinstock M, Plock JA, Solari MG, Venkataramanan R, Zheng XX, et al. Site-specific immunosuppression in vascularized composite allotransplantation: prospects and potential. Clin Dev Immunol. 2013;2013:495212.
31. Schneider M, Cardones AR, Selim MA, Cendales LC. Vascularized composite allotransplantation: a closer look at the banff working classification. Transpl Int. 2016;29(6):663–71.
32. Kaufman CL, Cascalho M, Ozyurekoglu T, Jones CM, Ramirez A, Roberts T, et al. The role of B cell immunity in VCA graft rejection and acceptance. Hum Immunol. 2019;80(6):385–92.
33. Wan SS, Ying TD, Wyburn K, Roberts DM, Wyld M, Chadban SJ. The treatment of antibody-mediated rejection in kidney transplantation: an updated systematic review and meta-analysis. Transplantation. 2018;102(4):557–68.
34. Padmanabhan A, Connelly-Smith L, Aqui N, Balogun RA, Klingel R, Meyer E, et al. Guidelines on the use of therapeutic apheresis in clinical practice - evidence-based approach from the Writing Committee of the American Society for Apheresis: the eighth special issue. J Clin Apher. 2019;34(3):171–354.
35. Xie P, Tao M, Peng K, Zhao H, Zhang K, Sheng Y, et al. Plasmapheresis therapy in kidney transplant rejection. Blood Purif. 2019;47(1-3):73–84.

36. Jordan SC, Toyoda M, Kahwaji J, Vo AA. Clinical aspects of intravenous immunoglobulin use in solid organ transplant recipients. Am J Transplant. 2011;11(2):196–202.
37. Lefaucheur C, Nochy D, Andrade J, Verine J, Gautreau C, Charron D, et al. Comparison of combination plasmapheresis/IVIg/anti-CD20 versus high-dose IVIg in the treatment of antibody-mediated rejection. Am J Transplant. 2009;9(5):1099–107.
38. Macklin PS, Morris PJ, Knight SR. A systematic review of the use of rituximab for the treatment of antibody-mediated renal transplant rejection. Transplant Rev. 2017;31(2):87–95.
39. Agarwal D, Allman D, Naji A. Novel therapeutic opportunities afforded by plasma cell biology in transplantation. Am J Transplant. 2020;20(8):1984–91.
40. Jordan SC, Choi J, Kahwaji J, Vo A. Complement inhibition for prevention and treatment of antibody-mediated rejection in renal allograft recipients. Transplant Proc. 2016;48(3):806–8.
41. Kaufman CL, Kanitakis J, Weissenbacher A, Brandacher G, Mehra MR, Amer H, et al. Defining chronic rejection in vascularized composite allotransplantation-The American Society of Reconstructive Transplantation and International Society of Vascularized Composite Allotransplantation chronic rejection working group: 2018 American Society of Reconstructive Transplantation meeting report and white paper Research goals in defining chronic rejection in vascularized composite allotransplantation. SAGE Open Med. 2020;8:2050312120940421.
42. Kumar V, Locke JE. New perspectives on desensitization in the current era - an overview. Front Immunol. 2021;12:696467.

Part II

Face Transplantation

Face Transplantation: Cleveland Clinic Experience

3

Nicholas R. Sinclair, Raffi Gurunian, Antonio Rampazzo, Bahar Bassiri Gharb, Brian Gastman, Risal Djohan, Frank Papay, and Maria Z. Siemionow

3.1 Introduction

The Cleveland Clinic Foundation (CCF) facial allotransplantation program began its Institutional Review Board (IRB) approval process in 2002. Two years later, the CCF Department of Plastic Surgery received the world's first IRB approval to perform facial allotransplantation on an experimental basis [1]. Due to its experimental status, funding was provided through the Cleveland Clinic Foundation (patient #1) and the Department of Defense Armed Forces Institute for Regenerative Medicine, grant number W81XWH-08-2-0034 (patients #2 and #3).

A recent review article [2] provides significant detail of the patient screening and evaluation process for potential face transplant candidates at CCF. Between 2004 and 2016, 200 patients were referred to CCF for transplant evaluation. Initial evaluation was performed by a transplant coordinator to ensure the patient met IRB inclusion criteria. The patient's tissue defect was characterized as proposed by our institution's classification system [3], which had been modified from Cordeiro and Santamaria [4]. Potential exclusion criteria included terminal illness, active cancer, preexisting immunosuppression, inability to travel, active substance abuse, or facial defect considered inappropriate for facial transplantation. During the 12-year period, 60 patients were deemed potential candidates and underwent a telephone interview. After review and discussion with the transplant team, 13 patients were invited for in-person evaluation. Subsequently, four patients at CCF have been listed for transplant, and three patients have undergone facial transplantation.

3.2 Case 1 [5, 6]

3.2.1 Patient Presentation

The patient was a 45-year-old female who sustained midface trauma from a close-range shotgun blast in September 2004. She was initially treated at an outside hospital and secondarily referred to CCF 2 months after the trauma. Her initial facial deformities included absence of the nose, including nasal lining and bone; subtotal palatal defect; contracted upper lip remnants; loss of orbicularis oris and orbicularis oculi function; lower eyelid scarring with ectropion; right-eye enucleation requiring eye prosthesis; and partial facial nerve deficit with lack of bilateral midface function. Prior to facial transplantation, she underwent 23 reconstructive procedures that included free fibula flap and split-calvarial/rib grafts for bony reconstruction; and anterolateral thigh free flap, temporalis muscle flap, paramedian forehead flap, radial forearm free flap, and multiple skin grafts for soft tissue reconstruction.

Unfortunately, she continued to have significant disfigurement and functional limitation after these procedures (Figs. 3.1 and 3.2). Thus, she was evaluated by the CCF Facial Transplantation team in 2008. After multidisciplinary clearance, including medical, psychosocial, and ethical, informed consent was signed, and she was listed with a local organ procurement organization in the third quarter of 2008. A summary of the patient's facial deformities at the time of transplantation can be found in Table 3.1.

3.2.2 Pretransplant Planning and Flap Design

A computed tomographic angiogram (CTA) was obtained to evaluate her vascular anatomy prior to transplantation

The original version of the chapter has been revised. A correction to this chapter can be found at https://doi.org/10.1007/978-3-031-21520-9_35

N. R. Sinclair (✉) · R. Gurunian (✉) · A. Rampazzo · B. B. Gharb
B. Gastman · R. Djohan · F. Papay
Department of Plastic Surgery, Cleveland Clinic, Cleveland, OH, USA
e-mail: GURUNIR@ccf.org; RAMPAZA@ccf.org; BASSIRB@ccf.org; GASTMAB@ccf.org; DJOHANR@ccf.org PAPAYF@ccf.org

M. Z. Siemionow
Department of Orthopaedics, University of Illinois at Chicago, College of Medicine, Chicago, IL, USA
e-mail: siemiom@uic.edu

© Springer Nature Switzerland AG 2023, corrected publication 2023

R. Gurunian et al. (eds.), *Reconstructive Transplantation*, https://doi.org/10.1007/978-3-031-21520-9_3

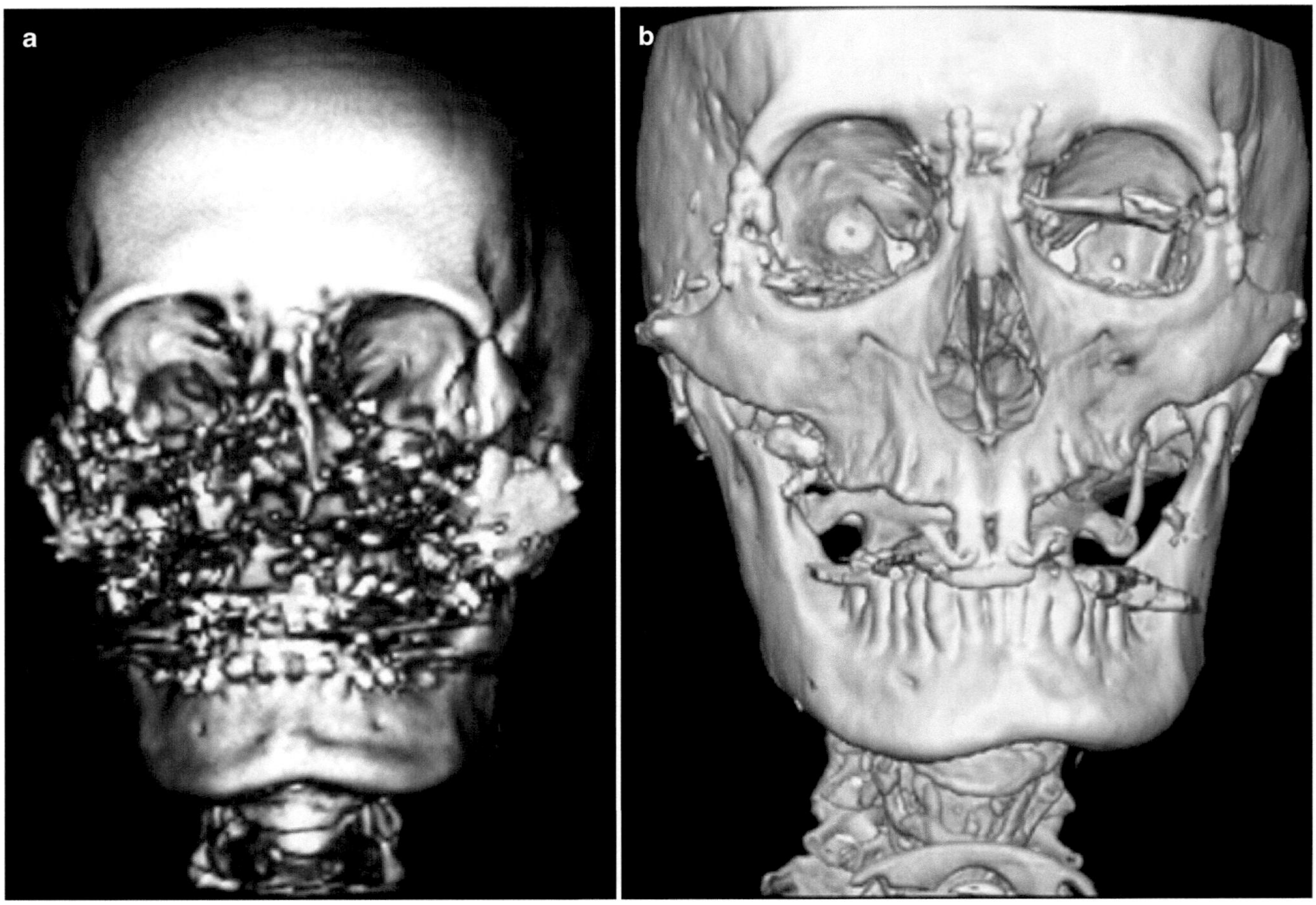

Fig. 3.1 Three-dimensional CT scan of patient 1. (**a**) Prior to reconstructive efforts, CT demonstrates near-total destruction of midface skeleton. (**b**) Three months after transplantation, CT demonstrates replacement of all missing bony components with the composite facial allograft from the donor

(Fig. 3.3). Her left external carotid artery (ECA) and facial artery (FA) systems were patent, as was the left internal jugular vein (IJV). On the right, the ECA was patent; however, the majority of its branches were compromised. Further, the right FA was absent at the level of the neck from prior free flap reconstruction. The right IJV was significantly stenotic. With the loss of midface vascular arcades connecting the upper and lower face arterial systems, the lower face was essentially supplied by the left FA while the upper face was supplied by the bilateral ECA systems.

Given the patient's defects and vascular anatomy, the ideal donor allograft would include bony support of the midface with adequate skin and soft tissue coverage. The planned allograft was based on a Le Fort III composite tissue design containing total nose, lower eyelids, upper lip, total orbital floor, bilateral zygomas, anterior maxilla, and the hard palate with alveolus and incisors. To restore mimetic function, the midface muscles and the facial nerve containing parotids would have to be included. The planned vascular pedicles for the allograft were the bilateral common FAs, bilateral EJVs, and the left posterior facial vein. To maintain perfusion to the native lower face, the native left FA would have to be preserved. A three-dimensional CT scan with life-size stereolithographic model and a facial moulage was created. Leading up to the actual transplant event, multiple mock fresh-cadaver dissections and transplants were performed by all participating surgeons.

3.2.3 Donor

The donor was a brain-dead woman who matched the patient in age, race, and skin complexion. Given the unique nature of facial transplantation, specific informed consent to recover and transplant the donor's face was obtained from the donor's family.

3.2.4 Immunologic Characteristics

The donor's blood group was A and the recipient's was AB. The donor and recipient shared two major human leukocyte antigens (HLA) (donor: HLA A 11,23; B 44,64; Cw 5,8; DR 7,16; DRw51; DQ5,9; recipient: HLA A 1,29; B 8,44; Cw 7,16; DR 7,17; DRw52; DQ2). The recipient had no anti-HLA reactive antibodies and retrospective cross-match was negative. The donor was cytomegalovirus (CMV) positive, and the recipient was CMV negative.

3.2.5 Operative Course

To facilitate simultaneous graft harvest and recipient preparation, eight surgeons were divided into two teams. To optimize communication and coordination, the two operating rooms were adjacent and connected by a substerile corridor. The duration of the entire procedure was 22 h. Prior to incision on either patient, a template of required tissues from the donor was created. The recipient team started first to ensure that the vascular territories were intact.

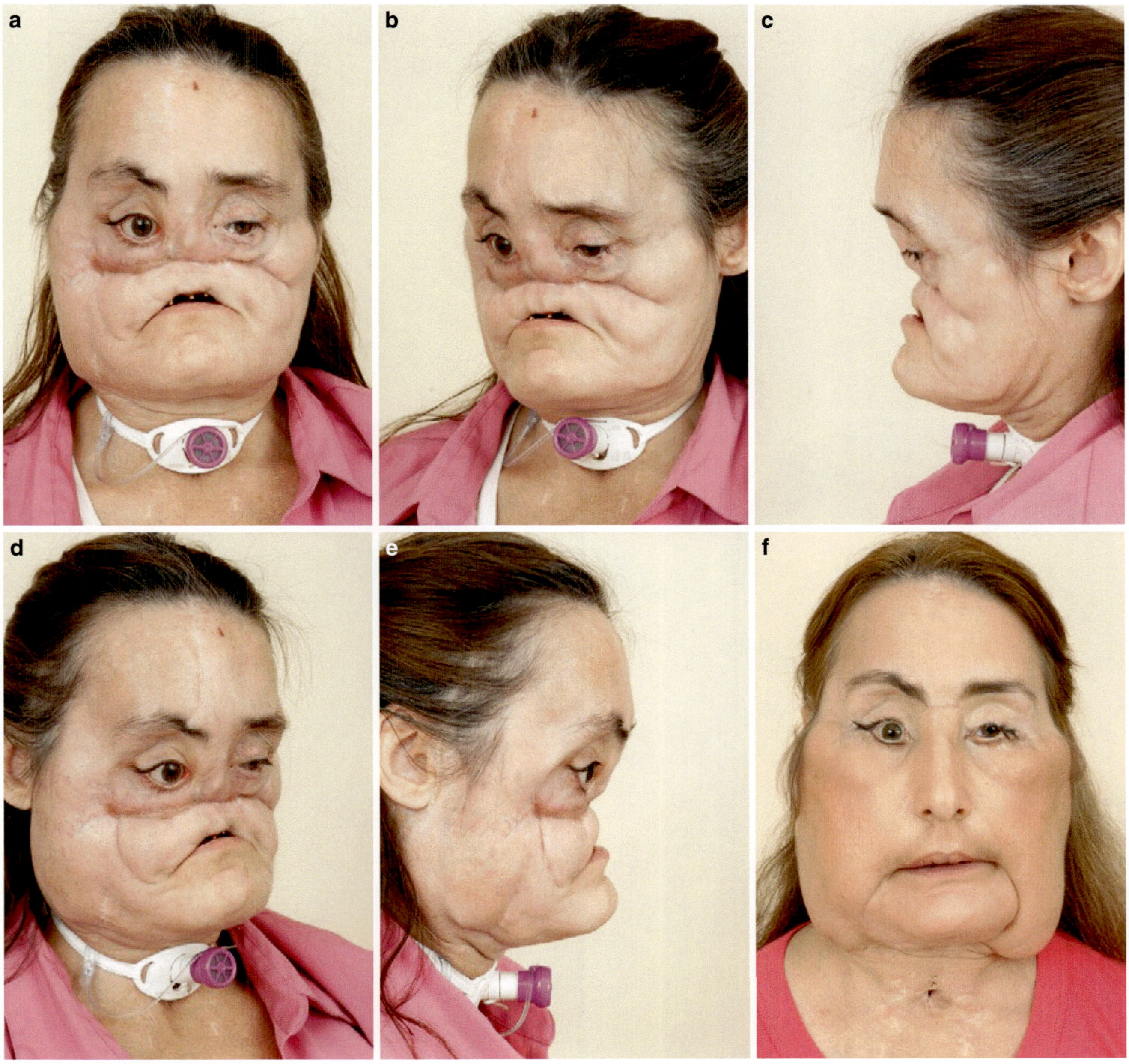

Fig. 3.2 Patient 1 before (**a**–**e**) and 6 months prior to face transplant (**f**–**j**). Preoperatively, one can appreciate severe facial concavity with absent nose, upper lip, and scarred lower eyelids. Maxilla-containing face transplant for successful reconstruction of the defect with restoration of functional and aesthetic subunits. Postoperatively, she did have increased bigonial width and laxity, which was eventually treated with a SMAS plication facelift

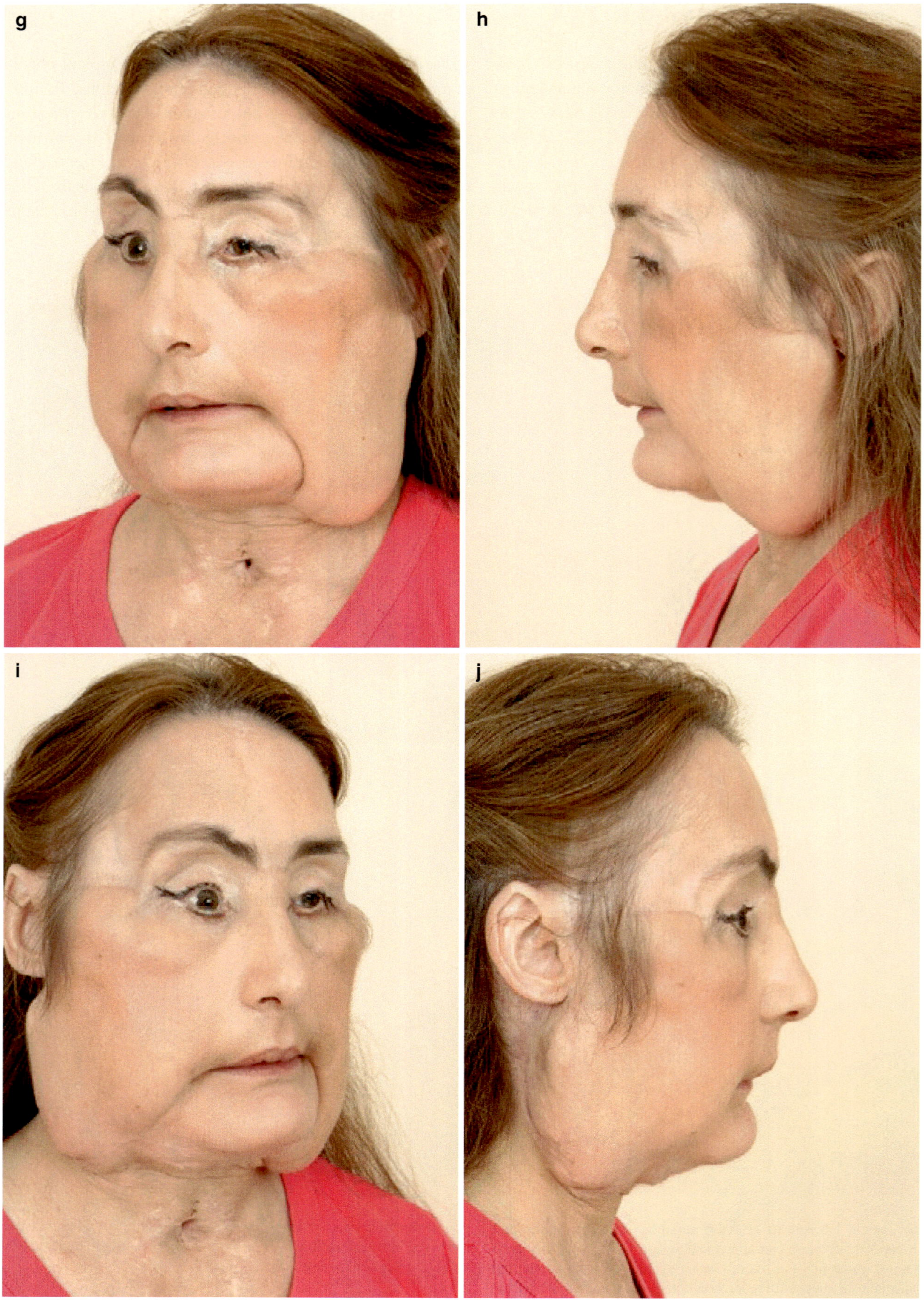

Fig. 3.2 (continued)

After an outline of the template was marked on the recipient's face, previous scars were incised to expose the bilateral ECAs, bilateral common carotid arteries, left FA, bilateral facial veins, bilateral EJVs, and bilateral IJVs. Both parotid glands were then dissected to expose the facial nerve trunks. The bone and soft tissue from previous reconstructions, as well as hardware, were all removed. The infraorbital nerves were not able to be identified, thus sensory reinnervation was not able to be performed as planned. After ensuring that the exposed vessels could accommodate the allograft while perfusing the native lower face and scalp, the donor team was notified and the harvest commenced.

Table 3.1 Craniofacial defects of patient 1 at the time of facial transplantation

1	Loss of total midfacial structure including absent nasal structure covered by a paramedian forehead flap, absent maxilla, zygoma, and orbital rims bilaterally
2	Loss of vertical facial height due to midface collapse and retrusion
3	Right eye enucleation with prosthesis
4	Telecanthus with bilateral eyelid shortening and loss of right medial and lateral canthal tendon attachments
5	Right brow malposition
6	Right temporal wasting
7	Excess right hemifacial bulk from previous ALT flap
8	Bilateral oral commissure descent secondary to loss midfacial mimetic musculature
9	Facial nerve deficits including total loss of midface mimetic muscles, unilateral right brow paralysis, and bilateral lower division weakness

Allograft harvest proceeded according to the defect template, which had been practiced during mock transplants in the cadaver laboratory. First, the neck vessels, including the common carotid arteries, ECAs, FA, IJVs, and EJVs were dissected. The retromandibular veins and IJVs were traced superiorly toward the parotid where the facial nerve trunk was then identified as proximally as possible. The intraoral mucosal incisions were then made. Osteotomies were then made following a Le Fort III pattern.

Once the recipient team confirmed that the wound bed and recipient vessels were ready, the allograft pedicles were divided and the graft was brought to the donor room. Prior to microvascular anastomosis, bony fixation was performed at five points, including the nasofrontal junction, the zygomatic arches, and the lateral orbital rims (Fig. 3.1). The left side anastomoses were done first. First, the left donor FA was anastomosed to the recipient ECA. The left donor facial vein and EJV were anastomosed to their recipient counterparts. The recipient left FA was left intact. After completing the left side vessels, the clamps were taken off to re-perfuse the allograft. Excellent perfusion was noted. The total ischemia

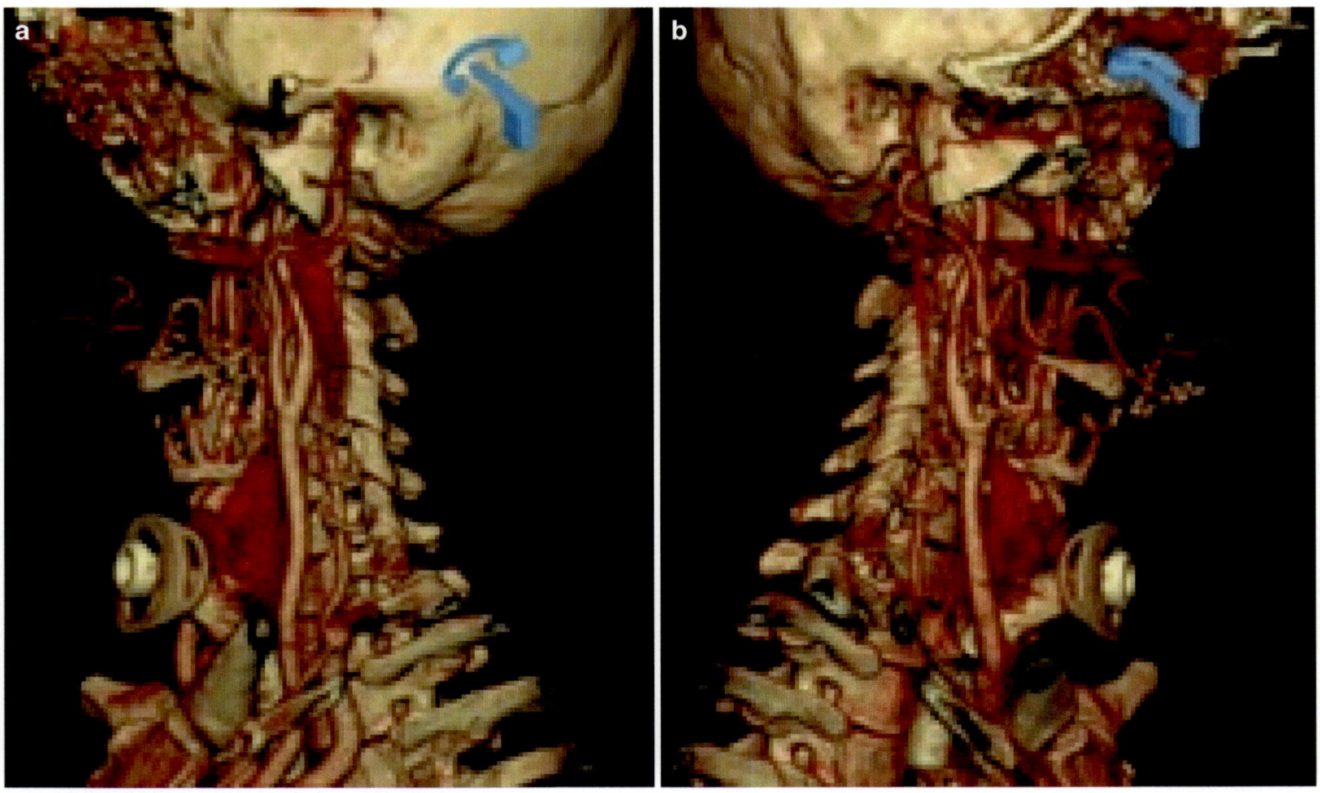

Fig. 3.3 Representative images from the computed tomographic angiogram of the left (**a**) and right (**b**) carotid systems

time for bony fixation and the left side microvascular anastomoses was 2 h and 40 min. Next, the right-side microvascular anastomoses were performed, consisting of donor FA to recipient FA and donor IJV to recipient IJV. The facial nerve coaptation was then performed. The recipient's right facial nerve upper division was connected to the donor main facial nerve trunk with an interposition graft taken from the donor's vagus nerve. The same procedure was performed on the left utilizing a nerve graft from the donor's hypoglossal nerve. Finally, the allograft was inset with approximation of muscle, mucosa, and skin. The patient was then taken to the Intensive Care Unit while being ventilated through a tracheostomy.

3.2.6 Immunosuppression

Induction of immunosuppression was achieved with rabbit anti-thymocyte globulin (1.2 mg/kg intravenously once a day for 9 days) combined with a 1000 mg bolus of intravenous methylprednisolone on the day of transplant. Bone marrow infusion, irradiation, nor phototherapy was used. The maintenance immunosuppression regimen consisted of tacrolimus, mycophenolate mofetil (MMF), and low-dose oral prednisone. Tacrolimus was dosed for a target blood trough level of 12–15 ng/mL for the first 3 months and 10–12 ng/mL thereafter. MMF dosage was determined by the patient's white blood cell count and was discontinued after 6 months.

Prophylaxis for cytomegalovirus and *Pneumocystis jirovecii* included ganciclovir (5 mg/kg intravenously twice a day) for 8 weeks followed by valganciclovir (900 mg twice a day) for 5 months, and trimethoprim-sulfamethoxazole (160 mg/800 mg three times per week) thereafter.

3.2.7 Initial Postoperative Course

The patient had an uneventful postoperative course. She was successfully discharged from the hospital 6 weeks after surgery. Prior to discharge she underwent intensive physical therapy, rehabilitation, and psychosocial care as detailed below.

3.2.8 Physical Therapy and Rehabilitation

Once daily physical therapy and speech therapy sessions commenced 48 hours after surgery. After 6 weeks of daily sessions, therapy sessions were continued three times per week. Rehabilitation consisted of supervised controlled passive and active motion exercises, assessment of mastication, speech exercises, swallowing of liquids and solid foods, facial expression exercises, and sensory re-education.

3.2.9 Psychosocial Care

Daily treatment sessions with a board-certified psychiatrist occurred during the first 6 weeks. Anxiety, depression, and quality of life were assessed and followed with the perception of teasing scale, Rosenberg's self-esteem scale, the body esteem scale for adolescents and adults, fear of negative appearance evaluation scale, physical appearance state and trait anxiety scale, and the body-self relations questionnaire (appearance evaluation subscale).

3.2.10 Functional and Neurosensory Outcome

Quantitative neurosensory testing was assessed with 2-point sensory discrimination of the facial skin by pressure-specified sensory device (Sensory Management Services LLC, Baltimore, MD, USA) and by clinical assessment. At 6 months posttransplant, sensory discrimination had returned to the entire face. The patient achieved excellent functional recovery with restoration of major functions, including sense of smell, ability to eat solid food, ability to drink from a cup, and intelligible speech.

3.2.11 Rejection Episodes and Long-Term Complications

Routine biopsies were performed intermittently, and the patient was followed closely for clinical signs of rejection. On posttransplant day 47, routine biopsy demonstrated Banff III/IV rejection of the graft mucosa without evidence of skin rejection. This was treated with a single 1-gram bolus methylprednisolone followed by an oral prednisone taper. Successful treatment of the episode was confirmed with biopsy 3 days later. For the next 4 years, routine biopsies consistently showed mild acute rejection (Banff scores I to II) without clinical signs of rejection. These findings were not treated. Approximately 4.5 years after transplantation, the patient was admitted to the hospital and treated for rejection after routine biopsy showed Banff III/IV rejection on the graft mucosa and skin. She was treated with 1 g of intravenous methylprednisolone followed by an increased dosage of oral prednisone. Her tacrolimus trough level was maintained at 10 ng/mL, and MMF was added back to her immunosuppression regimen. Repeat biopsies 1 month later demonstrated reduction in inflammation with a return to Banff I/IV rejection.

Approximately 9.5 years after transplantation, the patient was admitted to an outside hospital with pneumonia. She was subsequently transferred to CCF for care. She was successfully treated with intravenous antibiotics. Routine graft biopsies during that admission showed baseline Banff grade II/IV acute rejection with signs of mild chronic rejection. After multidisciplinary discussion, the decision was made to continue with an unchanged immunosuppression regimen. Six months later, she was admitted to the hospital with new cutaneous lesions of the allograft cheek. Biopsies of lesions showed suppurative ulceration with folliculitis and bacterial colonization. Biopsies of the unaffected skin and mucosa showed Banff II/IV rejection. The etiology of the lesions was thought to be secondary to skin picking. She was treated with local wound care and behavioral therapy to reduce skin picking. Her immunosuppression regimen was not changed.

Approximately 10.5 years after transplantation, the patient was admitted with worsening of the aforementioned cutaneous lesions. Biopsies now showed Banff III/IV acute rejection with severe chronic rejection. She was treated with a 1 g methylprednisolone bolus followed by an increase in her prednisone dosage to 20 mg with a gradual taper. Topical tacrolimus was added to her regimen. Her remaining oral immunosuppression regimen was left the same. Follow-up biopsies 1 month and 3 months later showed return to baseline Banff grade I to II rejection.

Approximately 11 years after transplantation, the patient presented with redness of the right cheek (graft tissue) as well as the native periorbital region. A CT scan showed preseptal cellulitis for which she was treated with intravenous antibiotics. Biopsies of the affected tissue and unaffected graft showed improving chronic B-cell rejection. Her redness improved with antibiotics and an unchanged immunosuppression regimen. She was eventually discharged on oral antibiotics.

In April 2020 (11 years and 4 months following transplantation), she was admitted to the medical ICU with acute pancreatitis, neutropenia, and respiratory distress. She was found to be SARS-CoV-2 negative but rhinovirus positive. She was treated with supportive care, filgrastim, and empirical intravenous antibiotics. Her immunosuppression regimen was maintained. After an 11-day hospitalization, she was discharged to a rehabilitation facility. Three months later she was transferred from the rehabilitation facility back to the medical ICU with hypoxemic respiratory failure requiring intubation and mechanical ventilation. She was found to have a fungal pneumonia on bronchoalveolar lavage. After 22 days in the ICU, she passed away from multiorgan failure secondary to an infection unrelated to her transplant. The patient passed away 11 years, 8 months, and 19 days after her facial allotransplantation. At that point, she was the longest living face transplant patient.

3.3 Case 2 [7–9]

3.3.1 Patient Presentation

The patient was a 44-year-old male who sustained bilateral combined Le Fort fractures from a motor vehicle collision in October 2011. The fractures were managed with open reduction and internal fixation (ORIF) at an outside hospital. He recovered uneventfully until March 2012 when he developed multiple episodes of necrotizing sinus and periocular inflammation that were refractory to antimicrobial treatment. He was treated with hardware removal and surgical debridement. By April 2013, his right globe had become exposed, and he was referred to CCF. He was found to have total blindness in the right eye. Thus, he was treated with wide debridement and right orbital exenteration. After multiple bouts of worsening inflammatory episodes, a large communication between his oral cavity, right orbit, and frontal sinus eventually developed. His orofacial communication was treated with a free rectus abdominis muscle flap, and his exposed skull was covered with a free latissimus dorsi muscle flap. After a brief period of quiescence, the inflammatory process again progressed. Frankly necrotic areas again necessitated further debridement. Given the progression of disease following surgical intervention, it became evident that aggressive debridement would not resolve the underlying issue. In August 2013, further histologic and immunologic workup revealed a diagnosis of granulomatosis with polyangiitis, formerly known as Wegner's granulomatosis. He was treated with corticosteroids, rituximab, and intravenous immunoglobulin. Within weeks of treatment initiation, his wounds stabilized; however, the existing craniofacial destruction was extensive (Figs. 3.4 and 3.5). Given his significant facial defects, persistent dural exposure, and impending bilateral loss of orbits with total blindness, facial allotransplantation was discussed with the patient. After systematic rheumatologic, psychosocial, medical, ethical, and surgical evaluation, the patient was listed for face transplant in March 2014. A summary of the patient's craniofacial defects at the time of transplant can be found in Table 3.2.

3.3.2 Transplant Preparation and Flap Design

Pretransplant CTA demonstrated patent bilateral ECAs, superior thyroid arteries, lingual arteries, maxillary arteries, and superficial temporal arteries. Both FAs had been used for previous free tissue transfers and were patent on CTA. Bilateral EJVs and IJVs were widely patent. Given the patient's defects, the planned allograft followed a Le Fort III pattern and included total replacement of the midface bony structures. Further, soft tissue harvest would include the entire midface, bilateral upper and lower eyelids, upper face, and anterior scalp. As granulomatosis with polyangiitis spares the lower face, the decision was made to leave the native lower face intact. Planned arterial supply for the allograft was the bilateral donor ECAs anastomosed to the recipient ECAs distal to the FA and lingual artery. Planned venous outflow included the donor IJVs anastomosed to the recipient IJVs. Given the destruction of peripheral facial nerve branches, we again planned to utilize interposition

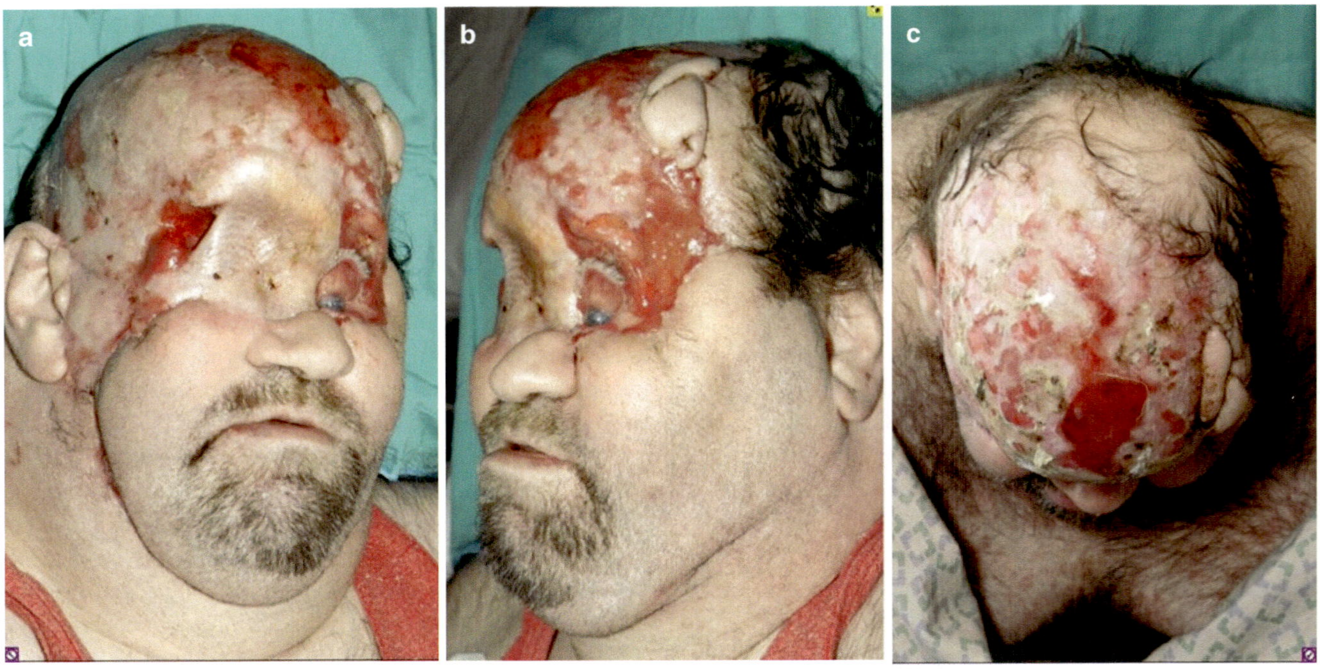

Fig. 3.4 (**a**) Right oblique view of the patient before transplantation. Note the extensive damage to the upper face soft tissues, which were replaced by unstable scarring. The right eye had been previously exenterated. The temporal scalp was absent and scarring of the preauricular and parotid regions extended to the neck. (**b**) Left oblique view of the patient before facial transplantation. Skeletal erosion had induced midface collapse. The left eye developed severe exposure keratopathy due to loss and scarring of the upper and lower eyelids. (**c**) View from above the head before transplantation. The anterior two-thirds of the scalp had been lost and replaced with unstable scarring

nerve grafts to perform a tensionless coaptation of the upper facial nerve divisions. With total destruction of the bilateral infraorbital and supraorbital nerves, no sensory reinnervation was planned. A three-dimensional CT scan with life-size stereolithographic model and a facial moulage were created. Leading up to the actual transplant event, multiple, mock fresh-cadaver dissections and transplants were performed by all participating surgeons. Facial transplantation was successfully completed in September 2014.

3.3.3 Donor

The donor was a 21-year-old male who was pronounced brain dead 48 h prior to transplantation after sustaining a near fatal gunshot wound. His craniofacial skeleton and soft tissues were intact and considered a good match for the recipient. Prior to transplantation, CTA demonstrated intact neck vessels including bilateral ECAs, FAs, IJVs, and EJVs.

3.3.4 Immunologic Characteristics

The donor's and recipient's blood groups were both A positive. The donor and recipient shared two major HLAs (donor: HLA A2; B18,60; Bw negative; Cw7,10; DR8,11; DRw52; DQ4,7; recipient: HLA A11,24; B27,63; Bw negative; DR4,4; DRw52; DQ8). The donor was CMV positive, and the recipient was CMV negative.

3.3.5 Operative Course

As with our previous face transplant, we utilized a two-team approach in adjacent operating rooms adjoined by a substerile corridor. Given the multiple available recipient vessels on CTA, the decision was made to start the allograft harvest first and ensure adequate progress prior to beginning the recipient preparation.

The allograft was harvested through a posterior scalp incision along the lambdoid suture curving along the upper helices of the ears to continue along the preauricular sulci to the neck. The central face incisions started at the subnasale and encircled the perioral region. The upper and lower eyelids were harvested with transconjunctival incisions. Vessels in the neck were dissected and traced superiorly toward the parotid. The facial nerve was identified and the facial nerve-containing parotid was included in the allograft. The superficial temporal anatomy was preserved in the allograft to maintain perfusion to the scalp. After soft tissue dissection, medical models were used to guide skeletal dissection and osteotomies. Donor enucleation and orbital osteotomies

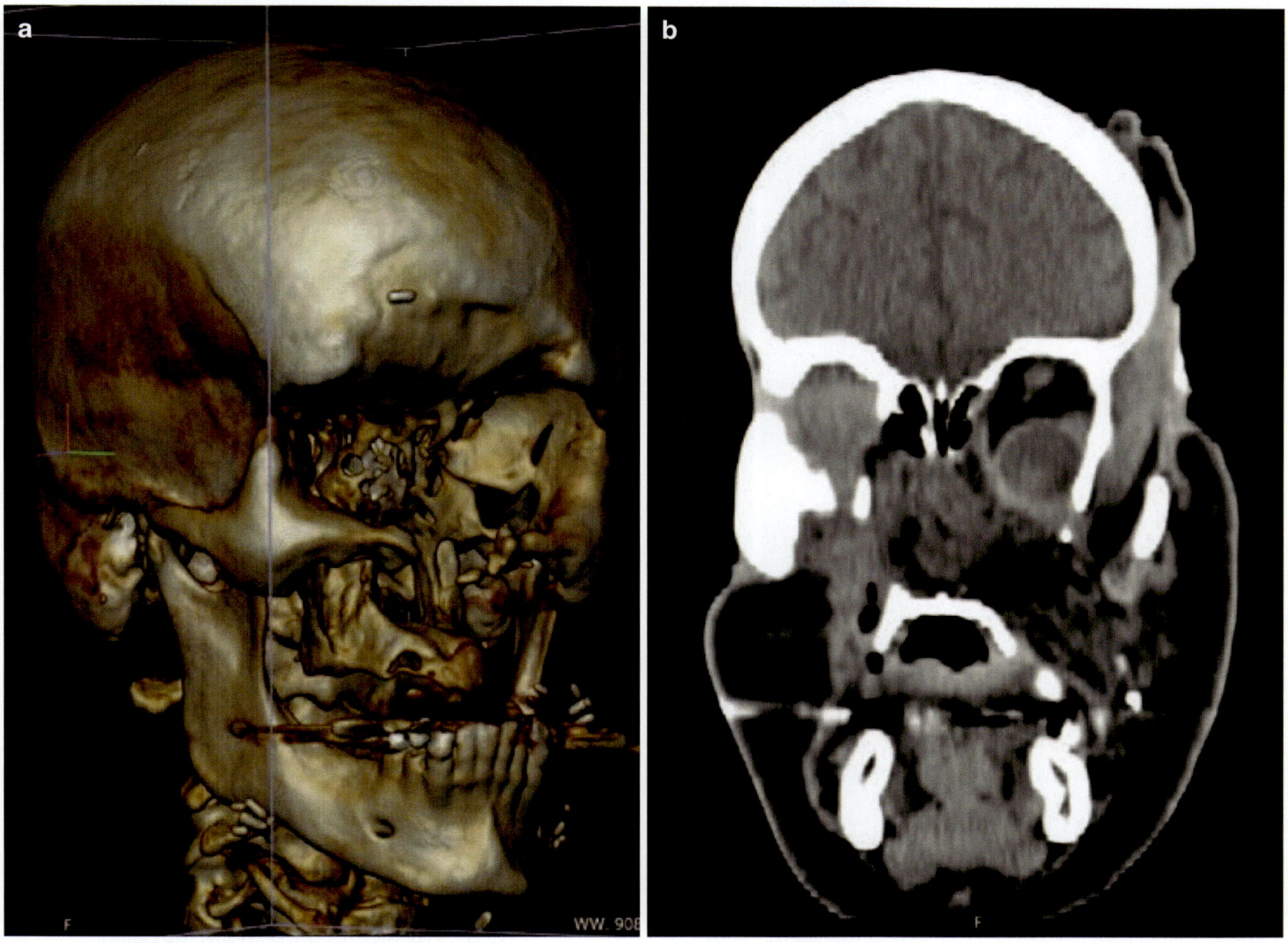

Fig. 3.5 (**a**) Three-dimensional reconstruction of craniofacial skeleton showing extensive bony loss of medial orbital walls; ethmoid air cells; orbital floor; nasal bones; nasal septum; and anterior, medial, and lateral wall of right and left maxillae, in addition to the alveolar process and all dental elements. Note the palatine process of the maxilla only remaining. (**b**) Coronal view of the craniofacial region showing downward migration of remaining left globe caused by loss of left orbital floor support. Note wide communication between sinonasal and both orbital cavities

Table 3.2 Craniofacial defects of patient 2 at the time of facial transplantation

1	Loss of frontal sinus tables and mucosa leading to dural exposure
2	Loss of medial supraorbital bar and glabella
3	Loss of midface structures: nasal bones, nasal septum, bilateral maxilla including orbital floors, primary and secondary palate, frontozygomatic junction
4	Loss of bilateral peripheral branches of facial nerve upper division
5	Loss of bilateral infraorbital nerve
6	Loss of bilateral supraorbital nerve

were performed. Craniofacial disjunction followed a Le Fort III pattern.

The recipient was prepared with radical resection of all midface and upper face skin, scarring, and fibrotic tissue (Fig. 3.6). Vessels in the neck were dissected and evaluation confirmed widely patent bilateral ECA systems, EJVs, IJVs. The perioral region and lower facial skeleton were left intact. After communication between the two teams confirming that the recipient was adequately prepared, the donor vascular pedicle was ligated and the allograft was brought to the recipient operating room.

First, 3-point skeletal fixation was achieved at the glabella and the bilateral zygomatic-frontal sutures (Fig. 3.7). The left-side microvascular anastomoses were done first, consisting of donor ECA to recipient ECA and donor IJV to recipient IJV. The ECA anastomosis was performed distal to the recipient facial and lingual arteries to maintain perfusion the native lower face. After finishing the left-side microvascular anastomoses, the vascular clamps were removed. Total ischemia time was less than 60 min. Next, the right-side microvascular anastomoses were done, consisting of donor ECA

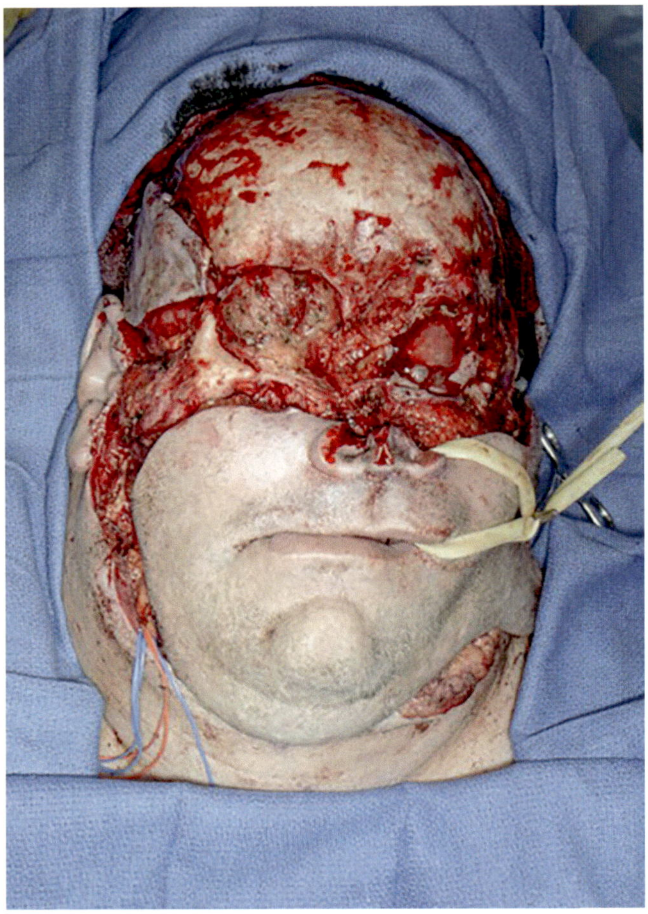

Fig. 3.6 Intraoperative photo of the recipient immediately before face transplant. In preparation of allograft inset, all unstable scarring and fibrosis involving the upper two thirds of the face were resected

to recipient ECA and donor facial vein to recipient EJV. The upper division of the facial nerves were coapted utilizing interposition nerve grafts with donor vagus nerve. Finally, inset of the allograft was undertaken with approximation of the facial muscles, mucosa, and skin (Fig. 3.8). The patient was taken to the SICU ventilated through a tracheostomy.

3.3.6 Immunosuppression

Six months prior to transplantation, the recipient had been started on tacrolimus to control his granulomatosis with polyangiitis. Mycophenolate mofetil (MMF) was added to his regimen immediately prior to transplantation. Following transplant, full immunosuppression was induced with rabbit anti-thymocyte globulin (1.2 mg/kg intravenously once a day for 9 days) combined with a 1000 mg bolus of intravenous methylprednisolone. Again, bone marrow infusion, irradiation, nor phototherapy was used. Following induction, his maintenance immunosuppression regimen consisted of tacrolimus, and oral prednisone. MMF was held postoperatively due to a *Methicillin-resistant Staphylococcus aureus* bacteremia. MMF was added back to his maintenance regimen 11 months posttransplantation. For the first month postoperatively, topical tacrolimus ointment was also utilized.

Prophylaxis for CMV and *Pneumocystis jirovecii* included ganciclovir (5 mg/kg intravenously twice a day) for 8 weeks followed by valganciclovir (900 mg twice a day) for 5 months, and trimethoprim-sulfamethoxazole (160 mg/800 mg three times per week) thereafter.

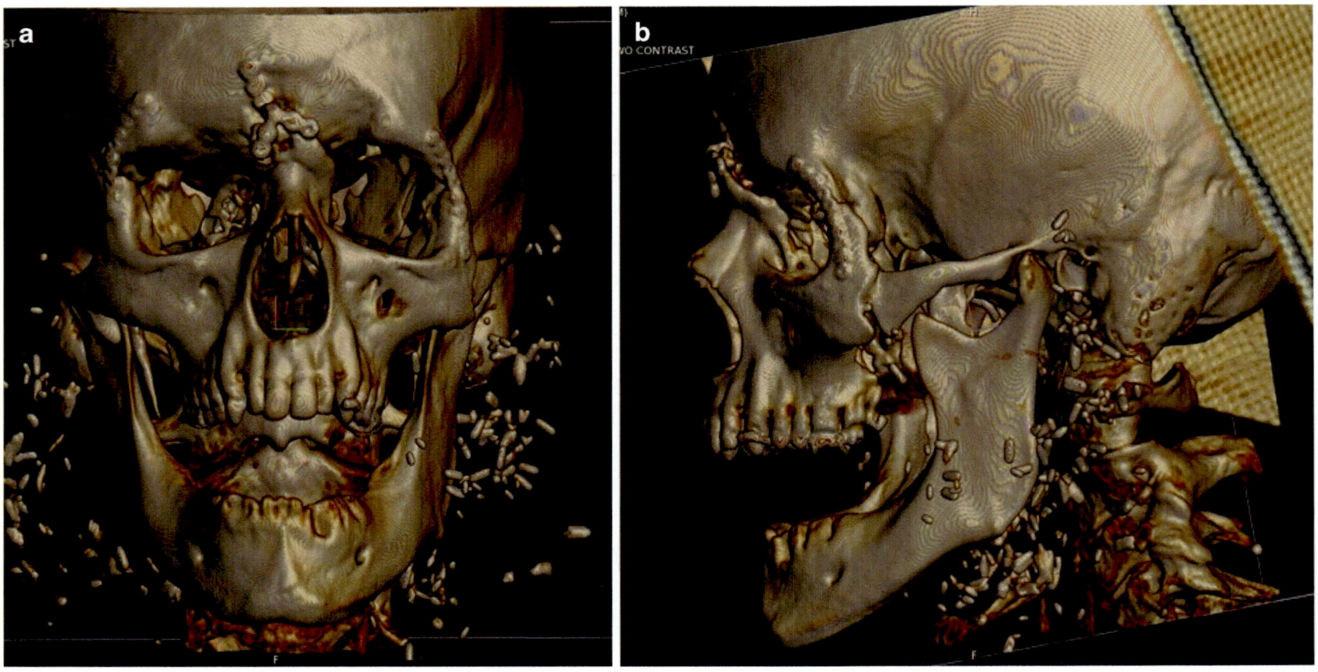

Fig. 3.7 Three-dimensional CT scan 12 months after facial transplantation showing the hybrid skeleton from a frontal view (**a**) and lateral view (**b**). (**a**) There is asymmetric loss of the caudal part of the frontal bone more on the left side. Despite the loss of all mandibular dentition to guide occlusion, there is an acceptable relationship between the donor's and recipient's skeleton. (**b**) Despite caudal frontal bone deficiency, the donor glabella has been placed in line with the intact cranial part of the recipient's forehead. Note the restoration of adequate mid-face projection and maxillomandibular relationship

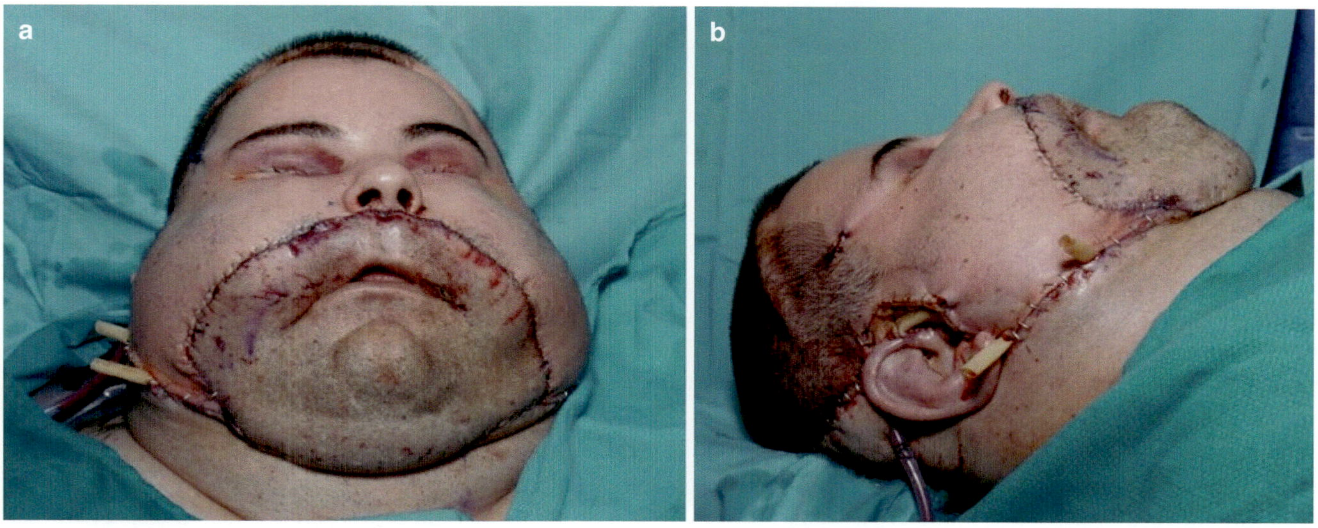

Fig. 3.8 Frontal-basal view (**a**) and right lateral (**b**) photographs of patient two immediately following transplant

3.3.7 Initial Postoperative Course

The patient's initial postoperative course was complicated by MRSA bacteremia which required treatment with intravenous antibiotics. On postoperative day 7, he developed a sialocele and his palatal incision dehisced. Treatment included operative debridement, intra-parotid injection of botulinum toxin, and culture-directed antimicrobials. On postoperative day 19, he developed an acute kidney injury (AKI) secondary to tacrolimus and amikacin. His AKI resolved with intravenous fluid support and re-titration of his tacrolimus dose. Five weeks after surgery, the patient was successfully decannulated (tracheostomy and gastric feeding tube). He was subsequently discharged to home 8 weeks after transplantation.

3.3.8 Physical Therapy, Rehabilitation, Psychosocial Care

Postoperatively physical therapy, rehabilitation, and psychosocial care followed the same regimen as previously described for case 1. This included daily treatment until discharge from the hospital and then treatment three times per week.

3.3.9 Functional and Neurosensory Outcomes

Following transplant, the patient's speech progressively improved and became intelligible with the aid of a palatal obturator. Within 5 weeks of transplantation, the patient was able to eat solid foods and drink liquids, which allowed for the removal of his gastric feeding tube. The patient's sensory recover has surpassed his motor recovery. Three years after transplantation, motor testing demonstrated symmetric strong cheek elevation, absent right eyelid blink with weak left eyelid blink, and absent scrunching of the nose. Sensory testing at that time demonstrated return of soft touch, heat, and cold to the entire allograft.

3.3.10 Rejection Episodes and Long-Term Complications

As with our previous transplant, he has been closely monitored for rejection with clinical exam and routine screening biopsies. One month after transplantation, routine biopsy demonstrated Banff grade III acute rejection. This was successfully treated with re-titration of his tacrolimus dose and a 1000 mg bolus of intravenous methylprednisolone followed by a taper back to his maintenance oral prednisone.

Approximately 4 months after transplantation, the patient was readmitted with fevers and methicillin-resistant *Staphylococcus epidermidis* bacteremia requiring intravenous antibiotics. Facial redness at that time prompted biopsy, which demonstrated Banff grade III acute rejection. This was treated with a re-titration of his tacrolimus and a pulse of intravenous methylprednisolone followed by a taper back to his maintenance oral prednisone. Both his bacteremia and rejection resolved, and he was discharged after a 7-day admission. One month later, however, he was readmitted with a soft tissue neck abscess that required a 5-day admission for intravenous antibiotics and incision and drainage.

Approximately 1 year following transplantation, routine biopsies again showed Banff grade III acute rejection. The patient was admitted. He again was treated with a re-titration of his tacrolimus and pulse dose intravenous methylprednisolone. During this episode, MMF was added back to his immunosuppression regimen. Repeat biopsies 5 days later demonstrated resolution of the rejection, and he was discharged. Two months later, however, routine biopsy re-demonstrated Banff grade III acute rejection requiring inpatient admission. He was initially treated with pulse dose intravenous methylprednisolone and a re-titration of his tacrolimus and his MMF. Given his multiple episodes of rejection to this point, thymoglobulin was also utilized. Though the rejection episode was successfully treated, he developed AKI and hemodynamic instability, thought to be secondary to thymoglobulin sensitivity. This required a prolonged ICU admission for hemodynamic support and intermittent renal dialysis. After a 62-day admission, the patient's renal injury and hemodynamic instability resolved, and he was discharged.

For the next 3.5 years, the patient did well. He experienced no further episodes of rejection, nor admission-requiring medical issues. Approximately 5 years following transplantation, however, he was admitted to an outside hospital with a bacterial pneumonia requiring intubation and mechanical ventilation. He was transferred to the Cleveland Clinic where further workup revealed a duodenal perforation. He was emergently treated with explorative laparotomy, abdominal washout, and a Graham patch duodenal repair. He subsequently developed an enterocutaneous fistula and required total parenteral nutrition (TPN). After a 3-month hospitalization, including a tracheostomy due to prolonged ventilation, he ultimately recovered and was discharged to a skilled nursing facility.

In April 2020, while still admitted to an outside skilled nursing facility, the patient developed respiratory distress and subsequently tested positive for SARS-CoV-2 (COVID-19). Given his declining respiratory function, he was admitted to an outside ICU. After a multidisciplinary discussion, the decision was made to transfer him to CCF for treatment with monoclonal antibody immunotherapy targeting IL-6 (tocilizumab). Upon arrival, he was hemodynamically unstable requiring vasopressors and mechanical ventilation. Initial COVID-19 treatment included tocilizumab, high-dose steroids, piperacillin/tazobactam, vancomycin, and hydroxychloroquine. Bronchoalveolar lavage cultures grew *Pseudomonas aeruginosa* and *Corynebacterium striatum*, for which he received sensitivity-directed ceftolozane/tazobactam, inhaled colistin, and vancomycin. By hospital-day 24, his hemodynamically instability, ventilatory requirements, and laboratory markers had improved sufficiently, so that he could be transferred to a skilled nursing facility. Throughout his COVID-19 admission and treatment course, immunosuppression was continued; however, his tacrolimus dosage was decreased. He did not develop clinical signs of rejection during the admission or after discharge. Since this admission, he has been doing well and has had no further episodes of rejection.

Due to pending IRB authorization, our third and most recent face transplant patient will not be discussed in this chapter. Future publications in peer-reviewed journals will provide full details of that case.

3.4 Lessons Learned

Since its outset, the Cleveland Clinic vascularized composite allotransplantation program has been at the forefront of facial transplantation. In 2004, our plastic surgery department received the world's first IRB approval for this experimental surgery [1]. In 2008, we performed the first successful near-total face and maxilla transplant in the United States [5, 6]. With our second case, we expanded facial transplantation from a functional and aesthetic surgery to a life and vision saving procedure [8]. Our third patient was the youngest person in the United States to receive a face transplant, which effectively replaced the entire maxillomandibular complex as well as all of the facial soft tissues [10].

Our ability to start and grow a facial transplantation program has been a product of the hard work and dedication of a multidisciplinary team, including plastic surgeons, otolaryngologists, transplant surgeons, psychiatrists, transplant coordinators, surgical intensivists, dentists, ophthalmologists, physical therapists, speech and language pathologists, and social workers. Equally as important, the long-term commitment and financial support of the Cleveland Clinic as an institution have made our success possible. Having now performed three facial transplants, we have defined protocols for preoperative planning, concurrent allograft harvest and recipient preparation in adjacent rooms, postoperative care in the SICU, and comprehensive postoperative rehabilitation. We feel confident in our ability to continue performing facial transplant surgery and advancing the field.

Progress and success, however, have not come without challenges and lessons learned. The first challenge after initiating a face transplant program is recipient selection. Though the majority of medical ethicists appear to support the notion of facial transplantation in medically optimized patients [11], which facial defects qualify for transplant consideration and when to list a patient is debated. Facial transplantation has traditionally been considered only after all conventional reconstructive modalities have been exhausted. There may exist certain instances, however, in which facial transplantation should be considered immediately following acute wound closure with simple methods. While classification systems [3, 4] have provided some guidance with regard to patient selection, consensus and early identification of patients who may benefit from transplant could yield improved outcomes.

Measured outcomes, however, tend to vary widely from center to center. While motor and sensory recovery can be quantified, many of the goals of facial transplantation are subjective in nature, including aesthetic outcome, functional status, and psychologic status. A retrospective study of pre- versus posttransplant FACES scores [12] did show a statistically significant improvement "aesthetic" and "exposed tissue" scores. "Functional status" and "co-morbidity" scores, however, showed no significant improvement following transplant. Further, the study noted a significant variability in how the scores were calculated between the patients. To yield better results in the future, measurements of functional, psychological, and aesthetic outcomes should ideally be validated and standardized.

Even if validated, functional and aesthetic outcomes require recipient compliance and realistic expectations. Functional result is largely dependent on a recipient's willingness to participate in intensive rehabilitation. In our experience, our first patient was fully committed to the rehabilitation program, whereas our second patient was not [13]. The potential lack of patient adherence to a rehabilitation protocol remains a challenge for any face transplant program. With regard to aesthetic results, patients must understand that although results will generally improve with time, facial transplantation will not restore their pre-injury appearance. Even with the best aesthetic outcome, the patient must be willing to accept a new appearance. When asked, our recipients have expressed acceptance of their new faces. In other cases, however, an inability to cope with a new appearance has led to severe emotional distress and suicide attempts [14, 15].

With regard to specific surgical technique, our experience has illustrated multiple points for future consideration. Our first patient's aesthetic result was marked by increased bigonial width secondary due to excessive parotid tissue in the allograft. In our second case, we attempted to limit the bulk of parotid tissue without violating the facial nerve branches. Alas, postoperative results again demonstrated excessive lower facial width. In both the cases, the initial postoperative result was improved with a secondary debulking and facelift procedure (Figs. 3.9 and 3.10). Moving forward, facial transplant surgeons should try to minimize the amount of glandular tissue but still should be prepared to perform secondary procedures.

Our second case highlighted an important vascular consideration in palatal containing allografts. Though studies have shown that the lower two-thirds of the face can be transplanted on a single facial artery [16, 17], our second patient suffered a wound dehiscence and partial necrosis of the transplanted palate. In this case, the internal maxillary arteries (IMAs) had been ligated. The literature suggests this a common occurrence when the IMAs are ligated with palatal containing allografts [18]. As such, we have developed a modified Le Fort III approach to preserve the IMAs and improve perfusion to the transplanted palate [18].

In allografts, such as ours, that contain maxilla and/or mandible, posttransplant occlusion is of particular concern, as poor outcomes may lead to problems with airway patency, speech, swallow, mastication, and facial aesthetics. A retrospective review of maxillomandibular-containing transplants found that all maxilla-only transplants developed skeletal deformities, and 66% of double-jaw transplants developed malocclusion with half of those patients requiring secondary orthognathic surgery [19]. Our first patient initially had Angle class II occlusion, which subsequently shift to class III over time. Our second patient maintained his postopera-

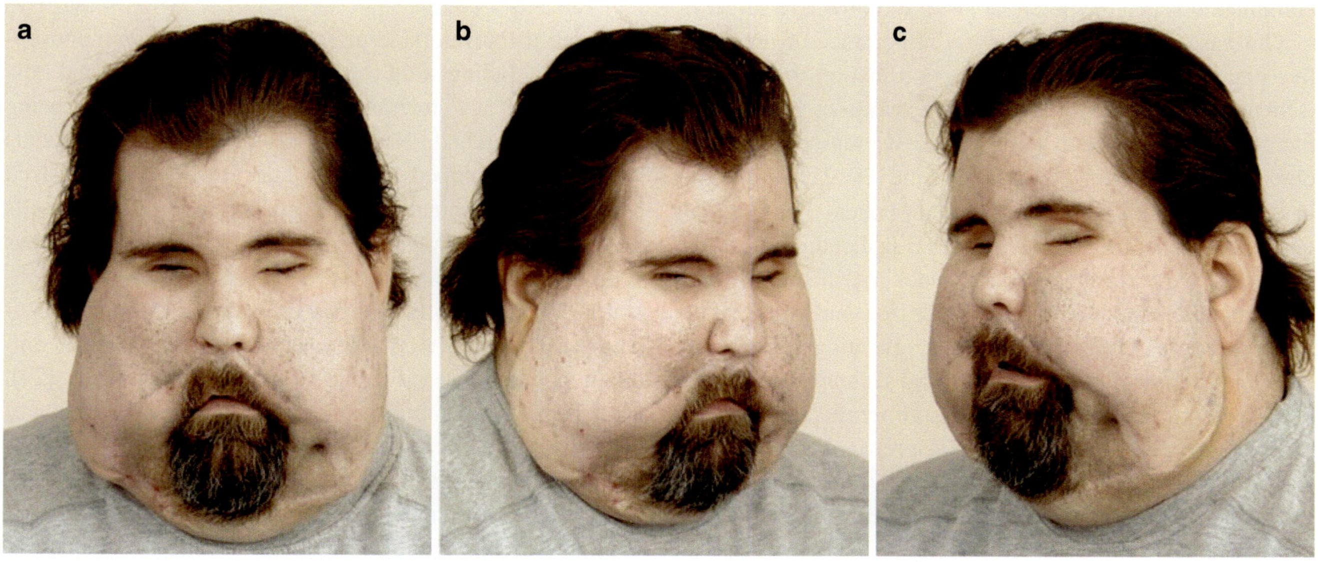

Fig. 3.9 Photographs of patient 2, 18-months after transplantation. (**a**) Frontal view demonstrates appropriate match in skin tone and skeletal proportions. The transplanted scalp demonstrates excellent hair growth. Excessive bigonial width is evident. (**b**) Right oblique view demonstrates excessive bulk in the parotid region. Additionally, excess skin was harvested along the lateral neck to accommodate post-operative swelling and to provide extra skin for postoperative sampling. (**c**) Left oblique view again demonstrates excess bulk in the parotid region

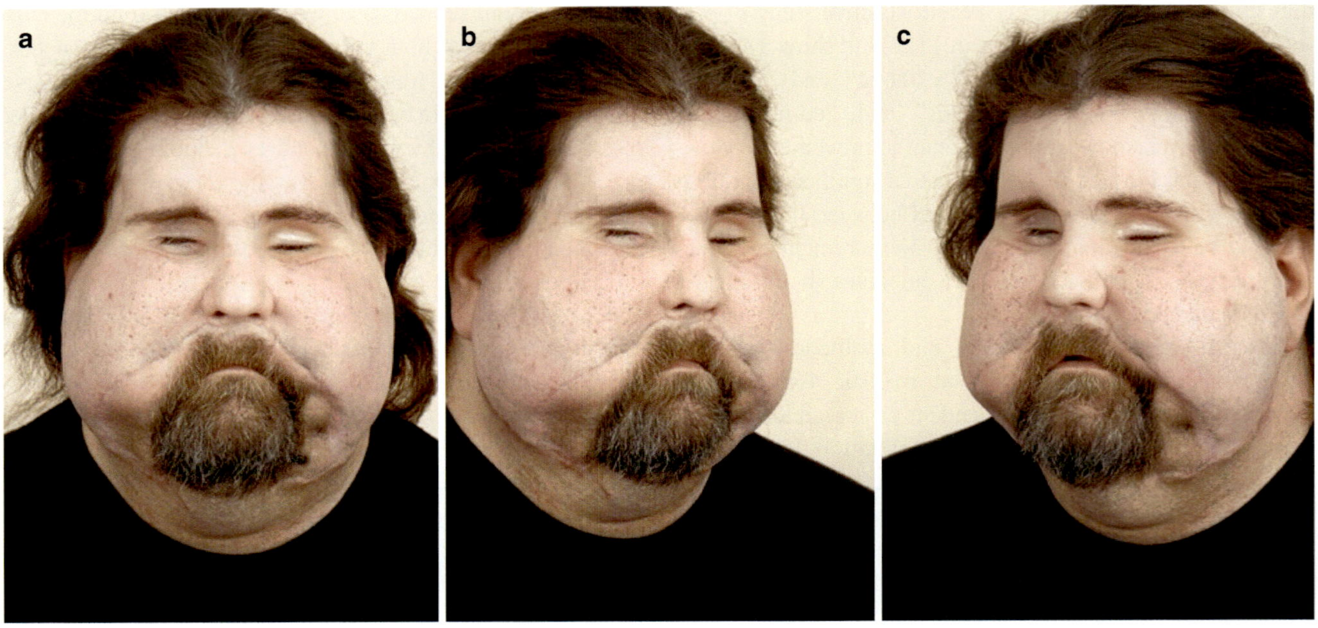

Fig. 3.10 Photographs of patient 2, 22 months after transplantation following revision with debulking of excess soft tissue and SMAS tightening. Frontal view (**a**), right oblique view (**b**), and left oblique view (**c**) demonstrate improved cervicofacial aesthetics following the revision surgery

tive class II occlusion. Our third patient initially had class I occlusion; however, within weeks a shift to class III occlusion was noted. This change was likely secondary to torque in the TMJ causing a loosening of screws and anterior movement of the mandible into a class III malocclusion. Fourteen months after transplant, she was treated with BSSO and 7 mm mandibular set back [19]. In the future, greater attention should be paid to dental and skeletal relationships with maxilla or mandibular containing transplants. Further, recipients should be counseled on the relatively high rate of dental complications and the potential need for corrective surgery.

Our cases also demonstrate the importance of preoperative planning and intra-operative coordination to minimize ischemia time and overall operative duration. Hand transplantation experience has suggested decreased functional outcomes with prolonged ischemia time [20, 21] though this has not been studied in face transplant patients. Throughout our cases, ischemia time was under 3 h. Leading up to the transplant, we performed frequent mock transplants with stereolithographic models to improve the flow and timing of the real procedure. Utilizing conjoined operating rooms with specifically trained nurses and surgical technicians afforded effective coordination to ligate the allograft pedicles only once the recipient wound was fully prepared. Moving forward, ex vivo VCA perfusion [22], as seen with kidney allografts, may allow another tool to minimize ischemia time and widen the donor pool.

Some of the largest challenges facial transplantation has encountered revolve around immunosuppression and rejection. In our first patient, we observed multiple episodes of subclinical grade I/II acute rejection on routine biopsies [23]. Though each episode was discussed at length among the multidisciplinary team, these low-level rejection episodes were usually not treated. With our subsequent cases, we decreased the frequency of routine screening biopsies and thus reduced the identified number of subclinical episodes of rejection. This allowed us to minimize the number of changes to the immunosuppression protocol and theoretically protect other organs from an increased immunosuppressive load. Despite the number of face transplants that have now been performed globally, no standardized immunosuppression regimen exists.

Given the severe side effects of long-term immunosuppression including solid organ damage, infections, and hospitalizations, new tolerance inducing protocols are being actively researched. New cell-based supportive protocols have been developed with the injection of donor-derived bone marrow, stromal vascular fraction, and CD34(+) cells to support VCA transplants [24–26]. Clinical benefit has been unclear, and widespread adoption has not been forthcoming. Consequently, we have investigated the induction of chimerism and therefore tolerance through the ex vivo combination of donor and recipient hematopoietic cells [24]. Models have shown promising results [26]. The induction of chimerism may represent the future of VCA immunosuppression.

To remove the challenges of immunosuppression entirely, advances in tissue-engineered facial scaffolds could ultimately render facial allotransplantation unnecessary. The use of bioengineered scaffolds that are then seeded by a patient's own stem cells have shown promising results in tracheal and laryngeal transplantation [27–29]. While this modality has not yet been applied to composite facial defects, it may represent the future of facial transplantation. Until that time, facial allotransplantation offers a viable solution to a subset of craniofacial defects that were previously untreatable.

3.5 Conclusion

In the past two decades, facial allotransplantation has grown from a theoretical surgical modality to a viable solution to previously untreatable craniofacial defects. Since the first face transplant in 2005, more than 40 of these experimental procedures have been done. Both our center's experience and the literature suggest that facial allotransplantation can improve function, quality of life, and craniofacial aesthetics for these patients. Though the field has made significant advances during this time, many challenges remain. The future of facial transplantation must optimize patient selection, standardize outcome measurements, develop new strategies for immunosuppression, and clarify funding.

References

1. Siemionow MZ, Gordon CR. Institutional review board-based recommendations for medical institutions pursuing protocol approval for facial transplantation. Plast Reconstr Surg. 2010;126(4):1232–9. https://doi.org/10.1097/PRS.0b013e3181ee482d.
2. Knackstedt R, Siemionow M, Papay F, Djohan R, Priebe D, Gastman B. Characterization of face transplant candidates evaluated at Cleveland clinic and algorithm to maximize efficacy of screening process. Ann Plast Surg. 2020;85(5):561–7. https://doi.org/10.1097/SAP.0000000000002466.
3. Gastman B, Djohan R, Siemionow M. Extending the Cordeiro maxillofacial defect classification system for use in the era of vascularized composite transplantation. Plast Reconstr Surg. 2012;130:419–22.
4. Cordeiro PG, Santamaria E. A classification system and algorithm for reconstruction of maxillectomy and midfacial defects. Plast Reconstr Surg. 2000;105(7):2331–46; discussion 2347-8. https://doi.org/10.1097/00006534-200006000-00004.
5. Siemionow M, Papay F, Alam D, Bernard S, Djohan R, Gordon C, Hendrickson M, Lohman R, Eghtesad B, Coffman K, Kodish E, Paradis C, Avery R, Fung J. Near-total human face transplantation for a severely disfigured patient in the USA. Lancet. 2009;374(9685):203–9. https://doi.org/10.1016/S0140-6736(09)61155-7.
6. Alam DS, Papay F, Djohan R, Bernard S, Lohman R, Gordon CR, Hendrickson M, Siemionow M. The technical and anatomical aspects of the World's first near-total human face and maxilla transplant. Arch Facial Plast Surg. 2009;11(6):369–77. https://doi.org/10.1001/archfacial.2009.80.
7. Gastman B, Hashem AM, Djohan R, Bernard S, Hendrickson M, Schwarz G, Gharb BB, Rampazzo A, Fernandez A, Zins J, Hoffman GS, Doumit G, Siemionow M, Papay F. Malignant pyoderma associated with granulomatosis with polyangiitis (Wegener granulomatosis) as a unique indication for facial vascularized composite allotransplantation: part I. Plast Reconstr Surg. 2016;137(6):1007–15. https://doi.org/10.1097/PRS.0000000000002162.
8. Hashem AM, Djohan R, Bernard S, Hendrickson M, Schwarz G, Gharb BB, Rampazzo A, Hoffman GS, Doumit G, Bergfeld W, Zins JE, Siemionow M, Papay F, Gastman B. Face transplantation for granulomatosis with polyangiitis (Wegener Granulomatosis): technical considerations, immunological aspects, and 3-year post-transplant outcome. Ann Plast Surg. 2019;82(3):320–9. https://doi.org/10.1097/SAP.0000000000001735.
9. Coombs DM, Kwiecien GJ, Koval C, Eghtesad B, Papay FA, Siemionow M, Gastman BR. Successful treatment of life-threatening COVID-19 infection in a face transplant recipient. Ann Plast Surg. 2021. https://doi.org/10.1097/SAP.0000000000002790.
10. How a face transplant transformed a young woman's life. https://nationalgeographic.com.
11. Suchyta MA, Sharp R, Amer H, Bradley E, Mardini S. Ethicists' opinions regarding the permissibility of face transplant. Plast Reconstr Surg. 2019;144(1):212–24. https://doi.org/10.1097/PRS.0000000000005748.
12. Chopra K, Susarla SM, Goodrich D, Bernard S, Zins JE, Papay F, Lee WP, Gordon CR. Clinical application of the FACES score for face transplantation. J Craniofac Surg. 2014;25(1):64–9. https://doi.org/10.1097/SCS.0b013e3182a2dda9.
13. Siemionow M. The past the present and the future of face transplantation. Curr Opin Organ Transplant. 2020;25(6):568–75. https://doi.org/10.1097/MOT.0000000000000812.
14. Coffman KL, Gordon C, Siemionow M. Psychological outcomes with face transplantation: overview and case report. Curr Opin Organ Transplant. 2010;15(2):236–40. https://doi.org/10.1097/MOT.0b013e328337267d.
15. Lemogne C, Bellivier F, Fakra E, Yon L, Limosin F, Consoli SM, Lantieri L, Hivelin M. Psychological and psychiatric aspects of face transplantation: lessons learned from the long-term follow-up of six patients. J Psychosom Res. 2019;119:42–9. https://doi.org/10.1016/j.jpsychores.2019.02.006.
16. Pomahac B, Lengele B, Ridgway EB, Matros E, Andrews BT, Cooper JS, Kutz R, Pribaz JJ. Vascular considerations in composite midfacial allotransplantation. Plast Reconstr Surg. 2010;125(2):517–22. https://doi.org/10.1097/PRS.0b013e3181c82e6f.
17. Nguyen JT, Ashitate Y, Venugopal V, Neacsu F, Kettenring F, Frangioni JV, Gioux S, Lee BT. Near-infrared imaging of face transplants: are both pedicles necessary? J Surg Res. 2013;184(1):714–21. https://doi.org/10.1016/j.jss.2013.04.039.
18. Bassiri Gharb B, Frautschi RS, Halasa BC, Doumit GD, Djohan RS, Bernard SL, Gastman BR, Siemionow MZ, Papay FA, Rampazzo A. Watershed areas in face transplantation. Plast Reconstr Surg. 2017;139(3):711–21. https://doi.org/10.1097/PRS.0000000000003130.
19. Coombs DM, Gharb BB, Tuncer BF, Djohan RS, Gastman GR, Bernard SL, Schwarz GS, Gurunian R, Siemionow MZ, Papay FA, Rampazzo A. Skeletal and dental outcomes after facial allotransplantation. Plast Reconstr Surg. 2022;149(4):945–62.
20. Herzberg G, Weppe F, Masson N, Gueffier X, Erhard L. Clinical evaluation of two bilateral hand allotransplantations at six and three years follow-up. Chir Main. 2008;27(2-3):109–17. https://doi.org/10.1016/j.main.2008.02.002.
21. Landin L, Cavadas PC, Garcia-Cosmes P, Thione A, Vera-Sempere F. Perioperative ischemic injury and fibrotic degeneration of muscle in a forearm allograft: functional follow-up at 32 months post transplantation. Ann Plast Surg. 2011;66(2):202–9. https://doi.org/10.1097/SAP.0b013e318206a365.
22. Fahradyan V, Said SA, Ordenana C, Dalla Pozza E, Frautschi R, Duraes EFR, Madajka-Niemeyer M, Papay FA, Rampazzo A, Bassiri GB. Extended ex vivo normothermic perfusion for preservation of vascularized composite allografts. Artif Organs. 2020;44(8):846–55. https://doi.org/10.1111/aor.13678.

23. Bergfeld W, Klimczak A, Stratton JS, Siemionow MZ. A four-year pathology review of the near total face transplant. Am J Transplant. 2013;13(10):2750–64. https://doi.org/10.1111/ajt.12379.
24. Siemionow M, Rampazzo A, Gharb BB, Cwykiel J, Klimczak A, Madajka M, Nasir S, Bozkurt M. The reversed paradigm of chimerism induction: donor conditioning with recipient-derived bone marrow cells as a novel approach for tolerance induction in vascularized composite allotransplantation. Microsurgery. 2016;36(8):676–83. https://doi.org/10.1002/micr.30041.
25. Siemionow M, Madajka M, Cwykiel J. Application of cell-based therapies in facial transplantation. Ann Plast Surg. 2012;69(5):575–9. https://doi.org/10.1097/SAP.0b013e31824803a5.
26. Hivelin M, Klimczak A, Cwykiel J, Sonmez E, Nasir S, Gatherwright J, Siemionow M. Immunomodulatory effects of different cellular therapies of bone marrow origin on chimerism induction and maintenance across MHC barriers in a face allotransplantation model. Arch Immunol Ther Exp. 2016;64(4):299–310. https://doi.org/10.1007/s00005-015-0380-8.
27. Gonfiotti A, Jaus MO, Barale D, Baiguera S, Comin C, Lavorini F, Fontana G, Sibila O, Rombolà G, Jungebluth P, Macchiarini P. The first tissue-engineered airway transplantation: 5-year follow-up results. Lancet. 2014;383(9913):238–44. https://doi.org/10.1016/S0140-6736(13)62033-4.
28. Hamilton NJI, Birchall MA. Tissue-engineered larynx: future applications in laryngeal cancer. Curr Otorhinolaryngol Rep. 2017;5(1):42–8. https://doi.org/10.1007/s40136-017-0144-6.
29. Kim IG, Park SA, Lee SH, Choi JS, Cho H, Lee SJ, Kwon YW, Kwon SK. Transplantation of a 3D-printed tracheal graft combined with iPS cell-derived MSCs and chondrocytes. Sci Rep. 2020;10(1):4326. https://doi.org/10.1038/s41598-020-61405-4.
30. Tasigiorgos S, Kollar B, Krezdorn N, Bueno EM, Tullius SG, Pomahac B. Face transplantation-current status and future developments. Transpl Int. 2018;31(7):677–88. https://doi.org/10.1111/tri.13130.
31. Lantieri L, Grimbert P, Ortonne N, Suberbielle C, Bories D, Gil-Vernet S, Lemogne C, Bellivier F, Lefaucheur JP, Schaffer N, Martin F, Meningaud JP, Wolkenstein P, Hivelin M. Face transplant: long-term follow-up and results of a prospective open study. Lancet. 2016;388(10052):1398–407. https://doi.org/10.1016/S0140-6736(16)31138-2.
32. Lemmens GM, Poppe C, Hendrickx H, Roche NA, Peeters PC, Vermeersch HF, Rogiers X, Lierde KV, Blondeel PN. Facial transplantation in a blind patient: psychologic, marital, and family outcomes at 15 months follow-up. Psychosomatics. 2015;56(4):362–70. https://doi.org/10.1016/j.psym.2014.05.002.

Orthognathic Outcomes and Technical Considerations in Vascularized Composite Facial Allotransplantation

4

Demetrius M. Coombs, Bahar Bassiri Gharb, Fatma B. Tuncer, Risal Djohan, Brian Gastman, Steven L. Bernard, Graham S. Schwarz, Raffi Gurunian, Maria Z. Siemionow, Frank Papay, and Antonio Rampazzo

4.1 Introduction

When viewed together, the worldwide facial vascularized composite allograft (VCA) experience consists of over 45 cases. The first facial VCA was reported in 2005, and since that point in time, the complexity of the procedure has increased precipitously [1, 2]. Following the success of initial facial transplantation procedures, plastic surgeons began to include maxillary and mandibular segments within the composite tissue allograft [3–5]. Including bony components, however, requires increased consideration of how the upper and lower jaws relate to the skull base of the recipient, bone healing, changes in dentition with time, ideal facial aesthetics and proportions, as well as consequences involving airway, speech, swallow, and mastication/bolus propulsion. This is reinforced by the fact that previous reports have documented considerable complications in facial allografts containing midfacial and mandibular bone—including impairments in phonation, dental cavities, trismus, and malocclusion [6–9].

4.2 Techniques for Cephalometric Analysis

A comprehensive examination of dental and skeletal outcomes following facial VCA with maxilla and mandible-containing composites requires a thorough understanding of donor and recipient characteristics, as well as the bony and soft tissue composition of the allograft. Cephalometric analysis may be performed using CT scans, MRIs, plain film lateral cephalograms, and when available, photographs or videos [10]. The latter, however, is expectedly less precise unless limiting the analysis to soft tissue cephalometrics. Virtual surgical planning (VSP) data, including computer-assisted design (CAD)/computer-assisted modeling (CAM) used for preoperative planning and intra-operative execution of the procedure may also facilitate understanding of the anticipated versus actual postoperative result.

Traditional cephalometric analysis is performed on either skeletal features or the facial soft tissue envelope. This represents an analysis of the sagittal relationship between the recipient's transplanted maxilla and mandible. Skeletal cephalometric analysis, as described by Riedel's classification, relates the A point to Nasion to B point forming the ANB angle [11]. Occlusion is therefore characterized as follows: class I ($1° < ANB < 4°$), class II ($ANB \geq 4°$), and class III ($ANB \leq 1°$) [12, 13]. Soft tissue cephalometric analysis, by contrast, describes the angle formed between the glabellar soft tissues, subnasale, and pogonion—the total facial angle. Using this relationship, class I occlusion refers to a total facial angle of 165–175°, while class II and III refer to angles less than 165° or greater than 175°, respectively [14].

Comparing facial levels across patients and over time remains integral to a rigorous cephalometric analysis in

D. M. Coombs (✉) · B. Bassiri Gharb · R. Djohan · B. Gastman
S. L. Bernard · G. S. Schwarz · R. Gurunian · F. Papay
A. Rampazzo
Department of Plastic Surgery, Cleveland Clinic, Cleveland, OH, USA
e-mail: coombsd@ccf.org; BASSIRB@ccf.org; djohanr@ccf.org; gastmab@ccf.org; bernars2@ccf.org; schwarg@ccf.org; GURUNIR@ccf.org; PAPAF@ccf.org; rampaza@ccf.org

F. B. Tuncer
Division of Plastic Surgery, University of Utah School of Medicine, Salt Lake City, UT, USA

M. Z. Siemionow
Department of Orthopaedics, University of Illinois at Chicago, College of Medicine, Chicago, IL, USA
e-mail: siemiom@uic.edu

© Springer Nature Switzerland AG 2023
R. Gurunian et al. (eds.), *Reconstructive Transplantation*, https://doi.org/10.1007/978-3-031-21520-9_4

facial VCA patients. With the pupils as the horizontal point of reference, reconstructive surgeons can compare the upper and lower canine levels as well as the jaw and chin levels. This allows identification of chin, jawline, and occlusal cants [14]. Although a variety of elaborate software programs exist that facilitate meticulous cephalometric analyses, the preference in our practice is to use Dolphin Imaging (Version 11.95, Dolphin Imaging and Management Solutions, Chatsworth, CA). In addition to the more routine cephalometric measurements mentioned above, we perform condylar analyses, take airway measurements pre- and postoperatively (which includes the nasal, oral, and superior sinus cavities) [15], track changes in specific craniofacial distances over time—opisthion to alveolus (at the level of the upper incisor cement–enamel junction (CEJ)), anterior to posterior nasal spine, and nasofrontal angle [16].

4.3 Skeletal Outcomes to Date

As of the writing of this chapter, the worldwide facial VCA experience has included 25 patients who received a composite allograft containing mandible, maxilla, or both. Of these patients, two grafts contained the mandible, seven included the maxilla, while 16 contained both [17].

4.3.1 Mandible-Only Transplantation

A closer examination of those patients who received a mandible-only containing allografts reveals that one patient developed trismus while the other developed class III malocclusion in the immediate postoperative period.

4.3.2 Midface-Only Transplantation

Among patients who received an allograft that included only the midface, the composite included a partial upper dental arch in two patients and the entire arch in five other patients. All seven patients eventually developed malocclusion: five patients demonstrated class II and two patients demonstrated class III.

4.3.3 Midface and Mandible Transplantation

Of the patients who underwent transplantation with an allograft containing both the maxilla and mandible, 15 patients received a midfacial segment that contained a full maxillary dental arch. One patient, by contrast, received a partial mandibular segment. Following the index transplantation, four patients achieved class I occlusion, while 66% of patients (eight) suffered from malocclusion—three patients with class III and five patients with class II.

Nonunion of the mandible was evident in three patients. A step-off at the hard–soft junction of the palate was also noted in three patients and attributed to significant size discrepancies in the relationship of the recipient and donor faces.

From the standpoint of corrective orthognathic surgery for posttransplant malocclusion, a variety of osteotomy choices exist and must be tailored to the deformity in question. In our analysis of the worldwide experience to date, two patients underwent BSSO, one Le Fort I and one Le Fort III, while one underwent an unknown osteotomy for orthognathic purposes. The timing of corrective orthognathic surgery following index transplantation ranged from 3 to 16 months and occurred at an average of 9.4 months. Two patients (40%) experienced recurrence of class II malocclusion despite the surgical correction. In summary, all patients who received a transplant containing both the maxilla and mandible developed at least one complication postoperatively.

Various craniofacial techniques for planning and execution of the transplant exist and depend largely on the preferences of the operative team. Virtual surgical planning (VSP) provides surgeons with an opportunity to pre-fabricate cutting guides. Based upon previous reports, this was used in multiple patients and relied upon recipient anatomy alone, or both donor and recipient anatomy. Additional reported adjuncts include CT-guided intraoperative navigation.

4.4 Dental Outcomes to Date

Of the 25 patients who received a composite allograft containing mandible, maxilla, or both, 40% developed periodontal disease and/or dental cavities. The need for tooth extraction was a relatively common occurrence—six patients underwent extraction of all teeth following the initial transplant procedure (mean 20 months, range 6–48 months).

4.5 The Cleveland Clinic Facial Vascularized Composite Allotransplantation Program

Since 2008, the Cleveland Clinic Facial Vascularized Composite Allotransplantation Program has successfully treated three patients with devastating facial injuries and disfigurements using midface and/or mandible containing allografts. Among these patients is the first facial VCA in the United States (patient 1) and the youngest patient in America to undergo such a procedure (patient 3). A detailed discussion of the indications for face transplantation in our patients is presented elsewhere within this textbook and is beyond the scope of this chapter. The skeletal and dental outcomes of these patients, including changes in the midfacial segments and airway volumes over time, are discussed in the following paragraphs.

Our first patient (patient 1; Fig. 4.1) received a midfacial composite allograft containing the maxilla. A change from skeletal class II malocclusion to class III was evident on cephalometric analysis performed at 2 weeks and 10.8 years, respectively. The ANB angle was +6.2° at the 2-week time point and changed to –4.6° by 10 years.

Our second patient (patient 2; Fig. 4.2) also received a midfacial composite allograft containing the maxilla. By 5.3 years postoperatively, skeletal class II malocclusion was maintained. This was evidenced by an ANB angle of 14.4° in the immediate postoperative period with a change to 10.5° at the 5-year time point. Of note, neither of these patients demonstrated significant changes in the temporo-mandibular joint (TMJ) with time.

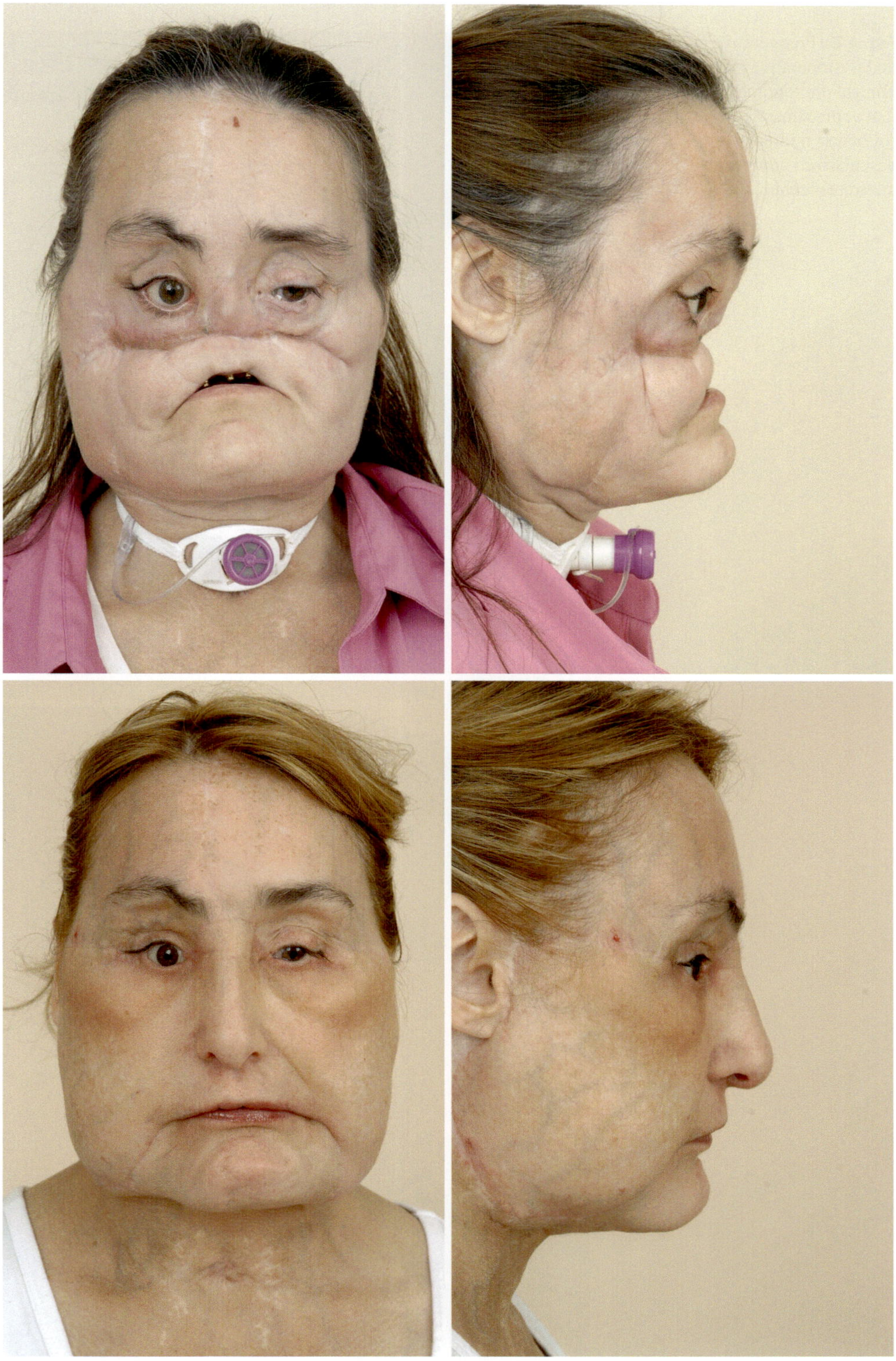

Fig. 4.1 Preoperative (above) and postoperative (below) clinical photographs of patient 1 at approximately 4 years following midfacial vascularized composite allotransplantation

Our third patient (patient 3; Fig. 4.3) received a double-jaw containing composite allograft that was accomplished via inclusion of a bilateral Le Fort 3 midfacial segment and a BSSO osteotomy to inset the tooth-bearing mandibular fragment. In the immediate postoperative period, class I skeletal and dental occlusion was achieved, however by approximately 1 week postoperatively, the patient developed trismus and class III malocclusion (Fig. 4.4). This was attributed in part to poor intercuspation and posterior instability at the level of the maxillary arch. In other words, preoperative occlusion in the donor was compromised by absent maxillary teeth. Posttransplantation radiographic analysis of the condyles revealed lateral rotation on the right and medialization on the left. Thus, the development of class III malocclusion shortly after surgery was additionally related to torque within the TMJs during the index transplant and screw loosening with return of the condyles to their native, torque-free position. Despite this rapid change

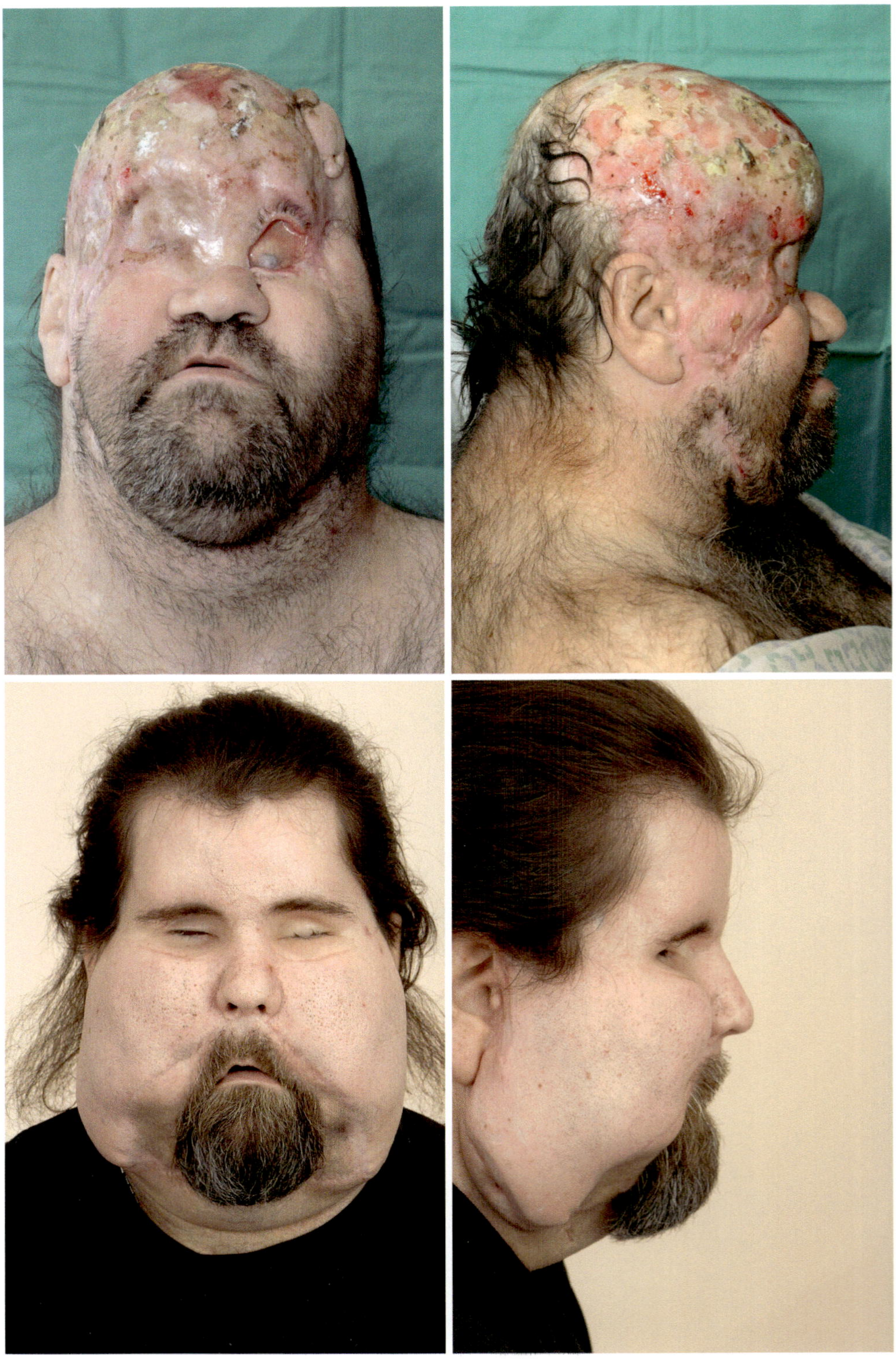

Fig. 4.2 Preoperative (above) and postoperative (below) clinical photographs of patient 2 at approximately 2 years following midfacial vascularized composite allotransplantation

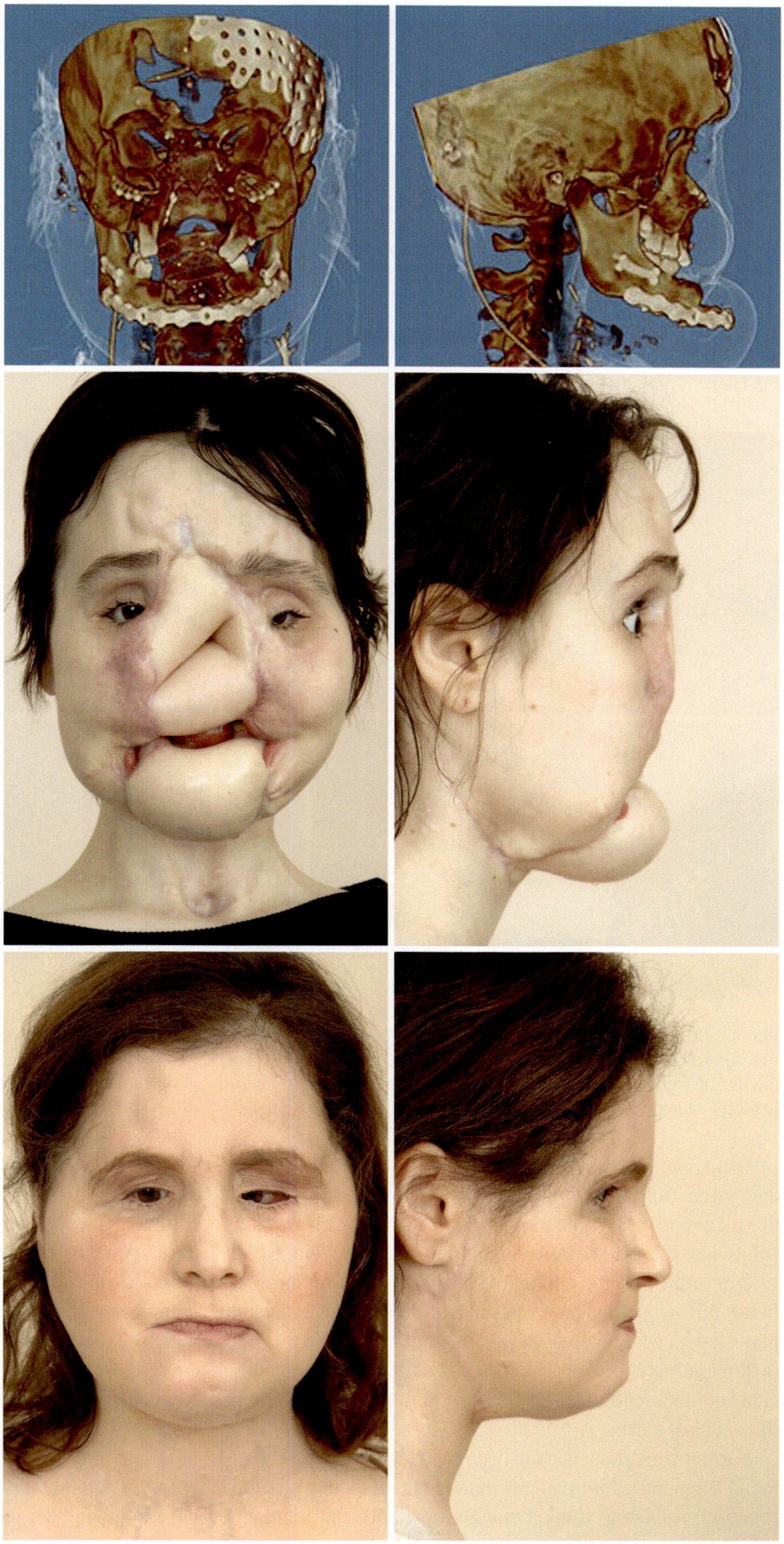

Fig. 4.3 Preoperative (middle) and postoperative (below) clinical photographs of patient 3 at approximately 2 years following double-jaw containing vascularized composite allotransplantation. The top images depict 3D renderings of preoperative CT scans with the soft tissues superimposed over the craniofacial skeleton. Refer to Fig. 4.4 for corresponding cephalometric images

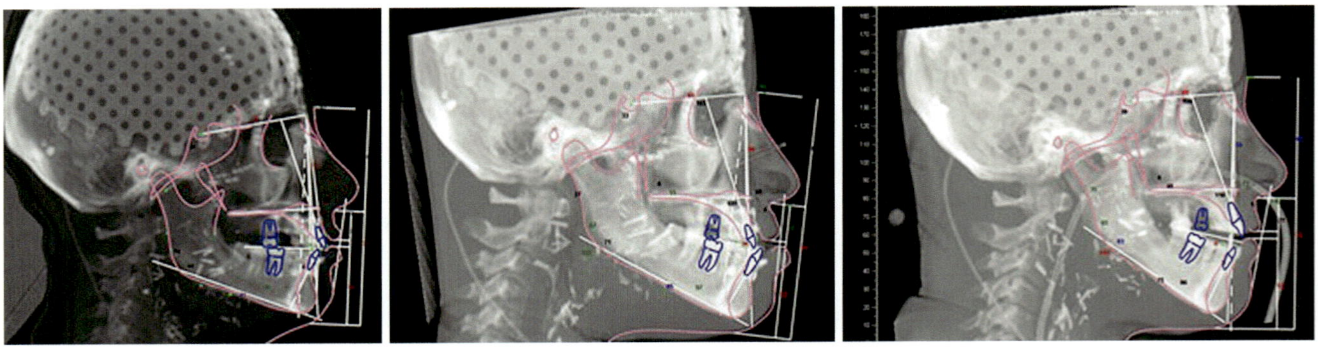

Fig. 4.4 Lateral cephalograms corresponding to patient 3 at the time of index transplantation (left), approximately 5 months postoperatively (middle) demonstrating class III malocclusion, and nearly 2 years postoperatively from the index transplantation but following revision bilateral sagittal split osteotomy with 7mm mandibular setback (right)

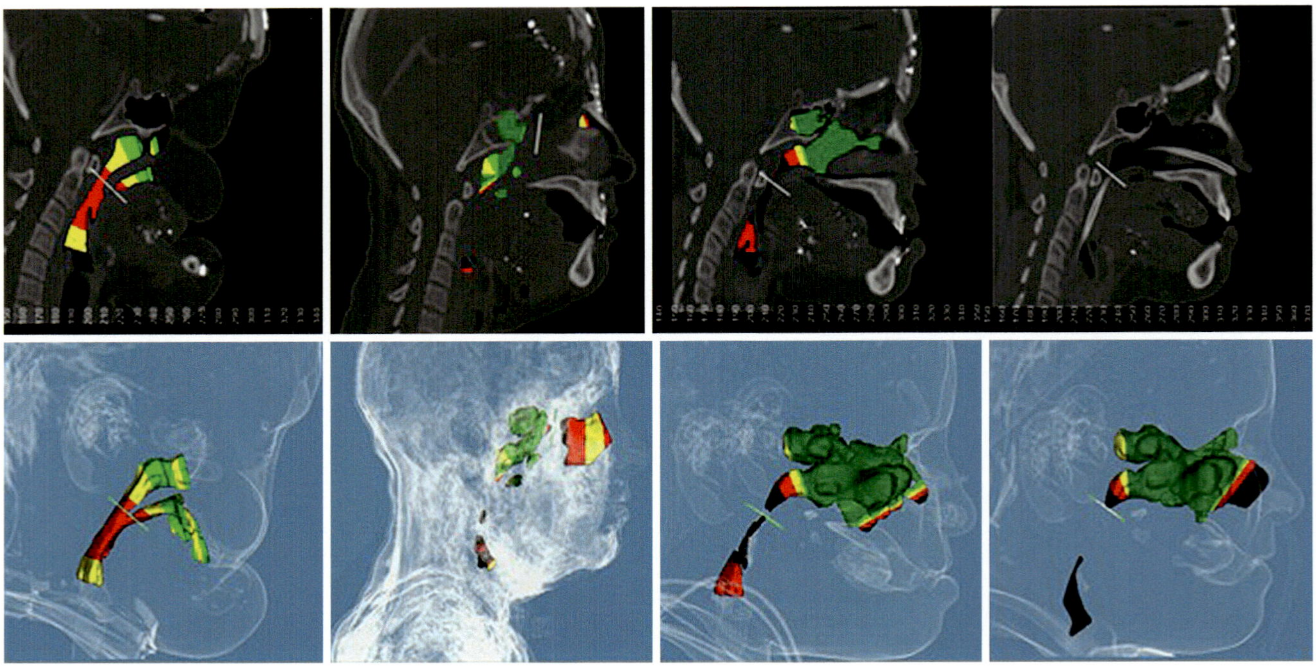

Fig. 4.5 Three-dimensional renderings of changes in airway volume over time corresponding to patient 3. Note the decrease in airway volume (second, third, and fourth columns) compared to the preoperative baseline (first column). The posterior positioning of the base of the tongue (top row, third image) was ultimately addressed by performing a tongue advancement procedure. These findings suggest that in addition to the effect on airway, the tongue, suprahyoid musculature, and contracture may also contribute to the development of malocclusion in these patients

in occlusion, however, the osteotomies healed without issue and over time, mandibular range of motion improved. Corrective orthognathic surgery was performed 14 months following the initial transplantation procedure via BSSO (7 mm setback of the mandible; Fig. 4.4). Despite improvement following this correction, dentofacial malocclusion persisted as evidenced by an ANB angle of 0.9°. By 1 year postoperatively, several teeth demonstrated substantial erosion into the dentin [18] and at least 2 mm loss of depth on the occlusal surfaces.

Further cephalometric analysis has revealed that the midfacial segments of all patients demonstrated clockwise rotation with respect to time. Among all patients, the following distances decreased: opisthion to CEJ (upper incisors) and anterior nasal spine to posterior nasal spine. The angle formed between the sella-nasion/palatal plane and frontonasal angle, by contrast, increased.

Following transplantation, all our patients demonstrated an increase in airway volume—33.6% in patient 1, 86.2% in patient 2, and 72.4% in patient 3. In patients 1 and 2, however, the overall gain in volume decreased slightly with respect to time: -4.8% in patient 1 and –15.1% in patient 2. In patient 3, by contrast, the overall decrease in airway volume was more substantial—34.3%. This was attributed to both the mandibular setback and retroposition of the tongue base following her index transplant procedure (Fig. 4.5).

4.6 Complications, Considerations, and Strategies for the Future

Severely disfiguring midfacial defect pose immense reconstructive challenges. In 2008, a Le Fort III-based composite tissue allograft was used to reconstruct a devasting ballistic injury that ushered in a new era in the management of complex craniofacial defects [3]. In the years that followed, at least 25 facial VCAs would be performed that included the maxilla, mandible, or both (double-jaw). Our review of these patients illustrates that all seven patients who received an allograft containing the maxilla experienced some degree of skeletal imbalance with time [17]. This is in part due to an unavoidable mismatch between the skeletal dimensions of the donor and recipient, and the fact that the pairing of recipient mandible with a total (or partial) donor maxilla results in a hybrid occlusion [19]. Among the general population, by contrast, the interplay between malocclusion and TMJ dysfunction remains to be further elucidated [20]. Interestingly, neither of our first two patients demonstrated any evidence of TMJ remodeling at 5 and 10 years follow-up, respectively. Furthermore, the lack of trismus during short follow-up suggests no detrimental effect on the TMJ.

Interestingly, the three face transplants from the Cleveland Clinic demonstrated clockwise rotation of the maxillary segment in relation to the skull base with respect to time. On cephalometric analysis, this was illustrated by changes in the following indices: increased nasofrontal angle, increased sella-nasion plane/palatal plane angle, and decreased distance between the caudal maxilla and skull base (posterior-inferior) [16]. This is in contradistinction to the counter-clockwise rotation following Le Fort III advancement surgery in both Apert's and Crouzon's patients previously reported in the literature [21–23]. It therefore seems that various events may play a role in the clockwise rotation we observed among our face transplant patients, including age, relapse, bony resorption, and perhaps chronic rejection. Surgical relapse may result from poor support to the posterior maxilla, tensioning forces, and scarring within the soft tissues, as well as fibrous unions where osteotomies were performed [24, 25]. Prior studies have demonstrated that resorption of craniofacial bone occurs with aging, and particularly in patients with a history of facial VCA [26, 27]. Although clockwise rotation of the maxilla was ultimately confirmed by Pessa, this phenomenon was originally described by Lambros and remains similar to the findings we observed [28, 29]. More specifically, we observed the following progressive occlusal changes (clockwise rotation) in our first face transplant patient—class II in early postoperative period, with transition to class I by 5 years, and finally, class III at 10 years postoperatively.

The ability to achieve a hybrid occlusion following facial transplantation cannot be underemphasized. Even though about a quarter of the patients who received transplants containing the maxilla, mandible, or both underwent extraction of all remaining teeth at a mean of 20 months postoperatively and that chronic rejection was evident in several patients by 10 years postoperatively, it appears that including the maxilla in midfacial segments for patients with an intact mandible represents an excellent reconstructive solution for devastating central facial defects. In other words, functional anatomy for feeding, phonation, and oral competence is preserved despite the occurrence of graft failure—early or delayed.

Double-jaw composites include the inherent benefit of maintaining ideal, or native occlusion from the standpoint of the donor tissues, however rates of trismus and malocclusion may approach 50% and 66%, respectively. Additionally, recurrence rates following corrective orthognathic surgery exceeds that of the general, nontransplant population and approaches 40% [30]. This may be a consequence of instability within the transplanted occlusal surface, size discrepancies in the recipience and donor craniofacial skeleton, inadvertent torque at the time of fixation resulting in displacement of condyles postoperatively, prior TMJ pathology, impaired proprioception, and imbalances within the masticatory/suprahyoid musculature.

When considering the United States population overall, rates of malocclusion approach two-thirds in pre-treatment adults [31]. Not surprisingly, stable intercuspation remains essential for bony healing and the maintenance of stable occlusion postoperatively [32]. For these reasons, double-jaw transplantation represents a surgery-first approach to orthognathic intervention [33]. Although the surgery-first approach has been reported elsewhere as an effective technique for the correction of class III malocclusion in non-transplant patients, the stability of this methodology over time requires further study [32, 34]. Essential components for establishing an overall stable occlusion include at least three contact points along the occlusal surface, no prior dental extractions, a stabilized occlusion posteriorly, coordinated midlines between the maxilla and mandible, and an absent or limited cross-bite [35, 36]. Once the aforementioned criteria is met, and the maxilla and mandible are appropriately oriented in surgery, occlusal stability and bony healing are optimized [33, 37]. Our third patient illustrates these considerations well—the occlusal surfaces in the donor maxilla and mandible demonstrated several prior tooth extractions, some of which involved the molar teeth, and only two contact points. This resulted in decreased occlusal stability postoperatively and considering the significant rates of malocclusion following double-jaw transplantation, may have plagued other patients. For these reasons, our practice prefers to implement orthodontic elastic treatment in the immediate postoperative period for both facial transplantation patients and those undergoing general orthognathic surgery [38, 39].

Accurately aligning the palate and orbital floor between the donor and recipient remains challenging if significant differences exist in both facial height and gnathic indices [40–42]. In our third patient, as well as in reports following face transplants in in the USA and Europe, step-off deformities were noted within the palate [7, 43]. This finding, in conjunction with the tenuous vascularity of the posterior palate after Le Fort osteotomies, may play a role in the observed rate of oronasal fistulas following facial VCA surgery—as high as 46% [44]. It is important to highlight that when fixating the mandibular segments, a considerable risk of ramus inclination (medial or lateral), torque along the axial plane, and sagging of the condyles exists. This is evidenced by a difference in minimum and maximum intercondylar distance of 30 mm [42, 45, 46]. In order to promote post-surgical stability and minimize untoward complications related to the TMJ, published recommendations include strict adherence to the native, preoperative position of the mandibular condyles as well as the ramus proximally [47–51].The consensus of our group is that without this crucial relationship the likelihood of posttransplant malocclusion and trismus increases substantially [39, 52–54]. Additionally, it would seem that trismus may be related to presurgical injuries involving the TMJ as well as posttraumatic scarring following ballistic injuries. Our recommendation includes addressing these factors prior to and after facial transplantation [7].

Following transplantation, multiple patients have required corrective orthognathic surgery involving the mandible or maxilla for treatment of malocclusion [39, 53, 55]. Both the techniques and timing of corrective orthognathic surgery depend on a variety of factors, including comprehensive skeletal cephalometric analysis, presence of fistulas, bone healing, speech deficits, and airway volumes. As many of these patients have undergone Le Fort osteotomies during their transplantation procedures, it remains important to consider the potential for injury to the vasculature supplying the allograft during any corrective operation [6]. A restricted oropharyngeal aperture, or inlet, represents an additional consideration when planning revision surgery. Of the patients who required corrective orthognathic surgery, one underwent correction of open bite with surgery limited to the mandible, while another required Le Fort I osteotomy [53, 55]. In our practice, we avoid performing Le Fort I osteotomies during revision surgery in these patients—primarily since the allograft relies on the facial vasculature rather than either the ascending or descending palatine or ascending pharyngeal arteries [56]. The clinical consequences of this osteotomy pattern include decreasing blood flow to the alveolus, which is of particular importance in patients with evidence of fistula. Ultimately, our review of published and institutional cases suggests that revision orthognathic surgery remains safe if performed between 3 and 16 months following the index transplantation. Our third patient developed class III malocclusion following corrective orthognathic surgery (BSSO with mandibular setback) even though the condyles remained in centric relation and without any appreciable torque at the time of fixation. Interestingly, a similar outcome was encountered by another facial VCA team within the United States, prompting us to realize that several factors may contribute to the relapse of dentofacial complications despite revision [57]. Such factors include a donor and recipient with discrepant intercondylar distances, facial heights, and gnathic indices, failing to take advantage of VSP, incomplete obliteration of bony interferences, and significant condylar torque at the time of fixation resulting in displacement of the recipient segments from the fossa. Additional considerations that could impart negative occlusal consequences include both retroposition of the tongue base and muscular imbalance (opposing forces between suprahyoid, medial pterygoid, and masseter muscles).

An analysis of the worldwide face transplant experience, with particular emphasis on patients receiving an allograft containing either the maxilla or mandible, reveals that following the index transplantation at least 40% of patients experienced dental caries and/or periodontal pathology, and at approximately 20 months postoperatively, 25% remained edentulous from necessary tooth extractions [17]. Numerous factors could account for these observations and several bear mentioning. First, in the last 15 years, we have witnessed an increasing number of donors that died following episodes of drug overdose or intoxication [58]. Second, when compared to the general population, patients suffering from substance abuse disorders have a greater risk of dental cavities and periodontal pathology [59]. Third, the importance of adequate salivary gland function cannot be underemphasized—optimal intraoral pH control protects and maintains tooth structure, as well as mineralization, cleansing, and antimicrobial defense [60]. Importantly, the literature indicates that hyposalivation is intimately associated with salivary gland denervation as well as immunosuppressive regimens over an extended period of time [61, 62]. This is further evidenced by the rate of tooth loss observed in patients with Sjogren's Syndrome—which is primarily attributed to xerostomia [63]. Perhaps similar events occur in our face transplant patients and ultimately lead to tooth loss. Our third patient suffered from significant tooth wear, which represents a precursor to exposure of the dental pulp and is facilitated by increased contact across the teeth as well as malocclusion [64]. It would therefore seem that the impaired viability of teeth following maxilla and mandible transplantation suggests both limited blood supply and sensory nerve input [65]. Although solid organ and facial VCA patients have received osseointegrated dental implants, more data is required to thoughtfully evaluate long-term success as well as whether or not such procedures alter the architecture of the composite with time [66]. Similarly, the mechanism and long-term implications of decreased airway volumes posttransplantation also represent an opportunity for further study.

4.7 Concluding Thoughts

Vascularized composite allografts involving the face represent powerful, life-changing options for severely disfigured patients with maxillary and mandibular defects. The primary goals of face transplant surgery involve re-establishing ideal facial harmony and projection of the craniofacial skeleton, stable occlusal relationships, and temporomandibular joint function to facilitate feeding and mastication, airway patency and phonation, as well as a less stigmatizing social appearance. Unfortunately, facial allografts containing single- or double-jaw constituents carry a considerable risk of dental and skeletal complications, often requiring revision surgery. Understanding dentofacial outcomes, ramifications, and strategies for mitigation will allow facial transplantation teams to optimally counsel candidates regarding this procedure and formulate evidence-based surgical plans. A truly comprehensive analysis of outcomes is limited due to the rarity of this procedure and the variability in reporting by primary transplant teams, however, we anticipate this to improve in the years to come and look forward to future discoveries.

References

1. Devauchelle B, Badet L, Lengelé B, et al. First human face allograft: early report. Lancet. 2006;368(9531):203–9.
2. Sosin M, Rodriguez ED. The face transplantation update: 2016. Plast Reconstr Surg. 2016;137(6):1841–50.
3. Siemionow M, Papay F, Alam D, et al. Near-total human face transplantation for a severely disfigured patient in the USA. Lancet. 2009;374(9685):203–9.
4. Sosin M, Ceradini DJ, Levine JP, et al. Total face, eyelids, ears, scalp, and skeletal subunit transplant. Plast Reconstr Surg. 2016;138(1):205–19.
5. Khalifian S, Brazio PS, Mohan R, et al. Facial transplantation: the first 9 years. Lancet. 2014;384(9960):2153–63.
6. Mohan R, Fisher M, Dorafshar A, et al. Principles of face transplant revision: beyond primary repair. Plast Reconstr Surg. 2014;134(6):1295–304.
7. Krezdorn N, Alhefzi M, Perry B, et al. Trismus in face transplantation following ballistic trauma. J Craniofac Surg. 2018;29(4):843–7.
8. Meningaud JP, Donsimoni JM, Lantieri L. Facial allograft transplantation and basal implantology (cortically anchored disk-design implants). Rev Stomatol Chir Maxillofac. 2009;110(6):353–8.
9. Van Lierde KM, Roche N, De Letter M, et al. Speech characteristics one year after first Belgian facial transplantation. Laryngoscope. 2014;124(9):2021–7.
10. Ploder O, Köhnke R, Winsauer H, et al. Skeletal-versus soft-tissue-based cephalometric analyses: is the correlation reproducible? Acta Odontol Scand. 2019;77(2):135–41.
11. Riedel RA. Esthetics and its relation to orthodontic therapy. Angle Orthod. 1950;20(3):168–78.
12. Eslamian L, Borzabadi-farahani A, Badiee MR, Le BT. An objective assessment of orthognathic surgery patients. J Craniofac Surg. 2019;30(8):2479–82.
13. Kim KJ, Park JH, Bay RC, Lee MY, Chang NY, Chae JM. Mandibular condyle bone density in adolescents with varying skeletal patterns evaluated using cone-beam computed tomography: a potential predictive tool. Am J Orthod Dentofac Orthop. 2018;154(3):382–9.
14. Arnett GW, Bergman RT. Facial keys to orthodontic diagnosis and treatment planning: part I. Am J Orthod Dentofac Orthop. 1993;103(4):299–312.
15. Fischer S, Wallins JS, Bueno EM, et al. Airway recovery after face transplantation. Plast Reconstr Surg. 2014;134(6):946–54.
16. Kim HJ, Kim BC, Kim JG, Zhengguo P, Kang SH, Lee SH. Construction and validation of the midsagittal reference plane based on the skull base symmetry for three-dimensional cephalometric craniofacial analysis. J Craniofac Surg. 2014;25(2):338–42.
17. Coombs DM, Gharb BB, Tuncer FB, et al. Skeletal and dental outcomes after facial allotransplantation: the Cleveland clinic experience and systematic review of the literature. Plast Reconstr Surg. 2022;149(4):945–62.
18. Kiliaridis S, Johansson A, Haraldson T, Omar R, Carlsson GE. Craniofacial morphology, occlusal traits, and bite force in persons with advanced occlusal tooth wear. Am J Orthod Dentofac Orthop. 1995;107(3):286–92.
19. Murphy RJ, Basafa E, Hashemi S, et al. Optimizing hybrid occlusion in face-jaw-teeth transplantation: a preliminary assessment of real-time cephalometry as part of the computer-assisted planning and execution workstation for craniomaxillofacial surgery. Plast Reconstr Surg. 2015;136(2):350–62.
20. Al-ani Z. Occlusion and temporomandibular disorders: a long-standing controversy in dentistry. Prim Dent J. 2020;9(1):43–8.
21. Meazzini MC, Mazzoleni F, Caronni E, Bozzetti A. Le Fort III advancement osteotomy in the growing child affected by Crouzon's and Apert's syndromes: presurgical and postsurgical growth. J Craniofac Surg. 2005;16(3):369–77.
22. Gibson TL, Grayson BH, Mccarthy JG, Shetye PR. Maxillomandibular and occlusal relationships in preadolescent patients with syndromic craniosynostosis treated by LeFort III distraction osteogenesis: 10-year surgical and phenotypic stability. Am J Orthod Dentofac Orthop. 2019;156(6):779–90.
23. Saltaji H, Altalibi M, Major MP, et al. Le Fort III distraction osteogenesis versus conventional Le Fort III osteotomy in correction of syndromic midfacial hypoplasia: a systematic review. J Oral Maxillofac Surg. 2014;72(5):959–72.
24. Gharb BB, Rampazzo A, Doumit G, et al. Skeletal changes of an osteomyocutaneous facial allograft five years following transplantation. J Craniofac Surg. 2017;28(2):352–8.
25. Hashem AM, Hoffman GS, Gastman B, et al. Establishing the feasibility of face transplantation in granulomatosis with polyangiitis. Am J Transplant. 2016;16(7):2213–23.
26. Karunanayake M, To F, Efanov JI, Doumit G. Analysis of craniofacial remodeling in the aging midface using reconstructed three-dimensional models in paired individuals. Plast Reconstr Surg. 2017;140(3):448–54.
27. Kueckelhaus M, Turk M, Kumamaru KK, et al. Transformation of face transplants: volumetric and morphologic graft changes resemble aging after facial allotransplantation. Am J Transplant. 2016;16(3):968–78.
28. Lambros VS. Personal communication. 1999.
29. Pessa JE. An algorithm of facial aging: verification of Lambros's theory by three-dimensional stereolithography, with reference to the

pathogenesis of midfacial aging, scleral show, and the lateral suborbital trough deformity. Plast Reconstr Surg. 2000;106(2):479–88.
30. Wu RT, Wilson AT, Gary CS, Steinbacher DM. Complete reoperation in orthognathic surgery. Plast Reconstr Surg. 2019;143(5):1053–9.
31. Asiri SN, Tadlock LP, Buschang PH. The prevalence of clinically meaningful malocclusion among US adults. Orthod Craniofac Res. 2019;22(4):321–8.
32. Soverina D, Gasparini G, Pelo S, et al. Skeletal stability in orthognathic surgery with the surgery first approach: a systematic review. Int J Oral Maxillofac Surg. 2019;48(7):930–40.
33. Gandedkar NH, Chng CK, Tan W. Surgery-first orthognathic approach case series: salient features and guidelines. J Orthod Sci. 2016;5(1):35–42.
34. Liao YF, Chiu YT, Huang CS, Ko EW, Chen YR. Presurgical orthodontics versus no presurgical orthodontics: treatment outcome of surgical-orthodontic correction for skeletal class III open bite. Plast Reconstr Surg. 2010;126(6):2074–83.
35. Baek SH, Ahn HW, Kwon YH, Choi JY. Surgery-first approach in skeletal class III malocclusion treated with 2-jaw surgery: evaluation of surgical movement and postoperative orthodontic treatment. J Craniofac Surg. 2010;21(2):332–8.
36. Liao YF, Lo SH. Surgical occlusion setup in correction of skeletal class III deformity using surgery-first approach: guidelines, characteristics and accuracy. Sci Rep. 2018;8(1):11673.
37. Kim JY, Park JH, Jung HD, Jung YS. Factors affecting total treatment time in patients treated with orthognathic surgery using the surgery-first approach: multivariable analysis using 3D CT and scanned dental casts. J Clin Med. 2020;9(3):641.
38. Sabri R. Orthodontic objectives in orthognathic surgery: state of the art today. World J Orthod. 2006;7(2):177–91.
39. Ramly EP, Kantar RS, Diaz-siso JR, Alfonso AR, Shetye PR, Rodriguez ED. Outcomes after tooth-bearing maxillomandibular facial transplantation: Insights and lessons learned. J Oral Maxillofac Surg. 2019;77(10):2085–103.
40. Celebi AA, Kau CH, Ozaydin B. Three-dimensional anthropometric evaluation of facial morphology. J Craniofac Surg. 2017;28(5):470–4.
41. Zacharopoulos GV, Manios A, Kau CH, Velagrakis G, Tzanakakis GN, de Bree E. Anthropometric analysis of the face. J Craniofac Surg. 2016;27(1):71–5.
42. Tradowsy M. Sex difference in intercondylar distance. J Prosthet Dent. 1990;63(3):301–2.
43. Roche NA, Vermeersch HF, Stillaert FB, et al. Complex facial reconstruction by vascularized composite allotransplantation: the first Belgian case. J Plast Reconstr Aesthet Surg. 2015;68(3):362–71.
44. Bassiri Gharb B, Frautschi RS, Halasa BC, et al. Watershed areas in face transplantation. Plast Reconstr Surg. 2017;139(3):711–21.
45. Eisenburger M, Haubitz B, Schmelzeisen R, Wolter S, Tschernitschek H. The human mandibular intercondylar angle measured by computed tomography. Arch Oral Biol. 1999;44(11):947–51.
46. Nunez-villaveiran T, Fahradyan V, Dalla Pozza E, et al. Full facial allotransplantation including the temporomandibular joints: a radiologic and anatomical cadaveric study. Plast Reconstr Surg. 2020;146(3):622–32.
47. Epker BN, Wylie GA. Control of the condylar-proximal mandibular segments after sagittal split osteotomies to advance the mandible. Oral Surg Oral Med Oral Pathol. 1986;62(6):613–7.
48. Arnett GW, Milam SB, Gottesman L. Progressive mandibular retrusion—idiopathic condylar resorption: part I. Am J Orthod Dentofac Orthop. 1996;110(1):8–15.
49. Moore KE, Gooris PJ, Stoelinga PJ. The contributing role of condylar resorption to skeletal relapse following mandibular advancement surgery: report of five cases. J Oral Maxillofac Surg. 1991;49(5):448–60.
50. Reyneke JP, Ferretti C. Intraoperative diagnosis of condylar sag after bilateral sagittal split ramus osteotomy. Br J Oral Maxillofac Surg. 2002;40(4):285–92.
51. Hackney FL, Van Sickels JE, Nummikoski PV. Condylar displacement and temporomandibular joint dysfunction following bilateral sagittal split osteotomy and rigid fixation. J Oral Maxillofac Surg. 1989;47(3):223–7.
52. Lantieri L, Grimbert P, Ortonne N, et al. Face transplant: long-term follow-up and results of a prospective open study. Lancet. 2016;388(10052):1398–407.
53. Barret JP, Serracanta J. LeFort I osteotomy and secondary procedures in full-face transplant patients. J Plast Reconstr Aesthet Surg. 2013;66(5):723–5.
54. Lassus P, Lindford A, Vuola J, et al. The Helsinki face transplantation: surgical aspects and 1-year outcome. J Plast Reconstr Aesthet Surg. 2018;71(2):132–9.
55. Meningaud JP, Hivelin M, Benjoar MD, Toure G, Hermeziu O, Lantieri L. The procurement of allotransplants for ballistic trauma: a preclinical study and a report of two clinical cases. Plast Reconstr Surg. 2011;127(5):1892–900.
56. Gauthier A, Lézy JP, Vacher C. Vascularization of the palate in maxillary osteotomies: Anatomical study. Surg Radiol Anat. 2002;24(1):13–7.
57. Plana NM, Malta Barbosa J, Diaz-siso JR, Brecht LE, Rodriguez ED. Dental considerations and the role of prosthodontics and maxillofacial prosthetics in facial transplantation. J Am Dent Assoc. 2018;149(2):90–9.
58. Mehra MR, Jarcho JA, Cherikh W, et al. The drug-intoxication epidemic and solid-organ transplantation. N Engl J Med. 2018;378(20):1943–5.
59. Baghaie H, Kisely S, Forbes M, Sawyer E, Siskind DJ. A systematic review and meta- analysis of the association between poor oral health and substance abuse. Addiction. 2017;112(5):765–79.
60. Sroussi HY, Epstein JB, Bensadoun RJ, et al. Common oral complications of head and neck cancer radiation therapy: mucositis, infections, saliva change, fibrosis, sensory dysfunctions, dental caries, periodontal disease, and osteoradionecrosis. Cancer Med. 2017;6(12):2918–31.
61. Frautschi R, Rampazzo A, Bernard S, Djohan R, Papay F, Gharb BB. Management of the salivary glands and facial nerve in face transplantation. Plast Reconstr Surg. 2016;137(6):1887–97.
62. Helenius-hietala J, Ruokonen H, Grönroos L, et al. Self-reported oral symptoms and signs in liver transplant recipients and a control population. Liver Transpl. 2013;19(2):155–63.
63. Maarse F, Jager DH, Forouzanfar T, Wolff J, Brand HS. Tooth loss in Sjögren's syndrome patients compared to age and gender matched controls. Med Oral Patol Oral Cir Bucal. 2018;23(5):545–51.
64. Pintado MR, Anderson GC, Delong R, Douglas WH. Variation in tooth wear in young adults over a two-year period. J Prosthet Dent. 1997;77(3):313–20.
65. Wall A, Bueno E, Pomahac B, Treister N. Intraoral features and considerations in face transplantation. Oral Dis. 2016;22(2):93–103.
66. Montebugnoli L, Venturi M, Cervellati F, et al. Peri-implant response and microflora in organ transplant patients 1 year after prosthetic loading: a prospective controlled study. Clin Implant Dent Relat Res. 2015;17(5):972–82.

Facial Composite Vascularized Allotransplantation: Barcelona Experience

5

Juan P. Barret

The program of facial composite vascularized allotransplantation at the Vall d'Hebron Barcelona Hospital Campus/Universitat Autònoma de Barcelona was founded in 2007. A working group of plastic surgeons, transplant surgeons, physicians, organ transplantation coordinators, and nursing staff joined together to put the basis of the clinical protocol and the administrative requirements to start clinical work. The first patient was assessed in 2007, but it was not until august 2009 that a final approval by the Catalan Organization for Transplantation (OCATT) and the National Organization for Transplantation (ONT) was obtained. The first donors were assessed as soon as August 2009, with different activations until the first world's full-face VCA was performed in March 2010 [1].

5.1 The Spanish Model of Accreditation

The face is currently treated as composite tissues according to the current Spanish Law on Organ, Tissues, and Advanced Cell Therapies. However, the process of accreditation and authorization follows the same principles that are in use for solid organ transplantation. The regional (OCATT) and national (ONT) transplantation organizations grant certification to VCA programs. However, after receiving full accreditation, each recipient must still be evaluated on a case-by-case basis by the Spanish Organ Transplantation Body (ONT), and the accreditation for any given face transplantation procedure is obtained on an individual basis only. Other requirements that any VCA program must fulfill include ethics committee approval and positive psychologic/psychiatric evaluation, and up-to-date accreditation of the center for solid organ transplantation.

J. P. Barret (✉)
Department of Plastic Surgery and Burns, Vall d'Hebron Barcelona Hospital Campus, Universitat Autònoma de Barcelona, Barcelona, Spain
e-mail: jpbarret@vhebron.net

5.2 Organization of Facial Tissue Donation at UHVH

Tissue donation in facial transplantation is much more difficult than the rest of the organs. Donation of facial structures is not invisible, and the overall process of organ donation becomes much more cumbersome. The psychological impact that the request for facial donation may pose on relatives should not be underestimated; therefore, a specific donation protocol when donation of facial tissues was contemplated was deemed appropriate in our institution. The overall goal of such protocol was to minimize requests to relatives and to protect the organ donation process from a negative impact. In general terms, transplant coordinators are informed of the general requirements of the recipient. Coordinators would contact the plastic surgery transplant team if any donor matched these requirements. Only after evaluation of any donor with a good match, relatives are approached.

5.3 Organ Procurement Protocol

A brain-death heart-beating donation is contemplated as the best option to obtain the facial tissues with intact circulation, safety, and to minimize bleeding after revascularization by means of a thorough and careful hemostasis during procurement.

The first part of the operation includes evaluation of the internal organs and cannulation without infusion. Synchronous in situ dissection of solid organs and face is then conducted until the face and solid organs are ready for final procurement. Cold Wisconsin solution is then infused with in situ cooling and procurement of heart and lungs. The operation is then completed by procuring the rest of the internal organs and the facial tissues [2].

As an alternative, a non-heart beating protocol has been also organized. In this situation, cold Wisconsin solution is infused as a continuous perfusion during procurement of

© Springer Nature Switzerland AG 2023

R. Gurunian et al. (eds.), *Reconstructive Transplantation*, https://doi.org/10.1007/978-3-031-21520-9_5

facial tissues. The operation may be performed at the end of a multiple organ donation procurement procedure or with simultaneous procurement of internal organs and facial tissues in case of a donation in asystole.

5.4 Funding of Programs

VCA programs receive economic support from the hospital budget and the regional Department of Health. They are considered as a specialized reconstructive technique and as such are included in the treatment portfolio of our Department of Plastic Surgery provided that the center has received the accreditation of the Hospital and the regional transplant organization body (OCATT). In addition, cases that have been approved by the national transplant organization of the Ministry of Health through the Interterritorial Commission are also reimbursed by the Ministry of Health of the Spanish Government. This reimbursement follows the same route of solid organ transplantation reimbursement scheme.

5.5 Program Development

Facial VCA program at the Vall d'Hebron Barcelona Hospital Campus received the OCATT and ONT accreditation in 2009. Since that date the program has been active, and Face and Hand VCA have been included in treatment protocols and techniques portfolio of the Department.

As such, Face VCA is contemplated as one of the rungs of the Reconstructive Ladder. When other traditional, including complex microvascular reconstructions, do not fulfill the functional requirements for patients or in cases of massive destruction of the face, a Facial-VCA is contemplated. Still, few cases have been considered as candidates for a face transplantation.

During the past 12 years of activity, more than 30 requests for face transplantation have been received at the Department. However, many of them had no indication whatsoever. Of all those, only eight patients were considered to have an indication for a face VCA. Eventually, six patients were fully screened and four were put in active search for donors. Table 5.1 summarizes the type of deformity and outcome of the screening.

Two patients have been transplanted so far. The program is active and open for requests.

There have been no obstacles for the development of the program, with support from all participating agencies. The only difficulty for the expansion of the program has been the lack of patients with an indication for facial transplantation [3].

Table 5.1 Outcome of face-VCA screening

	Type of deformity	VCA screening	Outcome
Patient 1	Lower third oncological deformity	Full	Not indicated for medical reasons
Patient 2	Severe traumatic deformity (gun shot)	Full	Transplanted
Patient 3	Neurofribromatosis	Full	Patient declined transplantation after long search for donor
Patient 4	Severe burn deformity	Only initial screening	Patient declined after full information received
Patient 5	Post-oncological deformity	Full	Patient declined after screening
Patient 6	Facial arteriovenous malformation	Full	Transplanted
Patient 7	Post oncological deformity	Full	Not indicated for medical reasons
Patient 8	Acquired endocrine deformity	Only initial screening	Patient declined after full information received

5.6 Patients

5.6.1 Patient 1

The first face transplant in our Institution was performed in March 2010. It consisted of a Full-Face Transplant including all facial bones. To our knowledge this was the first report of a full-face transplant [4]. He was a 30-year-old Caucasian male patient who suffered a severe facial disfigurement in 2005. The etiology was an accidental gunshot to the face. The patient presented with a deformity that included severe facial scars, traumatic hypertelorism, bilateral orbital dystopia, destruction of lacrimal apparatus and medial canthus ligaments, absence of the nose, destruction of the maxilla and both zygomatic bones, subtotal destruction of the mandible, and partial absence of the lips. Neurophysiology tests (EMG) showed intact nerve function with scarred and absent facial muscles. Sensation was normal in non-scarred areas. The functional impact of this deformity was very severe: the patient could not speak, breath, or eat normally. He required a permanent percutaneous gastrostomy tube feeding and a tracheostomy to preserve his airway.

Donation included the whole face and facial bones, heart, lungs, liver, pancreas, kidneys, and tissues. This was a heart beating multiple organ donation in a 41-year-old Caucasian male patient who died from a massive brain hemorrhage (massive bleeding from an arterial malformation).

The operation began with the preparation of a negative impression of the donor's facial features. Next, a facemask was fabricated to cover the facial raw area after completion of the graft procurement. The full facial allograft (Type VB)

[5] was harvested in a heart beating brain death donor. The procurement of the graft lasted 4.5 h. The last portion of the operation (osteotomies and separation of the floor of the mouth, anterior pillar of the pharynx and nasopharynx) was performed after the heart and lungs were procured. A running perfusion of Wisconsin solution at 4 °C was maintained to maximize the protection of the tissues under ischemia time. The facial allograft was harvested maintaining all retention ligaments of the face, and it was based on the vascular pedicles and nerves. All sensitive branches of the trigeminal nerve (supraorbital, infraorbital, and mandibular nerves) and the buccal, zygomatic, orbicularis oculi, and frontal branches of the facial nerve on each side were identified. The arterial inflow included both external carotid arteries. We dissected both external jugular veins and the anterior jugular vein on the right side and the retromandibular vein on the left side to provide venous outflow.

The graft included all skin and soft tissues of the face (from the frontal hairline to the mid part of the neck and from the right to the left preauricular crease, including all features of the face), the facial muscles, lachrymal ducts and cysts, eyelids, floor of the mouth, lips, upper and lower teeth, hard palate, all cheek mucosa up to the anterior pharyngeal pillar, the mandible from the right coronoid to left coronoid process, the maxilla, two thirds of both zygomatic bones, the nose (including cartilage and nasal bones and septum), turbinates, vomer, ethmoid bone, and maxillary sinuses. The facial allograft was preserved on cold Wisconsin solution. Total cold ischemia time was 2.5 h.

The second part of the operation began with the revascularization of the allograft on the recipient. Arterial revascularization was achieved with an end-to-end anastomosis between the right external carotid arteries. Venous outflow was provided with two end-to-end anastomosis between the external jugular veins and two end to side on the internal jugular. Complete perfusion of the whole allograft was achieved with active bleeding in all tissues. All deformed tissues and bone fragments on the recipient's face were removed, and the facial allograft was transplanted to the final position. The procedure followed with rigid fixation of the facial bones with titanium mini-plates and screws. The next step was a water-tight closure of the intraoral mucosa and hard and soft palate, end to end nerve neurorrhaphies of all sensitive and motor nerves, and suture of muscles, soft tissues, and skin. Excess of skin on the neck and the left preauricular area was preserved to allow for multiple skin and soft tissues biopsies for the control of the rejection.

Induction therapy included a slow infusion of thymoglobulin at 2mg/kg IV 2 h before the operation and 1 g of prednisone IV administered before the release of the arterial clamps.

Maintenance immunosuppression was performed with prednisone at 1 mg/kg/24 h IV with a taper to 10 mg overtime PO daily, tacrolimus to target levels of 10–15 ng/ml and mycophenolate mofetil 2 g PO daily. Infection prophylaxis included antibiotics for Gram-positive and Gram-negative bacteria, antifungal prophylaxis IV, Valganciclovir for CMV prophylaxis, and Co-trimoxazole for Pneumocystis prophylaxis.

The operation (procurement and transplantation) lasted 24 h. The patient required a total transfusion of 30 packed red cells. Half of the blood requirements occurred during revascularization, initial hemostasis, and resection of the recipient face. There was no major complication during surgery, and a complete revascularization and perfusion of the allograft was observed without any evidence of relative ischemia across the midline. The patient was fully awake and in spontaneous ventilation 24 h after the operation.

Postoperative complications included a thrombosis of the left venous anastomosis on day 3 after surgery (left external jugular and left retromandibular vein) due to edema and compression that required re-exploration and re-anastomosis. On day 17 posttransplant, the patient presented with an acute oro-cutaneous fistula after an episode of vomiting on day 17.

Our immunosuppression control protocol includes skin and mucosa biopsies on day 0, 3, 7 and at weekly interval thereafter during the first month. All but the last one showed grade I rejection without any clinical signs of rejection. These findings made us change our protocol to exclude biopsies unless a clinical suspicion of rejection arises.

The patient presented with three episodes of acute rejection in the first 12 months (day 28, day 75, day 180) that were treated with high-dose boluses of prednisone. The second episode also included thymoglobulin and inclusion for a few weeks of sirolimus in the regime.

The patient regained total sensation in the forehead, eyelids, cheeks, lips, and intraoral mucosa, active movement on all facial muscles (although the left side is still partially activated). The patient was able to recover his premorbid life condition (Fig. 5.1a, b).

5.6.2 Patient 2

The second patient transplanted in our institution was a 40-year-old Caucasian male patient who presented with a massive arteriovenous malformation in the neck, tongue, and soft tissues of the face. The patient had undergone several treatments in the past in other institutions, which included embolization, partial resections, ligation of external carotid artery in an emergency operation and antiangiogenic drug treatments with none or partial improvement. At the time of presentation, the patient had had several episodes of life-threatening massive hemorrhages.

The proposed surgical treatment included a resection of cervical and facial tissues with complete extirpation of the

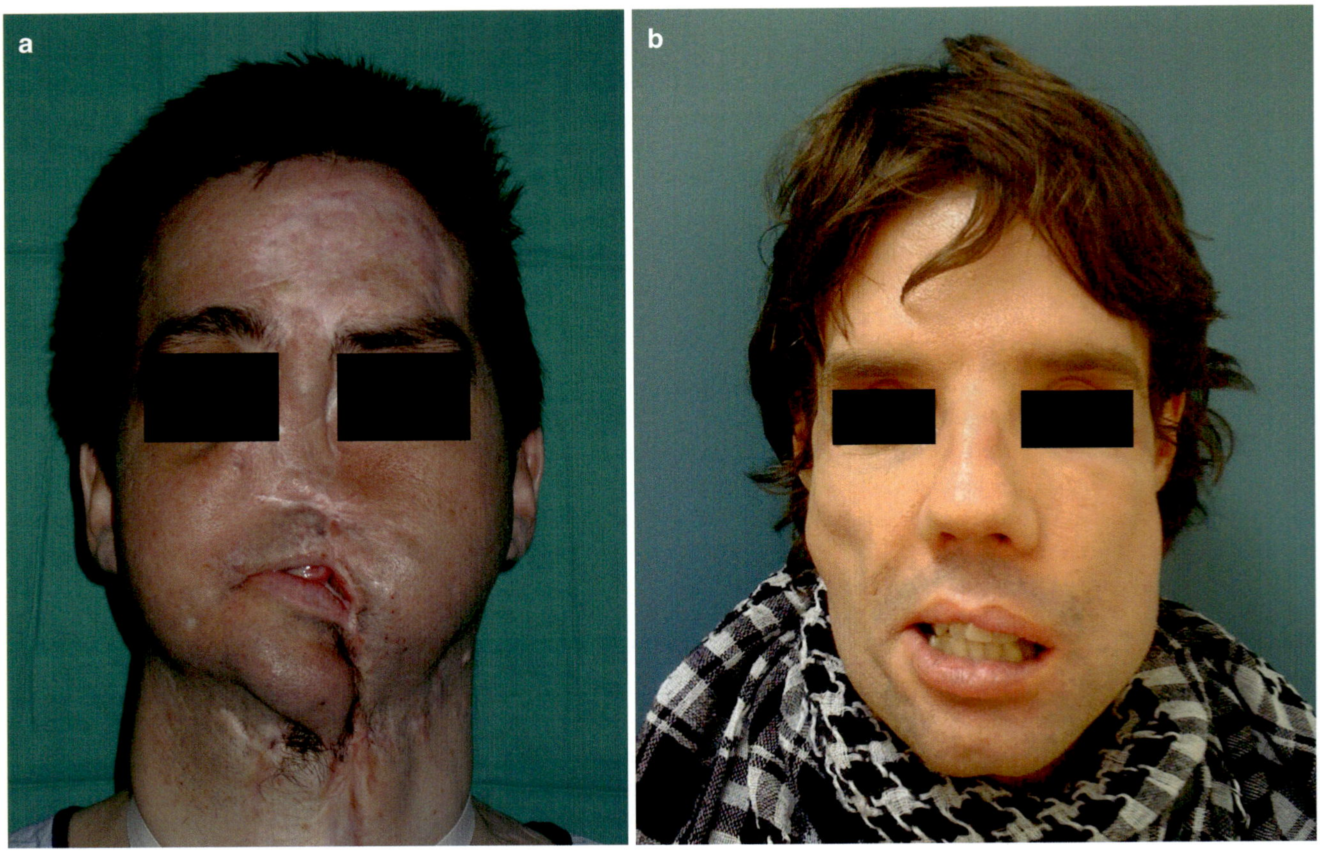

Fig. 5.1 (**a**) Posttraumatic deformity after gun-shot injury to the face. (**b**) Same patient after the first world's full-face facial transplantation

nidus and the whole arteriovenous malformation and reconstruction of a face transplant of the cervical skin and soft tissues, two lower thirds of the face and tongue.

The patient was transplanted in February 2015. Donor was a male Caucasian in his mid-40s who had suffered a massive brain hemorrhage. A controlled asystole multiple organ donation was performed, which included the face and a multiple internal solid donation. All big vessels were canulated and a controlled asystole was obtained. Once the death of the donor was documented and certified, cold Wisconsin solution was perfused at 4 °C with local cooling, and simultaneous procurement of face and internal organs started with running cold Wisconsin preservation fluids. The same procurement protocol as per patient 1 was followed. It included the procurement of the whole face, facial skeleton including mandible and tongue. The graft was pedicled on both common carotid arteries and the internal and external jugular veins. The procurement lasted for 4 h.

During the procurement of the facial graft, the recipient was embolized at the Interventional Neuroradiology Unit of the Hospital to minimize intraoperative bleeding. The AV nidus and all afferent vessels were embolized under general anesthesia. The patient was then transferred to the operating room where the transplantation began. The first step consisted in the identification of major neck vessels in the recipient and revascularization to assess graft vitality. The revascularization was performed with end-to-end external carotid artery to common carotid artery of the graft and external and internal jugular veins on both the sides. Total ischemia time was 90 min. Next, the arteriovenous malformation and the two lower thirds of the face were extirpated and the graft inset in a similar manner to patient 1. The graft included the tongue and the intraoral cavity to the anterior pillars. During the operation a total of 153 packed red cells were transfused.

The patient was transferred to the Burn ICU after the operation. During the first postoperative day, the patient presented with a right jugular thrombosis due to kinking of pedicle that required a new anastomosis. The thrombosis recurred 24 h later, and a third anastomosis was performed.

On day 4, the patient had a massive hemorrhage produced by uncontrolled hypertension that required exploration in theater. There were no other surgical complications thereafter and the patient was fully awake by day 7 postop.

Three weeks after the operation the patient presented with a grade 2–3 acute rejection. This episode occurred after a quick taper of prednisone. The acute rejection episode was resolved with three boluses of 1 g prednisone followed by a quick taper. The patient is now maintained with a low dose of tacrolimus and prednisone.

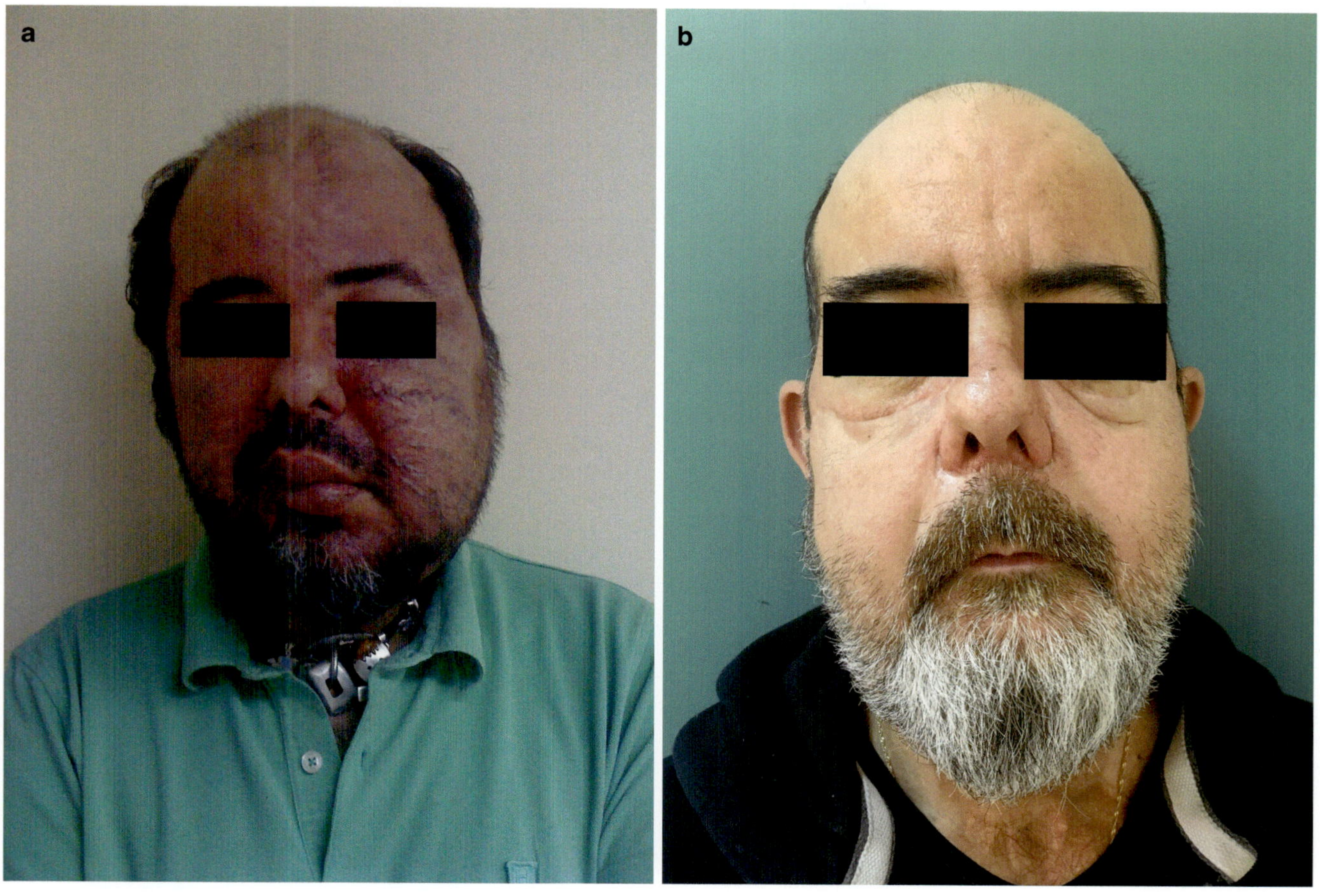

Fig. 5.2 (**a**) Facial deformity due to a massive arterio-venous malformation. (**b**) Same patient after a lower two-third facial transplantation

The patient gained full sensory recovery during the first year after transplant and full facial movement except for left frontalis after 18 months. Even though the tongue has maintained tone and trophism, the patient has not gained active tongue mobility. The patient has gained complete normal activities except for an inability to competency in swallowing. Percutaneous gastrostomy tube feeding had to be maintained. There is no recurrence of any arteriovenous malformation no new bleeding episodes have been encountered (Fig. 5.2a, b).

5.7 Lessons Learned

The introduction of the Face-VCA program in our institution has offered patients with extreme facial deformity an opportunity to restore them to their premorbid life condition. It allows the treatment team to offer patients in a tertiary plastic surgery department all techniques available for reconstruction.

The development of a Face VCA program in a tertiary hospital with a long and robust solid organ transplantation program has allowed us to implement efficient and safe protocols for composite vascularized allotransplantation. A multidisciplinary team approach is one of the strengths of the program. The tradition and success of donation through the OCATT and ONT system is another strength of the program, which warrants proper and efficient donation protocol standards and donation and transplantation surveillance and quality improvement.

Our inclusion criteria and face VCA indication were strict from the inception of the program. However, after screening of several candidates and the successful transplantation of two patients, functional and impact in quality of life are considered nowadays more important and relevant than anatomical deformity and severity of face destruction. Matching alteration of function and absence of quality of life (i.e., death as an alternative to current quality of life) is a must to perform a proper indication for face VCA.

In our initial surgical protocols only a heart beating procurement was contemplated. Reasons for this choice included the enhancement of surgical technique and improvement of vascularization of the graft, minimizing ischemia time. However, after our second transplantation, when procurement was performed under asystole with continuous cold Wisconsin i.v. perfusion, excellent graft perfusion and good hemostasis was achieved. Consequently, a non-heart beating donation is now considered a good and safe alternative.

The evolution of human transplantation has transported us from life-saving procedures (liver, heart, lung transplants) to life extending procedures (kidney transplantation) and life improving indication such as pancreas and small bowel transplantation. The next inevitable step was to achieve life normalizing transplantation, which merge lifesaving, extending, and improving, which is no doubt an overall normalization of quality of life. VCA programs fall in this last category and have produced an important move ahead for future explorations of modern treatments. Few patients have been operated on so far throughout the world. This indicates that this is an extremely complex procedure that should be reserved to few centers. The initial experience has been excellent, which signals that strict protocols and performing VCA in tertiary institutions with long and robust tradition in transplantation render predictive good results.

Results of Face VCA have proved to be superior than many traditional techniques in severe catastrophic facial deformity. However, the advent of new regenerative medicine strategies or hybrid techniques may make VCA in a not very far future obsolete.

References

1. Barret JP, Serracanta J, Collado JM, et al. Full face transplantation organization, development, and results—the Barcelona experience: a case report. Transplant Proc. 2011;43:3533–4.
2. Bueno J, Barret JP, Serracanta J, et al. Logistics and strategy of multiorgan procurement involving total face allograft. Am J Transplant. 2011;11(5):1091–7.
3. Barret JP, Tomasello V. Face transplantation: principles, techniques, and artistry. Berlin: Springer; 2015.
4. Barret JP, Gavaldà J, Bueno J, et al. Full face transplant: the first case report. Ann Surg. 2011;254(2):252–6.
5. Lengelé BG. Current concepts and future challenges in facial transplantation. Clin Plast Surg. 2009;36(3):507–21.

Facial Transplantation: First Canadian Experience

6

Eli Saleh, Jordan Gornitsky, and Daniel E. Borsuk

6.1 Introduction

Vascularized composite allotransplantation (VCA) is the culmination of advances in transplant immunology and refinement of surgical technique. In recent years, it has emerged as a ground-breaking reconstructive solution for patients with severely disfiguring facial injuries.

Overcoming the pitfalls of conventional reconstructive techniques, facial VCA allows simultaneous "like with like" restoration of both esthetic and functional deficits in a single-stage procedure with superior results.

Experience with facial VCA remains in its infancy. The need for lifelong immunosuppression, its adverse effects and potential for chronic rejection, has limited the procedure to only the most severe injuries. Despite these challenges, continued experience with honest and transparent reporting are instrumental for the long-term success of this procedure.

Our program's inception began in 2012 following the senior author's involvement with the facial transplantation performed at the R. Adams Cowley Shock Trauma Center in Baltimore, Maryland. Upon returning to Maisonneuve-Rosemont Hospital in Montreal, Canada, the program was officially launched, and a multidisciplinary team was established. Given that no previous facial vascularized composite allotransplantation had taken place in Canada, institutional review boards at the university hospital and organ procurement organization had to be appropriately addressed, in conjunction with health Canada and provincial ministry of health approval. Over a 3-year period, six full rehearsal procedures were performed on cadaveric specimens, allowing for the development and refinement of a systematic step-by-step approach.

The first transplant was partially funded through a research grant generously donated by Johnson & Johnson. Following the successful outcome of the 2018 facial transplant, an annual budget has been allocated to the VCA program by the government of the province of Quebec. Funding of the program is meant to cover all phases of the transplants including preoperative workup, peri-operative care, and postoperative long-term maintenance, including research and development.

The Quebec National VCA and innovative reconstruction program is currently active, and despite being in its infancy, expansion to include additional subtypes of vascularized composite allografts is underway. As of August 2021, a second potential face transplant recipient has completed their extensive preoperative workup and is awaiting a suitable donor match. The upper extremity VCA and targeted muscle reinnervation (TMR) branch of the program has been progressing quickly. A dozen unilateral amputation patients have undergone TMR, and six bilateral amputation patients have been evaluated for upper extremity bilateral VCA. The long-term mission of our program is to offer gold-standard treatment options for the most complex physical deformities. VCA in combination with TMR research and development will one day allow for the eventuality of surgically affixing biocompatible prosthetics or regenerated vascularized composite Homo-grafts.

To date, five facial, six upper extremity, and two abdominal wall patients have been screened. Including the first recipient, a total of two patients have been approved for facial vascularized composite allotransplantation. Approved candidates are required to complete rigorous medical and psychosocial evaluations.

Fortunately, there are few patients who would benefit from vascularized composite allotransplantation. Moreover, of those patients, only a small subset would qualify as suit-

E. Saleh · J. Gornitsky
Maisonneuve Rosemont Hospital, Montreal, QC, Canada
e-mail: Eli.saleh@umontreal.ca; Jordan.gornitsky@umontreal.ca

D. E. Borsuk (✉)
Maisonneuve Rosemont Hospital, Montreal, QC, Canada

Sainte-Justine University Healthcare Centre, Montreal, QC, Canada

Division of Plastic and Reconstructive Surgery, University of Montreal, Montreal, QC, Canada
e-mail: info@drborsuk.com

© Springer Nature Switzerland AG 2023
R. Gurunian et al. (eds.), *Reconstructive Transplantation*, https://doi.org/10.1007/978-3-031-21520-9_6

able recipients. A suitable patient must have a strong support system, be reliable, psychologically strong enough to withstand the arduous recovery and numerous potential complications, and have the capacity to completely understand the alternatives to VCA, and the great short-term and long-term risks of VCA. Despite the relative low volume of patients, we feel that surgical and medical innovation opportunities exist in this emerging field and that the clinical expertise and research discoveries will significantly contribute to the fields of transplantation and plastic surgery.

We report on the first Canadian (and 43rd worldwide) face transplant performed in May 2018 at the Maisonneuve-Rosemont Hospital in Montreal.

6.2 Patient

The recipient is a 64-year-old male who sustained a self-inflicted facial gunshot wound in 2011, resulting in severe mid and lower facial trauma (Fig. 6.1). Over the course of his treatment, he underwent five reconstructive procedures including a free fibula flap to restore the mandibular deficit and locoregional advancement flaps of the lips, mucosa, and tongue. He suffered from recalcitrant chronic pain in his reconstructed mandible and fibula donor site and refused any procedures requiring further facial scarring and donor site morbidity. The patient had refused prosthetic restorations and wanted the most normal appearance possible.

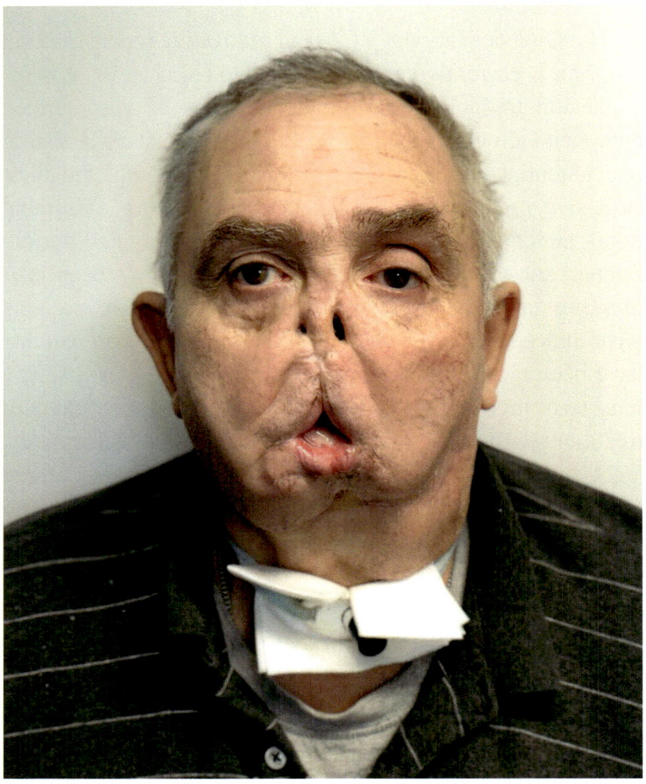

Fig. 6.1 A 64-year-old male who sustained a self-inflicted facial gunshot which resulted in severe mid and lower facial trauma

Functionally, loss of nasal architecture and upper airway obstruction caused by his glossoptotic tongue required a permanent tracheostomy. Peri-oral scarring coupled with tongue atrophy and hypomobility resulted in oral dysphagia. The temporomandibular joints showed no radiological signs of disease and were not painful despite a limited 25 mm functional opening. With precautionary measures such as drinking through an adapted straw, avoiding large boluses and mincing solids, feeding proceeded without aspirations. Despite several articulatory imprecisions and hypo-nasality, his speech was intelligible.

The patient was otherwise not known for any comorbidities. His preoperative workup was unremarkable. An extensive 3-year assessment was conducted by a clinical psychiatrist in order to establish the patient's motivation, to ensure his adherence to life-long immunosuppression therapy, and to confirm his mental fortitude to overcome any potential complications. He was informed of, and clearly understood, all non-transplant alternatives. Lastly, his support system was deemed as strong and reliable.

Upon initial consultation in 2015, the patient's goals included restoration of a normal facial appearance, oral function, de-cannulation, alleviation of chronic pain, and the ability to circulate in public without social stigmatization.

6.3 Donor

A compatible donor was identified 103 days after the recipient was placed on the VCA waitlist. He was a younger male with matching race, skin color, hair color, and bony morphology. His facial width was comparable, as determined by the precise fit of the recipient-based Le Fort III-level osteotomy cutting guide. His blood type was O Rh+; flow cytometry cross-matching revealed no B- or T-cell reactivity.

6.4 Preparation

Virtual surgical planning (VSP) and computer-assisted design (CAD) were used for this case. Le Fort III-level guides were manufactured based on the recipient's scan by Materialise solutions (Materialise N.V., Leuven, Belgium) and were used for both donor and potential recipient. A stereolithographic model of the recipient's facial skeleton following debridement was 3D printed. It would serve to pre-drill and pre-bend plates on the allograft in situ before vessel clamping, thereby minimizing ischemia time and improving accuracy.

6.5 Allograft Procurement

The facial allograft was procured from a multi-organ brain-dead beating-heart donor following placement of a tracheostomy and the creation of an anaplastologic facial mold. Cutaneous incisions were designed to include redundant skin at the lower eyelids and neck to help limit secondary ectropion and allow for postoperative skin biopsies, respectively. The procurement was grossly divided into the dissection of cervical vessels, facial nerve, intra-oral incisions, and osteotomies.

The procedure began with elevation of a sub-platysmal flap. Care was taken to identify the external jugular veins and preserve adequate length on the flap side. The posterior digastric muscles and hypo-glossal nerve were divided to allow for adequate exposure of the external and internal carotids, facial, and lingual trunks. All vessels were circumferentially dissected in anticipation for eventual division and flap transfer. Vessel loops were placed around the internal carotid arteries after their bifurcation for eventual ligation.

Next, a face-lift incision was made and sub-SMAS dissection carried until the anterior aspect of the parotid gland. The root of the facial nerve was identified using the Tragal pointer and all major branches were dissected in an anterograde fashion, resulting in removal of the superficial parotid gland. The nerve trunk was then tagged, cut as proximally as possible and elevated off of the deep parotid gland.

After completion of cutaneous incisions at the lower eyelids and nasal dorsum, osteotomy sites were prepared at the level of the nasion, orbital floor, zygoma, maxilla and mandible, bilaterally. The infra-orbital nerves were cut as proximally as possible within the orbits and reflected toward the skin. Intra-orally, incisions were carried at the soft palate as well as the tongue and floor of mouth.

Osteotomies began with bilateral sagittal split osteotomies performed via an external approach. Maximal length of inferior alveolar nerves was preserved on the anterior segment. The Le Fort III-level osteotomy was carried using prefabricated cutting guides at the level of the nasion and zygoma and continued posterior to the infra-orbital ridge (Fig. 6.2). Care was taken to preserve the infraorbital nerve. Following down-fracture and disjunction of the midface segment, the interior carotid arteries were ligated, and the flap isolated on its vascular pedicles. On the right, the pedicle consisted of the external carotid artery, facial and external jugular veins. On the left, the pedicle included the facial artery and facial vein. Administration of indocyanine green (ICG) and fluorescence angiography imaging confirmed adequate perfusion of the allograft on a single pedicle. After ligation of both pedicles, the flap was flushed with 3 L of Wisconsin solution and transported to the recipient's operation theater, located across the hall. Overall procurement time was 11 h and 15 min. Lastly, a realistic silicone replica of the donor's face was sutured over the wound.

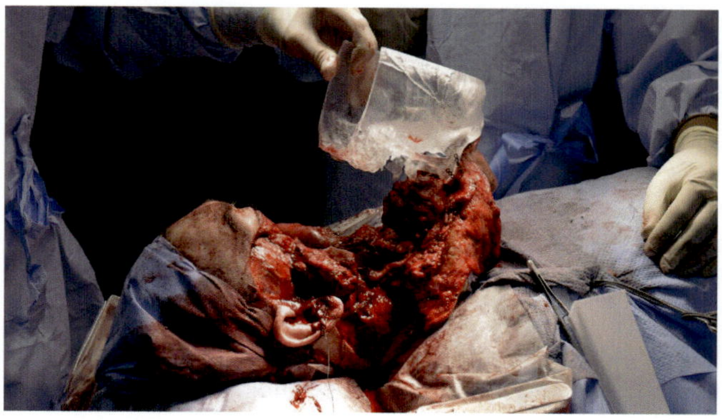

Fig. 6.2 Prefabricated model of the recipient's midface was used to pre-drill plates on the allograft in-situ

6.6 Recipient Debridement

Recipient debridement began 3 h prior in anticipation for difficult dissection in fibrosed tissues. A reverse face-lift dissection was carried in the subcutaneous plane. Care was taken to leave the orbicularis oculi muscles and their attachments on the recipient as well as preserve the parotid duct. Using a nerve stimulator and useful anatomic landmarks such as Zucker's point and an intra-orally cannulated Stenson's duct, the middle divisions of the facial nerve were identified as they exited the parotid glands medially. The zygomatic, buccal and marginal mandibular branches were then tagged and transected as proximally as possible. The branches innervating the native orbicularis oculi muscles were preserved.

Neck dissection followed by raising a sub-platysmal flap. The carotid, facial and lingual arteries, internal and external jugular veins, as well as the thyro-lingo-facial trucks were dissected bilaterally. The hypoglossal nerves were identified and preserved. The periosteum at the inferior margin of the mandible was incised and elevated over its lingual aspect.

In preparation for midface osteotomies, the periosteum over the nasion, inferior orbital rims, orbital floors, and zygomatic bodies was incised and elevated. The origin of the masseters lateral to the osteotomy sites were preserved. The lacrimal canals were carefully retracted from their fossae. The infra-orbital nerves were identified and transected as distally as possible within the orbit to preserve sufficient length for re-anastomosis.

Intra-orally, a standard BSSO approach was used to expose the mandible-fibula construct bilaterally. The cheek mucosa was incised anterior to Stenson's ducts until the maxillary dentition. The incisions connected superiorly over the hard palate. Sub-mucoperiosteal dissection was carried distally until the hard–soft palate junction, where attachments between these structures were released. The intra- and extra-oral incisions were joined anterior to Stenson's ducts. Finally, the mandible-fibula construct was completely dissected over its lingual and buccal surfaces until the transcervical dissection was reached. The insertions of the masseter muscles proximal to the osteotomy sites was left intact. Of note, as with the allograft procurement, intra-oral incisions were designed to incorporate wide soft tissue cuffs. However, the design was opposite, including additional soft tissue over the hard palate and placing the floor of mouth incision at the junction of the attached gingiva and lingual mucosa.

Osteotomies began at the BSSO level. Care was taken to preserve maximal length of the inferior alveolar nerve. Prefabricated cutting guide were used for Le Fort III-level osteotomies. Finally, osteotomies across the septum, maxillae and pterygoid plates were performed. Any remaining nasal soft tissue attachments were cut, completing the facial disjunction.

6.7 Allo-transplantation

Allo-transplantation consisted of bony rigid fixation, microvascular anastomoses, intra-oral closure, facial and infraorbital nerve coaptation, soft tissue resuspension, and skin closure. Reconstruction began with rigid fixation of the Le Fort III-level osteotomies. Bi-cortical lag screws were used for mandibular fixation. There was an excellent match in midface width and the allograft accurately fit into position. Osteosynthesis was facilitated by the presence of mid-facial plates, which were pre-bent and fixed onto the allograft with the stereolithographic model of the recipient during its procurement.

Microvascular anastomoses were performed bilaterally. (Right: external carotid artery (ECA), facial vein and external jugular vein (EJV) anastomosed to the recipient's ECA, internal jugular vein (IJV) and external jugular vein. Left: facial artery and facial vein anastomosed on the recipient's occipital artery and a branch of the IJV). Venous coupling devices in diameter were used for all venous anastomoses. Blood flow to the allograft was restored after unclamping of the right pedicle, marking a total ischemia time of 1 h 54 min (25 min of cold ischemia including Wisconsin solution perfusion and 1 h 29 min of warm ischemia during bony fixation and right side microanastomosis). Indocyanine green was injected intravenously and scanned by fluorescence angiography to confirm complete vascularization of the graft on a single pedicle. Despite excellent perfusion, the contralateral pedicle was anastomosed as a precautionary measure.

In order to correct the retro-pulsed and ptotic position of the recipient's tongue and increase the antero-posterior diameter of the oropharynx, the hyoid bone was resuspended anteriorly. The hyoido-pexy was performed by encircling, advancing, and anchoring the hyoid to the mental spine of the mandible using a bone anchor suture.

Due to severe ankylosis at both temporo-mandibular joints, the BSSO fixation had to be released to allow sufficient space for closure of intra-oral incisions. Upon secondary fixation, it was purposely decided to restore the donor's premorbid 3 mm anterior open bite and not to correct occlusion in order to compensate for the donor's trismus and facilitate postoperative oral feeding.

Bilateral coaptation of zygomatic, buccal, and marginal mandibular branches of the facial nerve was performed. The infra-orbital nerves were anastomosed inside of the orbit bilaterally. Anastomosis of the inferior alveolar nerve was not possible due to its location, limited oral opening and short length.

The midface soft tissues were resuspended on the periosteum of the zygomatic body to minimize ptosis and augment facial esthetics. Excess skin was trimmed, placing the incisions within the recipient's existing rhytids.

The allotransplantation procedure from beginning of ischemia time to skin closure lasted 15 h 28 min and the overall surgical time was of 30 h 17 min. The recipient's operative blood loss was 1900 cc. He received a total of 2 units of packed red blood cells, 500 cc of 5% albumin and 8800 cc of crystalloids. Hemoglobin at the end of the procedure was 96 g/L. There were no intra-operative complications.

6.8 Immunosuppression

The immunosuppression protocol was initiated on the day of the transplantation procedure. It consisted of rabbit antithymocyte globulin, a perfusion of tacrolimus to maintain blood levels between 10 and 15 ug/L, mycophenolate mofetil, and IV solumedrol.

In the maintenance phase, immunosuppression was administered via gastrostomy. Prednisone replaced IV methylprednisolone and was tapered over 5 weeks. Mycophenolate mofetil was continued at the same dose. Tacrolimus trough levels targets were set between 10 and 15 μg/L throughout the first 6 months and after each treated rejection episode. It was lowered to level to 8 μg/L starting week 34, when the patient underwent a Hartmann procedure for perforated diverticulitis.

6.9 Rejection Monitoring

Punch biopsies were harvested from the redundant neck skin weekly during the first 24 weeks and subsequently every 2–3 weeks until week 44. Specimens were taken irrespective of clinical signs of rejection and analyzed by an experienced dermato-pathologist. A total of 34 specimens were sampled between May 14, 2018 and July 9, 2019. Our two last biopsies were taken at weeks 44 and 60 postoperatively.

6.10 Prophylactic Antimicrobial Therapy

Prophylactic antibacterial and antifungal therapy was initiated on the day of the operation. Agents used were piperacillin-tazobactam, vancomycin and gancyclovir followed by valgancyclovir, Trimethoprim-sulfamethoxazole DS, and anidulafungin.

6.11 Postoperative Course

The patient remained in the intensive care unit for 7 days. De-cannulation was performed on postoperative day 38. He was discharged to a rehabilitation facility on postoperative day 59. Regular weekly outpatient follow-ups were conducted by the senior author.

6.12 Complications

6.12.1 Infectious

There were numerous infectious complications during the first-year posttransplantation. Minor complications included ventilator-associated pneumonia, clostridium difficile colitis, CMV esophagitis, and dacryocystitis. Major complications included two episodes of cutaneous mucormycosis, which presented as progression painful dark-purple lesions on the patients left posterior thigh. Microbiological analysis revealed non-septate hyphae corresponding to Lichtheimia species. Histopathological examination showed large filamentous fungal elements, broad and hyaline non-septate hyphae with right-angle branching, suggestive of a zygomycosis (mucormycosis) infection. Despite appropriate medical treatment and a wide local excision, the lesion recurred 6 weeks later, requiring a secondary wide excision with 1cm margins. Another major complication was a perforated diverticulitis requiring urgent laparoscopic lavage and Hartmann procedure. The colostomy was reversed laparoscopically on October 7, 2019.

6.12.2 Rejections

Evidence of Banff Grade I acute rejection was identified on numerous routine biopsies, all in the absence of clinical signs of rejection. Histological and immunohistochemical review of the intradermal vessels with a focus on lymphocytic vasculitis, intravascular fibrin, CD4 positivity, and inflammatory cell phenotyping was done on all specimens. No serological testing was performed with donor-specific antibodies. The decision to treat the acute rejection was based on vasculitis and not on perivascular lymphocytic infiltration alone. Initial management consisted of pulsed intravenous methylprednisolone, an increase of baseline oral prednisone and adjustment of tacrolimus dosage. Subsequent treatment consisted of Basiliximab and/or Solumedrol without changes to baseline prednisone due to recurrence of the lower extremity mycotic lesion and concerns over its association with the patient's significant immunosuppression.

6.12.3 Metabolic

The patient developed an acute kidney injury secondary to tacrolimus toxicity when trough levels exceeding 42 μg/L had occurred. This condition was treated conservatively, and renal function parameters returned to their baseline.

6.13 Functional Outcomes

Signs of sensory re-innervation appeared at 4 months post-transplantation. Over the course of the follow-up, evolution has been noted primarily over the infra-orbital distribution. In the inferior alveolar territory, re-innervation has been mitigated with lack of clinically significant findings (Fig. 6.3, Tables 6.1 and 6.2).

Signs of motor regeneration appeared at 4 months post-transplantation in all three re-anastomosed branches bilaterally. Nonetheless, at 18 months, overall facial movements remain moderately to severely compromised with the patient being unable to perform discernable facial expressions (Table 6.3). Involuntary blink on the right remains weak with a 5 mm of residual lagophthalmos. However, complete eye closure is possible with forceful contraction of his orbicularis. With regard to peri-oral animation, lateral displacement of the oral commissure during smiling efforts has been measured at 7 mm on the right and 4 mm on the left. Oral closure remains incomplete with 1cm of residual lip incompetence during forceful mouth closure.

At last follow-up, the patient is gastrostomy-free. However, deglutition is moderately-to-severely and moderately compromised, with regard to oral and pharyngeal phases, respectively. Five deglutition efforts are required for each 5 mL bolus of pureed or mixed consistencies. Clear fluids are more readily swallowed with 2–3 deglutition efforts per bolus. The patient is able to achieve 25 mm of mouth opening and full closure.

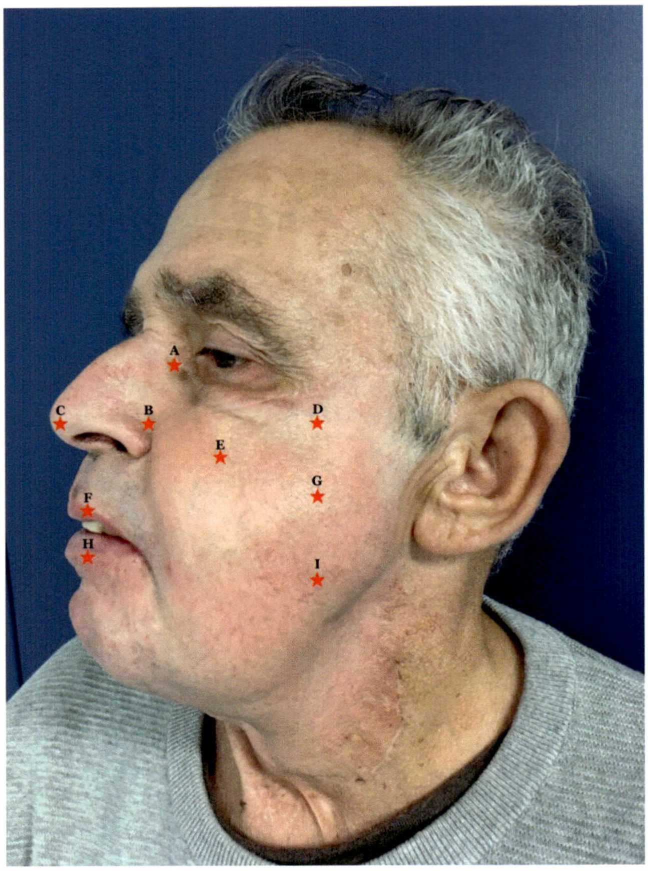

Fig. 6.3 Signs of sensory re-innervation appeared at 4 months post-transplantation. The letter points seen here can be correlated to the results in Tables 6.1 and 6.2

Table 6.1 Sensory evaluation of allograft at 6 and 18 months post-transplant (pressure perception threshold)

Trigeminal nerve branches	Reference points	Side	2018-11-12/13	2019-10-04/-11-15	Change[a]
V1	A	Right	9.7 g	1.1 g	↑8.6
		Left	25.0 g	2.2 g	↑22.8
	B	Right	1.9 g	3.3 g	↓1.4
		Left	45.6 g	2.1 g	↑43.5
	C	Right	7.8 g	4.6 g	↑3.2
		Left	36.8 g	28.7 g	↑8.1
V2	D	Right	2.5 g	0.7 g	↑1.8
		Left	81.3 g	1.8 g	↑79.5
	E	Right	3.0 g	2.5 g	↑0.5
		Left	7.6 g	2.4 g	↑5.2
	F	Right	1.5 g	1.7 g	Ø 0.2
		Left	31.3 g	8.0 g	↑23.3
V3	G	Right	7.5 g	18.6 g	↓11.1
		Left	202.5 g	No sensation at 300 g	↓
	H	Right	No sensation at 300 g	No sensation at 300 g	Ø
		Left	No sensation at 300 g	No sensation at 300 g	Ø
	I	Right	>300 g	>300 g	Ø
		Left	7.9 g	>300 g	↓

[a] ↑: Increase in sensation, ↓: Decrease in sensation, Ø: Little or no change

Table 6.2 Sensory evaluation of allograft at 6 and 18 months posttransplant (static 2-point discrimination)

Trigeminal nerve branches	Reference points		2018	2019	Norms	Change[a]
V1	Nasal sidewall (between points A and B)	Right	21 mm	18 mm	12 mm	↑3 mm
		Left	30 mm	12 mm		↑18 mm
V2	Infra-orbital (point E)	Right	Failure[b] 5/10	21 mm	10 mm	↑
		Left	25 mm	21 mm		↑4 mm
	Upper lip (point F)	Right	25 mm	25 mm	3 mm	Ø
		Left	Failure[b] 4/10	21 mm		↑
	Philtrum	Middle	18 mm	15 mm	2 mm	↑3 mm
V3	Parotid-masseteric (point I)	Right	25 mm	Failure[c]	10 mm	↓
		Left	Failure[c]	Failure[c]		Ø
	Lower lip (Point H)	Right	Failure[c]	Failure[c]	3 mm	Ø
		Left	Failure[c]	Failure[c]		Ø
	Chin	Right	Failure[c]	Failure[c]	10 mm	Ø
		Left	Failure[c]	Failure[c]		Ø

[a] ↑: Increase in sensation, ↓: Decrease in sensation, Ø: Little or no change
[b] Patient answered correctly less than 7 out of 10 times for a distance of 30 mm
[c] No sensation observed during the evaluation

Table 6.3 Muscle of facial expression functional evaluation

Muscles	Right side active range of motion (%)[a]	Left side active range of motion (%)[a]
Orbicularis oculi	Complete closure, persist weakness	Complete, good contraction
Zygomaticus	25	33
Risorius	25	25
Buccinator	75	50
Lower lip depressors	50	25
Depressor anguli oris	0	0
Mentalis	50	33
Orbicularis oris	0	0
Levator labii superioris	50	25

[a] Muscular amplitude expressed as percentage of normal expected values

As with deglutition, speech abilities are decreased due to incomplete labial closure, limited re-innervation of facial musculature and tongue hypo-mobility. The patient's speech has consistently been improving and is understandable, even during phone conversations.

Questionnaires assessing physical and social function were completed before surgery and at 16 months of follow up. The Performance Status for Head and Neck Cancer Patients (PSS-HN) questionnaire revealed pre- and postoperative scores of 250 and 90, respectively, reflecting deterioration in the spheres of normalcy of diet, public eating, and understandability of speech. Likewise, the Facial Disability Index (FDI) demonstrated physical function scores of 77 and 33, pre- and postoperatively, respectively. However, social function and quality of life scores on the FDI questionnaire revealed a decrease in disability scores from 76 to 40 postoperatively. Subjectively, the patient and his wife are extremely satisfied with the facial appearance, improved psychological well-being, and significant impact on social function.

6.14 Ancillary Procedures

In July 2019, the patient underwent a revision of his bilateral sagittal split osteotomy (BSSO) due to hardware loosening and non-union, which had caused a severe anterior open bite. An acute change in occlusion was noted shortly after the emergency abdominal surgery and was likely caused by traction exerted during endotracheal intubation. Using standard intra-oral BSSO incisions, all hardware was removed, and non-viable callus debrided. The mandible was fixed with load bearing reconstruction plates and was augmented using an iliac crest cancellous bone graft. TMJ function was consistently improving and had returned to the preoperative measurement of 25 mm of functional opening. A palatal splint and dental occlusion retainer were used during the first year postoperatively to assist in deglutition and mastication.

6.15 Lessons Learned

Facial VCA is a viable reconstructive option for severely disfigured patients, allowing simultaneous esthetic and functional restoration with outcomes superior to conventional autologous techniques [1]. In this report, we present the 18-month outcomes of a patient who underwent a sub-total face transplant for sequelae caused by a ballistic injury.

Successful facial allotransplantation requires careful patient selection, comprehensive multidisciplinary patient assessment and meticulous surgical planning. Despite an advanced age, his mental readiness and willingness to proceed were considered more important factors for patient selection, making him the oldest face transplant recipient at the time of surgery. Although an age limit for face transplantation has not yet been defined, solid organ transplantation literature favors physiologic age rather than chronologic age as a better predictor of posttransplant outcomes. Aduen et al. demonstrated that graft loss and mortality rates in liver transplant recipients aged 70 years or older were similar to those in recipients younger than 60 years of age [2].

Establishing a new facial VCA program required the joint expertise of a multidisciplinary team. Six full rehearsals procedures were performed on cadaveric specimens over a 3-year period, allowing the development of a systematic step-by-step approach. Despite the senior author's previous experience, cooperation with existing centers was instrumental. The advice, pearls, and pitfalls provided, helped flatten the learning curve and contributed to the overall success of our procedure, highlighting the importance of international cooperation.

Technology plays a pivotal role in modern facial VCA. VSP and CAD/CAM technology optimized all aspects of the operation, allowing accurate patient selection, minimizing ischemia time and optimizing osteotomies and dental occlusion [3–5].

Maxillo-mandibular occlusion can be a challenging step during facial VCA. The donor had a class I malocclusion with anterior open bite of 3 mm with bilateral premature contact of his molars. This anterior open bite was maintained with peri-transplant intermaxillary fixation, thereby preserving a 3 mm anterior open bite at the termination of the surgery. Unfortunately, the unstable occlusion led to hardware breakdown and a mandibular nonunion that required reoperation and bone grafting. Of note, correction of the open bite during re-operation was addressed through intra-oral incisions. A stable occlusion was achieved with the use of VSP and 3D printed occlusal splints. The patient had 25 mm of mouth opening and full functional occlusion at 18 months posttransplant and continues to improve with TMJ physiotherapy.

Despite some functional limitations with deglutition and sensorimotor re-innervation, at the time of last follow-up, the patient was gastrostomy and tracheostomy free. In addition, his social function and quality of life have significantly improved according to both patient and quality-of-life questionnaires. Similar findings have been described by numerous others, further supporting the potential positive psycho-social impact of this procedure, otherwise unachievable by autologous reconstructive means [6–9].

Immunosuppression remains the most challenging aspect of facial VCA. At therapeutic doses, a delicate balance and a significant overlap exist between rejection prevention and predisposition to infectious, metabolic, and neoplastic complications. Paucity of literature regarding ideal maintenance regimens, target trough levels, and thresholds for treatment of acute rejections further complicate the matter. As such, astute monitoring and early identification of complications are key. However, understanding the deleterious effects of over-treatment by erring on the side of caution cannot be overstated, particularly for first-time VCA teams.

When critically analyzing our case by plotting immunosuppression trough levels, episodes of acute rejections, and occurrence of complications, several interesting observations were made (Fig. 6.4). First, it was noted that all acute rejections were diagnosed histopathologically on routine biopsies taken weekly from a graft void of erythema. Serological testing and measuring of donor-specific antibody levels may have reduced the frequency of biopsies. Despite being Banff Grade I, several episodes were treated based on evidence of endotheliitis and its potential role in the pathophysiology of chronic graft rejection [10, 11]. The first rejection was managed aggressively with pulse dosing of solumedrol as well as a significant increase in baseline prednisone and tacrolimus. An additional pulse dosing of solumedrol was administered a week later due to persistence of findings on biopsy. The decision was likely influenced by concern of inadequately treating our first episode of rejection and fear of potentially losing the graft.

The second noteworthy observation relates to the timing of our first significant infectious complication. As seen on the graph (Fig. 6.4), the mucormycosis occurred shortly after the multi-modal management of consecutive acute rejections and likely stems from the profound immunosuppression it has precipitated. To our knowledge, this is the first report of a mucor infection in a face transplant recipient. The infection was managed with a short course of amphotericin B and a prolonged treatment with posaconazole. Due to the drug

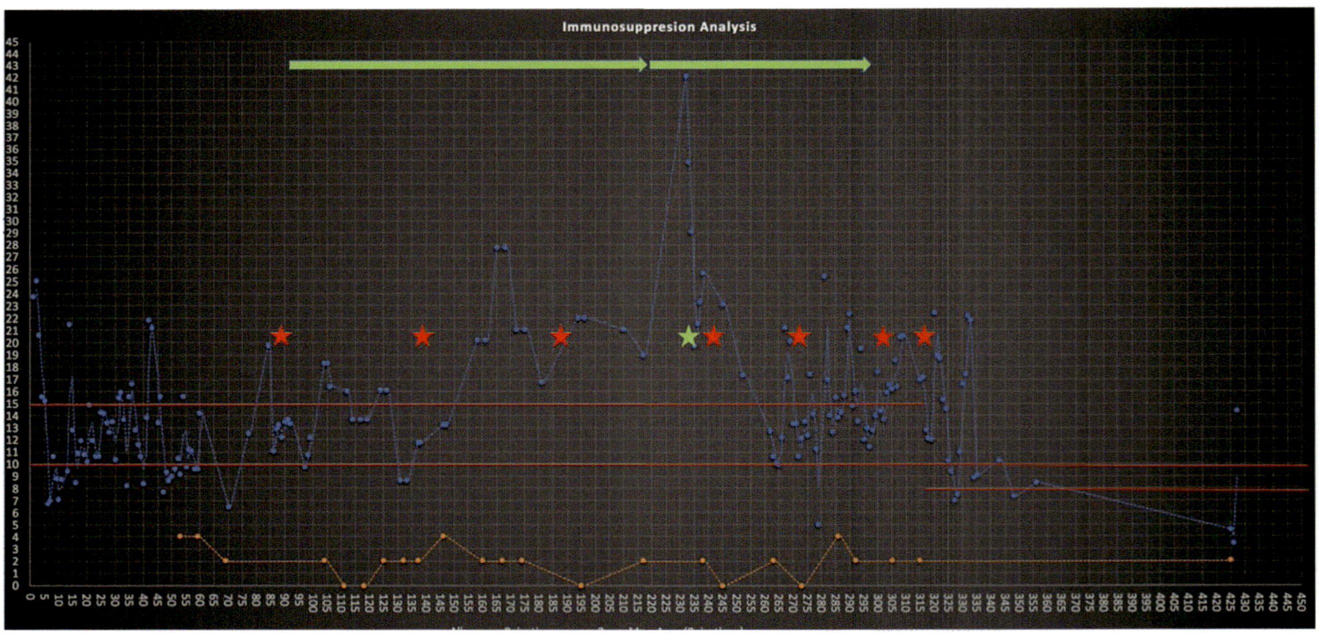

Fig. 6.4 Plotting of immunosuppression trough levels, episodes of acute rejections, and occurrence of complications. To be noted, as seen on the graph, the mucormycosis occurred shortly after the multi-modal management of consecutive acute rejections and likely stems from the profound immunosuppression it had precipitated. Red asterisks indicate infectious complications and the green the metabolic complications (the specific complications listed by number). The X axis represents postoperative days and the Y axis, the patients tacrolimus levels. So as can be seen in the graph, most times following pulses of tacrolimus the patient developed infectious complications

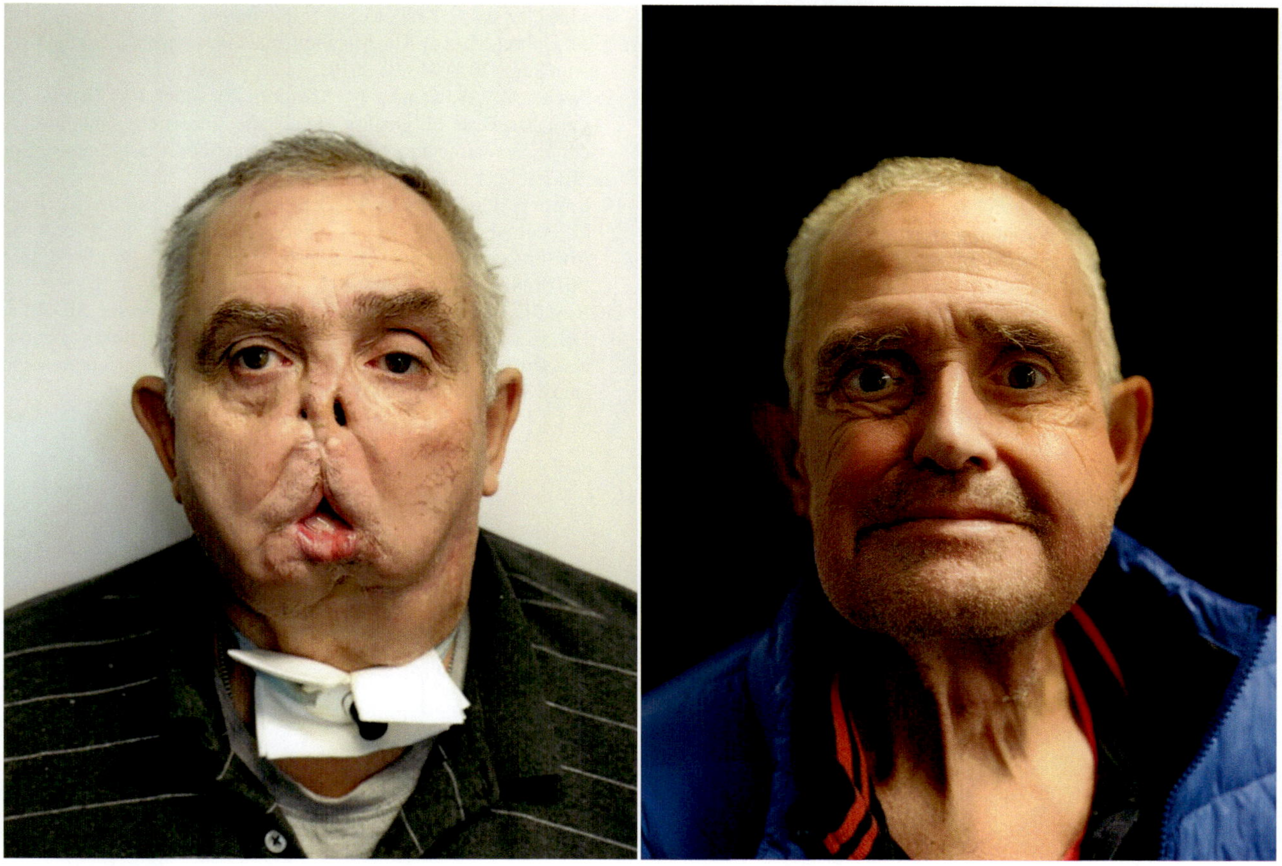

Fig. 6.5 Recipient at 16-months postoperative

interactions between posaconazole and tacrolimus, management of immunosuppression from that point forward proved extremely difficult and resulted in the series of infectious complications that ensued. Despite reduction of tacrolimus dosing by 50% in anticipation of disturbances, trough levels remained chronically high. An acute deterioration was noted in December when the posaconazole was changed from liquid format given via gastrostomy tube to solid tablets administered per os, resulting in an acute kidney injury.

Due to concern of over-treatment, the posaconazole was stopped and tacrolimus target trough levels were reduced to 8–10. Since these adjustments, the patient has been out of the hospital and complication free.

In summary, critical appraisal of our first VCA (Fig. 6.5) has taught us several lessons, which we ought to carry on to further procedures; (1) maintain a rigid but less frequent biopsy schedule augmented with serological testing; (2) treat grade I acute rejections with evidence of endotheliitis with caution, using pulsed solumedrol alone; (3) conservative baseline tacrolimus levels of 10–12 ng/mL in first 6 months, 8–10 ng/mL in following 6 months, and 6–8 ng/mL after 1 year; and (4) beware of drug interactions and their effects on tacrolimus levels.

The first Canadian facial VCA was a culmination of 7 years of work. The patient judges the surgery a complete success and says that he has "never been so happy in his life." Our judgment is far more critical however. Our limited experience and concern for rejection resulted in multimodal over-treatment and resulted in a multitude of opportunistic infections and complications. Critical appraisal of our experience has shed further light on these relationships and taught us important lessons which we ought to carry on to our future VCAs.

References

1. Cabrera AE, Kimberly LL, Kantar RS, Atamian EK, Manjunath AK, Rangel LK, et al. Perceived esthetic outcomes of face transplantation: a survey of the general public. J Craniofac Surg. 2018;29(4):848–51.
2. Aduen JF, Sujay B, Dickson RC, Heckman MG, Hewitt WR, Stapelfeldt WH, et al. Outcomes after liver transplant in patients aged 70 years or older compared with those younger than 60 years. Mayo Clin Proc. 2009;84(11):973–8.
3. Lassus P, Lindford A, Vuola J, Back L, Suominen S, Mesimaki K, et al. The helsinki face transplantation: surgical aspects and 1-year outcome. JPRAS. 2018;71(2):132–9.

4. Dorafshar AH, Bojovic B, Christy MR, Borsuk DE, Iliff NT, Brown EN, et al. Total face, double jaw, and tongue transplantation: an evolutionary concept. Plast Reconstr Surg. 2013;131(2):241–51.
5. Roche NA, Vermeersch HF, Stillaert FB, Peters KT, De Cubber J, Van Lierde K, et al. Complex facial reconstruction by vascularized composite allotransplantation: the first Belgian case. JPRAS. 2015;68(3):362–71.
6. Rodriguez-Lorenzo A, Audolfsson T, Wong C, Saiepour D, Nowinski D, Rozen S. Vascular perfusion of the facial skin: implications in allotransplantation of facial aesthetic subunits. Plast Reconstr Surg. 2016;138(5):1073–9.
7. Van Lierde KM, De Letter M, Vermeersch H, Roche N, Stillaert F, Lemmens G, et al. Longitudinal progress of overall intelligibility, voice, resonance, articulation and oromyofunctional behavior during the first 21 months after Belgian facial transplantation. J Commun Disord. 2015;53:42–56.
8. Maciejewski A, Krakowczyk L, Szymczyk C, Wierzgon J, Grajek M, Dobrut M, et al. The first immediate face transplant in the world. Ann Surg. 2016;263(3):36–9.
9. Aycart MA, Kiwanuka H, Krezdorn N, Alhefzi M, Bueno EM, Pomahac B, et al. Quality of life after face transplantation: outcomes, assessment tools, and future directions. Plast Reconstr Surg. 2017;139(1):194–203.
10. Lantieri L, Grimbert P, Ortonne N, Suberbielle C, Bories D, Gil-Vernet S, et al. Face transplant: long-term follow-up and results of a prospective open study. Lancet. 2016;388(10052):1398–407.
11. Roy SF, Krishnan V, Trinh VQ, Collette S, Dufresne SF, Borsuk DE, et al. Lymphocytic vasculitis associated with mild rejection in a vascularized composite allograft recipient: a clinicopathological study. Transplantation. 2020;104(7):208–13.

Facial Allotransplantation: Outcomes and Results of the Amiens/Lyon Team

7

Palmina Petruzzo, Jean Kanitakis, Sylvie Testelin, Stephanie Dapke, Bernard Devauchelle, Jean Michel Dubernard, and Emmanuel Morelon

7.1 Introduction

Facial allotransplantation has been performed in disfigured patients in order to restore the esthetic appearance and function when all the other conventional reconstructive techniques had failed or were expected to fail. The first facial allotransplantation [1] was performed in Amiens (France) in 2005 and became possible thanks to the collaboration of Amiens and Lyon teams. The teams received a national grant to perform a prospective study including five cases of facial allotransplantation. Up to now 22 patients have been screened and three patients have been transplanted. Table 7.1 outlines recipient and donor characteristics. At present no patient is in the waiting list because of the COVID-19 pandemic.

P. Petruzzo (✉)
Department of Transplantation, Hôpital Edouard Herriot, HCL, Lyon, France

Department of Surgery, University of Cagliari, Cagliari, Italy
e-mail: petruzzo@unica.it; palmina.petruzzo@chu-lyon.fr

J. Kanitakis
Department of Dermatology, Hôpital Edouard Herriot, HCL, Lyon, France
e-mail: jean.kanitakis@univ-lyon1.fr

S. Testelin · B. Devauchelle
Department of Maxillofacial Surgery, CHU Amiens-Picardie, Facing Faces Institute, Amiens, France
e-mail: Testelin.Sylvie@chu-amiens.fr; Devauchelle.Bernard@chu-amiens.fr

S. Dapke
UR-7516 CHIMERE, Amiens, France
e-mail: Dakpe.Stephanie@chu-amiens.fr

J. M. Dubernard
Department of Transplantation, Hôpital Edouard Herriot, HCL, Lyon, France
e-mail: jean-michel.dubernard@chu-lyon.fr

E. Morelon
Department of Transplantation, Hôpital Edouard Herriot, HCL, Lyon, France

Claude Bernard Lyon I University, Lyon, France
e-mail: emmanuel.morelon@chu-lyon.fr

Table 7.1 Recipient and donor characteristics

Patient	#1	#2	#3
Transplantation year	2005	2009	2012
Gender	F	M	F
Recipient age (years)	38	27	52
Donor age (years)	46	46	47
Year of disfigurement	2005	2008	2003
Cause of disfigurement	Dog bite	Explosion	Vascular malformation
Transplanted esthetic units	Nose Cheeks Lips Chin	Mandible Lips Cheeks Chin	Maxilla Mandible Cheeks Lips Tongue Chin
HLA mismatches	5	5	4

7.2 Patients

7.2.1 Pretransplant Evaluation

All the recipients underwent routine pretransplant investigations. Preoperative face magnetic resonance imaging (MRI) was done to study bones, muscles, vessels, nerves, and soft tissues; angiography was additionally performed in a patient with vascular malformations. Functional MRI was performed to study and compare cortical brain behavior in the face frontoparietal areas before and after transplantation.

Psychosocial evaluation plays an important role in the patients' selection criteria. A psychiatrist evaluated the patient's emotional state, behavioral trends, support structure, cognitive ability, coping skills, understanding of the procedure, and likelihood of medical compliance.

7.2.2 Transplantation

The transplant coordinators asked for the family's consent to harvest and transplant the donor's face. In all cases prior to surgery, bone marrow was collected from the donor's iliac crests. Half of the bone marrow cells were infused into the

© Springer Nature Switzerland AG 2023
R. Gurunian et al. (eds.), *Reconstructive Transplantation*, https://doi.org/10.1007/978-3-031-21520-9_7

recipients on days 4 and 11 after face allotransplantation, except in patient #2 who received only the first infusion.

In all the recipients a vascularized radial forearm flap was recovered from the donor for transplantation in the recipient's left submammary fold or abdominal wall. It was used as a sentinel graft for skin biopsies to spare the grafted facial skin.

After harvest, both facial allograft and sentinel flap were irrigated with IGL-1 (Institut Georges Lopez-1) organ preservation solution at 4 °C, then placed in double-plastic bags, in a standard ice box. The donor's face was always reconstructed with a colored silicone mask, custom-made inside a plaster cast molded on the face at the beginning of the procedure.

The immunosuppressive treatment included induction therapy (antithymocyte globulins during the first 10 days) and maintenance therapy including tacrolimus (targeted trough levels of 8–10 ng/mL), mycophenolate mofetil (MMF, 2 g/day), and prednisone (5 mg/day).

7.2.3 Rehabilitation Protocol

Rehabilitation therapy started 48 h after surgery, twice a day for the first 4 months, then once a day. The rehabilitation program included supervised controlled–motion passive and active facial exercises, mainly focused on the restoration of lip suspension and mouth occlusion.

Passive exercises were based on tactile stimulation in order to recognize the topography of the grafted regions, facilitating their integration. The stimulation was applied starting from the transplanted area close to recipient tissues with intact sensation, such as the area close to skin sutures, and the transplanted mouth region, which is located just above the recipient's gingival level. In addition, the tactile stimulation aimed at facilitating the recognition and contraction of the transplanted muscles.

The active exercises started asking the patient "to mind" all the different movements that he/she was unable to perform and using his/her muscles in order to facilitate contraction of the transplant muscles. The recipient has to repeat several times a day the same movements in order "to recognize" the transplant and to learn complex movements, such as chewing and swallowing, which became possible after the transplantation.

7.2.4 Follow-Up

The patient's general condition and functional results were evaluated at each anniversary of transplantation. Anti-HLA antibodies were monitored by LUMINEX and microchimerism by RQ-PCR (Taqman) analysis of DNA from blood, purified CD3+ cells, bone marrow, and purified CD34+ bone marrow cells. Biopsies of the oral mucosa and the skin (chin and sentinel skin graft) were taken at various time points of the follow-up (every week for 1 month, monthly for 4 months, and every 6 months thereafter) or during rejection episodes. The tissue specimens for histology were formalin-fixed and paraffin-embedded. Five-micrometer-thick sections were stained with hematoxylin-eosin-saffron and labeled immunohistochemically with antibodies detecting various lymphocyte subsets and cells present in normal skin.

After transplantation, ultrasound imaging and MRI of the face were performed yearly to study the tissues composing the transplant. Since 2015, flow magnetic resonance imaging (flow MRI) was performed in all the recipients [2]

Thermal tests (cold and hot) and Semmes-Weinstein test were performed at different time points of the follow-up. Motor recovery was evaluated using motion images, which were periodically captured by a video camera, and recording the phonetic exercises. The interaction among the upper and lower lip and jaw was studied repeating the same phonetic task, where the consonant was a bilabial stop consonant "*p*, *b*, *m*" and the vowels one of "*i*, *a*, *u*," while the labial tooth contact was studied repeating "*v*, *f*."

Psychological support was provided once a day during the first 4 postoperative weeks, twice a week for 4 months, then once a month or at the patient's request.

7.2.5 Patient #1

The first facial allotransplantation including nose, chin, part of the cheeks, and lips was performed on November 27, 2005. The recipient was a 38-year-old woman, who had been severely bitten by her dog on May 28, 2005 (Fig. 7.1a). The donor was a brain-dead 46-year-old woman; they shared the same blood group (0+) and 5 HLA antigens. Her skin complexion was similar to that of the recipient. The surgical procedure consisted in the revascularization of right and left facial arteries and veins, mucosal repair, bilateral anastomosis of infraorbital and mental sensitive nerves, joining of mimic muscles with motor nerve suture on marginal mandibular branch of the left facial nerve, and skin closure [1]. During the follow-up, the patient underwent transposition of the salivary duct (intraorally) and inferior blepharoplasty.

Since the eleventh posttransplant month [3], the immunosuppressive regimen consisted of prednisone, MMF, and sirolimus (because of increasing serum creatinine values). The patient developed two episodes of skin cellular acute rejection (AR) in the first posttransplant year (on days 18 and 214) that were successfully treated with steroid boluses. Thereafter, the patient did not show other clinical signs of AR, and the surveillance skin biopsies showed Banff [4] grades 0 or 1. The esthetic (Fig. 7.1b) and functional recovery was satisfactory [3, 5].

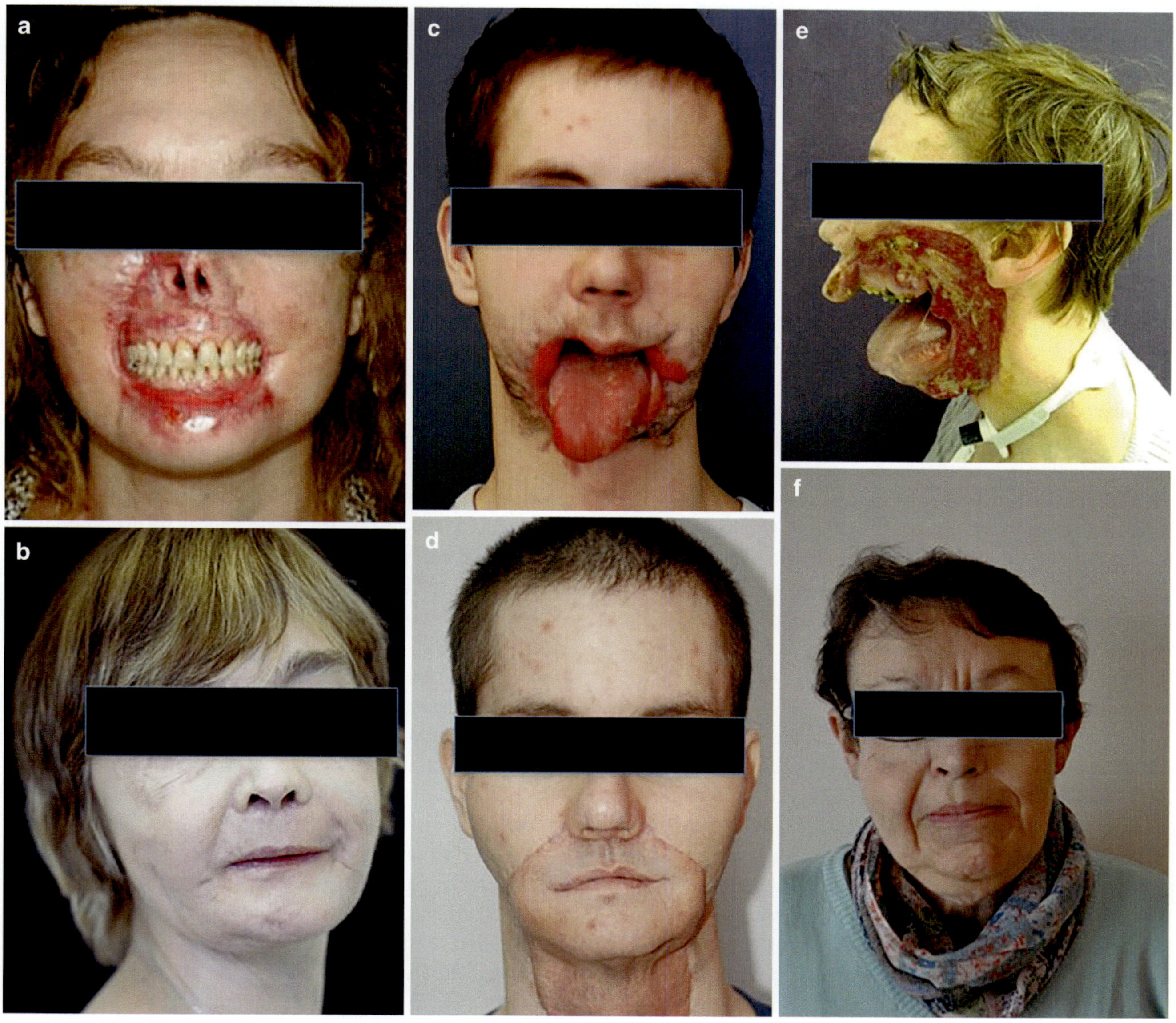

Fig. 7.1 (**a**) Patient #1 before the transplantation, following the dog bite. (**b**) Patient #1 3 years after the transplantation of nose, chin, part of the cheeks, and lips. (**c**) Patient #2 before the transplantation, following a pyrotechnic explosion. (**d**) Patient #2 some months after the transplantation of mandible, lips, chin, and the anterior part of the neck until the hyoid bone. (**e**) Patient #3: after the complete removal of the vascular malformation, few months before the transplantation. (**f**) Patient #3. Three years after the transplantation of maxilla, mandible, cheeks, lips, chin, and tongue

Ninety months after the transplantation, the patient developed de novo class II donor-specific antibodies (DSA), without clinical signs of rejection. Some months later, she developed several skin rejection episodes, which were treated with steroid boluses. Despite an immediate clinical improvement, 9 months later, the sentinel skin underwent necrosis due to graft vasculopathy (GV), as shown by microscopic examination [6, 7]. Skin biopsies of the facial skin showed C4d deposits on the endothelium of some dermal vessels, and flow MRI of the facial transplant showed a decrease in flow of the facial arteries at the distal level [2]. Despite the intensive treatment, necrosis of the lips and the perioral area developed, prompting surgical removal of the lower lip, labial commissures, and part of the right cheek on May 5, 2015. The patient underwent conventional facial reconstruction in January 2016 [6] but died on April 23, 2016 of small-cell lung cancer.

7.2.6 Patient #2

The recipient was a 27-year-old man who was disfigured by a pyrotechnic explosion on May 28, 2008 (Fig. 7.1c); this caused deficit of the upper and lower lip, chin, perioral area, and consequent unintelligible speech and necessity of feeding by jejunostomy. On November 27, 2009, he received an allograft including an edentulous mandible, upper and lower lips, cheeks, and chin (Fig. 7.1d).

The donor was a brain-dead 46-year-old man, sharing with the recipient the same blood group (0+) and 5 HLA mismatches. His skin complexion was similar to that of the recipient.

The surgical procedure consisted in transplanting the full mandible from angle to angle and soft tissue including the mouth floor, the whole thickness of the lips, the chin, and the anterior part of the neck until the hyoid bone. All sensitive nerve depending on the area were anastomosed (infra-alveolar and suborbital on both sides). The donor patient was edentulous and, consequently, no intermaxillary fixation was requested. No revisional surgeries were performed.

The patient developed a primary asymptomatic EBV infection on day 185. In April 2010 a posttransplant monoclonal B-cell lymphoma occurred and was treated with rituximab. Later on he developed hepatic EBV-associated posttransplant smooth muscle tumors, prompting a great reduction of his immunosuppressive therapy [8].

During the first posttransplant year, AR episodes were completely reversed with steroids [3, 5, 8]. Subsequently several episodes of AR that were characterized by lichenoid changes of the epidermis and appendages occurred. Since the second posttransplant year, the allografted facial skin and sentinel-skin graft became progressively sclerotic and presented pigmented macules on a background of hypopigmentation and telangiectasia, realizing a poikilodermatous aspect. These alterations resulted in a decreased mouth opening although lip closure was still possible allowing food intake. Skin biopsies showed epidermal and adnexal atrophy, basal cell vacuolization, and diffuse dermal sclerosis, in the absence of significant dermal cell infiltration. The dermal capillaries showed thickened walls and narrowed lumina, while the large vessels seemed less affected [8].

Anti-HLA class II antibodies (no donor specific) were detected transiently in January 2010.

The evolution of the hepatic EBV-associated posttransplant smooth muscle tumors led to liver transplantation in April 2017. The immunosuppressive treatment was based on tacrolimus, MMF, and steroids.

In June 2017 the first clinical signs of GV (partial necrosis of the upper lip) appeared, and it was also detected by flow MRI [2]. The patient died in October 2017 of pneumonia, sepsis, and consequent multiorgan failure.

7.2.7 Patient #3

The recipient was a 52-year-old woman affected by a high-flow hemorrhagic arterio-venous malformation of the face. In 2003 the patient underwent partial removal of the malformation and reconstruction using a latissimus dorsi flap. At that time, it was impossible to propose a complete removal including the mandible and tongue and reconstruction in one-time surgery. Then, not surprisingly, a large recurrence of the vascular malformation developed and a complete removal was decided because of the possibility to perform a face transplant. The decision was to realize surgery in two times: firstly the face was removed in February 2012 with consequent disfigurement (Fig. 7.1e) and impossibility to swallow, eat, drink (necessitating gastrostomy), and speech, then face transplantation was performed.

The patient received on June 13, 2012 an allograft including maxilla, mandible, cheeks, lips, chin, and tongue. The donor was a 47-year-old woman. They shared the same blood group (A+); 4 HLA mismatch existed with negative cross-match. The donor's skin complexion was similar to that of the recipient (Fig. 7.1f). The anastomoses were complicated because of the large amount of transplanted tissues. The arterial anastomoses were performed in a termino-lateral manner between the donor external carotid arteries and the recipient common carotids. Then, the facial nerve on the trunk and bilateral sensitive infra orbital and mandibular nerves on both sides were anastomosed. The maxilla was fixed with titanium miniplates and the mandible was positioned in the glenoid fossa on the left side because there was no more condyle available, and one plate on the right side on the remaining condyle. Intermaxillary fixation was performed, and it was useful during the first posttransplant year because of the bilateral facial palsy and the weight of the transplanted tissues. Nevertheless, tooth displacement occurred with some modification of the dental occlusion.

During the follow-up, the patient underwent inferior blepharoplasty and external canthopexy.

The patient developed only one episode of AR on postoperative day 12 which was easily treated with IV steroid bolus. She developed class II DSA (DR52: 1000MFI) since June 2018. At 5 years posttransplantation, there was no clinical evidence of chronic rejection or GV, while flow MRI showed a decrease in the distal arterial signal recovery and in 2017 the disappearance of the right lingual artery [2].

7.2.8 Patient and Graft Survival

Patient #1 died of small-cell lung cancer 11 years after the transplantation. Patient #2 died of pneumonia, sepsis, and terminal multiorgan failure 9 years after the face transplantation and 6 months after the liver transplantation.

The first patient with face transplantation lost part of her facial graft 10 years after transplantation because of GV manifesting with necrosis of the skin sentinel graft and of the lower lip, labial commissures and part of the right cheek, which had to be removed. Patient #2 did not accept the possibility to remove the grafted face despite the decrease in esthetic and functional recovery due to the chronic rejection process.

7.2.9 Acute and Chronic Rejection

Few episodes of AR occurred in all the recipients in the first posttransplant year (Table 7.2). They were macroscopically characterized by edema and erythema of the graft and histologically mainly by dermal infiltration with T cells, with occasional changes in the epidermis or the oral epithelium (basal cell vacuolization, lymphocytic exocytosis). They were easily reversed by steroid boluses [3, 5, 8].

In the long-term follow-up, chronic rejection developed in patients #1 and #2. Patient #1 developed de novo DSA seven years after transplantation. Several episodes of maculopapular lesions of the skin started 9 months later (Banff grade 3 acute cellular rejection with lichenoid features and occasional C4d deposits on the endothelium of dermal blood vessels). These changes were followed by GV (flow MRI showed a severe decrease in flow of the right facial artery distally, a decrease at its origin, and also a decrease at the level of the left facial artery, at the mandibular level). This process was considered a chronic antibody-mediated rejection [6, 8]. Despite treatment with steroid boluses, intravenous immunoglobulins, five sessions of plasmapheresis, Bortezomib and Eculizumab as rescue therapy, necrosis of the facial graft occurred, and this had to be partially removed [6].

After two easily treated AR episodes, patient #2 developed many episodes of AR with lichenoid aspect due to the significant decrease of his immunosuppressive treatment. Later, he developed signs of chronic rejection [7, 8], manifesting macroscopically with a sclerotic aspect of the graft, and histologically with dermal sclerosis and atrophy/effacement of skin adnexa, and histologically presence of dense dermal collagen bundles with hyalinosis, and atrophy/effacement of adnexa in the absence of significant inflammatory cell infiltration. The large vessels, such as facial arteries, were poorly involved while the dermal capillaries showed thickened, sclerotic walls and reduced lumina [8].

Table 7.2 Acute rejection episodes in face transplant recipients

Patient	No. AR episodes	POD	Banff score
1	6	23, 214, 3040, 3129, 343	2, 3, 3, 3, 3, 3
2	9	41, 112, 186, 239, 474, 527, 540, 931, 1795	3, 3, 2, 2, 3, 3, 3, 3, 3
3	1	12	3

AR acute rejection, *POD* postoperative day

After the liver transplantation in 2017, flow MRI detected signs of GV [2] and subsequently partial necrosis of the upper lip occurred clinically.

7.2.10 Functional Results

Functional results were impressive in all patients, although their ability was different on the basis of the lost units of the face and the possibility to perform the nerve repairs.

Patient #1 showed normal pain and cold sensation without dysesthesia and protective sensibility at 6 months. The Semmes-Weinstein test demonstrated sensitivity recovery of the graft at 1 year; discriminative recovery became normal 2 years after transplantation. Analysis of motion recovery showed a rapid and continuous improvement of muscle function. Labial closure was complete despite a slight asymmetry. The patient was able to eat, drink, chew, swallow, and smile, although there was a slight synkinesis on the left side and a mild contracture of some skin muscles, while pouting and kissing remained difficult. Phonation recovery was impressive, and the patient could talk intelligibly [3, 5].

From the beginning, the patient was satisfied of her new face, she took care of herself and had normal social interaction with the healthcare staff and her relatives.

The functional recovery in patient #2 was similar to that reported in patient #1. A progressive sensorimotor recovery of the transplant was evident by 6 months; mouth opening and lips motion were possible, although eating was difficult because of the edentulous status. Then, the chronic rejection process induced skin sclerosis and fibrosis with increasing difficulties to open the mouth and to eat [8].

The esthetic results in patient #3 were excellent with a perfect color-match and wound healing, which made almost "invisible" the difference between the transplant and the recipient's own face. The sensitive recovery was progressive and complete at 9 months. There was also a motor recovery, the mimic was progressively restored allowing eating, drinking and speaking. After 2 years recovery of taste was reported, although the tongue volume decreased and the speech was not very intelligible.

7.2.11 Complications

Patient #1 showed an increase in serum creatinine values in the early posttransplant period, which was well controlled introducing sirolimus and avoiding anticalcineurin inhibitors. Then, the patient developed arterial hypertension and increased gamma-GT values. She developed a basal-cell carcinoma on her native facial skin. She underwent a hysterectomy for uterine carcinoma. Then, she developed a small-cell lung carcinoma, which was unsuccessfully treated and caused her death [6].

In patient #2 the majority of complications were correlated to the posttransplant monoclonal B-cell lymphoma and later on to the hepatic EBV-associated posttransplant smooth muscle tumor [8]. These events led to a significant decrease in the immunosuppressive treatment, the occurrence of many AR episodes, the development of chronic rejection of the grafted face, and the necessity of a liver transplant. Moreover, the patient developed many herpes virus mucocutaneous infections and bilateral hip necrosis. Patient #3 developed a mild decrease in renal function and arterial hypertension.

7.3 Learned Lessons

Face transplantation proved to be able to significantly change the lives of terribly disfigured patients. However, the risks and benefits are continuously resketched from data collected from each patient [9]. In our experience, the esthetic and functional results were very encouraging, and the patients were satisfied of their "new face." Remarkably, patient #2 never considered the possibility of transplant removal prompted by the complications and the signs of chronic rejection.

However, the lack of standardization of outcome measures and quality of life should be addressed to better refine the risk/benefit ratio.

The long-term follow-up in our patients showed a high incidence of complications, which were more severe than those that occurred in our upper extremity transplanted patients. The immunosuppressive regimen, particularly the treatment of AR episodes, needs to be adapted to lower the incidence of these complications. The two patient deaths that occurred highlight the importance of patient selection, namely by avoiding serological mismatches (Epstein Barr) but also HLA sensitization as well as other medical comorbidities and psychosocial disorders. In our experience, as well as in that of other teams, the importance of the psychiatric/psychological follow-up in the majority of these recipients clearly emerged [10].

Two of our patients developed GV and chronic rejection leading to partial graft removal in patient #1 10 years after transplantation. Other teams reported that several face recipients at long-term follow-up showed histological changes that were rarely fully reversed by steroid therapy, suggesting a chronic rejection process [9, 11]. In the long-term follow-up, chronic rejection seems to be more frequent (or more easily detected?) in facial transplantation than in upper extremity allotransplantation.

A careful long-term monitoring is imperative to better understand the evolution of this type of transplantation [12]. On the other hand, face re-transplantation might be the next challenge.

In our experience the paucity of donors is the main obstacle to a faster development of our program. Moreover, the COVID-19 pandemic is currently an additional obstacle to the realization of VCA.

References

1. Devauchelle B, Badet L, Lengelé B, Morelon E, Testelin S, Michallet M, D'Hauthuille C, Dubernard JM. First human face allograft: early report. Lancet. 2006;368(9531):203–9.
2. Bettoni J, Balédent O, Petruzzo P, Duisit J, Kanitakis J, Devauchelle B, Lengelé B, Constans JM, Morelon E, Dakpé S. Role of flow magnetic resonance imaging in the monitoring of facial allotransplantations: preliminary results on graft vasculopathy. Int J Oral Maxillofac Surg. 2020;49(2):169–75.
3. Dubernard JM, Lengelé B, Morelon E, Testelin S, Badet L, Moure C, Beziat JL, Dakpé S, Kanitakis J, D'Hauthuille C, El Jaafari A, Petruzzo P, Lefrancois N, Taha F, Sirigu A, Di Marco G, Carmi E, Bachmann D, Cremades S, Giraux P, Burloux G, Hequet O, Parquet N, Francès C, Michallet M, Martin X, Devauchelle B. Outcomes 18 months after the first human partial face transplantation. N Engl J Med. 2007;357(24):2451–60.
4. Cendales L, Kanitakis J, Schneeberger S, Burns C, Ruiz P, Landin L, Remmelink M, Hewitt C, Landgren T, Lyons B, Drachenberger C, Solez K, Kirk A, Kleiner D, Racusen L. The Banff 2007 working classification of skin-containing composite tissue allograft pathology. Am J Transplant. 2008;8(7):1396–400.
5. Petruzzo P, Testelin S, Kanitakis J, Badet L, Lengelé B, Girbon JP, Parmentier H, Malcus C, Morelon E, Devauchelle B, Dubernard JM. First human face transplantation: 5 years outcomes. Transplantation. 2012;93(2):236–40.
6. Morelon E, Petruzzo P, Kanitakis J, Dakpé S, Thaunat O, Dubois V, Choukroun G, Testelin S, Dubernard JM, Badet L, Devauchelle B. Face transplantation: partial graft loss of the first case 10 years later. Am J Transplant. 2017;17(7):1935–40.
7. Morelon E, Petruzzo P, Kanitakis J. Chronic rejection in vascularized composite allotransplantation. Curr Opin Organ Transplant. 2018;23(5):582–91.
8. Petruzzo P, Kanitakis J, Testelin S, Pialat JB, Buron F, Badet L, Thaunat O, Devauchelle B, Morelon E. Clinicopathological findings of chronic rejection in a face grafted patient. Transplantation. 2015;99(12):2644–50.
9. Lantieri L, Grimbert P, Ortonne N, Lemogne C, Wolkenstein P, Hivelin M. Facial transplantation: facing the limits, planning the future. Lancet. 2017;389(10076):1293–4.
10. Bellivier F, Fakra E, Yon L, Limosin F, Consoli SM, Lantieri L, Hivelin M. Psychological and psychiatric aspects of face transplantation: lessons learned from the long-term follow-up of six patients. J Psychosom Res. 2019;119:42–9.
11. Krezdorn N, Lian CG, Wells M, Wo L, Tasigiorgos S, Xu S, Borges TJ, Frierson RM, Stanek E, Riella LV, Pomahac B, Murphy GF. Chronic rejection of human face allografts. Am J Transplant. 2019;19(4):1168–77.
12. Tasigiorgos S, Kollar B, Krezdorn N, Bueno EM, Tullius SG, Pomahac B. Face transplantation-current status and future developments. Transpl Int. 2018;31(7):677–88.

8 VCA in Head and Neck Region

Adam Maciejewski, Łukasz Krakowczyk, Daniel Bula, and Jakub Opyrchał

8.1 Introduction

Reconstructive and microvascular surgery involves a series of complex and often multistep techniques to recreate the structures of soft tissues, bones, vessels, and nerves. The aim of such operations is to obtain the following effects: anatomical, topographic, functional, and aesthetic, most similar to the physiological conditions. In microsurgery, several dozen kinds of free flaps (taken from distant parts of the body) have been defined and tested for usefulness, which can be routinely used for planned reconstructive procedures. Despite the numerous advantages of classic microvascular flaps, there is still a lack of ideal flap combinations which individually modified characteristics would ensure the best functional and aesthetic effects in facial reconstruction. The reconstruction of the complex bone-chondral-soft tissue complex of the nose, the correct shape and color of the lip vermilion, or the correct contour of the corner of the mouth is still one of the most difficult challenges for the reconstructive microsurgeon. The procedures mentioned above are extremely complex and rare worldwide; since the first face transplant in 2005 in France, around 50 reconstructive transplantation surgeries have been performed in this area so far. The fourth in the world and the first in the United States, such a transplant affected as much as 80% of the face, including the forehead and cheeks. The operation in the Cleveland Clinic was extremely difficult due to the need of transplanting the skin of the eyelids and their motor apparatus and turned out to be a breakthrough in world transplantation medicine [1]. The multidisciplinarity of face transplants, and in particular the introduction of stereolithography and neuronavigation in the planning and performance of procedures, significantly contributed to the spectacular improvement of the obtained outcomes, both functional and aesthetic, as exemplified by patients treated at the Langone Hospital NYU in New York by Eduardo D. Rodriguez [2, 3].

8.2 Face Transplantation (FTx)

8.2.1 Qualification and Preparation of Recipients

Organ transplantation is a complex therapy that requires extensive cooperation between the patient and the physician: the patient must not only show a strong will to survive and recover but also meet many recommendations related to pharmacotherapy regarding transplant rejection. If a potential recipient is not ready to comply with the rigors of postoperative treatment, he should be removed from the waiting list, as his treatment has no chance of success.

This issue is closely related to the patient's consent to the transplant procedure. In order to respect the dignity and autonomy of the recipient, the surgeon must obtain his consent, expressed in an appropriate form, prior to the procedure. The consent to transplant should be preceded by the patient getting to know and understanding all the conditions of the procedure: its course, chances of success, possible risks, side effects, etc. In the case of face transplantation, providing the recipient with full and understandable information is very important, because a failed procedure may result in serious complications, including the patient's death. In addition, the potential transplant recipient should understand that the postoperative treatment will last for the rest of his life, and consent to the surgery should be combined with the consent to further cooperation with the doctor [4, 5].

The basic criteria for selecting a face transplant recipient should be:

– A similar volume of facial tissues and the skin surface of the recipient and donor (these are the elements that directly affect the aesthetic effect, and thus the recipient's self-esteem and social acceptance),

A. Maciejewski · Ł. Krakowczyk · D. Bula (✉) · J. Opyrchał
Oncologic and Reconstructive Surgery, Maria Sklodowska-Curie, National Research Institute of Oncology, Gliwice Branch, Gliwice, Poland
e-mail: adammac@o2.pl; lukaszkrakowczyk@wp.pl

© Springer Nature Switzerland AG 2023
R. Gurunian et al. (eds.), *Reconstructive Transplantation*, https://doi.org/10.1007/978-3-031-21520-9_8

- Psychological tests aimed at excluding mental disorders and confirming the patient's ability to withstand the burdens of postoperative treatment (especially immunosuppression) and the possibility of returning to family and professional life. Psychological examination is especially important when preparing the recipient for facial transplantation: such a person must be aware of very significant changes in their appearance and mentally prepared for the assessment of other people.
- The urgency of transplantation may refer not only to the patient's health condition but also to his family (mother of young children) or social situation. A face transplant can make the patient reopen to others and restore abandoned contacts.

8.2.1.1 Detailed Psychological Qualification

Due to the strong correlation between physiological and psychological stresses and their shared mechanism involving biological behavior mechanisms, the main element in qualifying a patient to participate in such a burdensome experience as the process of facial transplantation is the psychological diagnosis of the patient's functioning.

Psychological qualification is based on the assessment of the patient's intellectual and personality abilities to make decisions about participating in this process. It takes place during a psychological interview—which is the basic diagnostic tool, and conclusions are formed on the basis of observations, analysis of existing medical records, and the interview with patient's family. Motivation, perseverance, resistance to stress, and readiness to bear the effects of the surgery are assessed (Fig. 8.1).

8.2.2 Donor Selection

The criteria for selecting a face transplant donor should be biological compatibility with the recipient, gender compatibility due to differences in facial morphology between male and female faces, and, as far as possible, similarity in appearance to the recipient. The most important element in the coordination of collection is to minimize the ischemic cold time. For this reason, the procedure of harvesting the face and preparation of the recipient takes place at the same time, in two different operating rooms. After the harvest, the face should be stored at a temperature of about 4 °C in a special liquid: ILG-1 (Institut Georges Lopez Organ Preservation Solution) or ViaSpan (University of Wisconsin Solution) with a high potassium content. The closing of the blood supply to the donated organ is planned at the very end of the

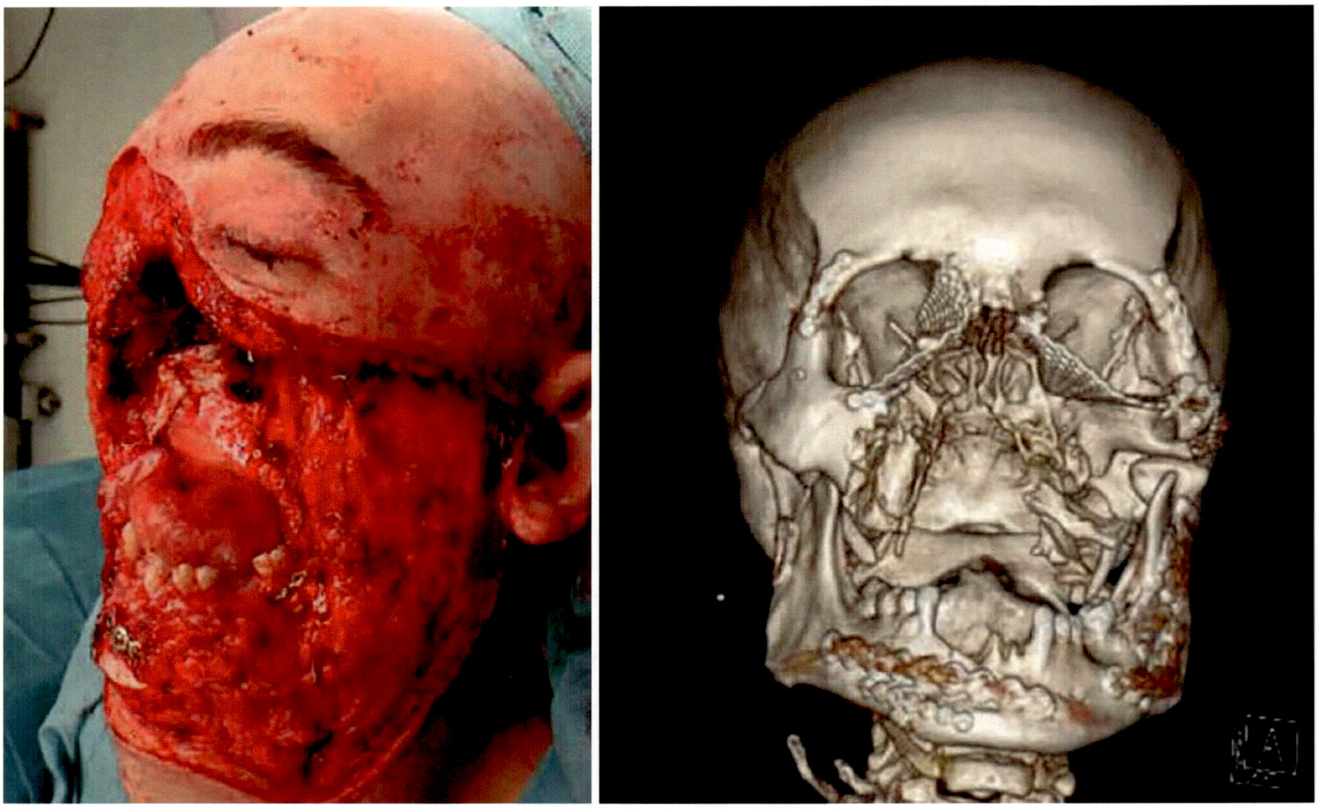

Fig. 8.1 Recipient after removal of previously applied skin grafts as biological dressings, removal of necrotic tissues, and preparation of vascular, nerve, bone, and mucosal structures

procedure as much as possible. For ethical reasons and to preserve the dignity of the donor and his family, the loss of face is replaced with a previously prepared and carefully made silicon mask. This minimizes visible changes after the tissues have been harvested. Close cooperation of transplant coordinators with the entire operating team is of great importance [6, 7].

8.2.3 Surgical Procedures

Not so long ago, facial transplantation was considered to be a proof of the extraordinary heroism of surgeons, bringing hope to regain the appearance of the face to all those who lost its previous shape, function, and aesthetics due to posttraumatic changes or genetic diseases. The face transplant procedure is controversial and has as many supporters as opponents. Its supporters argue that people with severely deformed faces are excluded from social life, frequently locking themselves into their own homes forever, unable to bear the humiliation and disgust shown by their environment. According to the opponents, face transplant does not save a person's life, but on the contrary, it poses a risk of transplant rejection and of the side effects of immunosuppressive drugs. Due to the introduction of modern techniques of microvascular reconstructive surgery to the standards of management and treatment of surgical diseases, more and more face transplant programs are appearing all over the world. Their creation is justified by the fact that for some people with deformed faces (extensive thermal and electrical burns, genetically determined diseases, e.g., neurofibromatosis), there is no other effective treatment option. Since the total area of the face is approximately 700 cm^2, no area of the body can be used to collect such a large part of the skin flap, which would cover the entire face, recreate the mouth, nose, cheeks, and eyelids, and most of all restore proper functionality and aesthetics. The largest free flap that can be collected is only 60% of the face area, and the lack of the possibility of its reinnervation and the color of the skin other than in the area of the face do not meet the standards of today's reconstructive surgery. Several possible variants of the scope and location of the face transplant have been determined, depending on the damaged structures of the recipient's face—from partial face transplant involving only soft tissue elements (reconstruction of the nose, cheeks, lips, chin, and chin area), to complete face transplantation with bone elements. It is necessary to assess the surface of the transplanted face, its shape, skin tightness, and the number and location of vascular and nerve elements intended for anastomosis. The surgical procedure must be preceded by a detailed imaging diagnosis of the recipient in order to determine the scope of the reconstruction, identify the recipient's vessels, and locate any damage to the peripheral nerves. For the proper planning of the allotransplant, it is necessary to select the donor appropriately, taking into account the anatomical and morphological conditions of the recipient—in terms of sex, age, body weight, tissue compatibility, and comorbidities of both the recipient and the donor. The surgical technique of harvesting and implanting a face graft depends on the size of the donor's face skin and consists in identifying vascular and nerve elements, dissecting them in the distal section and harvesting the allotransplant along with the following elements: cartilage, muscle, subcutaneous tissue, mucosa, and skin. The elements of the allotransplant are attached to the recipient's tissues in the following order: vessels, nerves, muscles, mucosa, subcutaneous tissue, skin.

The scope of the reconstruction includes nose, cheeks, upper and lower lips, mouth vestibule, and chin area. The facial vessels serve as donor vessels, the motor innervation comes from the marginal branches of the facial nerves, and the sensory innervation—from the mental nerves. Each of these allotransplant structures is combined with the anatomical structures of the recipient under the microscope according to the rules of microsurgery (the recipient's facial arteries and veins are connected with the donor's facial arteries and veins, the mental nerves and marginal branches of the donor's facial nerve—with the recipient's corresponding nerves).

From a technical point of view, face transplants can be divided into full and partial. Due to the small number of such procedures performed worldwide, this nomenclature was introduced arbitrarily. Currently, the transfer of soft tissues of all three complete levels of the face, including the bone and cartilage frame of the middle level and the anterior part of the mandible, qualifies as a full face transplant. The type of neurovascular structures may vary and does not affect the nomenclature. The content of the eye sockets is usually not included in the graft. Thus, any allotransplantation of less than the above-mentioned extent in terms of soft tissues should be qualified as partial. There are a number of variants of partial allotransplantation depending on the extent of the recipient's tissues to reconstruct. The use of a specific type of transplant is associated with the necessity to solve each time different technical problems resulting from the different anatomy of each transplant and the operation plan of the operating team. These problems include, among others, proper selection of the shape of the bone fragment(s), sensory and motor innervation, dental restoration, chewing, swallowing and speech functions, airway restoration, vascular issues, immunological issues, and finally recipient identity issues (Fig. 8.2).

8.2.3.1 Planning of Bone Components

The bone structure supports the more superficial tissues, hence its proper adjustment to the recipient's defect allows for obtaining the correct contours and face profile. Additionally, it is one of the key elements influencing the

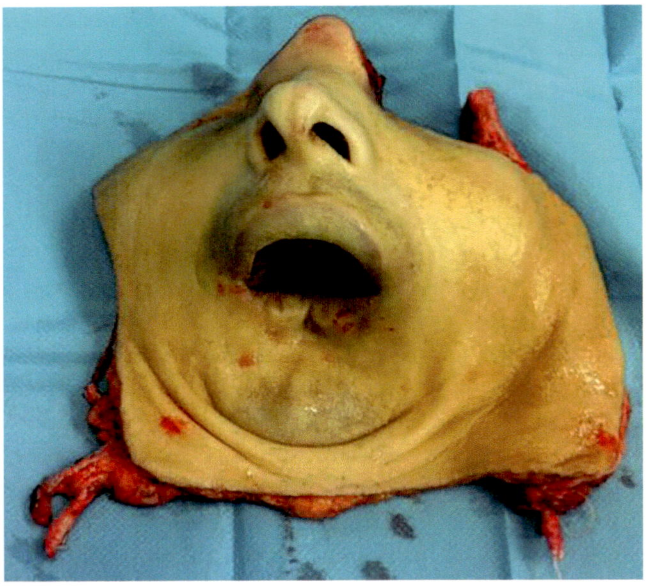

Fig. 8.2 Face graft harvested from a donor

distant aesthetic effect of the transplant. In addition, the proper spatial orientation of bone elements is an absolute condition for the reconstruction of the respiratory tract, and thus obtaining the desired functional effect. Bone fragments are fixed using conventional maxillofacial surgery techniques.

8.2.3.2 Sensory and Motor Innervation

Anatomically, four bilateral pairs of nerves are responsible for the sensory innervation of the face: auricular nerve, an orbital nerve, an infraorbital nerve, and a chin nerve. In practice, however, any trauma that justifies a face transplant most often damages most of these nerves, and it is sometimes impossible to find them intraoperatively in scar tissue. The infraorbital nerve runs in the bone structures that are transferred during transplantation; hence, in order to maintain its continuity, it would have to be anastomosed "backwards" from the jaw, which is technically difficult and does not guarantee the return of its function. In the case of partial facial transplantation involving the soft tissues of the middle and lower levels of the face, the identification of the mental nerve is most likely, and it is possible to anastomose it. The extent of innervation of the great ear nerve is functionally insignificant to justify searching for it and possible anastomosis. The facial nerve and its branches are responsible for the motor innervation within the face. The extent and manner of potential motor reinnervation depends on the level of damage to the nerve in question. It is possible to collect the sublingual and vagus nerves from the donor along with the tissue content of the graft, which can be used as bridges in the reinnervation of the facial nerve branches. The experience of many authors shows that the effective restoration of the neural pathway of even one branch of the facial nerve translates into a much better psycho-social effect and is of great value for the patient. If it is not possible to obtain a facial nerve adequate for reinnervation, the motor fibers of the trigeminal nerve (running to the masseter muscle) can be used, which is usually not included in the scope of transplantation.

8.2.3.3 Chewing Function Restoration

To obtain the chewing function, two conditions must be met—the mandible should be moved by the innervated muscles and the temporomandibular joint must function properly. If the stumps of the temporal and/or masseter muscles remain innervated after the resection, they can be connected with the corresponding muscles carried with the graft. Restoring motor function may be difficult due to the limitations described previously.

8.2.3.4 Speech and Swallowing Function Restoration

Even slight changes in the anatomy and innervation of the oropharynx can lead to a marked impairment of the functions of speech and swallowing. The restoration of these functions in the case of face transplantation will depend on the possibility of innervation of the transplanted muscles and intensive voice rehabilitation.

8.2.3.5 Continuity of the Respiratory Tract Restoration

In the case of face allotransplantation with bone elements, the appropriate matching of the structures of the midface of the donor's and recipient's faces is a key element in maintaining the continuity and patency of the airways. Transplantation of only soft tissues with appropriate planning of the shape and structure of the allograft should not pose technical difficulties in the reconstruction of the respiratory tract.

8.2.3.6 Vascular Aspect

As shown by experimental studies, even a large volume of facial soft tissues covering all three floors, along with some bone elements, can be adequately vascularized through the branches of the external carotid artery. The very use of the facial vessels allows the vascularization of all three levels of soft tissues, the anterior part of the maxilla, the mandible, the anterior part of the sphenoid bone, ethmoid bone, and the zygomatic arches. Even if some of the bone tissues are not revascularized, they will serve as structural/support elements, as is the case with nonvascularized autologous bone grafts. If a part of the mandible is transplanted, its periosteal vascularization (facial vessels) is sufficient without the need for anastomosis of the inferior alveolar vessels.

The stages of face transplant surgery include:

1. Preparation of the recipient (resection of damaged tissues, deepithelialization of the deformed and damaged facial skin, localization of recipient vessels and nerves) (Fig. 8.3).
2. Simultaneous preparation of the allotransplant in another operating room (harvesting a transplant of an appropriate size, including vessels and nerves, and placing it in a suitable fluid for transport) (Fig. 8.4).
3. Transferring the allotransplant into the recipient's tissue defect, performing microvascular (arterial and venous) and nerve anastomosis under the microscope (Fig. 8.5).
4. Connecting the muscle, fascial and dermal elements of the allotransplant with the appropriate recipient structures (Fig. 8.6).

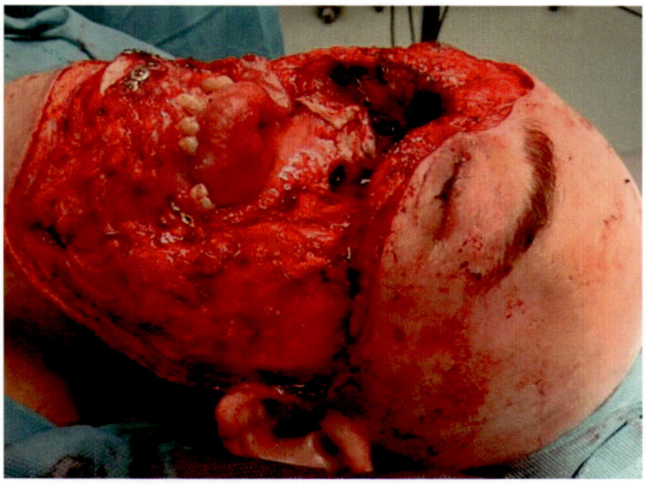

Fig. 8.3 Preparation of the recipient for the face transplant

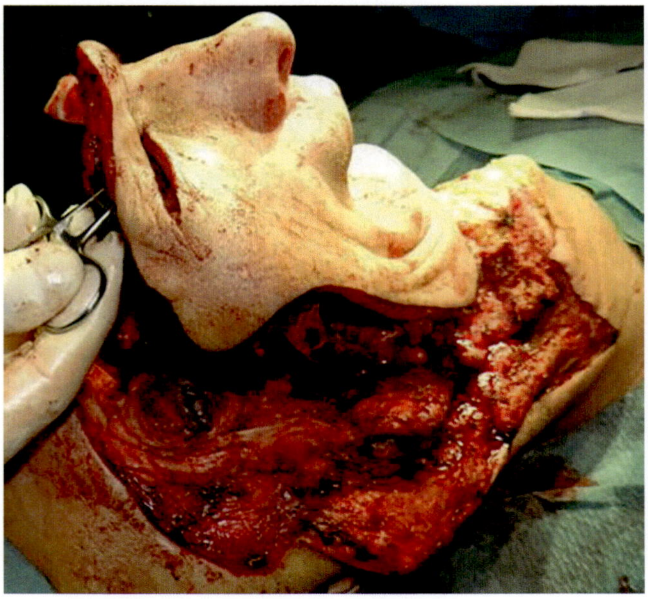

Fig. 8.4 Harvesting the allograft

8.2.4 Postoperative Management

After the surgery, the patient goes to the intensive care unit, where he spends about 14 days, depending on his condition. That is where intensive physical therapy begins. After the

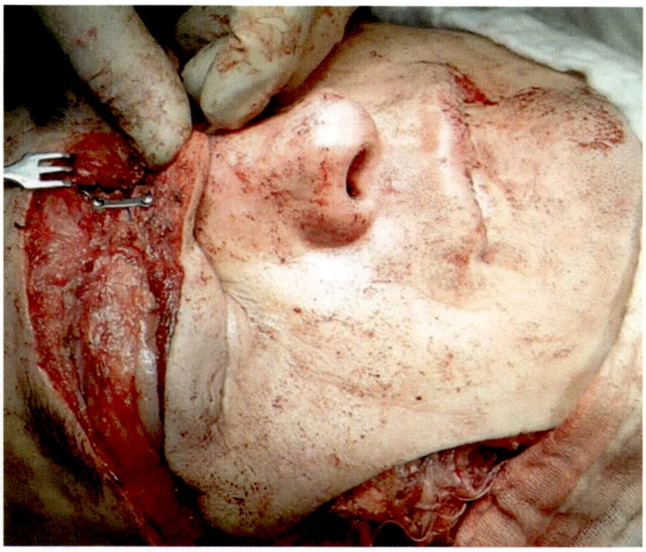

Fig. 8.5 Transferring the allograft

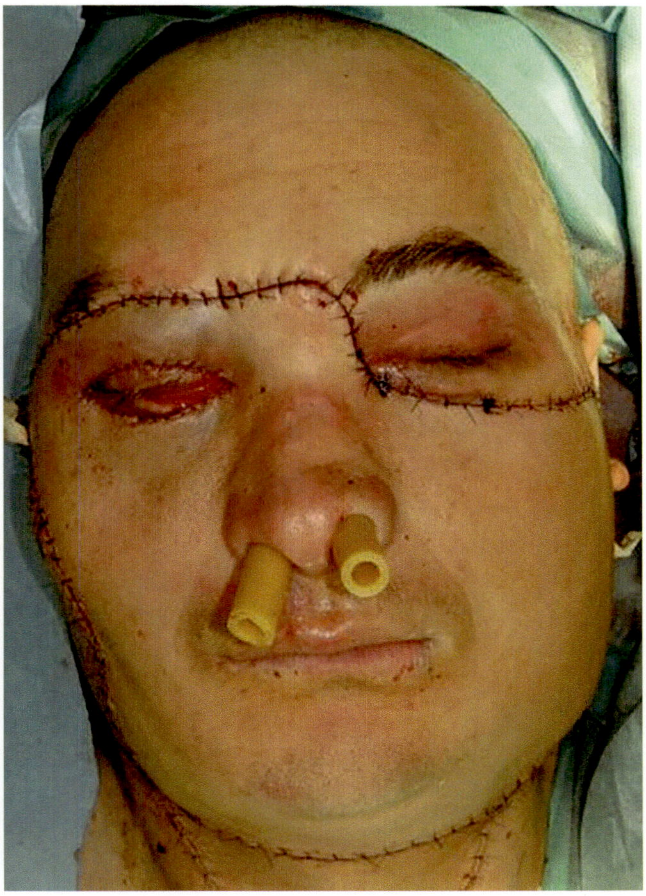

Fig. 8.6 Recipient after the face transplant is completed

tracheostomy and the gastric tube are removed, the patient is transferred to the transplant department. Over the next few weeks, patients after face transplant are slowly getting used to their new image. It is very important to maintain the privacy of patients, especially in the first weeks. Patients should absolutely be under the care of a psychologist who monitors their condition from the first hours after waking up. The main mission of physiotherapy in this period is to work on the functioning of the muscles supporting the structure of the face (static part) and to gradually increase the range of oral cavity closing (dynamic part).

8.2.5 Immunosuppression and Pharmacotherapy

In the case of VCA involving a large area of the skin (limbs, face), tacrolimus, mycophenolate mofetil, and steroids are administered as long-term treatments. In addition, in the immediate perioperative period, i.e., 2 h before the procedure and 4 days after it, to prevent acute rejection, immunosuppression is induced with an intravenous preparation (basiliximab). The immunosuppressive induction in the form of anti-thymocytic globulin should be administered for 7 days at a dose of 1.25 mg/kg/24 h. Tacrolimus should be administered in such a way that the plasma concentration is maintained at 12–15 ng/mL. Mycophenolate mofetil is administered in a dose of 2 g daily. Regarding glucocorticoid therapy, the following methylprednisolone treatment regimen should be followed (Table 8.1).

In the stage of maintaining immunosuppression, the tacrolimus dose should be reduced to plasma levels of 7–10 ng/mL and mycophenolate mofetil to 1 g daily. Maintaining the appropriate level of these pharmaceuticals in the blood is possible thanks to outpatient controls of the recipient. Over time, treatment is adjusted so that the patient receives the minimum doses of drugs that allow the transplant to survive.

8.2.6 Managing Patients After the Face Transplant

Histopathological inspection of the transplanted organ includes tissue biopsy followed by microscopic examination.

Table 8.1 Methylprednisolone treatment regimen

Clinical situation	Dosage
Day 0	10 mg/kg
Day 1–2	5 mg/kg
Day 3–4	3 mg/kg
In the stage of maintaining immunosuppression	4 mg/24 h
In the case of a rejection episode	2 mg/kg/24 h

A biopsy can be performed in any case where a change in the appearance of the transplanted organ (face) suggests rejection, but most biopsies are elective, independent of symptoms. Their frequency is highest when the risk of rejection is highest, i.e., in the first year after transplantation, and particularly in the first 3 months after surgery.

Due to the very long recovery time of patients, it is necessary to carefully educate patients about the rate at which tissue regeneration takes place and what consequences are associated with it. Patients also need to know how to recognize early signs of transplant rejection in order to notify their physician as soon as possible.

8.2.7 Complications After Face Transplant

Face transplantation belongs to a broad spectrum of the group of composite tissue grafts (allografts). This means that the graft includes embryologically heterogeneous tissues such as skin, blood vessels, nerves, muscles, and bone parts, along with the bone marrow. Changes in graft rejection vary considerably between cases, but always depend on the severity of the phenomenon. They mainly affect the dermis, and then, as the rejection progresses, they are transferred to the subcutaneous tissue and epidermis. It should also be remembered that the skin and mucosa of all types of tissue will change first. The cells of the immune system responsible for the damage to the allograft are mainly T lymphocytes (CD3, CD4, CD8), monocytes (CD 68), and, to a lesser extent, eosinophils. In order to examine the changes, a biopsy should be taken at a depth of minimum 4 mm at the site of the most erythematous, but still living skin. Other common postoperative complications were wound healing disorders, Stensen's duct stenosis, ptosis, and eyelid eversion (ectropion). The most serious complications associated with face transplants are those resulting from immunosuppressive therapy. These include, among others, drug toxicity leading to metabolic disorders, opportunistic infections, and increased risk of neoplasms. Despite rigorous antibacterial and antiviral prophylaxis, face transplant patients developed at least one opportunistic infection. The most common are Cytomegalovirus (CMV), Herpes simplex, Herpes zoster, *Candida albicans*. To this date, there have been a few deaths in facial transplant patients. The first patient who, in addition to the face transplant, received a bilateral hand transplant died as a result of graft infection with a multiresistant *Pseudomonas aeruginosa* strain, which resulted in an extended stay in the intensive care unit. The consequence of the developing bacterial infection was pneumonia and sepsis, which led to the patient's death. A second death in a facial transplant patient was described in China, where the patient died 27 months after the operation. His death was probably due to improper immunosuppressive therapy. The third known case concerns a patient whose cause of death was recurrent, aggressive squamous cell carcinoma of the tongue and HIV infection. Cases of death of patients with accompanying infections and immunodeficiencies show how important it is to properly qualify people for the face transplant program. In the case of psychological complications, so far there is no evidence of problems in patients after face transplants; however, there are isolated reports of an increased risk of alcohol addiction. In addition, highly satisfactory cases have been described where patients obtained higher scores on quality of life (SF-36 scale) and mental health (MOS-SF 12 scale) than before face transplant [8].

8.2.8 Results of the Face Transplant Program in Poland

So far, two face transplant surgeries have been performed in Poland. Both the first and the second were successful. It is worth mentioning that both were conducted by the team of the Department of Oncological and Reconstructive Surgery of the National Institute of Oncology in Gliwice. The first face transplant was performed in 2013 [9]. A 31-year-old patient had an accident at work on a construction site with a stone cutting machine. After being transported to the hospital, an attempt was made to replant the cut off part of the face in the first place, but it was not successful. The team unanimously decided to perform a face transplant. The surgery itself took place 10 days after the accident. The donor turned out to be a man a year younger, of similar weight and height. The surgery to harvest and transplant the face was performed simultaneously in two operating theaters and took the surgical team a total of 27 h. After the surgery, the patient spent 2 weeks in the intensive care unit, where from the first days he was subjected to intensive logo- and physiotherapy. After being transferred to the transplant department for the next 21 days, the patient was able to get used to his new face and all issues related to its functional state. The patient underwent rehabilitation twice a day. It included static and dynamic facial muscle exercises focused on restoring proper opening and closing the mouth. The superficial sensation started to return relatively quickly, in the eighth week, and already in the 12th week after the surgery, it covered the entire face, all the way to the tip of the nose. Motor activity, on the other hand, was first observed at week 10. The patient's further stay in the hospital was uneventful and after 14 weeks he was discharged home, where he could return to the rest of the world. It is worth adding that this operation was innovative on a global scale. It was the world's first life-saving face transplant. The second patient qualified for the face transplant program was a 28-year-old woman suffering from type I neurofibromatosis (von Recklinghausen's disease) confined to the head region [10]. Over the past 24 years, the patient

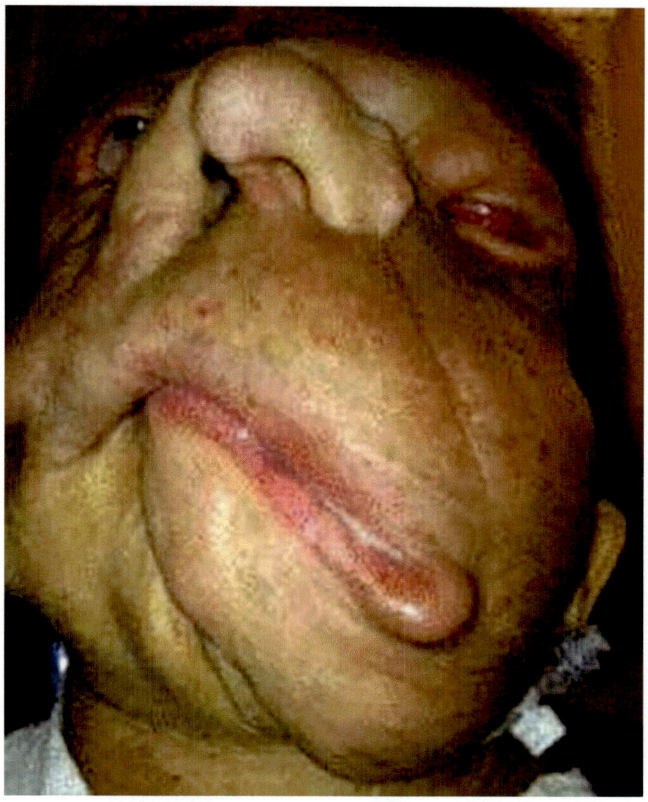

Fig. 8.7 The appearance of the patient before the face transplant

has undergone over 35 surgeries (Fig. 8.7). Due to the deteriorating visual and functional condition of the face for 3 years, a decision was made to qualify the patient for a face transplant. Additionally, the patient suffered from left-sided hemi and right-sided partial paralysis of the facial nerve function, most likely due to a huge neurofibroma compressing the peripheral part of the nerve.

The operation was carried out in 2014. The donor was a 19-year-old woman who died as a result of a car accident. As was the case with the first transplant, the procedure was performed simultaneously in two operating rooms. One team harvested the face and the other prepared the recipient by resection of the tumors and preparing the nerves and blood vessels for the anastomosis with the graft. Due to the high blood supply to the lesions, the patient's blood loss was high, which was replaced with 27 blood units, which was a real challenge for the anesthetic team. Ultimately, due to the extensive neoplastic process, 75% of the face surface had to be replaced. The entire procedure took 24 h (Fig. 8.8).

After the surgery, the patient's condition was stable, and no postoperative complications were observed. The tracheostomy was removed on the eighth day after surgery, and a week later, attempts were made to start an oral diet. On the ninth day after the surgery, the patient had the opportunity to see her new face for the first time. No negative psychological effects related to such a significant change in life have been

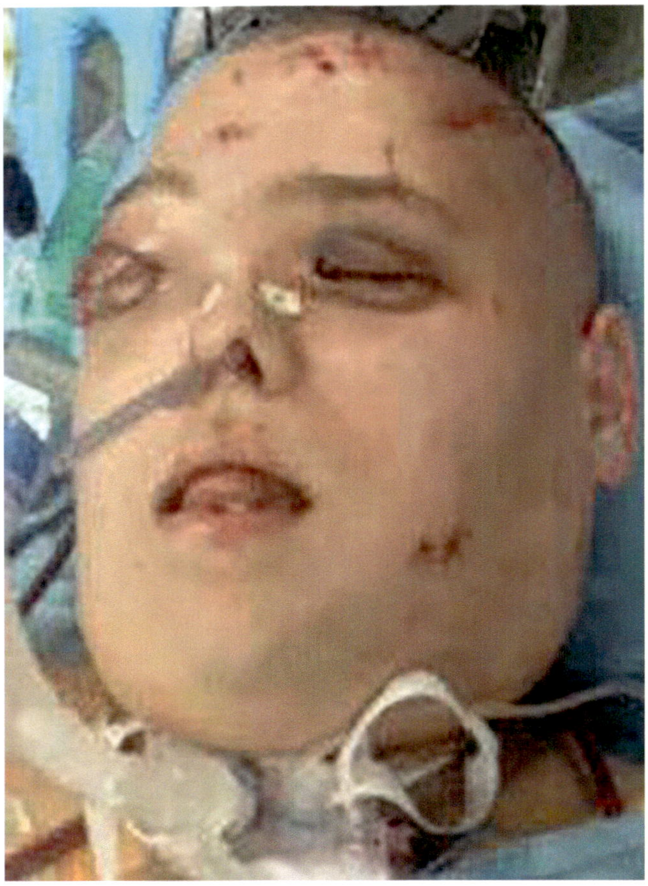

Fig. 8.8 The appearance of the patient immediately after the face transplant

observed. For 34 months after the operation, there was no sign of rejection. Physiotherapy and rehabilitation began relatively quickly, already on the third and fifth day after the transplant. Superficial feeling began to return in the second month, and by week 9, it was almost the entire face (90% on the Semmes-Weinstein test). Motor activity was returning much more slowly. The first signs were observed at week 16, and the patient was able to smile and close her mouth to 75% by 1 year after the procedure.

8.3 Neck Organ Transplantation (NTx)

8.3.1 Qualification and Preparation of Recipient

Although the group of patients after laryngectomy among patients diagnosed with laryngeal cancer is extensive, there are still no specific indications nor qualification protocol for allotransplantation of this organ, which significantly limits the group of potential recipients. Predictable anatomy, sufficient length of vessels and nerves supplying the organs of the neck as well as repetitive technique of the procedure should be sufficient arguments for these procedures to become commonly performed. Unfortunately, this procedure is not life-saving and "only" aims to improve the quality of life; hence, the ethical issues related to perioperative risks are often the main reason for discussion regarding its legitimacy. Another aspect of concern is the immunosuppression required after allotransplantation and its potential consequences. Cases treated at the Department of Oncological and Reconstructive Surgery to some extent were selected in terms of the latter aspect, because most of the patients qualified for complex neck organ allotransplantation were already treated with immunosuppression due to the previous solid organ transplantation, so another allograft had not brought new risks or additional burdens [11]. The main aspect qualifying the candidates for this procedure was the extremely low quality of life, resulting from the lack of a fragment of the upper alimentary as well as respiratory tract and i.a. subsequent infections. This was often the result of an extended laryngectomy due to laryngeal cancer, complicated by fistulas, treated with mediocre effect by both surgical and conservative methods, or by chemical burns of both the upper respiratory upper gastrointestinal tract (Fig. 8.9) [12, 13].

8.3.2 Selection of Donors and Coordination of Donation

The criteria for selecting a neck organ transplant donor should be:

- Tissue compatibility with the recipient.
- Gender compatibility.
- Similar morphology of the cervical tissues of the donor as well as recipient.

It should be kept in mind that a complex neck organ transplant is much more sensitive to a prolonged period of ischemia in comparison to commonly transplanted solid organs. Thus, the most important part of coordinating organ donation is the simultaneous collection of the allotransplant and preparation of recipient site, so that the cold time of ischemia is shortened as much as possible. Efficient cooperation of national transplant coordinators with the surgical teams is also of paramount importance [14].

8.3.3 Surgical Procedure

The procedure usually takes about 12–14 h. The allograft contains larynx, cervical part of trachea, pharynx with esophagus, thyroid and four parathyroid glands, hyoid bone with anterior bellies of digastric muscle, part of infrahyoid muscles as well as the anterior wall of the neck. This vast

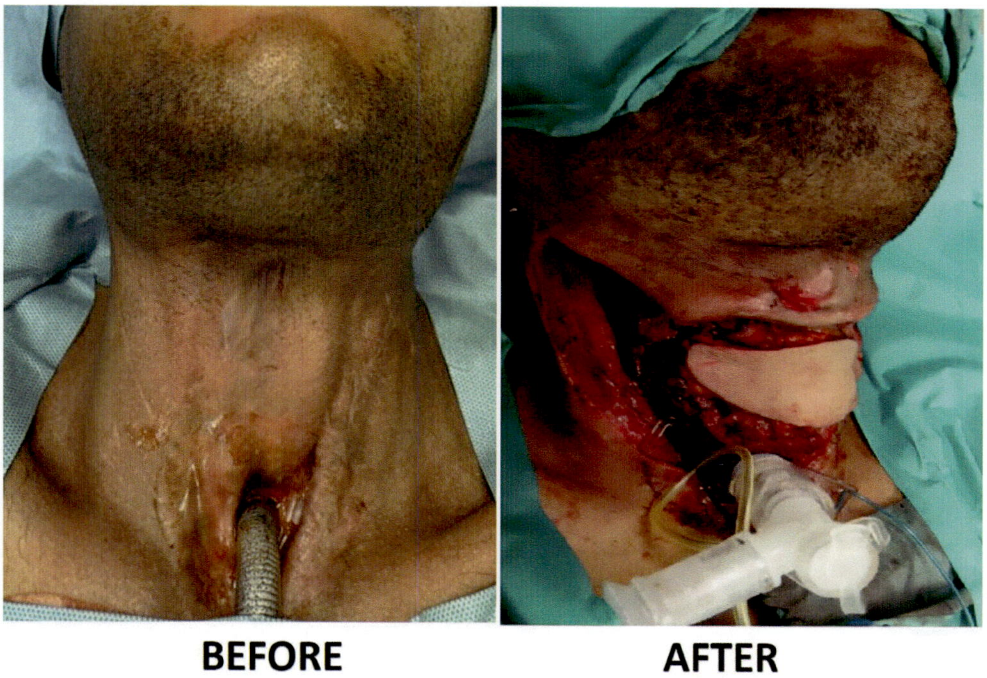

Fig. 8.9 Comparison of the anterior neck wall before allotransplantation and at the procedure's final stage

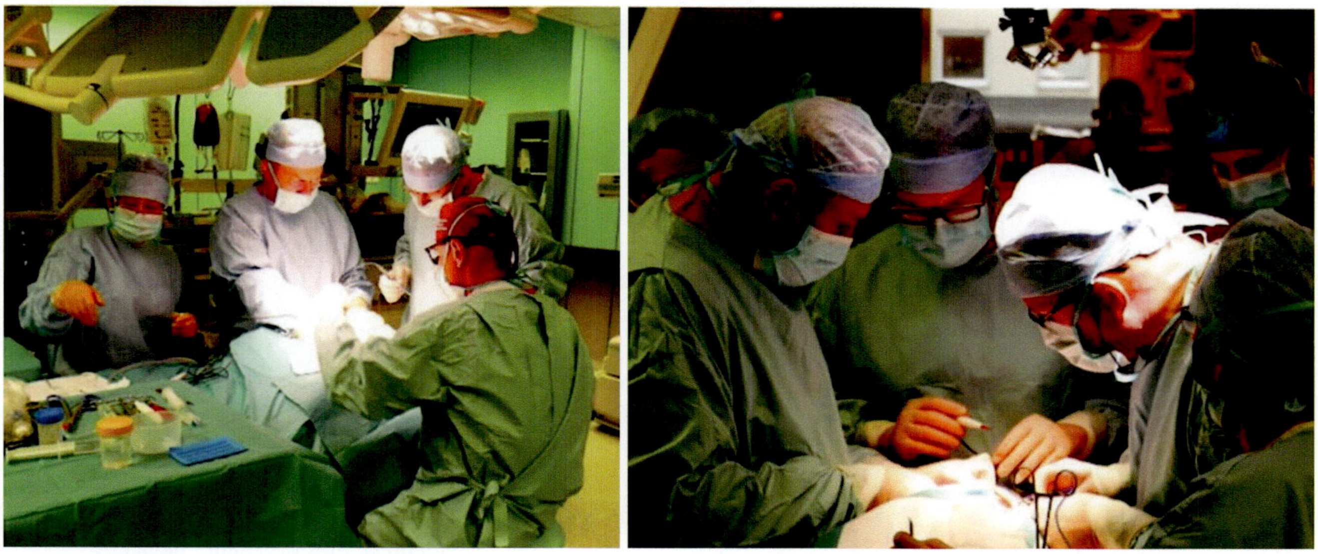

Fig. 8.10 Both donor (left) and recipient (right) were prepared simultaneously in two adjacent operating rooms

complex is supplied by four arteries (two superior and two inferior thyroid arteries), four accompanying veins, two anterior jugular veins, as well as four nerves (two superior laryngeal and two recurrent laryngeal nerves).

The donor and the recipient are operated simultaneously in two adjacent operating rooms by two surgical teams. In the donor, the skin paddle is planned corresponding to the defect expected in the recipient. Consecutively, neurovascular bundles as well as distal stumps of esophagus and trachea are exposed, dissecting proximally to the level of hyoid bone. Additionally, as long as possible portions of the donor vessels and nerves are prepared (Fig. 8.10).

In the recipient, the neck is explored by resection of scar tissues, fistulas, and part of the anterior cervical wall. The corresponding recipient vessels and nerves are dissected. In some cases, due to the lack of part of the arteries, as a result of previous treatments, branches of external carotid and supraclavicular arteries can be used. Additionally, in case of inaccessibility of laryngeal nerves, the sublingual, phrenic, and vagus nerves can be used as a recipients for end-to-side anastomoses to suitable nerves of allograft (Figs. 8.11 and 8.12).

After receiving the information that recipient site is prepared, the trachea and esophagus are detached at the level of

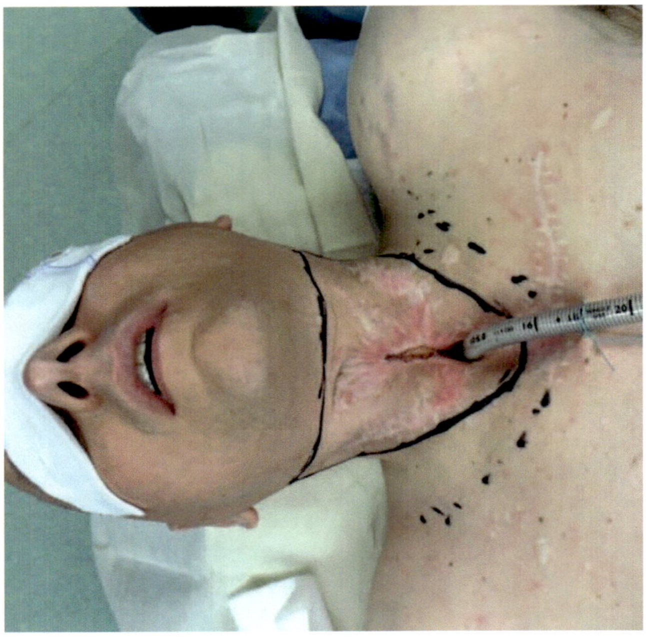

Fig. 8.11 Recipient before complex neck organ allotransplantation with marked resection range

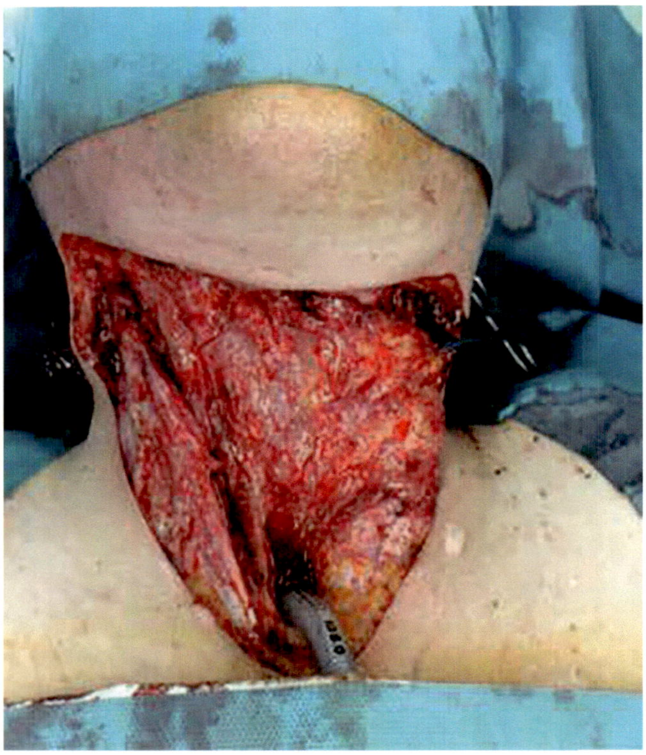

Fig. 8.12 Neck exploration and preparation of vascular structures, nerves, digestive tract, and tracheal stump

the jugular notch of sternum, the pharynx at the level of the base of the tongue, as well as bilateral vessels and nerves are cut, which completes the harvest of the allotransplant. After detachment of the transplant, it is perfused for 30 min with preservation fluid (Celsior) which aims not only to remove residual blood stagnation, but also to slow down the metabolism of the transferred graft cells. Then the transplant is transferred to the recipient's defect (Figs. 8.13 and 8.14).

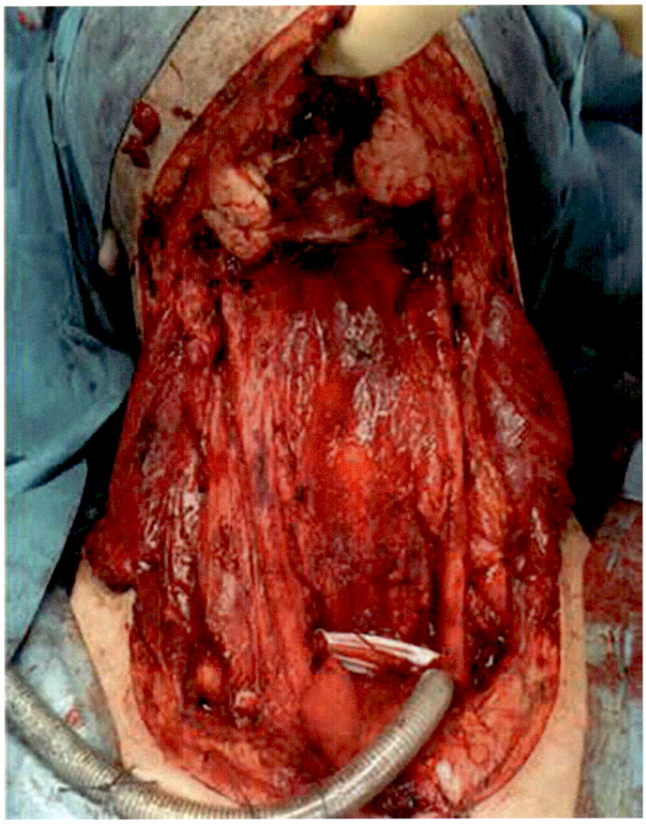

Fig. 8.13 Donor after harvesting a complex neck organ transplant

The implantation stage begins with four arterial microanastomoses between superior and inferior thyroid arteries (if available), then venous microanastomoses—four between accompanying veins and two between anterior jugular veins. Finally the superior laryngeal nerves as well as recurrent laryngeal nerves are anastomosed. All anastomoses are performed using 10.0 nylon sutures or coupler devices of appropriate diameters (Fig. 8.15).

The next step is to restore the aerodigestive tract continuity. Proximally, the transplant's pharynx is sutured at the level of the edge of base of the tongue and distally—the stumps of both esophagus and trachea are sutured in an end-to-end manner. Implantation stage is completed with the dynamic suspension of the hyoid bone, suturing the donor's digastric muscles to their stumps in the recipient, placement of numerous suction drains as well as subcutaneous tissue and skin suturing (Fig. 8.16).

For ethical purposes and to preserve the dignity of the donor and his family, the defect after allograft harvest is replaced with a silicone prosthesis. This minimizes the visible deficiencies in the neck area.

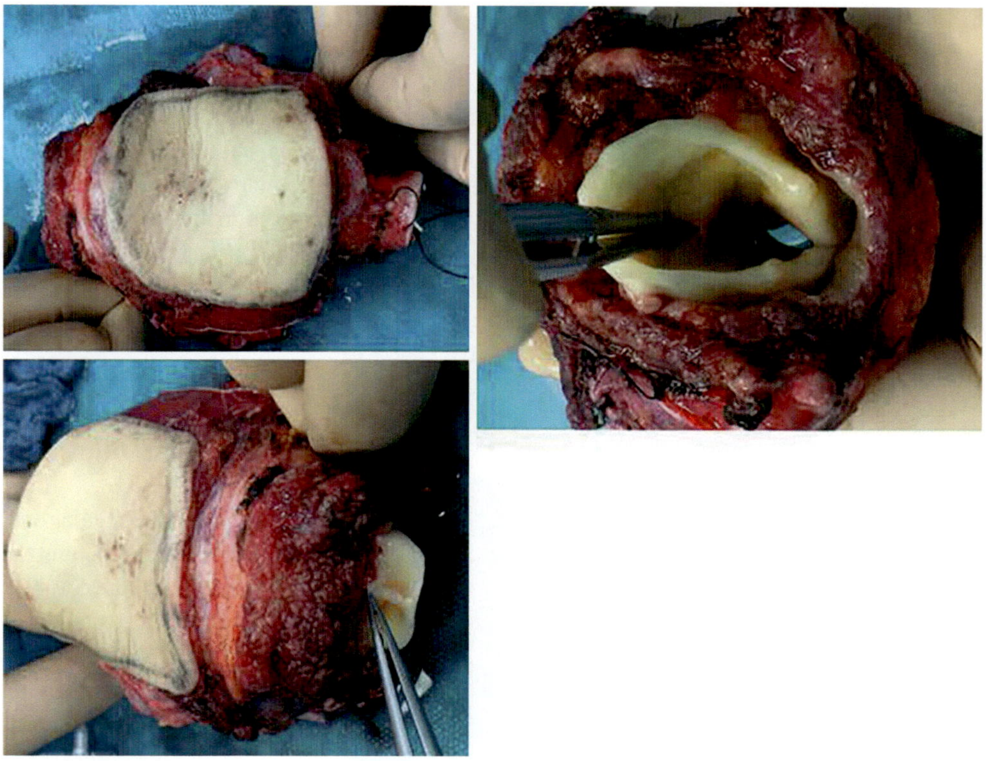

Fig. 8.14 Complex allotransplant of neck organs. Subsequent projections of the harvested graft including the larynx, pharynx, esophagus, thyroid gland, parathyroid glands, hyoid bone, neck muscles, and skin paddle

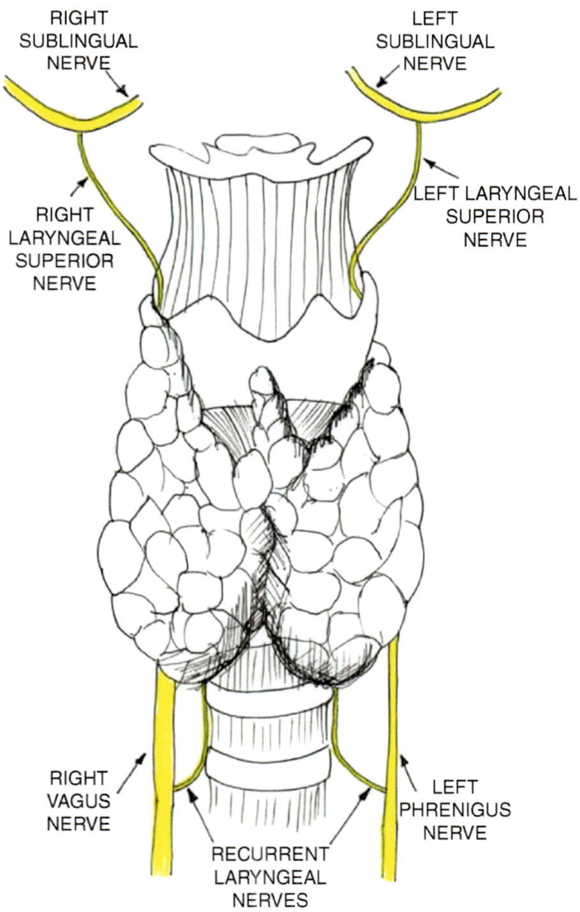

Fig. 8.15 Scheme of example nerve anastomoses (in case of unavailability of corresponding nerves)

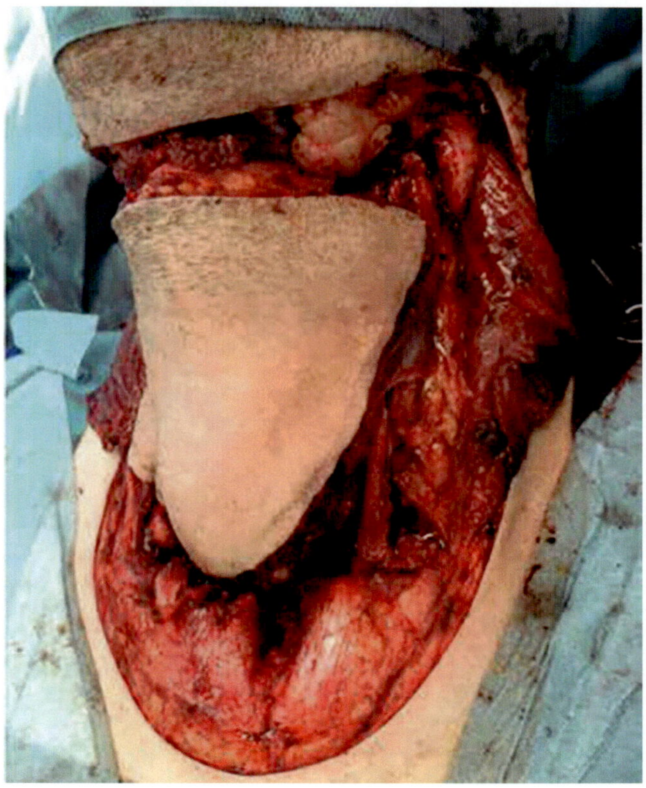

Fig. 8.16 Inset of the allotransplant into the recipient site

8.3.4 Postoperative Management

Patients stay in the intensive care unit for about a week. Based on endoscopic examinations, they have a tracheostomy removed on the tenth postoperative day and then a gastrostomy, which allows for full oral nutrition and breathing with the restored respiratory tract (initially with an indirect positioning of the vocal cords). In the following weeks, they are able to utter individual words quietly, yet clearly. Thanks to further intensive rehabilitation and exercises, their speech increasingly reflects the physiological state, which is directly related to endoscopic examinations—a change to the lateral position of the vocal cords can be observed (Figs. 8.17 and 8.18).

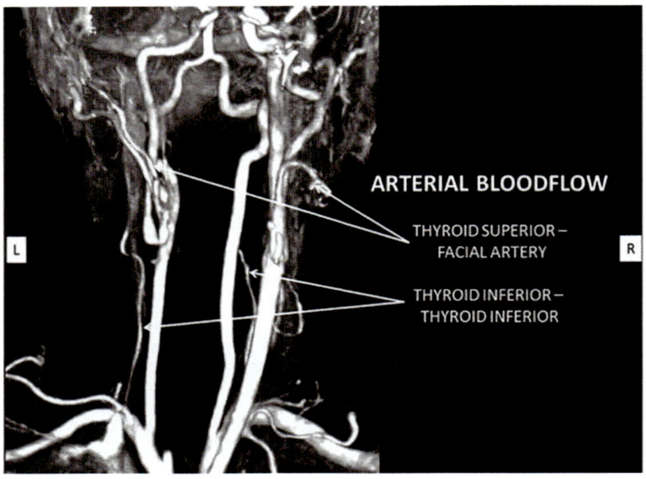

Fig. 8.17 Postoperative CT angiography showing normal perfusion provided by all four arterial anastomoses

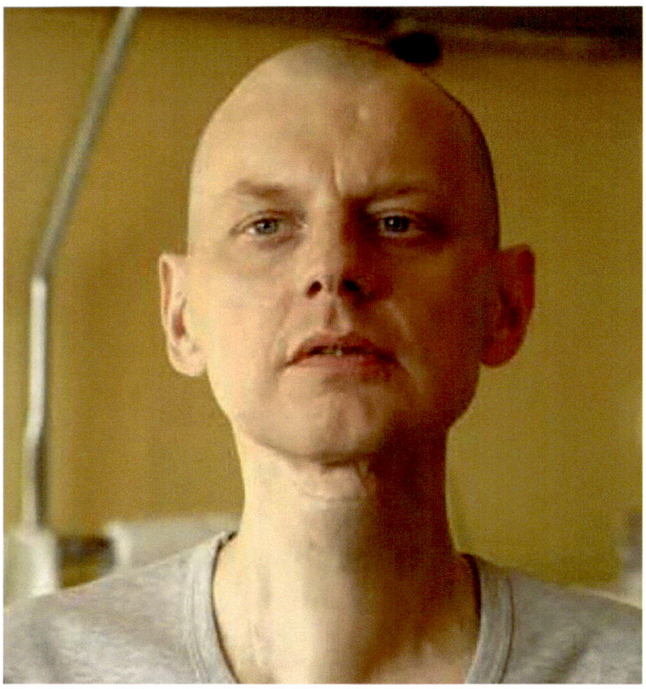

Fig. 8.18 Aesthetic outcome 4 months postoperatively

8.3.5 Immunosuppression and Pharmacotherapy

The scheme of drug treatment for the prevention of allotransplant rejection (immunosuppression) is the same for most complex tissue grafts and is fully described in Sect. 8.2.5. Additionally, bronchodilators as well as inhaled steroids play an important role in neck organs transplantation—in addition to improving ventilation after surgery, they also facilitate the rehabilitation process (Fig. 8.19).

8.3.6 Managing Patients After Complex Neck Organ Allotransplantation

In addition to the regular endoscopic examinations described above, taking into account the fact that most patients received hormonal and calcium substitution before the procedure, the levels of thyroid-stimulating hormone (TSH), triiodothyronine (T3), thyroxine (T4), calcium, and phosphorus are being checked regularly. After the treatment, they gradually return to reference values. During the 2-year follow-up period, there was no rejection episode, and after the initial intensification of immunosuppression, patients return to pre-neck organ allotransplantation regimens. During the long-term observation, the physiological act of swallowing was demonstrated, as well as the normal function of the transplanted endocrine glands. The restoration of skin sensation within the anterior neck wall was observed (Fig. 8.20).

8.3.7 Complications After Complex Neck Organ Allotransplantation

The main complications after allotransplantation and the most common at the same time are transplant rejection as well as side effects of immunosuppression, which are thoroughly described in Sect. 8.2.3.

When it comes to complications specific for the transplanted organ and the surgical site, in the case of complex neck organ allotransplantation, one of the most serious complications is severe postoperative edema. In the case of the NTx, it can lead to obstruction in the alimentary or respiratory tract, which may be a direct threat not only to the viability of the transplant but also directly to the patient's life. Additionally, complications within the reconstructed alimentary tract are an important issue. Theoretically, there is a risk of leakage within the anastomosis between esophagus of the donor and recipient in the early postoperative period. In this case, the treatment of choice is a temporary gastrointestinal stenting, performed by an experienced endoscopist. Due to the four microanastomoses supplying the transplant, even in the case of failure of one or two of them, the perfusion of the graft should not

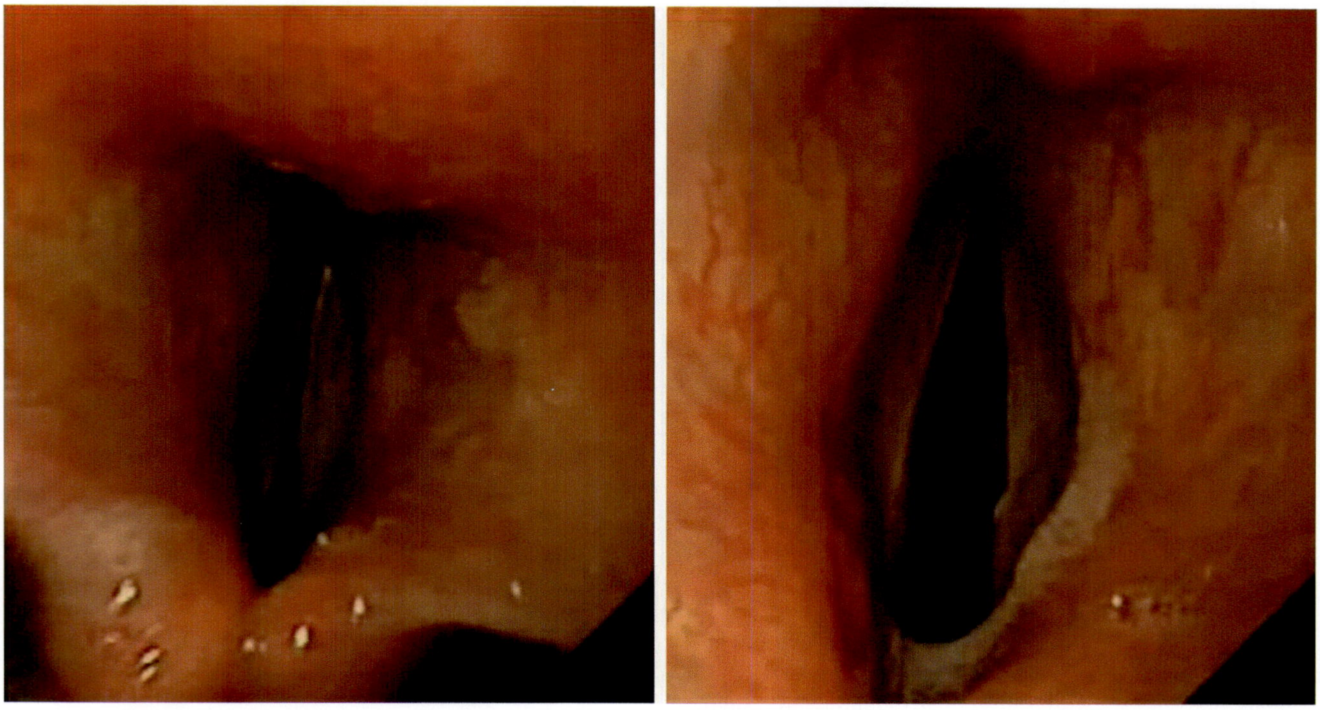

Fig. 8.19 Postoperative endoscopy (1 month after allotransplantation) presenting the mobility of the vocal cords

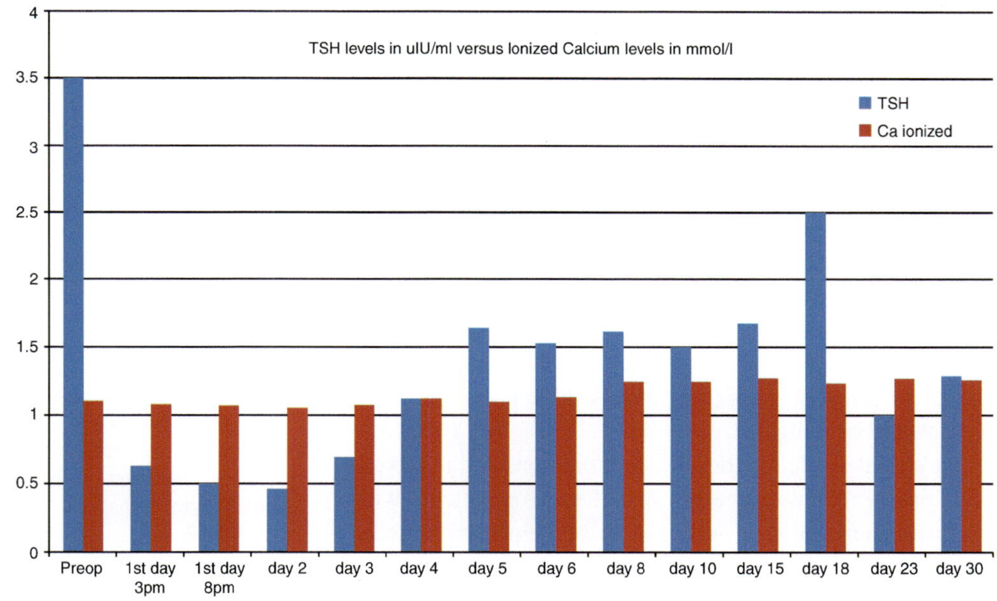

Fig. 8.20 TSH and calcium levels graph

be significantly impaired. In the material of our clinic, we did not observe any impairment of the blood supply of the transplant in the postoperative period.

8.3.8 Outcomes of the Neck Organ Transplant Program

So far, five complex allotransplantations of neck organs have been performed in the world. All of them were conducted by the team of the Department of Oncological and Reconstructive Surgery of the National Institute of Oncology in Gliwice [15].

During late postoperative check-ups (after a period of at least 2 years), the vocal cords of the patients function properly, they are able to communicate with the environment in an understandable way and to breathe freely through the mouth and nose without tracheostomy. A fully healed skin paddle recreating the front wall of the neck provides a satisfactory aesthetic outcome. The transplanted endocrine glands (thyroid and parathyroid glands) became fully functional within about 3 weeks after the procedure, and this function has been maintained to this day. Blood TSH, FT3, FT4, PTH, and calcium levels are within the reference values and supplementation is not required.

8.4 Perspectives of the Development of the Face and Neck Organ Transplantation Program

Due to the high complexity of surgery as well as related pharmacotherapy, technological advances will make a significant contribution to the development of the face transplant program. The development of crafting objects on 3D printers is already helping surgeons prepare for the procedures significantly, and the advent of the VR (virtual reality) era is likely to revolutionize the way we look at preoperative planning. There are also high hopes for printing organs from living cells. Research in this direction is already being carried out, but we must remember that we are dealing with a human face—the only human "organ" that is so complicated in terms of shape and contour, which additionally significantly changes over time. Many years will pass before the technology will allow us to print organs in such a way that they do not differ from their archetypes. The benefits of such solutions are invaluable. Immunotherapy would be unnecessary, which would allow to qualify patients at high risk of neoplasms and with impaired immune system. The role of society in the development of the program should also be emphasized. The main purpose of a face transplant is to allow patients to return to normal functioning. The role of society in the development of the program cannot be overemphasized. The main purpose of a face transplant is to allow patients to return to normal functioning. The best determinant of this would be, e.g., a return to work in the pre-accident or disease profession. With the increased number of people after face transplantation, the risk of so-called stigmatizing patients in their own environment would be mitigated.

Face transplantation, despite its limitations and relatively high risk, will always be the only hope for patients with extensive facial defects, who cannot be helped by conventional reconstructive surgery. It seems that this procedure has as many supporters as opponents. But it seems that all their doubts will be dispelled by more and more experienced centers and the incoming evidence of the need to develop this specialized branch of transplantology.

Taking into account all the facts and expectations mentioned above, we have great hope that in the near future face transplantation will become a standard procedure performed and commonly accepted in many centers around the world.

Composite tissue allografts from deceased donors, apart from justification in the case of directly life-threatening situations, can also be considered for diseases that significantly shorten life time and considerably impair its quality or prevent from normal functioning in the society. However, especially in these cases, the indications should be carefully assessed, individually due to the risk of various complications related to both the surgery and the consequence of immunosuppression [16, 17].

References

1. Iske J, Nian Y, Maenosono R, Maurer M, Sauer IM, Tullius SG. Composite tissue allotransplantation: opportunities and challenges. Cell Mol Immunol. 2019;16(4):343–9. https://doi.org/10.1038/s41423-019-0215-3.
2. Ramly EP, Kantar RS, Alfonso AR, Diaz-Siso JR, Rodriguez ED. Preclinical animal models in facial transplantation. Plast Reconstr Surg Glob Open. 2019;7(9):e2455. Published 2019 Sep 23. https://doi.org/10.1097/GOX.0000000000002455.
3. Molitor M. Transplantation of vascularized composite allografts. Review of current knowledge. Acta Chir Plast. 2016;58(1):18–28. Indexed in Pubmed: 27873528.
4. Caplan A, Purves D. A quiet revolution in organ transplant ethics. J Med Ethics. 2017;43(11):797–800. Indexed in Pubmed: 28424230. https://doi.org/10.1136/medethics-2015-103348.
5. Prabhu V, Plana NM, Hagiwara M, et al. Preoperative imaging for facial transplant: a guide for radiologists. Radiographics. 2019;39(4):1098–107. https://doi.org/10.1148/rg.2019180167.
6. Palmer WJ, Nelms L. Face transplantation for massive mandibular defects: considerations for allograft design and surgical planning. Plast Aesthet Res. 2020;7:2. https://doi.org/10.20517/2347-9264.2019.34.
7. Kantar RS, Ceradini DJ, Gelb BE, et al. Facial transplantation for an irreparable central and lower face injury: a modernized approach to a classic challenge. Plast Reconstr Surg. 2019;144(2):264e–83e. https://doi.org/10.1097/PRS.0000000000005885.
8. Kollar B, Rizzo NM, Borges TJ, et al. Accelerated chronic skin changes without allograft vasculopathy: a 10-year outcome report after face transplantation. Surgery. 2020;167(6):991–8. https://doi.org/10.1016/j.surg.2020.01.010.
9. Maciejewski A, Krakowczyk Ł, Szymczyk C, Wierzgoń J, Grajek M, Dobrut M, Szumniak R, Ulczok R, Giebel S, Bajor G, Półtorak S. The first immediate face transplant in the world. Ann Surg. 2016;263(3):e36–9. https://doi.org/10.1097/SLA.0000000000001597.
10. Krakowczyk Ł, Maciejewski A, Szymczyk C, Oleś K, Półtorak S. Face transplant in an advanced neurofibromatosis type 1 patient. Ann Transplant. 2017;22:53–7. https://doi.org/10.12659/aot.900617.
11. Jo HK, Park JW, Hwang JH, et al. Risk acceptance and expectations of laryngeal allotransplantation. Arch Plast Surg. 2014;41(5):505–12. Indexed in Pubmed: 25276642. https://doi.org/10.5999/aps.2014.41.5.505.
12. Krishnan G, Du C, Fishman J, et al. The current status of human laryngeal transplantation in 2017: a state of the field review. Laryngoscope. 2017;127(8):1861–8. https://doi.org/10.1002/lary.26503.
13. Sakallıoğlu Ö. Laryngeal transplantation: a review. Turk Arch Otorhinolaryngol. 2015;53(3):128–32. Indexed in Pubmed: 29391994. https://doi.org/10.5152/tao.2015.999.
14. Shipchandler TZ, Lorenz RR, Lee WT, et al. Laryngeal transplantation in the setting of cancer: a rat model. Laryngoscope. 2008;118(12):2166–71. Indexed in Pubmed: 18948827. https://doi.org/10.1097/MLG.0b013e3181855108.

15. Grajek M, Maciejewski A, Giebel S, et al. First complex allotransplantation of neck organs: larynx, trachea, pharynx, esophagus, thyroid, parathyroid glands, and anterior cervical wall: a case report. Ann Surg. 2017;266(2):e19–24. Indexed in Pubmed: 28463895. https://doi.org/10.1097/SLA.0000000000002262.
16. Lott DG. What is the future of "organ transplantation" in the head and neck? Curr Opin Otolaryngol Head Neck Surg. 2014;22(5):429–35. Indexed in Pubmed: 25101936. https://doi.org/10.1097/MOO.0000000000000087.
17. Lorenz RR, Strome M. Total laryngeal transplant explanted: 14 years of lessons learned. Otolaryngol Head Neck Surg. 2014;150(4):509–11. Indexed in Pubmed: 24436467. https://doi.org/10.1177/0194599813519748.

Face Transplantation by Ozkan Team (Turkey)

9

Özlenen Özkan, Mustafa Gökhan Ertosun, and Ömer Özkan

9.1 Introduction

In Turkey, discussions were started with the government in 2005 to obtain a special permission for hand transplantation. During this process, the infrastructure of the necessary legislation for face transplantation was created. In terms of composite tissue transplants, the first hand transplant was performed in our country in 2010 [1]. In addition, the first cadaveric uterus transplant in the world was performed by our team in 2011 [2, 3]. After receiving the necessary government permits for the first face transplantation in 2012, Turkey's first face transplantation was carried out by our team (Table 9.1).

9.2 Status of the Program

The face transplantation program is still active in our hospital.

9.3 Screening Process

After the first successful face transplantation, more than 40 applications were received from all over the world. When facial deformities were thoroughly examined clinically and using imaging methods, face transplantation was not indicated in half of the applicants. The number of eligible patients further decreased when comorbidities, mental health, and the legal age limit were considered.

There are currently six patients on the waiting list. In parallel with the growth of the transplantation program, patient lists are constantly revised and made ready for donations.

Ö. Özkan · M. G. Ertosun · Ö. Özkan (✉)
Department of Plastic, Reconstructive, and Aesthetic Surgery, Akdeniz University School of Medicine, Antalya, Turkey

9.3.1 Obstacles to the Expansion of the Program

As with other transplantations, the main obstacle in face transplantation is the low number of cadaveric donations. Transplantation of kidney and liver from a living donor has enabled this type of transplant to become widespread. In most composite tissue transplants such as face transplants, the major hurdle is the requirement for the donor pool to be only cadaveric [4]. When death by cessation of brain activity occurs for any reason, the first-degree relatives of the potential donor are not willing to donate organs. Especially women and young people's relatives are very reluctant to donate a face.

9.4 Patients

Proper donor selection is of utmost importance. Medical history and comorbidities as well as age of the donor should be thoroughly investigated. The age difference between the recipient and the donor must be about 10 years. The existing comorbidities of the donor before death could affect the tolerance to ischemia and healing process of the tissue to be transplanted. The age range of our donors was 19–42 years. The sex of the donors was matched with the recipient [5]. Suicide and traffic accidents were the most common causes of death (Table 9.1).

Recipients' age range was similarly 19–54 years. The most common causes were burn and gunshot injury, resulting in significant functional limitations. Inability to breathe through nose, failure of oral feeding and absence of facial expression were the most frequent problems (Table 9.1). Due to these limitations, they had undergone ten or more surgical operations in other centers before face transplantation. After physical examination, psychological assessment, and necessary lab tests, patients were added to the waiting list for face transplantation.

© Springer Nature Switzerland AG 2023

R. Gurunian et al. (eds.), *Reconstructive Transplantation*, https://doi.org/10.1007/978-3-031-21520-9_9

Table 9.1 Summary of our patients

	Date of TX	Donor age	Recipient age	Recipient current age, sex	Indication	Allograft components	Facial nerve neurorraphies	Sensory neurorraphies	Total allograft ischemia (hours)	Duration of operation (hours)	Episodes of rejection
Patient 1	21.01.2012	37	19	27, M	Burn, 1 yo	Facial skin and facial musculature, with exception of eyelids and nasal bones	Bilateral facial nerve's frontal branches, buccal branches, and marginal mandibular branches	Bilateral infraorbital, supraorbital and mental nerves	4h	9h	Grade 0 P/CS: 1/2 Grade 1 P/CS: 7/12 Grade 2 P/CS: 3/20 Grade 3 P/CS: 1/3
Patient 2	15.05.2012	19	35	43, M	Burn, 3 yo	All facial skin and facial musculature, together with eyelids, nasal bones, the anterior half of the hair bearing scalp, and the right auricle	Inferior alveolar and facial nerve trunk	Bilateral infraorbital nerves	4h	9h	Grade 0 P/CS: 4/3 Grade 1 P/CS: 7/7 Grade 2 P/CS: 1/3 Grade 3 P/CS: 0/0
Patient 3	18.07.2013	42	26	33, M	Gunshot injury-6 years before TX	All facial skin and facial musculature, the upper and lower jaws and nasal bones	Facial nerve trunk	Bilateral infraorbital, supraorbital and mental nerves	5h	11h	Grade 0 P/CS: 3/0 Grade 1 P/CS: 7/0 Grade 2 P/CS: 2/2 Grade 3 P/CS: 0/0
Patient 4	23.08.2013	31	54	Ex(PTLD)	Gunshot injury-4 years before TX	All facial skin and facial musculature, both eyelids, nasal bones, maxilla, part of the mandible, base of tongue, and the anterior part of the scalp	Buccal and marginal mandibular branches, inferior alveolar nerve	İnfraorbital and inferior alveolar nerves	5h	15h	Grade 0 P/CS: 4/2 Grade 1 P/CS: 2/2 Grade 2 P/CS: 0/0 Grade 3 P/CS: 0/0
Patient 5	28.12.2013	34	22	29, M	Gunshot injury-4 years before TX	The entire nose and upper lip	None	None	4h 20 min	11h	Grade 0 P/CS: 6/0 Grade 1 P/CS: 5/0 Grade 2 P/CS: 1/0 Grade 3 P/CS: 0/0

P protocol, *CS* cause specific

The selection of appropriate face transplant candidates is necessary for long-term success of the procedure. Face transplantation candidates are selected among those whose facial defect cannot be repaired conventionally, and whose mental status and physical condition are optimal. In addition, mental stability and psychological maturity should be confirmed in order to support compliance with lifelong use of immunosuppressants and social problems. In addition, it is very important that the recipients did not have a history of malignancy.

Choosing the appropriate donor is also important for the success of the operation. Full HLA compliance is not required, as in kidney transplantations. But face transplantation includes other primary criteria. Having the same gender, and similar skin color with the recipient is one of the criteria. It is stated in the literature that the age difference can be tolerated for up to 10 years due to the limited number of donations [6].

In addition to imaging studies such as 3D computed tomography, chest radiography, echocardiogram, blood tests (liver and kidney function tests, CMV, EBV, other viral markers, etc.), psychiatric evaluation was performed before the operation. Specific tests may be requested to observe the problems that we may encounter regarding the age and sex of the patient. Examples of these specific tests are the screening mammography in female individuals and age-appropriate colonoscopy in the both sexes and the level of prostate-specific antigen in men.

Transplantation procedures were carried out by our team after finding a suitable donor. In our center, five face transplantations were performed, four of which were full-face and one of them was midface.

9.4.1 Patient 1

Our first patient was 19 years old when the transplant was performed. Facial deformity was caused by a burn injury at the age of 1 year. The patient had functional limitations caused by involvement of the entire nose and upper lip. In addition to these findings, there was no facial expression. To resolve these functional limitations, face transplantation was performed. Facial skin and facial musculature, except for eyelids and nasal bones, were transplanted on January 21, 2012. The patient underwent antibody screening for viral infections such as CMV and EBV before transplantation. The ischemia time was about 4 h, and the transplantation procedure took about 9 h. During the surgery, 5 units of packed red blood cells were transfused. After the operation, the patient was kept intubated and followed up in the intensive care unit. On the third postoperative day, the patient was extubated.

Neutropenia below 100/mL developed in the early postoperative months, which required GM-CSF. The MMF (mycophenolate mofetil) dose was adjusted according to the severity of neutropenia, with maximum of 500 mg twice a day. Nonspecific findings were detected in bone marrow biopsy, and the problems resolved spontaneously 3 months after surgery.

The first rejection episode occurred at the twelfth month and scored Grade 2 according to the BANFF classification. Following this rejection episode, multiple grade 1 and grade 2 rejection episodes were observed (Table 9.1). One of the reasons for the frequent occurrence of acute rejection was patient noncompliance with the immunosuppressive medications, especially in the first 2 years. The rejection episodes were responsive to treatments. All grade 1 rejections resolved with topical use of tacrolimus and an increase in tacrolimus dose. Grade 2 rejections were treated with administration of steroids together with a temporary increase in tacrolimus dose.

The first patient suffered a severe infection at the 24th month postoperatively. The patient developed severe viral pneumonia and required intensive care unit admission. No agent was isolated from samples, and immunosuppressive dosages were reduced, together with the administration of empiric antibacterial, antifungal, and antiviral prophylaxis (Fig. 9.1a). At the end of the treatments, the patient recovered successfully.

9.4.2 Patient 2

Our second patient had functional limitations such as no facial expression and inability to close the eyes due to burn injury. The patient underwent a face transplant on May 15, 2012. The operation was carried out in 9 h. The allograft ischemia time was 4 h. The transplanted tissues included facial muscles and skin, eyelids, tear ducts, nasal bones, the right auricle, and half of the hair bearing scalp. The patient was extubated on postoperative day (POD) 2 and the tracheostomy was decannulated on POD3.

The patient underwent levator muscle plication surgery for ptosis correction in the second postoperative month. In addition, lower eyelid surgery was performed for ectropion correction (Fig. 9.1b). The first rejection episode (Grade 2) occurred 12 months postoperatively.

9.4.3 Patient 3

Patient 3 had sustained a gunshot injury at the age of 20, which resulted in inability to breathe through nose, incomprehensible speech, lack of facial expression, and inability to close his mouth. When the patient reached the age of 26, a face transplant was performed in our center. All facial muscles and skin, the lower and upper jaws, and nasal bones were transplanted.

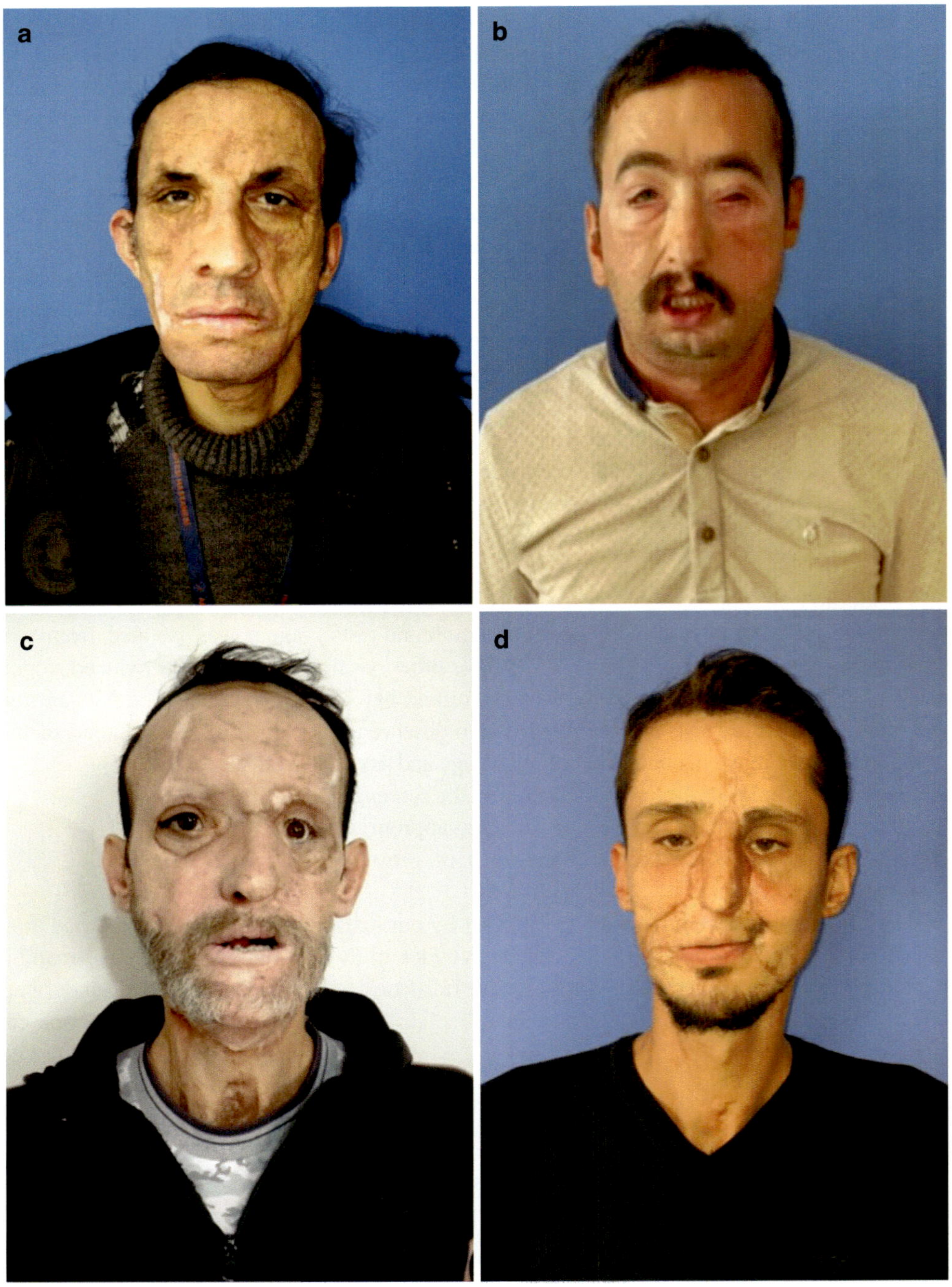

Fig. 9.1 Current photos of our face transplant patients. (**a**) Patient 1. (**b**) Patient 2. (**c**) Patient 3. (**d**) Patient 5

Total allograft ischemia time was 5 h, and the duration of the operation was 11 h. During the operation, 13 units of pRBCs were transfused. The patient was kept intubated with a tracheostomy for 5 days after the surgery and was transferred to the floor on the eighth day, postoperatively. The tracheostomy was closed on the 26th day.

Patient underwent orthognathic surgery 3 months postoperatively to provide better occlusion. At 6 months, he required drainage of an abscess and removal of hardware in the right infraorbital region (Fig. 9.1c).

The patient's first rejection episode (grade 2) occurred in the fifteenth month. This episode resolved with administration of steroids and a temporary increase of tacrolimus dose.

9.4.4 Patient 4

This patient was a 54-year-old man with significant disfigurement of the entire face following an accidental gunshot injury 5 years earlier. His large facial defect involved the maxilla, the mandible, and mid-face. These deformities were causing functional limitations, such as not being able to breathe through the nose, severely impaired speech, no facial expression, inability to close the mouth, drooling, and malodor. The patient was fed by jejunostomy and had tracheostomy. The transplantation duration was approximately 11 h, and all facial skin and facial muscula- ture, both eyelids, the nasal bone, the maxilla, part of the mandible, the base of the tongue, and the anterior part of the scalp were transplanted. The patient required transfusion of 13 units of pRBCs during the operation. After surgery, the recipient was transferred to the intensive care unit, where he was monitored for 2 days. He was transferred to the floor once his vital signs had been stabilized.

At post-op 5 months, two small ulcerative lesions appeared on the left hand's dorsum and the right pretibial regions [7]. Biopsy specimens identified both lesions as squamous cell carcinoma, and wide excision with split-thickness skin graft was performed. One month later (6 months postoperatively), the patient presented a rapidly growing 2×2 cm ulcerative nodule (lymph node) in the left preauricular region. Total excision of the mass was performed, and histopathological examination revealed a CD-20(+) diffuse large B-cell lymphoma. The patient was diagnosed with Stage IIIA non-Hodgkin lymphoma (NHL). Treatment was commenced with a reduction of immunosuppressive therapy and R-CHOP regimen (rituximab, cyclophosphamide, vincristine, adriamycin, and prednisolone). A low level of tacrolimus was administered, maintaining a blood level of 2–3 ng/mL, with 5 mg of prednisolone. Although rapamycin had been started to reduce the tacrolimus dosage and benefit from its antitumor effect, this was discontinued 1 week later because of pulmonary complications such as dyspnea on exertion and dry cough.

Nine months postoperatively, aspergillosis was diagnosed, and liposomal B was started, the dose was adjusted based on increasing creatinine levels [7]. Wide spectrum antibacterial antibiotics were administered together with antifungal treatment. Control PET/CT scanning revealed a highly active area in the right cerebellum. Magnetic resonance imaging (MRI) was performed for confirmation of diagnosis, and a 1-mm lesion was identified close to the pons Following consultation with the neurology and neurosurgery, it proved impossible to take a biopsy sample from the lesion because of its location. The lesion was thought to represent cerebellar aspergillosis.

The patient presented ataxia, concordant with the cerebellar lesion. All immunosuppressive agents used were completely stopped. Face transplant was monitored with serial biopsies from the skin and oral mucosa as well as by clinical observation.

Ten months postoperatively, biopsy specimens revealed grade 2 rejection. To prevent further progression of rejection and in view of adverse effects of immunosuppressive medications, the facial allograft was removed and the defect reconstructed with a free flap [7]. Two teams worked simultaneously. The pedicles of the flap, external carotid arteries, and internal jugular veins were located. Facial allograft pedicles were ligated bilaterally. Allograft's skin, subcutaneous layers, muscle, parotid glands, and mucosa, as well as bony parts of the maxilla, mandible, nose, and zygomatic arch were removed. All surrounding soft tissues and tooth segments were removed on the table. These were then placed in their original locations as bone grafts. Soft tissue coverage was performed with a large free anterolateral thigh (ALT) flap. The flap was harvested on four separate perforators based on a main vascular pedicle. Incisions were made to reconstruct the orifices of the eye, nose, and mouth. Anastomoses were performed in an end-to-end manner to the external carotid artery and in an end-to-end manner to the internal jugular vein. The whole procedure lasted 5 h.

The patient died despite a prolonged attempt at cardiopulmonary resuscitation on posttransplantation month 11. Autopsy was recommended for differentiation between aspergillosis and lymphoma, but the family refused. A biopsy examination of the removed transplanted tissue revealed grade 1–2 rejection.

9.4.5 Patient 5

This patient was referred to our center at the age of 21 for a mid-face defect caused by gunshot injury 4 years earlier. Physical examination revealed functional limitations such as inability to breathe through the nose, speech disorder, lack of facial expression, and inability to close the mouth. At the age of 22 (2013), a face transplant involving the entire nose and upper lip was performed. During the 11-h operation, there was no need for blood transfusion, and the patient's duration of intubation time was 1 day. On POD 3, the patient was transferred to the floor. Minimal scar revision surgery was performed after 1 year (Fig. 9.1d).

The treatment of the first rejection episode at 24 months was similar to the treatment of the other patients.

9.5 Surgical Technique

One team harvested the face allograft. All allografts were perfused with University of Wisconsin solution and transported in an ice-water slurry. The prosthodontist on the donor team prepared a mask prior to allograft recovery. This mask was applied after allograft removal to preserve donor body integrity. Simultaneously with the donor operation, another team removed the scarred remnants of recipient skin and facial tissue and prepared all necessary motor and sensory nerve branches and neck vessels.

All facial allografts exhibited full perfusion after transplantation, and neural repair was performed when needed. End-to-end arterial anastomoses were performed between external carotid arteries in all four full-face transplantations. Bilaterally venous anastomoses were performed between the external jugular veins in an end-to-end manner and internal jugular vein matches in an end-to-side manner. In the case of partial face transplantation, arterial anastomoses were performed between the external carotid artery on one side and between the facial arteries on the other side. End-to-side venous anastomoses were performed between the external jugular vein on one side and between the internal jugular veins on the other side.

Facial nerve coaptations and sensory neural repair were performed in four cases, excluding partial face transplant. In the first two full-face and partial (patient 5) transplant patients, only the nasal bones were fixed for skeletal reconstruction, while in the third and fourth patients, both Le-Fort III segment fixation and central mandibular segment fixation were performed.

Patients were initially treated in the intensive care unit for a few days and then transferred to the surgical floor until discharge. In our four cases, the donor tissue was obtained from various centers located quite far from our own institution. Cold ischemia time ranged from 1 to 3 h, and total ischemia time ranged from 2 to 6 h.

9.5.1 Immunosuppression Protocol

Initial induction treatment: Anti-thymocyte globulin and prednisolone were administered. Anti-thymocyte globulin was initiated intraoperatively at a dose of 2.5 mg/kg per day. Prednisolone was started on the day of surgery, at 1000 mg and tapered down to 20 mg, 1 week postoperatively. On post-op day 4, tacrolimus (0.2 mg/kg Prograf per day with blood levels 15–20 ng/mL) was started. Anti-thymocyte globulin was stopped on day 7–10, depending on the blood CD3 level and the achievement of the desired tacrolimus blood levels.

Maintenance treatment: Prednisolone (20 mg/day) tapered to 10 mg/day 6 months postoperatively, tacrolimus (blood levels between 15 and 20 ng/mL for the first 3 months, tapered to 7–10 ng/mL 6 months postoperatively), and mycophenolate mofetil (MMF) (2 g/day) represented the maintenance regimen.

Treatment of acute rejection: The dose of tacrolimus was increased, and topical tacrolimus treatment was initiated in addition to systemic tacrolimus. We also used a steroid bolus during acute episodes.

9.5.2 Monitoring Protocol

Mucosal biopsies were scheduled every 2 weeks for 3 months in the transplanted oral mucosa, and then monthly for 6 months. Skin biopsies close to incision scars were performed every month for the first 6 months and then every 3 months from the most inconspicuous area. Biopsy samples were analyzed according to the Banff 2007 classification.

9.5.3 Rehabilitation Protocol

The face has an important role for speech, communication skills, eye protection, expression of emotional states, and vital activities such as eating [8, 9] and psychological and social significance as 2/3 of our communication takes place through nonverbal facial expressions. Therefore, the facial rehabilitation protocol includes three main domains. These are speech therapy, range of motion exercises, and sensory recovery training. Both the patient and the transplant team need to understand the roles of this therapy in recovery [8, 9].

Facial transplantation rehabilitation focuses on sensory and motor function restoration, speech, breathing, and swallowing. It is very important to regain independence in activities of daily living. Thus, the therapeutic effects of face transplantation, such as social reintegration and alleviation of psychosocial barriers, will also emerge. It should not be forgotten that the overall goal of face transplantation is to restore facial function and movement. As a result of the successful face transplant, the patient's physical, emotional, social, and spiritual independence will increase [10].

The physiotherapy program should start after the patient is stabilized. It is one of the most important posttransplantation steps of the transplantation that the patient and family should be informed about. Treatment steps to be followed during rehabilitation [8]:

1. Assessment of function and dysfunction.
2. Establish long- and short-term goals.
3. Development and application of treatment methods.
4. Monitoring and reassessment of the progress toward the goals.

The first assessment should include passive and active range of motion in the cervical region, temporomandibular joint movements, upper and lower extremities muscle strength, flexibility and endurance, sensory functions of the face, daily life activity performance, and especially facial movements and function observations. Functions of the facial muscle groups in the facial expression should be a focus for the physical therapist.

Treatment methods commonly used in facial neuromuscular rehabilitation can be summarized as patient education, facial muscle physiotherapy techniques (muscle relaxation techniques, stimulation, mirror exercises, facial muscle training), speech and swallowing training, smell and odor training, daily life activities, and psychosocial support.

In our center, respiratory support and positioning were provided in the intensive care unit for the first 5 days. When the patients were transferred to the ward, motor and sensory studies were performed to support eating and drinking functions. More emphasis was placed on breathing exercises. Attention was paid to the position of the head and neck when sitting, lying, and standing. Mobilization was provided as early as possible. During this early period, the synergistic movements of the head, neck, face, and extremities were observed, and the patient and family were informed. The compliance of the family and the patient with the treatment was important for the post-surgical protection and continuity of the treatment. Initially protective approaches were gradually be replaced by more controlled movements and then daily life activity.

From the first month to the third month, functionality and rehabilitation were planned more actively. The patients were more active; active/active assisted face and lip exercises, swallowing and breathing exercises, adaptation exercises for daily life activities, strengthening and mobility exercises for face and facial muscles. At these stages, the patient's psychological state was considered, and it was not forgotten that socio-cultural adjustment problems affected rehabilitation.

In this time period mirror exercises, electrical stimulation, proprioceptive neuromuscular facilitation techniques, and sensory training were used intensively.

Self-massage and passive stretching techniques were demonstrated to restore normal muscle length and improve facial muscle tone.

Stimulation techniques were used in the appropriate period when the facial muscles were hypotonic and by considering the postoperative measures and protocol. Electric stimulation was used with caution. It was noted that it did not cause problems such as burns and synkinesia due to loss of sensation.

The independence of patients, who were discharged from hospital at approximately 4–6 months, increased. This was the most important psychological period of the patient. The physiotherapist worked for the patient to become the most independent in their functions such as safety, mobility, compliance with daily life activities, speaking, and eating. The aim of the entire rehabilitation process was to achieve maximum independence in this period when reintegration is achieved.

Sensory trainings, muscle training, strengthening techniques, electrical stimulations, and motor point stimulations continued through in this process.

9.5.4 Unique Problems or Challenges Encountered

Squamous cell carcinoma developed in one of our patients (patient 4) on the fifth month after transplantation, and post-transplant lymphoproliferative diseases (PTLD) developed a month later [7]. The dose of immunosuppressant drugs was reduced, and R-CHOP treatment was started. However, pulmonary and cerebellar aspergillosis developed. Immunosuppressant drugs were discontinued and the transplant was followed up by serial biopsies. At the tenth month after transplantation, grade 2 rejection occurred. Transplanted face was removed and replaced with ALT flap at tenth month. The patient died 11 months after the transplantation.

9.6 Lessons Learned

9.6.1 Challenges

Malignancy is one of the most important catastrophic complications of immunosuppressant agents used at transplant patients. We lost one of our patients due to malignencies, which is one of the most important challenges that can be encountered [11]. Posttransplant lymphoproliferative disorder [12, 13] is less responsive to conventional treatment, and outcomes are often poor. Although reduction or withdrawal of immunosuppression is the first step in treatment and has great prognosis in solid organ transplants, we do not have adequate experience in patients undergoing vascularized composite tissue transplants.

Another factor that complicates the progression of the composite tissue transplant program is the side effects of the immunosuppressants and opportunistic infections. In particular, unlike solid organs, the large interaction area of face transplants with the environment increases the possibility of infection. Opportunistic infections may specifically create potential foci in facial allografts containing paranasal sinuses. Exposure to direct mechanical and surgical trauma, including postoperative manipulative procedures such as irrigation and gastrointestinal tube insertion, is other possible predisposing factors for opportunistic infections.

Fungal infections are life-threatening opportunistic infections. The presence of clinically nonspecific symptoms makes early diagnosis difficult. They are generally well disseminated when diagnosed, and associated mortality rates are around 90%.

9.6.2 What Did You Change Over Time?

We are not accepting donors from long distance centers. This decision was taken for reasons related to circulation and tissue perfusion.

9.6.3 What Will You Not Repeat in the Future?

We lost one of our patients due to malignancy. If a face transplant patient develops a malignancy, we plan to remove the transplanted face without wasting time.

9.6.4 How Do You See the Future of VCA?

The development of modern immunosuppressant agents will enable the advancement of composite tissue transplants as well as solid organ transplantations. In addition to developing immunosuppressant agents, some centers are working on some modified immunosuppressant protocols to reduce the side effects of these drugs used in transplantations. Structuring of the recipient's immune system by transplanting the donor's bone marrow is one of these trials. As a result of these trials, the groups working in Pittsburgh/Johns Hopkins declared that they could control the transplantation process by using only one agent [14]. Although this protocol constitutes a chimeric structure, it seems that there is no complete tolerance protocol, since it cannot eliminate alloreactivity. Despite this mentioned study, data obtained from composite tissue transplantation studies performed in animal experiments show that the most realistic possibility for composite tissue transplantation tolerance is the creation of stable mixed chimerism, at least for the near term. There are studies in the literature where reliable induction of skin tolerance has been demonstrated across MHC barriers [15]. Leonard et al. demonstrated the long-term chimerism in composite tissue transplants increasing the skin survival time [15]. However, the transplantation protocol used in this study cannot be directly pertinent for clinical applications. However, study findings still encourage the development of clinically feasible protocols for composite tissue allografts.

In addition to chimerism studies, studies have shown that mesenchymal stem cells not only suppress inflammation and acute rejection in composite tissue transplantation but also modulate T-cell regulation and related cytokine expression [16, 17]. It has been shown that adipose-derived stem cells increase the life span of the skin content as a result of suppressing the Th-17 immune response [18]. This result indicates that stem cell therapies can be used in auxiliary and/or main treatment protocols to increase the survival time of composite tissue transplantations, which are rich in skin contents.

Three-dimensional modeling (3D printing), from patients' radiological imaging, will be of great importance in planning the surgery. Thus, possible complications during surgery can be prevented. Also, the operation time is shortened as a result of an exercise on a three-dimensional model before the operation. Thus, complications such as ischemia caused by long surgery time can be decreased. Besides, 3D printing is essential to show patients the planned surgery.

As the field of composite tissue transplantation continues to evolve, alternative options are also being explored. In the future, significant advances in autologous tissue engineering, better facial prostheses, or traditional methods may offer results that eliminate the need for composite tissue transplants and reduce patient morbidity [19]. However, the development of the three-dimensional structure necessary for the formation of tissues and the stratification of different cell origins present significant challenges. Therefore, autologous tissue engineering is still far from widespread therapeutic use. As a result, due to the presence of more than one tissue in composite tissue transplantation, it seems complicated for tissue engineering to replace composite tissue transplantations in the near future.

Funding Surgical procedure and postoperative immunosuppression therapy associated with face transplants are very costly. However, transplant costs for Turkish citizens with social security in our country are covered by the state. Similarly, the costs of face transplantation are covered by the state.

References

1. Ozkan O, Demirkan F, Ozkan O, Dinckan A, Hadimioglu N, Tuzuner S, et al. The first (double) hand transplantation in Turkey. Transplant Proc. 2011;43(9):3557–60.
2. Ozkan O, Akar ME, Erdogan O, Ozkan O, Hadimioglu N. Uterus transplantation from a deceased donor. Fertil Steril. 2013;100(6):e41.
3. Ozkan O, Akar ME, Ozkan O, Erdogan O, Hadimioglu N, Yilmaz M, et al. Preliminary results of the first human uterus transplantation from a multiorgan donor. Fertil Steril. 2013;99(2):470–6.
4. Ozkan O, Ertosun MG, Ozkan O. Technical, immunological, and ethical similarities and differences between vascularized composite allotransplantation and solid organ transplantation in current practice. Transplant Proc. 2018;50(10):3775–82.
5. Ozkan O, Ozkan O, Ubur M, Hadimioglu N, Cengiz M, Afsar I. Face allotransplantation for various types of facial disfigurements: a series of five cases. Microsurgery. 2018;38(8):834–43.
6. Aflaki P, Nelson C, Balas B, Pomahac B. Simulated central face transplantation: age consideration in matching donors and recipients. J Plast Reconstr Aesthet Surg. 2010;63(3):e283–5.
7. Ozkan O, Ozkan O, Dogan U, Yilmaz VT, Uysal H, Undar L, et al. Consideration of difficulties and exit strategies in a case of face allotransplantation resulting in failure. Microsurgery. 2017;37(6):661–8.
8. Dixon PL, Zhang X, Domalain M, Flores AM, Lin VWH. Physical medicine and rehabilitation after face transplantation. In: The know-how of face transplantation. Cham: Springer; 2011. p. 151–72.
9. Siemionow M. The decade of face transplant outcomes. J Mater Sci Mater Med. 2017;28(5):64.
10. Gulbetekin E, Bayraktar S, Ozkan O, Uysal H, Ozkan O. Face perception in face transplant patients. Facial Plast Surg. 2019;35(5):525–33.
11. Kanitakis J, Petruzzo P, Gazarian A, Testelin S, Devauchelle B, Badet L, et al. Premalignant and malignant skin lesions in two recipients of vascularized composite tissue allografts (face, hands). Case Rep Transplant. 2015;2015:356459.
12. Diaz-Siso JR, Sosin M, Plana NM, Rodriguez ED. Face transplantation: complications, implications, and an update for the oncologic surgeon. J Surg Oncol. 2016;113(8):971–5.
13. Piselli P, Verdirosi D, Cimaglia C, Busnach G, Fratino L, Ettorre GM, et al. Epidemiology of de novo malignancies after solid-organ transplantation: immunosuppression, infection and other risk factors. Best Pract Res Clin Obstet Gynaecol. 2014;28(8):1251–65.

14. Schneeberger S, Gorantla VS, Brandacher G, Zeevi A, Demetris AJ, Lunz JG, et al. Upper-extremity transplantation using a cell-based protocol to minimize immunosuppression. Ann Surg. 2013;257(2):345–51.
15. Leonard DA, Kurtz JM, Mallard C, Albritton A, Duran-Struuck R, Farkash EA, et al. Vascularized composite allograft tolerance across MHC barriers in a large animal model. Am J Transplant. 2014;14(2):343–55.
16. Kuo YR, Chen CC, Goto S, Huang YT, Wang CT, Tsai CC, et al. Immunomodulatory effects of bone marrow-derived mesenchymal stem cells in a swine hemi-facial allotransplantation model. PLoS One. 2012;7(4):e35459.
17. Ertosun MG, Ozkan O, Ozkan O. Effects of different tacrolimus doses on adipose-derived stem cells. Exp Clin Transplant. 2021;19(7):723–31.
18. Larocca RA, Moraes-Vieira PM, Bassi EJ, Semedo P, de Almeida DC, da Silva MB, et al. Adipose tissue-derived mesenchymal stem cells increase skin allograft survival and inhibit Th-17 immune response. PLoS One. 2013;8(10):e76396.
19. Susarla SM, Swanson E, Gordon CR. Craniomaxillofacial reconstruction using allotransplantation and tissue engineering: challenges, opportunities, and potential synergy. Ann Plast Surg. 2011;67(6):655–61.

Facial Transplantation: Nonimmune-Related Hyperacute Graft Failure

10

Fabio Santanelli di Pompeo and Benedetto Longo

10.1 Introduction

Face transplantation is a new surgical experimental technique that represents one of the most prominent areas of vascularized composite allotransplantation (VCA). It allows replacement of severely compromised or lost specialized portions of the face overcoming limitations of conventional autologous free flap procedures [1–6]. Since the first facial allograft transplantation performed in France in 2005, a total of 48 (including Italy's first case) partial and full facial allograft transplantations (FAT) have been performed worldwide. Despite the advent of innovative immunosuppressive drugs and the commitment of skilled surgeons, this innovative technique raised many questions regarding the acceptable risk-benefit ratio, indications, and alternative salvage procedures to perform in case of eventful outcomes [7]. Risks, side effects, and health implications associated with the need for life-long immunosuppression to prevent graft rejection may result in adverse outcomes such as facial graft loss and patient's death. A negative outcome, such as this, highlights the experimental status of this procedure. An accurate examination of the previous medical history should be performed by the transplantation team, as well as a comprehensive psychological evaluation should be conducted prior to transplantation surgery to exclude any contraindication to the procedure [8]. Both patient and physician have the duty and responsibility to discuss the best treatment options and acceptable risks before proceeding with the inclusion on the waiting list for facial transplantation. Patient and families should also be carefully advised about the media attention to this procedure and pressure that some reporters could put on for exclusive interviews. In our center, facial transplantation program was carefully evaluated and then approved by the multidisciplinary team of Sant'Andrea Hospital, by the Italian National Transplant Center and National Ethical Committee. Then the comprehensive experimental protocol was submitted to the Ministry of Health in 2014 (DGPRE 0034369-P-23/11/2015) by the principal investigators (Fabio Santanelli di Pompeo and Benedetto Longo) and eventually approved in 2015 [9]. As with organ transplantations, the costs of facial transplant program were completely covered by the Italian National Healthcare System which provides universal coverage to citizens and residents. Actually, the program is still active, and we do have two patients on the waiting list. One is a female NF1 patient who is indicated to facial retransplantation because of first partial face transplantation failure and salvage procedure with autologous flap, while the other is a male patient affected by Sturge-Weber Syndrome with a giant hemangioma of the inferior and central face. The main problem we are facing in managing these complex patients is the process of donation that requires long time to find an available donor. Consent to and authorization of face tissues procurement are constant elements of psychological distress or conflict with the families. In our first experience, it took almost 4 years to find an available donor and get the consent from her relatives. In Italy, the process to express individual consent is an opting-in system in which consent to donation has to be explicitly obtained. As face transplantation is considered a life-improving procedure, such a regulation makes the donation process more difficult and provided us with the first donor after long time. Although Competent Authorities allowed the possibility of living organ donation and recognized vascularized composite allotransplantations as "organs," unfortunately there can-

F. S. di Pompeo (✉)
Division of Plastic Surgery, Sant'Andrea Hospital, NESMOS Department, School of Medicine and Psychology, "Sapienza" University of Rome, Rome, Italy
e-mail: Fabio.santanelli@uniroma1.it

B. Longo
Division of Plastic and Reconstructive Surgery – Breast Unit, Tor Vergata University Hospital, Department of Surgical Sciences, School of Medicine and Surgery, Tor Vergata University of Rome, Rome, Italy
e-mail: Benedetto.longo@uniroma2.it

© Springer Nature Switzerland AG 2023

R. Gurunian et al. (eds.), *Reconstructive Transplantation*, https://doi.org/10.1007/978-3-031-21520-9_10

not be a living face donor because of the intrinsic unique properties of facial tissues. In this time of restrictions for health resources, economic issues are becoming more important. In our experience, logistics, human resources, procedure costs, and lifelong cost of immunosuppression are becoming prohibitive and sustainable only in very few cases. Moreover, in our country, the system of Diagnosis-Related Group (DRG), which is used by regional healthcare systems to reimburse the hospitals for each medical and surgical procedure, does not appropriately cover the expenses for routine microsurgical procedures, negatively affecting the application and development of such methods in advanced plastic surgery centers.

10.2 Patient

Consent for facial tissue donation was obtained following consent for solid organs donation. The donor was selected based on matching of gender, skin color, age, and facial anthropometrics. A 21-year-old Caucasian female, brain-dead, heart beating donor with compatible blood group and negative cross match was selected.

A 49-year-old female patient affected by NF1 with a giant neurofibroma involving the whole left hemiface and defacing the ipsilateral eyelids, nose, upper and lower lips, malar and maxilla-mandibular bones was selected for facial transplantation. Even though she had undergone several previous surgeries, she still suffered severe functional and aesthetic deformity with left facial nerve palsy, epiphora, and lagophthalmos of the left eye, recurrent sinusitis associated with obstruction of left nasal airway, inability to chew solid food due to difficult mastication cause nonfunctional residual remnants of maxilla and mandible, and incomplete lip closure. The patient was blood group A, rhesus positive, and had a negative panel reactive antibody (PRA) status. She was also negative for cytomegalovirus and Epstein-Barr virus, HCV and HBV, HTLV 1, Treponema screening, and HIV. The patient was also affected by multiple sclerosis (MS), and her candidacy to FAT was carefully assessed by the multidisciplinary team of Sant'Andrea Hospital, by the National Ethical Committee and Italian National Transplant Center, and eventually approved by the Ministry of Health (DGPRE 0034369-P-23/11/2015). Psychological evaluation by two clinical psychologists was assessed over a 2-year period examining her capability to give informed consent and eventually positively considered to be a recipient for FAT. Relatives were also fully informed about all the risks, postoperative course, and possible sequelae. Preoperative computer tomography angiography (CTA) with three-dimensional reconstruction models, and magnetic resonance imaging were performed to outline bony, soft tissue needs, and vascular anatomy for surgical planning.

Simulations of the intraoperative steps were performed by all members of surgical teams. Donor and recipient cadaveric rehearsals in a real-time, simultaneous two-team approach were performed at the Department of Plastic Surgery and Hand Surgery, University Hospital Zurich, Switzerland, and Department für Anatomie, Histologie und Embryologie, Section Klinisch Funktionelle Anatomie, Innsbruck Medical University, Austria. Donor mask production has also been simulated twice on cadaver and volunteer at University Hospital Zurich and Ronchetti & Ronchetti Laboratories of Rome, respectively.

The surgical preoperative plan was aimed to restore the whole left hemiface including the auricle, all skin and soft tissues from the temporal region, under the eyebrow, periorbital region, including the lateral three fourth of the upper and lower eyelid together with orbicularis oculi, and the levator muscles and conjunctival mucosa up to the level of the cornea. In our preoperative dissection studies emerged that the three major branches of the anterior auricular arteries and their anastomotic networks provided good blood supply to the entire auricle including the external auditory meatus (Fig. 10.1). The planned facial allograft would also include:

- Lateral orbital wall
- Infraorbital nerve
- Entire nasal skin with upper lateral cartilage
- Alar cartilages and anterior part of the nasal septum and mucosa
- Maxillary process of the zygomatic bone
- Left hemimaxilla (harvested by hemi Le Fort I osteotomy)
- Mouth
- Hemimandible from contralateral parasymphysis to the incisura mandibulae

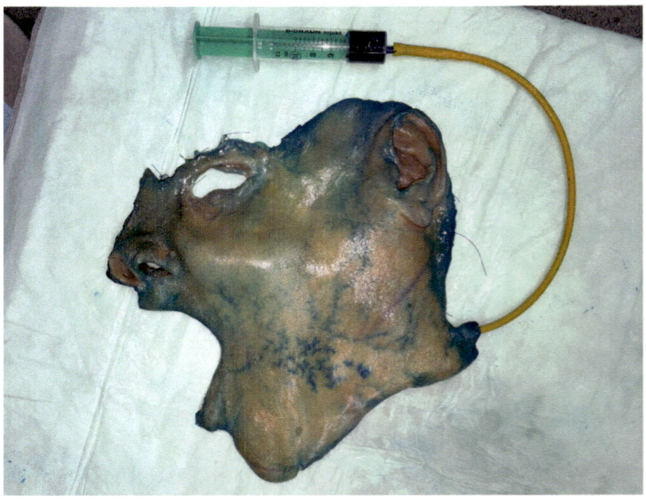

Fig. 10.1 Evaluation of perfusion to auricle based on the anterior auricular arteries, dissection study

- Anterior floor of the mouth muscles and overlying mucosa
- Whole left intraoral cheek mucosa up to the anterior tonsillar pillar
- Parotid gland including its superficial and deep portions with facial nerve main trunk and its bifurcation, and Stenson's duct

The lingual-facial trunk and submandibular gland were preserved and the left external carotid artery and internal and external jugular veins were then dissected. The facial allograft was detached and perfused on a back table with Celsior cold solution and transported in ice water slurry, then all organs were perfused with cold Celsior solution. The facial allograft harvest took 6 h.

The dissection and radical debridement of recipient's malformation were performed simultaneously as the procurement. This started with the placement of a percutaneous endoscopic gastrostomy (PEG) and tracheostomy. The recipient vessels were first dissected including left external carotid artery, internal and external jugular veins, while completion of malformation debridement proceeded and was finalized once the donor facial allograft was confirmed to be well perfused before detachment of the FAT. The main trunk of left facial nerve at the level of the stylomastoid foramen was located and preserved, left hemi Le Fort I and hemimandibulectomy were performed to remove maxillary and mandibular remnants which were involved with the neurofibromas. Anterior floor of the mouth along with left lateral and central facial skin and soft tissues including all poor-quality tissue were removed. Fragments of the orbicularis oculi, upper and lower eyelids, orbital process of the maxillary bone along with miniplates and screws from previous surgeries were also removed. The recipient patient's debridement took 10 h.

After perfusing the allograft with heparin solution on a back table, because of the short ischemia time (125 min), the transplantation procedure started with an end-to-end interrupted stitches venous anastomosis between the left internal jugular vein of recipient and donor, then proceeded with an end-to-end interrupted stitches arterial anastomosis, between both external carotid arteries. After the first two anastomoses, perfusion of the facial allograft was excellent to the entire transplant, and a second end-to-end interrupted stitches venous anastomosis between external jugular veins of donor and recipient was performed to enhance venous outflow. The facial allograft was then tailored and inset into the recipient defect, starting with the maxillary and mandibular osteosyntheses fixing both bones into place, followed by facial nerve coaptation between the donor and recipient nerve stumps. Five hours after allograft's reperfusion, the flap became whitish with absence of arterial inflow. The arterial anastomosis was inspected and a massive thrombosis, predominantly extending into the donor external carotid artery, was found. After flushing and washing the allograft's carotid artery with heparin solution, an arterial end-to-end interrupted stitch anastomosis was done again. The arterial inflow remained robust for approximately 30 min, and then the artery thrombosed again. It was then decided to shorten also the donor artery, by discarding the terminal portion of the wall close to blood clots, lumens were washed again with heparin solution, and third arterial anastomotic attempt was performed still in an end-to-end interrupted fashion. Following the arterial pedicle shortening, the venous anastomoses were also revised to avoid venous kinking. The perfusion was restored again, even though still reduced compared to previous ones, but because the FAT was still perfused, all the team decided to proceed with the allograft inset.

Facial restoration took 10 h, while the total surgical time was 26 h, and the whole procedure from notification of a potential donor to completion of surgery was 38 h. The recipient operative blood loss was 380 ml, and two units of packed red blood cells were transfused. There were two intraoperative arterial thromboses that were promptly solved with new anastomoses and sufficient, albeit diminished flap perfusion. Kidney and liver transplants were successfully completed.

Induction immunosuppression involved rabbit antithymocyte globulin (1.5 mg/kg) for 4 days, and tacrolimus-based triple therapy (target 10–12 ng/ml) with mycophenolate mofetil and methylprednisolone (500 mg iv) with tapering doses. The antibiotic protocol included clindamycin, ciprofloxacin, micafungin, ganciclovir (5 mg/kg), and trimethoprim/sulfamethoxazole. Postoperative low molecular weight heparin (4000 IU bid) was also administered.

On postoperative day 2, the allograft became very pale with suspected arterial occlusion. Skin biopsies were performed and showed balloon degeneration and pyknosis of the epidermal basal layer and skeletal muscle, confirming diffuse microcirculatory thrombosis. Therefore, the patient was taken back to the operative room for exploration, confirming the FAT was not perfused. It was then decided to remove the allograft and reconstruct the recipient site with a composite left latissimus dorsi-serratus anterior flap whit meshed skin graft. The procedure took 6 h, and despite the small size of thoracodorsal artery and vein, the flap was well vascularized with uneventful post-op. The immunosuppressive medications were immediately discontinued as well as the antiviral and antifungal prophylaxis. On postoperative day 15 patient showed a noticeable reduction of glomerular filtration rate but maintained estimated glomerular filtration rate (eGFR) higher than 60 ml/min. The degree of loss of eGFR was thought to be due to slightly compromised preoperative renal function and perioperative medications. The patient had fever and a pulmonary infection with pseudomonas aeruginosa between postoperative day 75 and 110 treated with appropriate antibiotic therapy.

Histological examination of the facial allograft specimen showed a normal structure of external carotid arterial wall, with no signs of blood extravasation or severe acute inflammation of a hyperacute rejection. Nevertheless, the vascular lumen appeared clogged with blood laying directly in contact with the internal elastic lamina, indicating a complete loss of intimal layer. The microscopy of the peripheral skin of the cheek showed an absence of hyperacute rejection signs but demonstrated thrombosis of vasculature with integrity of vascular walls and loss of intimal layer.

The patient was discharged on postoperative day 125 with tracheostomy and PEG, and she is currently on the waiting list to undergo a second transplant procedure.

10.3 Lesson Learned

After the world's first partial face transplant was performed in Amiens in northern France in 2005, this experimental procedure and its accompanying ethical issues released a worldwide "media tsunami." Since then, face transplants became a concrete object of medical attention and morbid fascination symbolized in the face of first patient, a 38-year-old woman who had been mauled by her dog. The transplant was a surgical revolutionary procedure that dramatically improved the patient's appearance but placed her directly and somewhat uncomfortably in the media and public spotlight [10]. Every time a face transplant is performed worldwide, patient and surgical teams are squarely put in the public news, making the medical event as one of the most read and discussed. In our experience, the media could unveil and cover the news on the first Italian face transplant, when we were still in the operating room performing the surgical procedure, revealing some personal details of both the donor and the recipient with sensationalistic titles [11]. This caused a further psychological distress among all surgical team while we were facing the complicated situation of recurrent thromboses and revisions of vascular anastomoses.

While most transplants are not readily observable, face transplants are the most visible form of transplantation. Every time a face transplant recipient looks in a mirror, he or she sees the result of his or her surgery, a highly evident reminder of what has been lost and gained. Face transplants are also firmly bound up in psychological issues involving personal identity. Because the face represents its own personal identity, it has been called unquestionably the most important aesthetic anatomical feature of the human body, face transplants present bioethical issues not raised by other transplants. Will face transplantation recipients look like their former selves, the donor, or some hybrid? What if the patient does not accept the new "organ" as part of himself or herself? What if a rejection process or a complication pushes the surgeon to remove the transplanted tissues? Who should be approached to donate a face, how, and when?

Physicians and ethicists agree that physical and psychological risks and benefits of face transplantation need to be weighed carefully. The most obvious risk is surgery that fails: there is an estimated 10% chance of rejection within the first year and a 30–50% chance in 2–5 years. Nevertheless, recently the first US face transplant died of an unspecified infection after 12 years from surgery [12]. This suggests that, even after many years, a potentially fatal complication due to the immunosuppressive medications can happen. A failed face transplant could be devastating both to a patient and surgeons as well. The transplant must be removed, leaving an extensive facial wound that would require moving other tissues from elsewhere on the patient's body by further microsurgical procedure, shortly extra stressing patient and team. As of today, two patients have undergone second face transplant procedure for chronic rejection of transplanted tissues [13].

In case of suspected and critical situations, surgical solving strategies in vascularized composite tissue transplantations are particularly challenging. Salvage procedures may be required and should be accurately planned before surgery, in case of acute complications such as failures due to technical or early immunological and ischemic conditions. They may also be needed if the recipient patient is not psychologically compliant, or in conditions where the immunosuppressants need to be withdrawn due to severe infections [14], malignancies, or chronic rejection [15, 16]. In our first case of facial transplantation, the allograft was unfortunately removed on the second postoperative day, and a salvage procedure with a skin-grafted, combined autologous latissimus dorsi and serratus anterior muscle free transfer [1] was performed. Pathological findings of the allograft's biopsy did not show classical signs of hyperacute rejection confirmed by the negativity of C4d staining. A general and diffuse thrombosis of both the vascular components involved the entire allograft. We hypothesized that the complete loss of the endothelial and subendothelial glycocalyx of the intima, further confirmed by the accumulation of the platelet endothelial cell adhesion molecule-1 (PECAM-1), was activated by the clotting cascade, leading to irreparable hypoxic damage of the allograft with subsequent need to remove all transplanted tissues. Appropriately, our face transplantation failure appeared to be affected by vascular impairment rather than immunological rejection. Focusing on possible causes that disrupted the intimal layer and endothelial/subendothelial glycocalyx of the vascular walls, we tried to identify the reason of such complication.

In the organ transplantation scenario, the possible role of endothelial glycocalyx breakdown in graft failure has already been described on ex vivo lung perfusion [17], ischemic reperfusion injury [18, 19], and rejection in lung transplantation [20]. Based on the findings of solid organ transplants, catecholamines could primarily negatively interact with the vasculature of composite allograft. Moreover, administration of exogenous catecholamines for maintenance of circulatory stability in brain-death patients can even increase their detrimental effects on the vascular system [21]. In our donor, a young girl involved in a fatal motorcycle accident, a heavy dose of epinephrine and norepinephrine was administered before surgery (0.04 and 0.7 μg/kg/min, respectively), and it was even higher during the facial and organs procurement procedure (0.10 and 1.10 μg/kg/min, respectively) (Table 10.1). According to the catecholamine-induced damage hypothesis, the facial allograft vasculature could have had a preexisting latent endothelial dysfunction that was possibly enhanced indirectly by cold ischemia [22, 23] and further worsened by perfusion of cold preservation solution. This could explain the arterial thrombotic events that we experienced some hours after the allograft reperfusion, followed by the development of venous and diffuse capillary thrombosis found in the face allograft specimen. In our case, endothelial dysfunction cannot be directly attributed to an ischemia-reperfusion injury as warm and cold ischemia times were 53 and 38 min, respectively. Our donor received an amount of norepinephrine and epinephrine which is up to 10 times higher than the normal dose as to maintain systolic pressure ≥100 mmHg, and that, along with her autonomic storm produced in response to brain death (which typically increases endogenous catecholamine levels to about 7–8 times the normal concentrations), resulted in a marked rise of these vasoactive hormones. At present, catecholamine patterns in brain-death donors are a key parameter in heart [24] and lung transplantation [16, 25, 26], and the neuroendocrine effects of brain death are still under investigation in liver [27] and intestine transplantation [28]. In organ transplantation the mechanical injury to the vascular endothelium by manual [29] and hypothermic machine perfusion [30] has already been widely reported. The mechanism of perfusion injury is considered the causing factor of microvascular disturbances similar to classical vascular rejection in the absence of lymphocytic infiltrates, suggesting a "barotrauma" physical insult rather than pure immunological rejection [31]. Curtis et al. [32] reported a typical "hyperacute rejection" occurred in kidneys with the absence of immunological pathogenetic mechanism in the non-transplanted organs, identical signs of "hyperacute rejection" were observed in the organs' vasculature, finally reporting this phenomenon as syndrome of "hyperacute graft failure" secondary to non-immunologically mediated perfusion injury. These histological findings led the authors to assume that these preexisting endothelial damages were the preliminary factors with machine perfusion then compounding this injury [33]. Typically, perfusion injuries to the intimal layer are histologically described as fragmented, segmental or cut-like since they are produced by both vessel wall excessive distension and chemical trauma of saline solutions [34, 35], and likely accountable for the mechanism of platelet activation and early thrombotic complications. Our allograft showed such an extensive loss of the intimal layer from major arteries up to small veins, including parotid capillaries, that a multiple effect of several variables has been supposed. Though this is a single transplant, our adverse outcome has led us to suggest a working hypothesis of the possible damaging effect of very high levels of catecholamines (endogenous and administered) on endothelial surfaces. This phenomenon can be further impaired by cold ischemia with allograft perfusion, which eventually may permanently damage the endothelium leading to thrombosis and graft failure.

Table 10.1 Vasoactive amines administered to the donor

Day	Ward	Time	Norepinephrine (γ/kg/min)	Epinephrine (γ/kg/min)	Dopamine (γ/kg/min)
16-Sept	Emergency unit	3:26 am	0.5		
	ICU	5:30 am	0.5		
		10 am	0.10		
		1 pm	0.70		
		4 pm	0.90		5
		5 pm	1.00		5
		7 pm	1.00		10
17-Sept	ICU	1:30 am	1.00		5
		4 pm	0.80		
		9 pm	0.50		
18-Sept	ICU	10 am	0.40		
19-Sept	ICU	9 am	0.30		
		12 am	0.35		
		5 pm	0.40		
20-Sept	Neurosurgery	4 am	0.40		
	ICU	7 am	0.50	0.11	
		2 pm	0.50	0.08	
21-Sept		2 am	0.60	0.04	
22-Sept	ICU	1 am	0.70	0.04	
	Procurement surgery	2 am	1.10	0.10	

Now in our protocol, high doses of catecholamines administered to the donor for a long time preoperatively represent a relative exclusion criterion for face donation since then. Ideally, donor eligibility criterion for face transplant is low inotropic support (no epinephrine of norepinephrine). Face transplantation is still an experimental procedure, and restrictions in selection criteria for a successful result are of outmost importance for both recipients and donors.

Although composite allografts are not recognized as vital organs, the loss of the graft in the context of face transplantation is considered disastrous for both the recipient and the surgeons. Graft removal and replacement with autologous flap represent the best way to approach the salvage reconstructive procedure and to preserve patient's life. In this case, the facial defect following FAT failure was successfully reconstructed with a skin-grafted composite latissimus dorsi-serratus anterior free tissue transfer [1] allowing us to give the patient a reasonable temporary reconstruction and to put her again on the waiting list for a second face transplantation.

Accurate evaluation of the patient, proper donor selection, weighting risks and benefits of the procedure and following long-life administration of immunosuppressive medications with their biological implications will be the key to success of this exciting and very complex procedure in the near future.

Disclosure The authors declare no conflicts of interest. The authors declare no funding received for this work.

References

1. Longo B, Laporta R, Pagnoni M, et al. Skin grafted latissimus dorsi flap for reconstruction of lateral aesthetic units of the face. Microsurgery. 2015;35(3):177–82. https://doi.org/10.1002/micr.22305.
2. Longo B, Nicolotti M, Ferri G, et al. Sagittal split osteotomy of the fibula for modeling the new mandibular angle. J Craniofac Surg. 2013;24(1):71–4. https://doi.org/10.1097/SCS.0b013e318271018b.
3. Longo B, Paolini G, Belli E, et al. Wide excision and anterolateral thigh perforator flap reconstruction for dermatofibrosarcoma protuberans of the face. J Craniofac Surg. 2013;24(6):597–9. https://doi.org/10.1097/SCS.0b013e3182a238c1.
4. Longo B, Belli E, Pugliese P, Ferri G, Santanelli F. Bilobed skin paddle fibula flap for large oromandibular defects. J Craniofac Surg. 2013;24(4):327–30. https://doi.org/10.1097/SCS.0b013e31828a7856.
5. Longo B, Ferri G, Fiorillo A, Rubino C, Santanelli F. Bilobed perforator free flaps for combined hemitongue and floor-of-the-mouth defects. J Plast Reconstr Aesthet Surg. 2013;66(11):1464–9. https://doi.org/10.1016/j.bjps.2013.06.058.
6. Longo B, Pagnoni M, Ferri G, et al. The mushroom-shaped anterolateral thigh flap for subtotal reconstruction. Plast Reconstr Surg. 2013;132(3):656–65. https://doi.org/10.1097/PRS.0b013e31829acf84.
7. Shanmugarajah K, Hettiaratchy S, Butler PE. Facial transplantation. Curr Opin Otolaryngol Head Neck Surg. 2012;20(4):291–7.
8. Pomahac B, Nowinski D, Diaz-Siso JR, et al. Face transplantation. Curr Probl Surg. 2011;48(5):293–357.
9. Santanelli di Pompeo F, Longo B, Giovanoli P, et al. Facial Transplantation. Nonimmune-related hyperacute graft failure – the role of perfusion injury: a case report. Ann Plast Surg. 2021;86(4):469–75.
10. Azadeh Ansari SA. First face transplant patient, Isabelle Dinoire, dies at 49 CNN News2016 [CNN Official website]. Available https://edition.cnn.com/2016/09/06/health/france-face-transplant-patient-dies/index.html. Accessed 1 April 2020.
11. Al Sant'Andrea di Roma il primo trapianto di faccia in Italia. Available at https://www.iltempo.it/roma-capitale/2018/09/22/news/primo-trapianto-di-faccia-in-italia-in-corso-al-sant-andrea-1084621/. Accessed 25 Aug 2021.
12. Fay Bound Alberti, Victoria Hoyle. First US face transplant recipient dies, leaving an important legacy. Available https://theconversation.com/first-us-face-transplant-recipient-dies-leaving-an-important-legacy-144522. Accessed 25 Aug 2021.
13. The Associated Press. For the first time, a woman in the U.S. gets a second face transplant. Available https://www.nbcnews.com/health/health-news/first-time-woman-u-s-gets-second-face-transplant-n1236172. Accessed 25 Aug 2021.
14. Meningaud JP, Benjoar M, Hivelin M, et al. Procurement of total human face graft for allotransplantation: a preclinical study and the first clinical case. Plast Reconstr Surg. 2010;126(4):1181–90.
15. Morelon E, Petruzzo P, Kanitakis J, et al. Face transplantation: partial graft loss of the first case 10 years later. Am J Transplant. 2017;17(7):1935–40.
16. Kristova V, Krista M, Canova R, et al. Endothelial changes following repeated effect of vasoconstrictive substances in vitro. Acta Physiol Hung. 1993;81:363–70.
17. Soccal PM, Gasche Y, Poche J-C, et al. Matrix metalloproteinases correlate with alveolar-capillary permeability alteration in lung ischemia-reperfusion injury. Transplantation. 2000;70(7):998–1005.
18. Soccal PM, Gasche Y, Miniati DN, et al. Matrix metalloproteinase inhibition decreases ischemia-reperfusion injury after lung transplantation. Am J Transplant. 2004;4(1):41–50.
19. Yano M, Omoto Y, Yamakawa Y, et al. Increased matrix metalloproteinases 9 activity and mRNA expression in lung ischemia-reperfusion injury. J Heart Lung Transplant. 2001;20(6):679–86.
20. Beeh KM, Beier J, Kornmann O, et al. Sputum levels of metalloproteinase-1, and their ratio correlate with airway obstruction in lung transplant recipients: relation to tutor necrosis factor-a and interleukin-10. J Heart Lung Transplant. 2001;20(11):1144–51.
21. Ullah S, Zabala L, Watkins B, Schimtz ML. Cardiac organ donor management. Perfusion. 2006;21(2):93–8.
22. Lüscher TF, Barton M. Biology of the endothelium. Clin Cardiol. 1997;20:3–10.
23. Tousoulis D, Kampoli AM, Tentolouris C, et al. The role of nitric oxide on endothelial function. Curr Vasc Pharmacol. 2012;10:4–18.
24. Pérez López S, Otero Hernández J, Vázquez Moreno N, et al. Brain death effects on cathecolamine levels and subsequent cardiac damage assessed in organ donors. J Heart Lund Transp. 2009;28(8):815–20.
25. Vink H, Constantinescu AA, Spaan JA. Oxidized lipoproteins degrade the endothelial surface layer: implications for platelet-endothelial cell adhesion. Circulation. 2000;101:1500–2.
26. Makhmudov RM, Mamedov Y, Dolgov VV, Repin VS. Cathecolamine-mediated injury to endothelium in rabbit perfused aorta: a quantitative analysis by scanning electron microscopy. Cor Vasa. 1985;27:456–63.
27. Van der Hoeven JA, Moshage H, Schuur T, et al. Brain death induces apoptosis in donor liver of the rat. Transplantation. 2003;76(8):1150–4.

28. Koudstaal LG, Hart NA, Ottens PJ, et al. Brain death induces inflammation in the donor intestine. Transplantation. 2008;86(1):148–54.
29. Sheil AG, Drummond JM, Boulas J. Vascular Thrombosis in machine-perfused renal allograft. Transplantation. 1975;20(2):178–9.
30. Hill GS, Light JA, Perloff LJ. Perfusion-related injury in renal transplantation. Surgery. 1976;79(4):440–7.
31. Wilson CH, Gok MA, Shenton BK, et al. Weight increase during machine perfusion may be an indicator of organ and in particular vascular damage. Ann Transplant. 2004;9(2):31–2.
32. Curtiss JJ, Bhathena D, Lucas BA, et al. "Hyperacute rejection" due to perfusion injury. Clin Nephrol. 1977;7(3):120–4.
33. Hearse DJ, Bolli R. Reperfusion induced injury: manifestations, mechanisms, and clinical relevance. Cardiovasc Res. 1992;26(2):101–8.
34. Harjula ALJ, Mattila S, Järvinen A, et al. Endothelial cell damage following crystalloid cardioplegic solution infusion. Arch Surg. 1984;119:946–9.
35. Ramos JR, Berger K, Mansfield PB, et al. Histologic fate and endothelial changes of distended and nondistended vein graft. Ann Surg. 1976;183:205–28.

The Helsinki Vascularized Composite Allograft Program

11

Patrik Lassus

11.1 Building the Helsinki Vascular Composite Allotransplantation Program

11.1.1 Program Setup

The Helsinki Vascular Composite Allotransplantation (VCA) program was started in 2011 in the Department of Plastic Surgery, Helsinki University Hospital (HUH). The program was started by Patrik Lassus and strongly supported by the concurrent head of the department, Erkki Tukiainen. The setup of Helsinki program is explained in detail in a publication in 2018 [1].

11.1.1.1 Finnish National Solid Organ Transplantation Center

All organ transplantation activities are in Finland centralized to Helsinki University Hospital by legislation. Therefore, Helsinki is the only University that is allowed to perform VCAs, and Helsinki VCA program can be called the National Finnish VCA program. In Helsinki, the Solid Organ Transplantation (SOT) Center is in close connection with the national Organ Procurement Organization (OPO), and they operate in joint facilities. Helsinki VCA program is coordinated from the Department of Plastic Surgery but with close connection with the SOT Center.

11.1.1.2 Legal Issues

In 2011, there existed no national legislation concerning vascular composite allografts. At that time, the European Commission was preparing recommendations for national laws concerning VCAs. In 2012, European Commission recommended that VCAs should be categorized as organ transplantations. After that the Ministry of Health classified VCAs as "organs" in Finland, all VCA activities were subjected under organ transplantation legislation. This facilitated legal permission to be granted also by the National Supervisory Authority for Social Welfare and Health (Valvira) and the Finnish Medicines Agency (Fimea).

11.1.1.3 Helsinki University Hospital Permission

For the University Hospital permission, HUH required that the new VCA program should be aligned with the solid organ transplantation (SOT) team. In 2012, the VCA team started working on programs for face transplantation (FT), upper extremity transplantation (UET), abdominal wall transplantation (AWT), and laryngeal transplantation (LT). The main issue that concerned the SOT team was to ensure the safety of the vital solid organ harvesting during a multiorgan procurement that included an additional vascular composite allograft procurement. FT procurement was decided to be performed in a heart-beating donor, and a detailed multiorgan procurement algorithm was prepared (Table 11.1).

Table 11.1 Multiorgan procurement algorithm

1. Tracheostomy	VCA team
2. Abdominal organ inspection	SOT team alone
2. Simultaneous abdomen and upper face dissection	VCA and SOT teams together
3. Lower face and neck alone (until osteotomies)	VCA team alone
4. Thorax organ dissection	Cardiac team alone
5. Simultaneous perfusion[a]	VCA, SOT, and cardiac teams together
6. Thx organ detachment	Cardiac team alone
7. Osteotomies and face detachment	VCA team alone
8. Abdominal organ detachment	SOT team alone

VCA vascular composite allograft, *SOT* solid organ transplantation
[a]Face perfused via aortic arch

Supplementary Information The online version contains supplementary material available at https://doi.org/10.1007/978-3-031-21520-9_11.

P. Lassus (✉)
Department of Plastic Surgery, Helsinki University Hospital, University of Helsinki, Helsinki, Finland
e-mail: patrik.lassus@hus.fi

© Springer Nature Switzerland AG 2023
R. Gurunian et al. (eds.), *Reconstructive Transplantation*, https://doi.org/10.1007/978-3-031-21520-9_11

11.1.1.4 Organ Donation

By birth, each person in Finland is a presumed organ donor. In 2019, there were 141 brain-dead organ donors in Finland (25.6 per million population). In Helsinki, the only transplant center in Finland, 453 solid organ transplants were performed in 2019. In order not to jeopardize public opinion toward organ donations, a decision was made that a VCA-specific permission for VCA donation needs to be asked from the kin. A donor consent process and a specialized consent form for facial transplantation were formulated with the SOT team and OPO. Consent for facial tissue donation was decided to be approached only after consent for solid organ donation had been agreed. For a donor, only hemodynamically stable brain dead organ donor without a significant need for vasoactive inotropic medication, without previous facial morbidity, appropriate gender and ethnicity, age >18 years, and with blood group compatibility would be considered. Donor facial procurement was decided to be restricted to the Helsinki region in order to minimize the logistic challenges in spite of the reduction in the donor pool.

11.1.1.5 Ethical Issues

The hospital also required an ethical analysis on FT due to the anticipated public interest and potentially controversial nature of the program. An analysis on the ethical implications was performed by a medical ethicist Samuli Saarni. The analysis was divided into general aspects including evidence in support of this still experimental treatment, serious risks versus benefits of this non-life-saving treatment, autonomy, and requirements for truly informed patient decision-making. The other aspect was FT-specific aspects such as differences to other non-visible organ transplants, esthetic vs. medical goals, and the potential social reactions to FT program and recipients' perception of these.

11.1.1.6 Financial Issues

The program had two possibilities for financing it. First would have been to base it on a scientific grant. The other option was to apply an experimental care status. That enabled the program to be financed by the national healthcare system. The VCA program was evaluated by the Helsinki and Uusimaa health municipality region before granting permission to proceed. The cost for the face transplantation first posttransplant year was estimated to be €150,000. After the agreement from the HUH municipalities to finance the program and SOT team approval, the hospital granted permission to start the VCA program. The first patient was placed on the waiting list for FT in November 2015 almost 5 years after the start of the program.

11.1.2 Helsinki VCA Team

The HUH is a tertiary care academic university hospital with referral area of 1.9 million inhabitants. It covers one third of the Finnish population. About half of the facial and head & neck (H&N) microvascular reconstructions in Finland are performed in Helsinki, and the number of these free flaps is currently approximately 120/year. The Department of Plastic Surgery has 35 senior consultant plastic surgeons, making it one of the largest centers in Europe.

11.1.2.1 Surgical Team

Since FT is a complex surgical treatment including microsurgery, a large number of surgeons capable of facial and microsurgery were included in the team. The program was led by the Plastic Surgery unit and included six plastic surgeons capable to perform facial and microsurgery. In addition, two maxillofacial microsurgeons and an ENT H&N specialist joined the surgical team. All these surgeons were in senior position and capable to perform complex H&N surgery. Every surgeon had a special task in the surgery depending on each expertise. Surgeons in charge of each phase were clearly named.

11.1.2.2 SOT Team

FT is organ transplantation, and collaboration with the SOT team is vital for success. Collaboration enables full access to the multiple clinical specialties necessary in solid organ transplantation. These include immunology, infectious diseases, psychiatry, rejection pathology, internal medicine as well as the OPO. The FT program was built in close contact with the SOT team, and all of the abovementioned medical specialties were involved in the design of the FT protocol.

11.1.2.3 H&N Cancer Team

The third leg of the FT team was constructed with incorporating the specialists from the Helsinki Head and Neck Cancer Center into the program. These included H&N radiologists, dental specialists, and several therapists (oral physiotherapy, physiotherapy, speech therapy, nutritional therapy) as well as a social worker. For FT, the complex issues in design of the surgery and rehabilitation require the expertise from these specialists. In addition, the team includes dedicated operation nurses who prepare detailed operation checklists for both the donor and the recipient procedures (Table 11.2).

Table 11.2 Multidisciplinary VCA team

Surgical team
• Plastic and reconstructive surgery
• Oral and maxillofacial surgery
• ENT/head and neck surgery
• Anesthesiology
• Dedicated OR nurses
Organ transplantation team
• Transplant surgery
• Immunology
• Infectious diseases
• Psychiatry/pyschology
• Rejection and skin pathology
• Internal medicine
• Organ procurement organisation
Head and neck team
• Radiology
• Dentistry
• Oral physiotherapy
• Physiotherapy
• Speech therapy
• Nutritional therapy
• Social worker

11.2 Face Transplantation Patient Evaluation

11.2.1 Patient Selection and Screening

11.2.1.1 Indications and Contraindications

In Helsinki, an indication for an FT is a severe functional facial deficiency that cannot be reconstructed with conventional techniques. Our indications do not differ from the indications from other teams [2, 3]. This includes functional loss of oral or periocular sphincters or significant loss of midfacial structures. Absolute contraindications include non-compliance, recent malignancy (<5 years), psychiatric lability, or a severe chronic illness. As FT is not a life-saving treatment, the patient's perspective is of fundamental importance, and factors such as poor quality of life and social impairment affect the final decision. It is important to notice that a plan is needed also for those patients who are not suitable for FT, since these patients also need help for their symptoms, support, and follow-up.

11.2.1.2 Facial Analysis

Candidate's facial disfigurement is analyzed by evaluating the affected facial anatomical zones. For this we have used 10 facial zones including forehead and scalp, periorbital, nasal, perioral, cheek and ears, chin, neck, intraoral, maxilla, and mandible. Concerning facial function, the functions most often affected and considered most important for quality of life are evaluated (breathing, mouth opening, dentition, mastication, swallowing, speaking, labial competence, eyelid function). Mimic muscle function is tested using the Sunnybrook facial scale analysis [4]. It is not perfect for the analysis since Sunnybrook scale compares the affected side to the healthy side and in FT candidates often both sides are affected. Sensory function is assessed with light touch discrimination using a static monofilament and 10 mm two-point touch discrimination.

11.2.1.3 General Checkup

After the patient is evaluated to be a candidate for FT, several examinations are needed to find potential contraindications for the treatment. Most common malignancies need to be ruled out (age dependently). A chest X-ray, colonoscopy, gastroscopy, prostate-specific antibody for males, and gynecological examination and mammography as well as breast ultrasound for females are done. An internal medicine specialist consultation with wide laboratory analysis and cardiac echography are performed to every patient.

11.2.1.4 Microbial Examinations

Many of the severely facially disfigured patients have chronic infections, and it is important to evaluate potential microbial colonization. In Helsinki, cytomegalovirus (CMV) is evaluated, and the length of the valgansiclovir prophylaxis depends on both recipient and donor CMV status. In Epstein-Barr virus (EBV)-negative recipients, EBV-positive donors are contraindicated. Other tests include Hepatitis A, B, and C, HIV, toxoplasma, varicella, and herpes simplex. Concerning virus status for the recipient, our policy is that HAV+: only acute infection is a contraindication, HBVcAb+ (earlier cured infection) and or HBVsAb (vaccinated): not a contraindication, HCV+: not a contraindication if cured, HIV+: not a contraindication (medication will need adjustments due to immunosuppression), Toxoplasma+ and VZV+ not a contraindication. For the donor, HBVsAb+ (vaccinated): accepted and HBVcAb and HBVsAB (earlier cured infection) may possible be accepted, HCV+ accepted if cured, HIV+: not accepted, Toxoplasma+ and VZV+: accepted.

11.2.1.5 Immunological Evaluations

Recipient is analyzed for blood type and low-resolution type for HLA-A, -B, and -DR. A panel reactive antibody test is performed to evaluate potential immunization. HLA antibodies are determined using Luminex before the transplantation. Before the final decision for FT, a crossmatch between donor blood T- and B-cells is performed using the complement-dependent cytotoxicity method. In addition, a virtual crossmatch is performed. Postoperatively HLA antibodies are checked to detect potential development of donor-specific antibodies.

11.2.1.6 Psychiatric Evaluation

The aim of the evaluation is to ensure that the candidate has sufficient psychological and social resources to cope with the whole transplantation process. The other aim is to ensure the compliance for lifelong immunosuppressive medication, rehabilitation, and follow-up.

In order to evaluate capability to give informed consent, the patient's capability to receive and process information is assessed. A semistructured interview by a clinical psychologist on three or more occasions aims to evaluate the candidate's preparedness for the operation and to predict potential psychological reactions or possible risk factors. Test patterns are designed individually since some of the candidates may have preexisting brain damage or organic brain illness.

11.2.1.7 Health-Related Quality of Life (HRQoL)

In Helsinki, the candidate's HRQoL is measured using a generic 15D scale, SF-36, and the European Organization for Research and Treatment of Cancer Quality of Life Questionnaire Head and Neck Module (EORTC QLQ-HN35) [5–7]. 15D is chosen for Finnish patients since it is well validated in Finnish population and has the potential to compare candidate's 15D score to age and sex adjusted normal score in Finland [8]. EORTC QLQ-HN35 is chosen because many of the problems FT candidates have resemble the problems patients with oral cancer have.

11.2.1.8 Social Impairment

The effect of facial disfigurement on social well-being of the facial disfigurement and functional deficit is also evaluated [9, 10]. The Sheehan Disability Scale (SDS), a patient-rated measure of functional disability in work, social, and family life, is used [11]. These three items added together provide a global impairment score that ranges from 0 (unimpaired) to 30 (highly impaired).

11.2.1.9 Esthetic Evaluation

FT is not performed because of esthetic reasons. The appearance of many of the FT candidates is very abnormal which has great impact on their social and psychological well-being. Many of the candidates have expressed their wish to look normal. Therefore, one of the goals for FT is to restore normal and if possible attractive appearance. In Helsinki, FT candidate's esthetic appearance is evaluated by the FT team members using an observer-rated disfigurement scale for head and neck cancer patients, a patient group similar to FT candidates in relation to appearance [12].

11.2.1.10 Decision-Making for FT

The aim for candidate screening and evaluation is to have an objective estimation for the severity of the facial disfigurement. Factors that we take into account are an analysis of the affected facial regions, functional facial deficiencies, impact on quality of life, social impairment, and esthetic disfigurement. If these parameters show a severe overall impact of the facial injury, the candidate is more likely to be suitable for FT. The aim for other screening is to rule out potential contraindications such as noncompliance or psychiatric disorders or malignancies, illnesses, preimmunization, or infections that would possess a risk for the forthcoming FT (Table 11.3).

Table 11.3 Face transplantation candidate evaluation chart

Demographic data		
	Gender (M/F)	
	Age (years)	
	Age at injury (years)	
	Mechanism of injury	
	Number of reconstructions	
Affcted facial regions		(Severity 0–2)
	Maxilla	
	Mandible	
	Forehead and scalp	
	Periorbita	
	Nose	
	Lips	
	Cheek and ears	
	Chin	
	Neck	
	Intraoral	
	Other affected body areas	
Functional impairment		(Severity 0–2)
Oral	Mouth opening	
	Labial competence	
	Teeth	
	Mastication	
	Swallowing	
	Breathing	
	Speech	
Periorbital	Eyelid function	
	Visus	
Sensation	Forehead and scalp	
	Periorbital	
	Perioral	
	Cheeck and ears	
	Chin	
Mimic muscles	Forhead wrinkle	
	Anger	
	Smile	
	Mouth pucker	
Sunnybrook	Left	
	Right	
Esthetic disfigurement score (0–9)		
Social impairment score (0–30)		
QOL	EORTC HN-35	
	15D	
	SF-36	
Immunological status	Blood type	
	PRA	
	HLA-ab	
Contraindications		

11.2.2 Radiology and 3D Planning in FT

Composite FT creates an additional three-dimensional challenge for the reconstruction: the bone alignment. Patients receiving a composite FT have usually very disfigured bony midfacial anatomy, and it would be very difficult to plan the surgery without using radiology and 3D modeling. Patients usually miss many of the normal bony landmarks, or they are in wrong position. In order to visualize and understand patient's bony disfigurement and the goals for restoration, we have used extensively 3D planning. We perform a facial CT angiography scan with thin slices (0.65 mm) and without tilt as well as a high-resolution MRI. The angiography is taken to verify neck and facial vessel anatomy for planning the vascular anastomoses. MRI is taken to analyze the soft tissue anatomy including remnant facial musculature. CT scan is used to perform 3D planning, and we have collaborated with Planmeca Oy, a Helsinki-based company specialized in 3D imaging and computer-aided design and manufacturing software to produce customized osteotomy guides [13].

11.2.2.1 3D Planning for the Recipient

Aim for the planning was to remove as much of the damaged bones as possible without removing normal bone and to restore normal facial height and symmetry when the donor maxilla and mandible would be transplanted (Video 11.1). In our two recipients, we used nasion as the reference point for planning since it was the only normal facial landmark. The osteotomies that followed the principles of Le Fort II osteotomy lines removed most of the damaged midfacial bony tissues. We simplified the maxilla osteotomy to have only two straight planes (Video 11.2). Sagittal osteotomy lines were designed from mandibular angle to angle to remove the damaged central mandible. After we had decided the osteotomy lines, we printed customized cutting guides for the recipient (Fig. 11.1).

11.2.2.2 3D Planning for the Donor

It is very difficult to plan ahead the required osteotomy lines for the donor since the size and shape of the donor maxilla and mandible are not known ahead. By using the recipient osteotomy planning, we incorporated that data to random normal 3D imaged skulls. We performed several attempts on different sized and shaped skulls and produced a generic donor osteotomy cutting guides that would help us in the procurement (Video 11.3). We simplified the osteotomy by creating two straight planes that were at the same angle with the recipient osteotomy lines (Videos 11.4, 11.5, and 11.6). With this design, the size discrepancy between recipient and

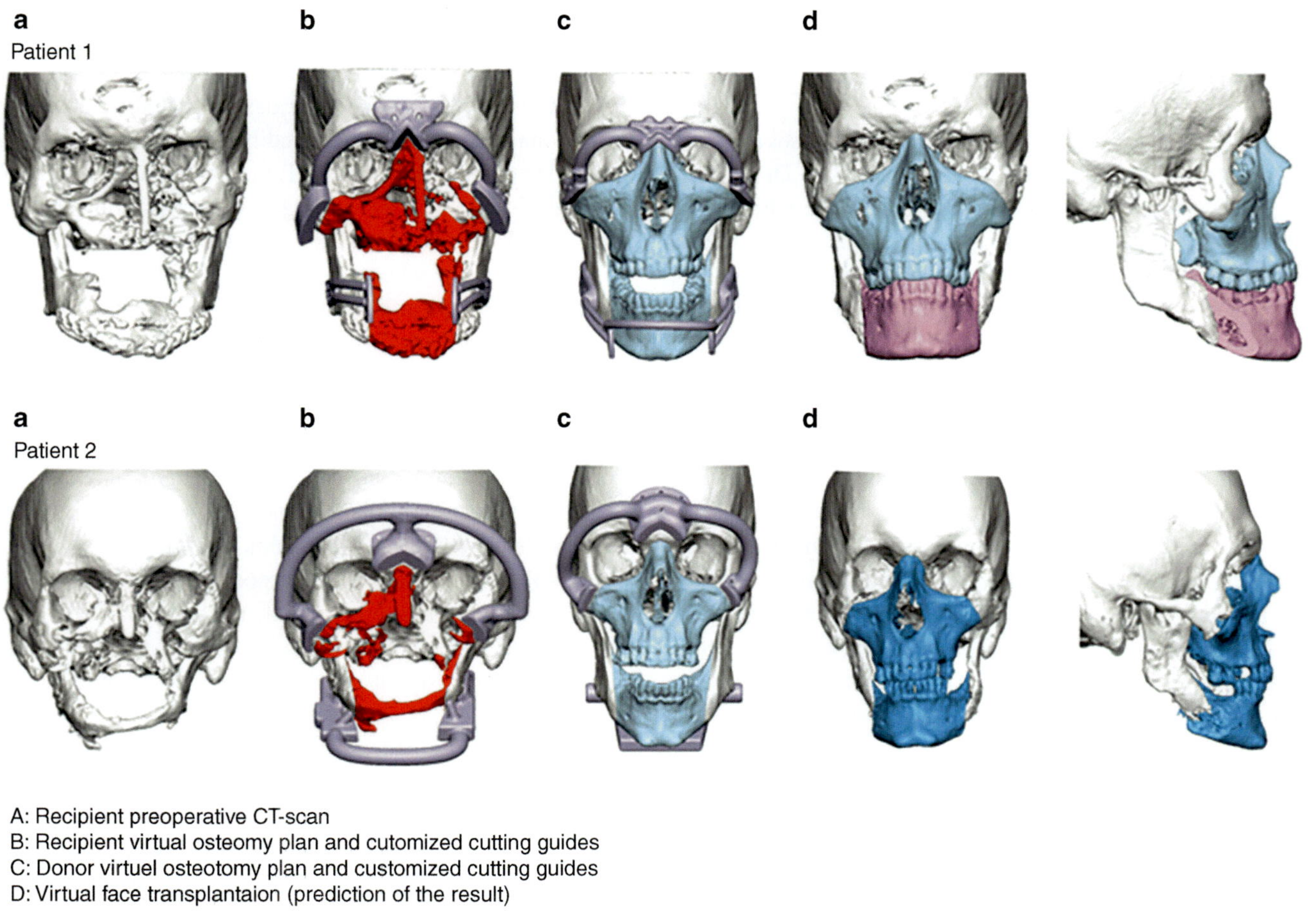

Fig. 11.1 Virtual 3D planning, customized cutting guides, and virtual face transplantation (made by Planmeca Oy)

donor maxilla does not matter because if the donor maxilla is bigger, it will just be inserted more anteriorly and if smaller more posteriorly. The orbital rim will be at the same level (Video 11.7).

However, during both face transplantations before the surgery, we were able to obtain facial CT scan from the donor and were able to 3D print customized osteotomy cutting guides for the real donors as well. These guides were used in both FTs for the recipients and the donors [13] (Fig. 11.1).

11.2.2.3 Donor Funeral Mask

The procurement leaves a significant facial defect for the donor. In case the kin wish to see the donor after organ harvest, there is a need to restore donor's facial appearance as closely as possible. For this purpose, we used 3D digital methods to produce a 3D printed donor facial mask. The donor was photographed from different angles using standard digital camera. The data was sent to the Helsinki Technical University where a 3D model was constructed from the photographs (Agisoft Photoscan, AgiSoft LLC, Russia). The physical mask was printed from this data using a binder jetting method with a full color complement (ZPrinter 450 or 650, 3D Systems Corp, USA). The whole process took 15.5 h, and the mask was ready before the organ procurement was finished [14].

11.2.3 FT Candidates in Helsinki

We have screened a total of 11 patients with a severe facial disfigurement and potential FT candidates in the Department of Plastic Surgery in Helsinki since 2013. The patient geographical distribution represents roughly the distribution of Finnish population. Of the patients, eight are male and three female, and the age range is between 26 and 66 years. The etiology of the injury has been burn in five, ballistic in three, blast in two, and neurofibromatosis 1 in one patient. All patients have had several previous reconstructive surgeries (range 4–34).

All the 11 patients had central facial deficiencies, and six patients had eight or more injured facial regions. Facial function was affected in at least some parameters in all patients. Mouth opening was affected in 8/11, labial competence in all 11, and eating was compromised in four patients. Breathing was impaired in seven patients with loss of the nasal airway and speech in five patients. Eight patients had suffered an injury that impaired their lid function, most commonly causing an ectropion. In this patient group, impaired sensation most commonly affected the midface in comparison to the forehead and neck. All patients had at least some missing facial mimic function. All patients had medium to severe esthetic disfigurement when analyzed by the team. Seven of the 11 patients had medium to severe social impairment. All patients had lowered quality of life and in five it was markedly impaired.

None of the patients was significantly preimmunized. Interestingly, none of the major burn patients had performed HLA antibodies. Five patients had significant contraindications for FT (psychiatric issues, alcohol abuse, and liver cirrhosis). Of the 11 patients, six were considered to have enough severe facial disfigurement that affected patient's social life and quality of life to justify FT. Of the six, three had contraindications for FT leaving three potential candidates for FT. Of these three patients, two have had an FT and one patient is not willing to go for the treatment.

11.3 Helsinki Face Transplantation Patients and Transplantation Surgery

We have performed two FTs in Helsinki, the first in February 2016 and the second in March 2018. Both the patients wish to remain anonymous, and their photographs cannot be published.

11.3.1 First Helsinki FT Patient (Transplanted in 2016)

Our first FT patient was a 34-year old male who had had a self-inflicted facial gunshot injury 17 years earlier. He had suffered loss of his midface soft tissues including nose and loss of maxilla and central mandible. He was completely blind after the injury. Prior to FT, the patient had undergone 28 surgical procedures including five microvascular reconstructions. The main reason for repeated problems and failures after surgery where due to persistent, recurrent soft tissue and hardware infections. The patient had central facial injury involving all 10 facial zones. He had limited mouth opening, impaired lip closure, and he was edentulous. His tongue projection was limited due to an absent tip and floor of the mouth scarring. He had difficulties in eating, and his speech was unclear. He suffered from absent nasal breathing. He had no sensation in his lips and chin. His mimic muscle movements were stiff, and he couldn't produce all emotions with his facial mimics. He had a poor score in the esthetic analysis, showed social impairment, and had a marked reduction in the HRQoL scoring. CT scan showed significant loss of facial height (estimated to be 30 mm less than average facial height).

The patient was otherwise healthy, blood group O rhesus positive and immunologically had a panel reactive antibody (PRA) status of 33%. Serological status included cytomegalovirus (CMV) and Epstein-Barr virus (EBV) positivity. In psychological evaluation, he was found to be suitable for

FT. While the patient was strongly motivated for the treatment, he was also fully informed about all the risks, postoperative course, and possible sequelae 1 [3].

11.3.2 Second Helsinki FT Patient (Transplanted in 2018)

The second patient was a 60-year-old male at the time of FT who had suffered a self-inflicted ballistic injury 20 years earlier, resulting in a severe facial disfigurement including defects in all ten facial zones especially in his mandible, maxilla, midface, nasal, and periorbital regions. He had had over 20 surgical revisions and reconstructions before FT. He had limited mouth opening and lip incompetence. He was edentulous and was limited to a soft diet only. He had no nasal breathing and was dependent on tracheostomy. He had unclear speech. His anterior mandible was reconstructed with fibula and his maxilla with a large titanium implant which had to be removed due to chronic infection. He had severe enophthalmos, lower lid ectropion, and lagophthalmos resulting in left eye dryness. He had limited facial mimic expression and impaired midfacial muscle activity including orbicular oris muscle. The left lower eyelid was fixed and had no movement. He had a poor score in the esthetic evaluation, and he had problems with social interaction especially because of continuous drooling due to incomplete lip closure. He had a severely reduced quality of life score.

The patient was otherwise healthy, and in the psychological evaluation, he was assessed to be emotionally stable and compliant. The patient had some Class II preformed HLA antibodies and a panel reactive antibody (PRA) score of 12%. The patient was strongly motivated to have FT even after knowing the potential risks and life-long medication [1].

11.3.2.1 Donors

Due to the Finnish organ transplantation legislation, it is not possible to publish any individual data concerning the donors. After the OPO had made the decision that the brain-dead deceased patient will be an organ donor and was the same blood-type and sex as the FT recipient on the waiting list, they contacted the FT team. After the FT team member had approved that the deceased could also be a facial tissue donor, the OPO had a separate discussion with the kin, and they asked for a specific permission to donate facial tissues. The first FT recipient had to wait for 2 months, and the kin for the first suitable donor approved the donation. The second FT recipient had to wait for 15 months and the kin for the fourth suitable donor approved the donation. In this small cohort, 40% of the kin approved the facial tissue donation.

After the decision for FT, a facial CT angiography was done for 3D planning, photographs were taken for funeral mask, and the immunologists were informed on the transplant to perform T- and B-cell and virtual crossmatch. Members of the surgical team were alerted. Donor facial donation surgery and recipient surgery were performed in the same hospital but in different buildings.

11.3.3 Face Transplantation Surgery

Very detailed checklists were made for all components of face transplantation. Surgery was planned ahead in great detail. Roles for every surgeon were defined and also a replacement person for each so that during the long surgery everyone could have breaks. A detailed plan was also made how to coordinate the separate recipient and donor operations in which the timing was also dependent on the SOT teams (Fig. 11.2).

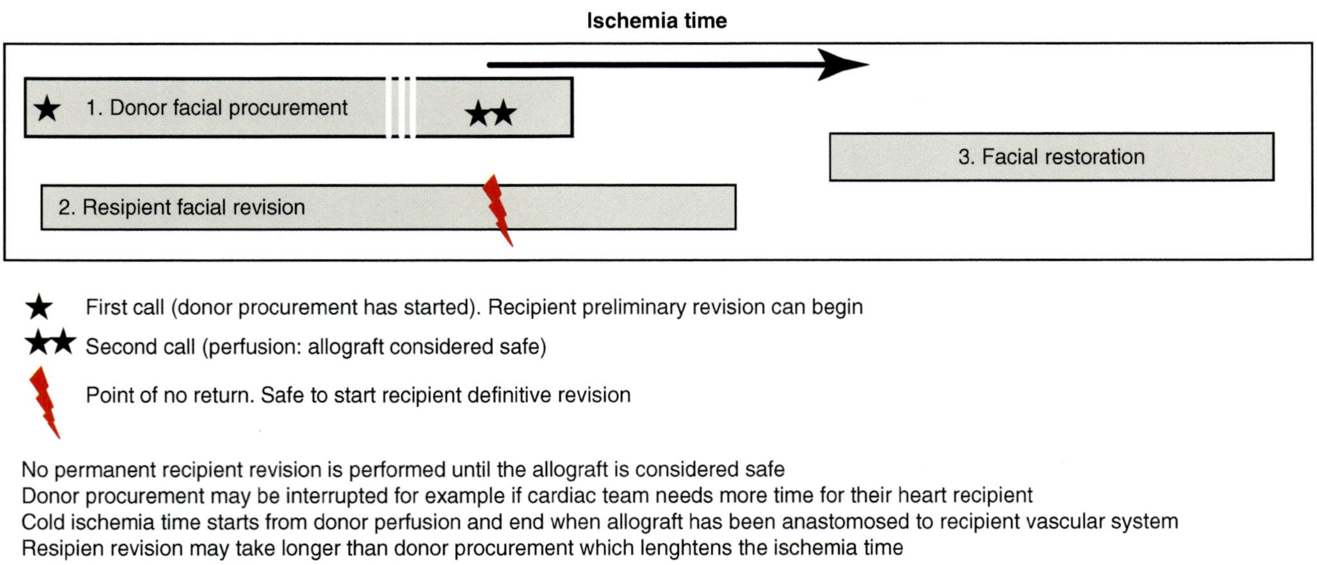

Fig. 11.2 Timing of different phases of face transplantation in multiorgan procurement

Both our patients had a relatively similar FT. The first FT was a composite allograft that included 2/3 facial and neck soft tissues as well as anterior mandible and Le Fort II type of maxilla. Intraorally it included all oral mucosa and anterior tongue. The second FT was otherwise similar but it included all facial soft tissues including lids (Fig. 11.3).

11.3.3.1 Face Donation Surgery

Face procurement was practiced in cadaver dissections and standardized to be performed with same principles in all cases. Both face donations were on a brain-dead, beating heart multi-organ donation including heart, lungs, liver, kidneys, and pancreas. The advantage of beating heart donation is better control for the hemostasis and shorter ischemia time but disadvantage is that the order of surgeries needs to be planned well because of the complexity of the procedure unless face procurement can be performed before other surgery.

A detailed algorithm was agreed on the order of different procedures (Table 11.1). The procedure started with tracheostomy and continued with the inspection of visceral organs by transplant surgeons. Then the FT team started the dissection from upper face simultaneously with the abdominal organ transplant surgeons. After the transplant surgeons finished, the FT team continued alone for 2–3 h until everything was ready except osteotomies and palatal separation. Maxillary osteotomy guides were fixed in place to the nasal radix and medial orbital margins as well as both zygomatic maxillary processes. The infraorbital nerves were identified in the inferior orbital fissure, buccal nerves in the buccal fat

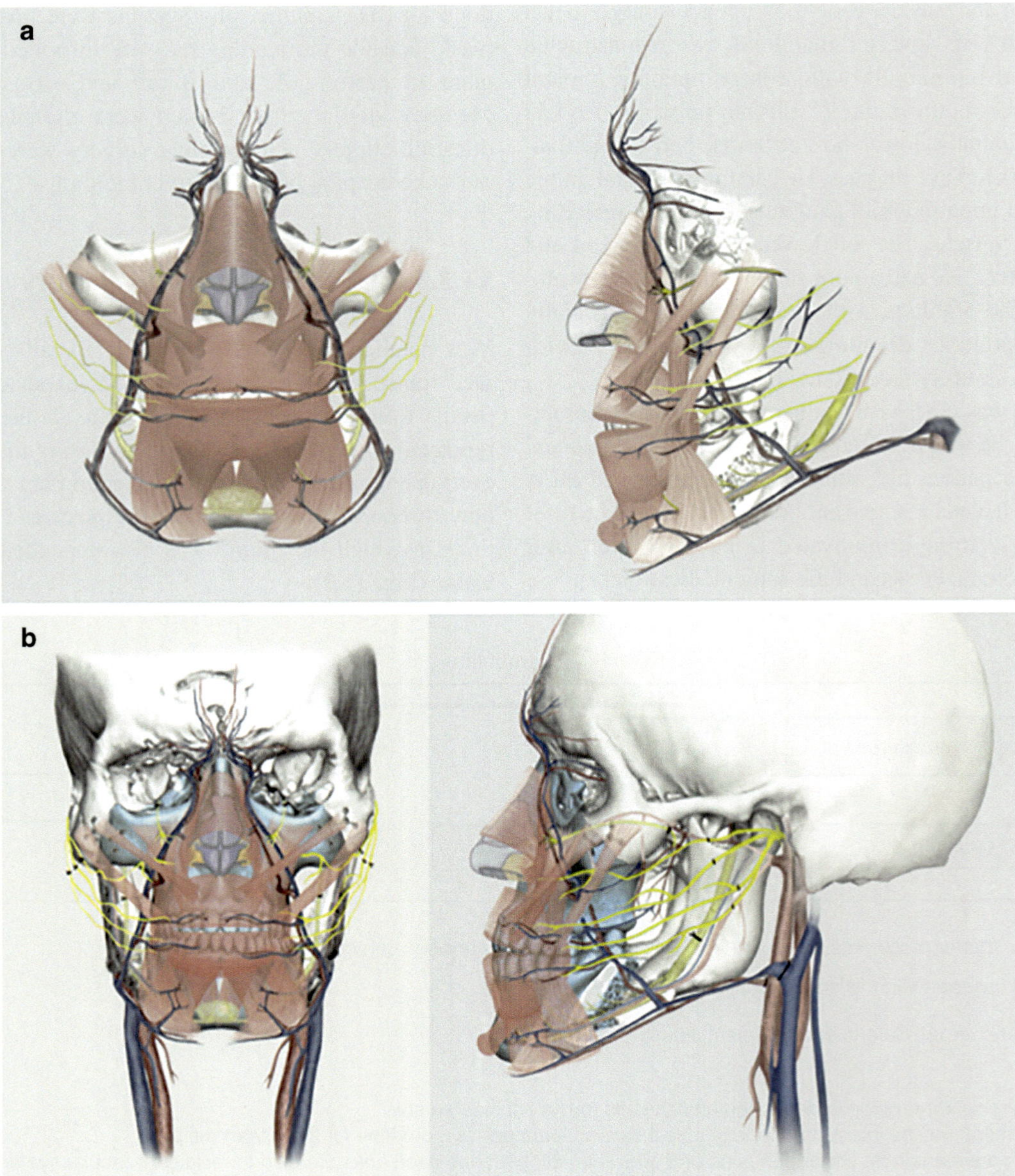

A: Allograft showing transplanted bones, muscles, nerves, and vascular structures
B: Allograft transplanted to the recipient

Fig. 11.3 Schematic presentation of the face allograft (drawn by Heidi Kuivaniemi-Smith)

pad, and alveolar nerves through the neck incision. Facial nerve was separated from parotid gland and dissected to the common trunk level and hypoglossal nerve was identified. The external carotid arteries and internal and external jugular veins were dissected bilaterally, with preservation of the facial vessels and submandibular glands within the allograft. The hyoid bone and anterior floor of the mouth muscles were also included in the allograft as well as intraoral cheek mucosa up to the anterior tonsillar pillars, ventral portion of the tongue, and hypoglossal nerves.

The FT team had a break when cardiac transplant surgeons dissected heart and lungs. After that all organs were perfused simultaneously. Face was perfused via cannula that was placed in aortic arch. For perfusion, we used cold University of Wisconsin solution. It is important to perfuse the graft with gentle pressure and not to over-perfuse it in order not to damage the vascular intima in the graft. After the perfusion, ascending ramus mandibular osteotomies were then performed on both the sides with inclusion of the inferior alveolar nerves. Maxillary osteotomies were performed with the aid of customized cutting guides (Videos 11.3, 11.4, 11.5, and 11.6). Nasal septum was divided caudally, and the palate divided between soft and hard palate. The facial allograft was then isolated on the vascular pedicles which were divided. Simultaneously, a right radial forearm flap was also harvested to act as a sentinel flap. Grafts were transported in ice water slurry. After procurement of other organs, venous, arterial, fascial, and nerve grafts were harvested in case they were needed. In the end the 3D manufactured face mask was attached to the donor facial defect.

11.3.3.2 Recipient Face Debridement

Since the donor team and the recipient team worked in separate buildings, it was important to keep both the teams informed on progress in the other hospital. Two time-points were defined. First point was the time the donor had a tracheostomy. That was a sign for the recipient team to start preliminary face debridement. The team identified neural and vascular structures and placed the customized cutting guides but avoided doing anything permanent in case the face allograft would fail. The second time-point was when the donor face allograft was being perfused and considered safe. After that the recipient team commenced definitive debridement and removed all damaged tissues. Le Fort II maxillary and central mandible segments were removed using customized osteotomy guides (Videos 11.1 and 11.2). All poor quality soft tissue and central facial skin were removed as well as the anterior floor of the mouth and ventral scarred tongue.

For recipient vessels, internal and external jugular veins bilaterally, external carotid artery on one side and facial artery on the other were dissected. Facial nerve branches were dissected as distally as possible along with bilateral hypoglossal nerves and buccal nerves. For the second patient, supraorbital and alveolar nerves were identified additionally. Remnants of the orbicularis oris muscle with scar tissue attached to it was split in the midline and left in situ with its own neurovascular supply intact. In addition, remnants of the zygomatic muscles were spared for subsequent attachment.

11.3.3.3 Restoration of the Face

The recipient debridement took longer time than the face procurement in both the cases. Before restoration phase, mandible sagittal osteotomies were performed on the side table using 3D printed custom-made donor osteotomy guides. The donor facial maxilla and central mandible were first fixed into place. This took only a short time since customized cutting guides were used for both the donor and the recipient and only minor adjustments were needed (Video 11.7).

Arterial anastomoses were performed between external carotid arteries and facial arteries on the other side. In the first patient, a venous graft was needed for the external carotid anastomosis. Venous anastomosed involved donor allograft facial vein to a branch of the internal jugular vein on both the sides and all possible smaller veins available. After that facial nerves were anastomosed on the branch level as distally as possible and hypoglossal nerves bilaterally end-to-side. For the first patient, of the sensory nerves only buccal nerves were connected. For the second patient, recipient supraorbital nerves were connected to donor infraorbital nerves and recipient alveolar nerves were connected to donor alveolar nerves with donor nerve allografts.

In order to support the lips and to avoid allograft sagging, the recipients divided medial ends of the orbicularis oris muscle and scar tissue were tunneled subcutaneously within the donor allograft's upper and lower lip tissue and sutured about 2 cm medial to the contralateral commissures. The remnants of the patient's zygomatic muscles were attached to the equivalent muscular region in the allograft. Excess skin in the neck and preauricular regions was preserved to allow for post-op swelling. Simultaneously, transplantation of the sentinel (radial forearm) flap was performed to the right lateral thigh using the lateral femoral circumflex vessels as recipient vessels.

Cold ischemia time was 3 h 15 min for the first and 4 h for the second FT. The total surgical time was 19 h for the first and 22 h for the second FT. The entire procedure from notification of a potential donor to completion of surgery took a total of 32 h for the first and 36 h for the second FT.

11.4 Follow-Up Protocol

11.4.1 Immunosuppression Protocol

Helsinki immunosuppressive protocol is based on thymoglobulin induction (1.5 mg/kg for 4 days; if CD3-positive cells are found after fourth day, continuation of thymoglobulin is considered). Mycophenolate mofetil (MMF) 1 g and tacrolimus 0.1 mg/kg are given before induction. Maintenance therapy is based on tacrolimus, MMF, and methylprednisolone. Tacrolimus target levels are 13–16 μg/L for the first months, 10–13 μg/L for the first 6 months, 8–10 μg/L for the first year, and if there are no signs of rejection, the long-term target level is 5–7 μg/L. MMF is given 1 g two times a day. Methylprednisolone is started 3 mg/kg/day, and the dosage is tapered so that after 1 month, it is 0.3 mg/kg/day and the long-term dosage is targeted to be 4–6 mg/day. Tacrolimus level is checked on every clinical control and MMF levels occasionally.

11.4.2 Rejection Monitoring Protocol

11.4.2.1 Biopsies

Rejection monitoring is based on punch biopsies in addition to clinical monitoring. We have used sentinel flaps and biopsies have been taken every time from both facial allograft and sentinel allograft. We have used 4 mm biopsies and include also subcutaneous tissue in the biopsy. Routine biopsies have been taken weekly for the first month, monthly for the first 6 months, every 3 months for the first 2 years, and every 6 months after that. An additional biopsy was always taken when rejection was suspected. Rejection diagnostics is based on histological analysis and immunohistochemical stainings are used when needed. We use Banff 2007 VCA grading [15].

11.4.2.2 HLA Antibodies

In order to detect possible donor-specific antibodies, HLA antibodies are checked 1 month postoperatively and after that every 6 months.

11.4.3 Antimicrobial Protocol

Antibiotic prophylaxis is targeted to treat potential chronic bacterial colonizations. Even though there is no evidence for the practice, we have used 1 week antibiotic prophylaxis. For CMV prophylaxis, we have used Valgansiclovir 900 mg. Treatment has continued for 3 months if both recipient and donor are CMV negative, 6 months if recipient is CMV positive, and 12 months if recipient is CMV negative and donor CMV positive. Trimetoprim-sulfametoxazol is continued for 6 months to prevent pneumocystis and toxoplasma infections. The patients are also given Caspofungin for 1 week to prevent *Candida* or *Aspergillus* infections. CMV and EBV antibodies are checked on every clinic follow-up to detect possible viral activation.

The patients received low molecular weight heparin treatment for 4 weeks and continued with permanent low dose acetylsalicylic acid.

11.4.4 Rehabilitation Protocol

11.4.4.1 Early Recovery Period

During the early recovery period, tracheostomy and all invasive catheters are removed as early as possible as being potential infectious sources. The allograft is monitored clinically as any conventional free flap monitoring. We have used oral chlorhexidine flushing for 2 weeks. Enteral feeding is started on first postoperative day unless retention. The patient is allowed to drink clear fluids as soon as possible. Soft nutrition is allowed after 2 weeks and normal diet after 6 weeks if possible. For the recovery period, the diet has been designed by our nutritional therapist. The patient is mobilized as soon as possible. Oral physiotherapy is started as soon as the patient is capable to do it. Our occupational therapist has designed a customized face-lift masks for the swelling period lasting approximately 3 months and guided the normal scar prevention treatment.

11.4.4.2 Psychological Support

The patients are allowed to see their new faces as soon as they want. Early psychological supportive therapy is given to the patient, and it is tailored to meet the needs. The patients have routine psychologist controls, and they are being followed with structured tests. The quality of life is recorded with 15D, SF-36, and EORTC QLQ-HN35 tests routinely. Social worker is involved in the period that the patient is being discharged from the hospital.

11.4.4.3 Surgical Controls

The patients need to be controlled frequently in the beginning because of potential early complications such as fistulas, infections, wound problems, or bone healing problems. In Helsinki, the routine follow-ups are organized by the plastic surgeon in charge. In the beginning, follow-ups are held weekly and reduced to monthly follow-ups when there are no more acute matters. In the long-term, follow-ups occur twice a year. Maxillofacial surgeons and ENT specialists will also see the patient depending on the needs. Speech therapy is started already before discharging the patient from the ward and continued depending on the needs.

11.4.4.4 Dental Follow-Up

The patients with composite allograft will need frequent dental follow-up. Caries prevention should be taken into account from the early period. The patients develop easily gingival and dental problems due to reduced salivary flow and possibly due to dental innervation. Our patients meet cardiologists, periodontists, orthodontists, and prosthodontists depending on the need.

11.5 Results

Both the patients stayed in the ICU for 9 days and Patient 1 in the ward for 8 weeks and Patient 2 for 6 weeks. Early recovery period went without major problems. Patient 1 lives 1-h drive from the hospital, and his follow-ups were organized to HUH. Patient 2 lives 4-h drive from HUH, and the follow-ups were organized between HUH and the local hospital.

11.5.1 Functional Outcomes

11.5.1.1 Motor Recovery

First allograft movements on both the patients were seen in the floor of the mouth muscles innervated by hypoglossal nerve at 3 months. For both the patients, facial muscle activity was first seen at 4–5 months, and it increased rapidly during the first year. For patient 1, improvement in fine midface muscular movements has been seen even 4 years after transplantation. At 4 years for Patient 1 and 2 years for Patient 2 post transplantation, motor activity is visible in all of the facial muscle groups confirmed by EMG in both the patients (Table 11.4). Patient 1 is able to show most common emotions with his face, he is able to have lip competence but small part of the right lower lip orbicular oris muscle is not activated. Patient 2 is able to show spontaneous emotions with his face, he has a good lip competence and symmetrical movements on his face.

11.5.1.2 Sensory Recovery

First signs of sensory recovery were seen at 3 months for both the patients. Patient 1 to whom we only connected buccal nerves showed steady increase of sensation in the whole allograft within 1 year. However, the sensation is only protective and not spatially very accurate and 2-point discrimination is seen only in lateral cheeks [13]. For Patient 2 we connected buccal nerves, mental nerves to alveolar nerves with an allograft, and infraorbital nerves to supraorbital nerves with an allograft. He showed more rapid improvement in sensory recovery reaching the whole allograft within 9 months. He has good sensation in his lips and at 1 year also 10 mm 2-point discrimination in the cheeks and chin. At 2 years, he has adapted to feel his upper lip as upper lip instead of forehead. We conclude that sensory recovery is possible without nerve anastomosis probably via facial nerve, but the recovery is slower and less precise. Supraorbital to infraorbital nerve coaptation is recommended to perform when recipient infraorbital nerves are not available (Fig. 11.4).

Table 11.4 Electromyography results 18 months post transplantation

Patient 1		Patient 2	
Muscle	Right/left	Muscle	Right/left
Orbicularis oculi[a]	++/++	Orbicularis oculi[a]	++/+
Nasalis[a]	+/+	Nasalis[a]	+/0
Zygomaticus major[a]	+/++	Zygomaticus major[a]	++/+
Orbicularis oris[a]	++/++	Orbicularis oris[a]	+/++
Genioglossus[b]	+/–	Genioglossus[b]	+++/+++

[a]Innervated by facial nerve
[b]Innervated by hypoglossal nerve

11.5.1.3 Oral Recovery

After 3 months, both the patients had good mouth opening (>30 mm). Both the patients obtained labial competence after 9 months and have not had problems with drinking or drooling after that. Eating improved for both the patients after obtaining teeth with the allograft. Patient 1 showed no aspiration in the FEES examination and videofluorography (VGF). Patient 2 developed an aspiration pneumonia at 18 months post transplantation and VGF showed minimal aspiration. The patient had a temporary gastrostomy. For both the patients, there has been minor improvement in eating after FT. Patient 1 is able to eat normal food, whereas patient 2 is still on a soft diet. Speech intelligibility decreased in the beginning after FT for both the patients but improved during the follow-up. During the follow-up, both the patients' speech acceptability improved to moderately impaired. Patient 1 had speech improvement surgery (posterior pharyngeal flap) at 30-months post FT which improved the patient's speech (unpublished results).

11.5.1.4 Breathing

Neither patient had nasal breathing prior to FT, and patient 2 had a tracheostomy. After FT, both obtained unobstructed nasal breathing, and the tracheostomy for patient 2 was removed 3 months post FT. Both the patients declared that they had no smell before the FT. Six months after FT, both the patients told that they can smell strong smells such as gasoline and cigarette, etc. In the Sniffin' Sticks® 12-point smell test, patient 1 scored 2/12 and patient 2 scored 4/12 showing some recovery in olfactory function [16].

11.5.1.5 Dental and Intraoral Recovery

In both the patients, salivary flow was compromised after FT, partly due to several medications. Recipient's own parotid glands were spared but malfunctioned postoperatively possibly due to ductal obstruction. Patient 1 has had gingival problems. Both the patients have had teeth extracted due to caries lesions. Dental implants have been placed in the transplanted

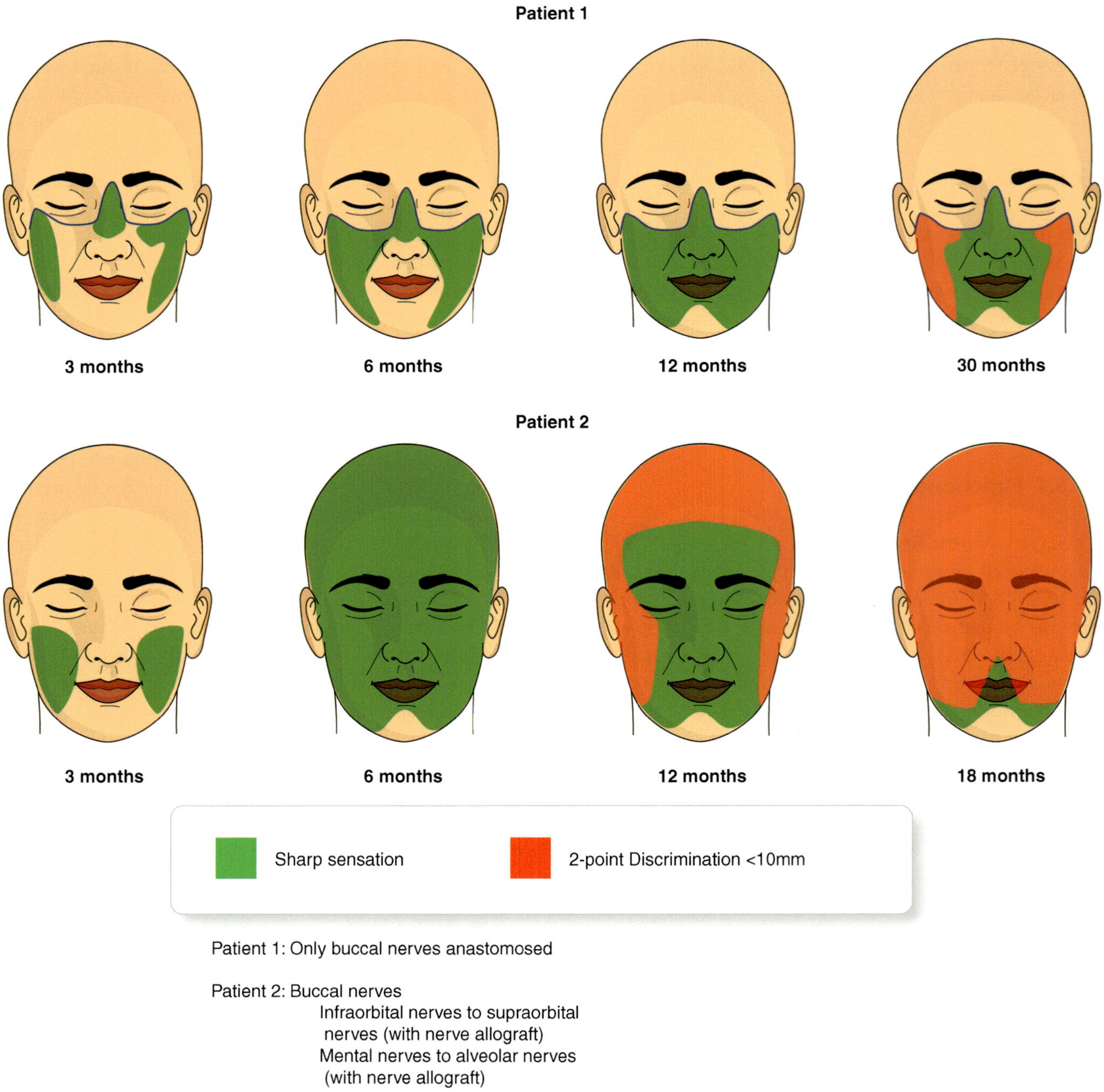

Fig. 11.4 Development of sensory recovery

jaws of patient 2 with successful osseointegration. Both the patients obtained Angle class 1 occlusion, but both had an occlusal discrepancy in the beginning. Temporomandibular joints have functioned normally on both the patients.

11.5.1.6 Eyelids

Patient 1 was blind but had his eye globe left on the right side. An early postoperative ectropion was corrected on the right side [13]. Patient 2 was extremely enophthalmic after FT. He has had canthal repositing on both the sides and repeated fat transfers on the left side to get the lid into contact with the globe.

11.5.1.7 Bone Ossification

Patient 1 developed nonunion on the left sagittal mandible osteosynthesis. After revision and replating also that side ossified. Patient 2 had ossification of both maxilla and mandible without problems.

11.5.2 3D Planning, Prediction, and Bone Stability

We performed for both the patients a virtual FT on the day of transplantation in order to produce cutting guides for the donor and the recipient. In a 3D analysis from postoperative CT scans, we found that we could obtain near to predicted positions for maxilla and mandible. There were 0.1–5.6 mm discrepancies in bone position in comparison with the prediction and the result. The postoperative relationship between maxilla and mandible was almost identical in comparison with the prediction. The obtained early result in bone position has been very stable, the maxilla to mandible relationship has not changed during the 3-year follow-up. We have noticed that the total volume of the transplanted bone diminished 4% in patient 1 and 11% in patient 2 in 2-year follow-up (unpublished results) (Fig. 11.5).

11.5.3 Psychosocial Results

Both the patients have coped well with their new face after FT, and they have expressed their satisfaction for choosing to go for the treatment. Neither patient has shown any signs of depression or other psychological symptoms. Both the patients have been compliant with the rehabilitation and medication. Patient 1 has had some changes with his friends, some of them have not been able to cope with the new situation. Both have returned to their normal daily activities and hobbies. In HRQoL measurements, 15D shows mild improvement in quality of life but not to the level of their age and sex-matched Finnish population. In esthetic analysis, team of professionals evaluated that patient 1 has had significant esthetic improvement and patient 2 looks near to normal person (unpublished results).

11.5.4 Immunological Results

The donors had four mismatching HLA-antigens for patient 1 and six for patient 2. Cytotoxic crossmatches between the donor and recipient were negative for both T- and B-cells in both the patients. Patient 1 had preoperatively developed antibodies against B7 HLA antigen (MFI 1967), thus the virtual crossmatch was positive. This finding was considered an increased risk but not contraindication for FT. Early postoperatively, patient 1 increased HLA immunization (Class I PRA increased from 33% to 98%), and he developed additional donor specific antibodies. These findings were transi-

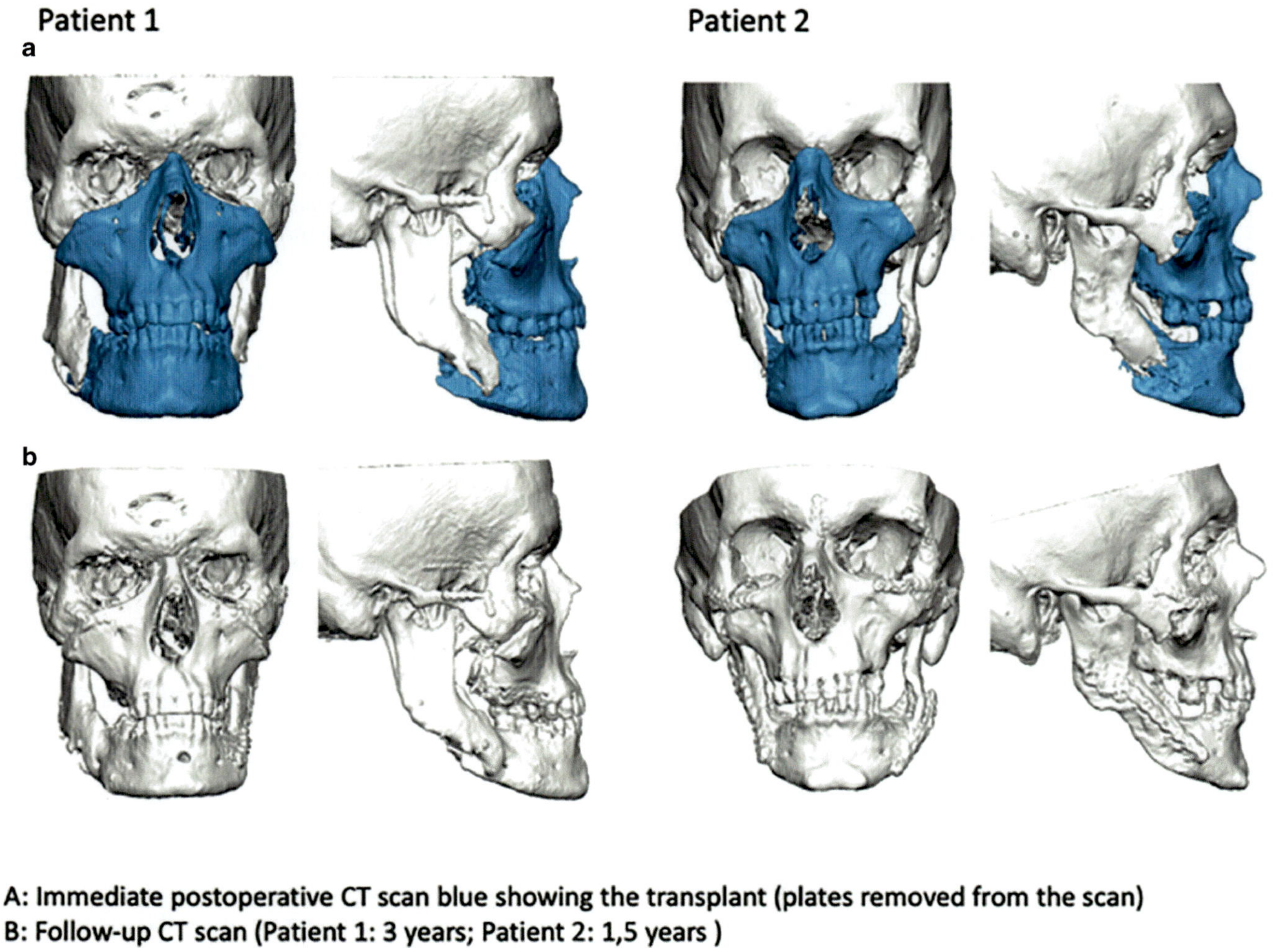

Fig. 11.5 Osseous stability in follow-up

tory, and at 1 year post transplantation and after that, the HLA antibody levels had almost returned to the preoperative level. Patient 2 has not developed donor-specific antibodies.

Neither patient has had an acute rejection during the follow-up (patient 1, 4 years and 7 months and patient 2, 2 years and 6 months). No signs of chronic rejection has been seen clinically or in the biopsies. The transplanted faces have not yet shown signs of accelerated aging (unpublished results).

11.5.5 Complications

11.5.5.1 Surgical Complications

Patient 1 developed on day 7 an oronasal fistula which required three surgical attempts until closure at 14 months. The fistula supposedly resulted from compromised vascularity in posterior hard palate of the allograft. The patient developed an early sialocele on his right parotid gland and in the transplanted submandibular gland. Both resolved without surgery. The patient had a non-union on the right mandible osteosynthesis which required revision and re-plating at 3 months post FT. An ectropion was corrected 4 months post FT [13].

Patient 2 developed also an early oronasal fistula due to small necrosis in the hard palate which required surgical revisions. He also developed unilateral sialocele which resolved. Due to severe enophthalmos, he had marked lower lid ectropion on both sides which required canthal repositions. Patient had an aspiration pneumonia at 14 months post FT (unpublished results).

11.5.5.2 Immunosuppression-Related Complications

Patient 1 had transient steroid-induced type 2 diabetes for the 3 first months after FT which required insulin treatment. He has needed treatment for hypertension since the week 5 post FT. The patient developed kidney insufficiency during the first month post FT. Creatinine levels have been permanently increased, but the level has been steady during the follow-up being 1.5 mg/dL at the moment [13].

Patient 2 became neutropenic 16 months post FT. After reduction of MMF to 1 g/day, the neutropenia resolved slowly.

11.5.5.3 Infections

Patient 1 developed a candida infection in his right maxilla 5 months post FT which was confirmed with sterile bone biopsy. Three molars had to be removed due to the infection. The patient has had repeated oral candida infections which have required topical treatments. The patient developed 3 years post FT a bacterial infection which had started from an infected incisor. The infection required surgical revision.

Patient 2 had symptomless cytomegalovirus infection at 5 months post FT. He developed herpes zoster infection in the right neck and cheek 8 months post FT (unpublished results).

11.6 Lessons Learned

11.6.1 Program Update

The Helsinki VCA program started 9 years ago and the first FT was performed 4.5 years ago. We have examined 11 FT candidates, but there is no patient on the waiting list at the moment. The program is active and open. The Helsinki UET program was approved in 2019, and we have at the moment two patients under evaluations for candidacy for UET. We have also started our laryngeal transplantation program with the ENT unit, and the protocol is under preparation.

11.6.2 Strengths of Helsinki VCA Team

One of the strengths of Helsinki VCA team is that we are one of the largest plastic surgery units in Europe, and we have a long history of reconstructive microsurgery. Our consultants are subspecialized, and several seniors focus their work on facial and head & neck reconstructive surgery and microsurgery. Since VCAs are still experimental, rare, and extremely complicated procedures, it is important to have a large unit with wide expertise in order to minimize complications and to produce best possible results. It is also an advantage to have strong additional units such as maxillofacial surgery, ENT, oculoplastic surgery, and others especially if the VCA team plans to perform several types of VCAs.

The other positive aspect in Helsinki is that Finland has centralized all organ transplantation activity to Helsinki. This results in close collaboration and incorporation of the SOT team with the VCA team. VCA's are organ transplantations. It is extremely important to have strong support from SOT specialists.

One reason for success in Helsinki is that we did thorough preparation for 5 years and tried to minimize all potential hazards during the procedure and planned all aspects of the rehabilitation in advance.

We have been very strict with the selection of our patients. It is most important that the patient is motivated, committed, and compliant. One common potential factor for failure is patient related [17].

11.6.3 Obstacles to Expansion of the Program

Since VCAs are still experimental, they are strictly regulated and followed, which restricts the rapid expansion of the field. On the other hand, during this early period, it is important not to rush and perform VCAs in centers that have not prepared the program well enough or which do not have the necessary infrastructure. Failures during this period will damage the image of VCAs and might result in restrictions in other centers.

Helsinki VCA program is funded by the public healthcare system, and the finance is basically permanent. Finance is the one potential risk factor for the future of VCA. Grant-based programs are at risk for discontinuation of the grant. For the future, it is important to try to get steady and long-term solutions for finance in different countries until these treatments are no more classified as experimental.

The catchment area for Helsinki VCA program is 5.5 million, the Finnish population. Since the number of patients benefitting from VCAs is really small, the catchment area should be at least five times larger. For Helsinki center that would mean the population of Scandinavia which is approximately 25 million. There is a need for small countries to collaborate and centralize these extremely rare procedures. Centralization is recommended also for larger countries in order to at least in some units to gain experience.

11.6.4 The Future of VCAs

We are at the end of the beginning of VCA era. Now is the time to shift the attitude from experimental and unique operations into standardized and commonly accepted procedures. The number of VCAs will never be large due to the fact that there are not many patients who will benefit from them when all the risks are taken into account. These procedures will always be complicated and laborious and require expertise. Therefore, the future will be in centralized large centers that cover several different types of VCAs. The variety of VCAs will increase in the future. An interesting approach is the spare part transplantation concept. There are several SOT patients who have missing or malfunctioning body parts. A patient who already has immunosuppression could benefit from VCA without marked additional morbidity.

References

1. Lindford AJ, Mäkisalo H, Jalanko H, Lauronen J, Anttila VJ, Juteau S, et al. The Helsinki approach to face transplantation. J Plast Reconstr Aesthet Surg. 2018;7(2):132–9.
2. Pomahac B, Diaz-Siso JR, Bueno EM. Evolution of indications for facial transplantation. J Plast Reconstr Aesthet Surg. 2011;64(11):1410–6.
3. Carty MJ, Bueno EM, Lehmann LS, Pomahac B. A position paper in support of face transplantation in the blind. Plast Reconstr Surg. 2012;130(2):319–24.
4. Neely JG, Cherian NG, Dickerson CB, Nedzelski JM. Sunnybrook facial grading system: reliability and criteria for grading. Laryngoscope. 2010;120(5):1038–45.
5. Sintonen H. The 15D instrument of health-related quality of life: properties and applications. Ann Med. 2001;33(5):328–36.
6. Brazier JE, Harper R, Jones NM, O'Cathain A, Thomas KJ, Usherwood T, et al. Validating the SF-36 health survey questionnaire: new outcome measure for primary care. BMJ. 1992;305(6846):160–4.
7. Sherman AC, Simonton S, Adams DC, Vural E, Owens B, Hanna E. Assessing quality of life in patients with head and neck cancer: cross-validation of the European Organization for Research and Treatment of cancer (EORTC) quality of life head and neck module (QLQ-H&N35). Arch Otolaryngol Head Neck Surg. 2000;126(4):459–67.
8. Alanne S, Roine RP, Räsänen P, Vainiola T, Sintonen H. Estimating the minimum important change in the 15D scores. Qual Life Res. 2015;24(3):599–606.
9. Furr LA, Wiggins O, Cunningham M, Vasilic D, Brown CS, Banis JC Jr, et al. Psychosocial implications of disfigurement and the future of human face transplantation. Plast Reconstr Surg. 2007;120(2):559–65.
10. Bramstedt KA. A lifesaving view of vascularized composite allotransplantation: patient experience of social death before and after face, hand, and larynx transplant. J Patient Exp. 2018, Jun;5(2):92–100.
11. Sheehan DV, Harnett-Sheehan K, Raj BA. The measurement of disability. Int Clin Psychopharmacol. 1996;11(3):89–95.
12. Katz MR, Irish JC, Devins GM, Rodin GM, Gullane PJ. Reliability and validity of an observer-rated disfigurement scale for head and neck cancer patients. Head Neck. 2000;22(2):132–41.
13. Lassus P, Lindford A, Vuola J, Bäck L, Suominen S, Mesimäki K, et al. The Helsinki face transplantation: surgical aspects and 1-year outcome. J Plast Reconstr Aesthet Surg. 2018;71(2):132–9.
14. Mäkitie A, Salmi M, Lindford A, Tuomi J, Lassus P. 3D printing for restoration of the donor face: a new digital technique tested and used in the first facial allotransplantation patient in Finland. J Plast Reconstr Aesthet Surg. 2016;69(12):1648–52.
15. Cendales LC, Kanitakis J, Schneeberger S, Burns C, Ruitz P, Landin L, et al. The Banff 2007 working classification of skin-containing composite tissue allograft pathology. Am J Transplant. 2008;8(7):1396–400.
16. Rumeau C, Nguyen DT, Jankowski R. How to assess olfactory performance with the sniffin' sticks test. Eur Ann Otorhinolaryngol Head Neck Dis. 2015;133(3):203–6.
17. Bunzel B, Laederach-Hofmann K. Solid organ transplantation: are there predictors for posttransplant noncompliance? A literature overview. Transplantation. 2000;70(5):711–6.

Part III

Laryngeal Transplantation

Laryngeal Transplantation, I

12

David G. Lott and Robert R. Lorenz

12.1 Introduction

Human laryngeal transplantation was first studied in animal models in the 1960s by Boles [1], Ogura [2], and Silver [3]. The first subtotal laryngeal transplant was performed by Kluyskens and Ringoir [4] in 1969 in the setting of reconstruction after cancer extirpation. No neuronal or microvascular anastomoses were performed, and the recipient perichondrium was preserved as the blood supply to the transplanted cartilage. Unfortunately, the cancer quickly recurred while on immunosuppression, causing interest in laryngeal transplantation to wane for the next two decades.

There are barriers to overcome for laryngeal transplantation to become a viable option for a large cohort of patients. First, the larynx is considered a nonvital organ since it is possible to survive following its removal. The ethics of subjecting patients to the potential complications of transplantation for a nonvital organ are of primary concern. This topic is discussed thoroughly in a publication by Genden and Urken [5]. Second, transplantation requires lifelong immunosuppression which can have many known adverse side effects. Most notably, the relative risk of developing a malignancy while on immunosuppression has been estimated to be up to 400 times that of the general population [6]. This concern currently prohibits laryngeal transplantation in cancer patients. Despite this risk, 75% of surveyed laryngectomy patients said they would accept a larynx transplant if offered [7]. Patient desire to restore larynx functionality, and the possibility to restore one's individuality, puts into question the "non-vital" classification. Lastly, restoring vocal fold motion is in its infancy with some successes reported to date.

In 1987, Marshall Strome began to investigate the potential of laryngeal transplantation, focusing on reinnervation, revascularization, immunosuppression, and the ethics of laryngeal transplantation. A rat laryngeal transplantation model was developed to investigate the maximum tolerated total ischemia time [8], preservative solutions, stages of histologic rejection [9], and immunosuppressive regimens [10]. Once the research supported the feasibility, the first human total laryngeal transplantation was performed on January 4, 1998 by a multidisciplinary team at the Cleveland Clinic led by Strome, the details of which were later reported in a New England Journal publication [11].

12.2 The First Human Composite Laryngeal Transplant

Following extensive interviews, counseling, and testing, a 40-year-old man with a dysfunctional larynx secondary to trauma was chosen. A motorcycle accident 20 years earlier caused a crush injury to his larynx and pharynx. Despite multiple attempts at another institution to reconstruct his larynx, he remained aphonic and tracheotomy dependent.

The donor was a 40-year-old brain dead man from a ruptured cerebral aneurysm. He met all the predetermined criteria for acceptance in regard to HLA matching (4 of 5) and serum virology. The donor organ harvest included the entire pharyngolaryngeal complex, including six tracheal rings and the thyroid and parathyroid glands (Fig. 12.1). The organ complex was stored in solution during transport until revascularization 10 h later.

Cyclosporine, azathioprine, and methylprednisolone were administered to the recipient prior to surgery. Perfusion was

Supplementary Information The online version contains supplementary material available at https://doi.org/10.1007/978-3-031-21520-9_12.

D. G. Lott
Division of Laryngology; Otolaryngology-Head and Neck Surgery, Mayo Clinic Arizona, Phoenix, AZ, USA

Head and Neck Regenerative Medicine and Transplantation Program, Mayo Clinic Arizona, Phoenix, AZ, USA
e-mail: Lott.David@mayo.edu

R. R. Lorenz (✉)
The Head and Neck Institute, Cleveland Clinic, Cleveland, OH, USA
e-mail: lorenzr@ccf.org

© Springer Nature Switzerland AG 2023

R. Gurunian et al. (eds.), *Reconstructive Transplantation*, https://doi.org/10.1007/978-3-031-21520-9_12

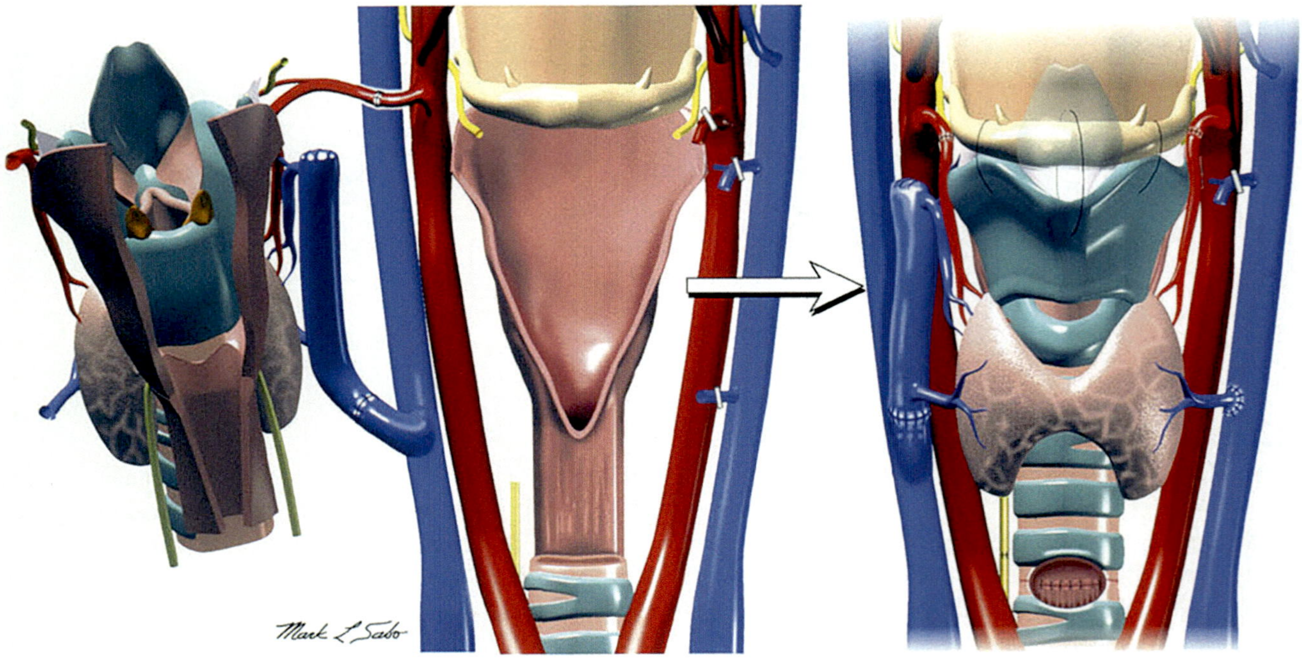

Fig. 12.1 Surgical technique of the first successful composite total laryngeal transplant. Vascular anastomoses included the donor right internal jugular vein to the recipient right facial vein, donor left middle thyroid vein to recipient left internal jugular vein, donor superior thyroid arteries to the recipient superior thyroid arteries. Nerve anastomoses included both superior laryngeal nerves and only the right recurrent laryngeal nerve. (Reprinted with permission, Cleveland Clinic Center for Medical Art & Photography © 2015. All Rights Reserved)

re-established to the donor organ as the first step of the transplant. The donor's right superior thyroid artery was anastomosed to the same artery of the recipient. The proximal end of the donor's right internal jugular vein was anastomosed to the patient's right common facial vein. Blood flow through the transplanted thyroid gland, six tracheal rings, larynx, and pharynx was observed within 30 min of clamp release.

Once perfusion was established, a narrow field laryngectomy was performed on the recipient. His thyroid lobes were kept in situ but lateralized. The hyoid bone was left in place. A majority of the donor's pharynx was utilized to widen the patient's stenotic pharyngoesophageal complex. The donor laryngeal cartilage was sutured to the hyoid bone to create fixed, laryngeal elevation which maximized future swallowing capabilities. Five of the donor's tracheal rings were sutured to the recipient tracheostoma. The stoma was left open as a safety mechanism, given that bilateral vocal fold paralysis in the cadaveric position was anticipated.

The left-sided vascular anastomoses were then completed, which included the donor's superior thyroid artery to the recipient's superior thyroid artery and the donor middle thyroid vein to the recipient internal jugular vein. Both superior laryngeal nerves were located and reanastomosed. Only the recipient's right recurrent laryngeal nerve could be located for reinnervation to the donor's right recurrent laryngeal nerve. The donor's left recurrent laryngeal nerve was allowed to remain free within the soft tissues of the neck and not connected to a recipient nerve. A gastrostomy tube was placed for perioperative nutrition.

The immediate postoperative immunosuppression regimen included muromonab-CD3, cyclosporine, methylprednisolone, and mycophenolate mofetil. Initial aspiration episodes were controlled with glycopyrrolate and atropine, which were later discontinued. After observation in the hospital for 1 month, the patient's transplanted trachea was noted to be slightly edematous on endoscopy but showed no signs of rejection on biopsy. Three months posttransplant, the supraglottis and vocal folds became sensitive to touch. Purposeful swallowing, taste, and smell returned. Subsequent barium swallows revealed no aspiration. To evaluate thyroid function, a 4-h uptake of iodine-123 demonstrated 83% activity in the transplanted thyroid lobes, as well as 17% in the patient's native thyroid. The transplanted parathyroid glands were assumed to be nonfunctional given the extended ischemic time.

Posttransplant voicing first occurred on the third postoperative day. Endoscopy at 1 month revealed that both true vocal folds were in a lateral (cadaveric) position, creating a breathy voice. The right fold (the side of the recurrent nerve anastomosis) was midline at the 4 months endoscopy. By 6 months posttransplant, the left had medialized. Neither vocal fold demonstrated abduction, but rather appeared to be synkinetic. Electromyographic (EMG) measurements confirmed reinnervation of both thyroarytenoid muscles and bilateral volitional cricothyroid function [12] (Fig. 12.2a, b). It was postulated that the innervation on the left was likely due to "field-reinnervation," in which the left thyroarytenoid muscle is supplied by surrounding motor nerves. Subjective

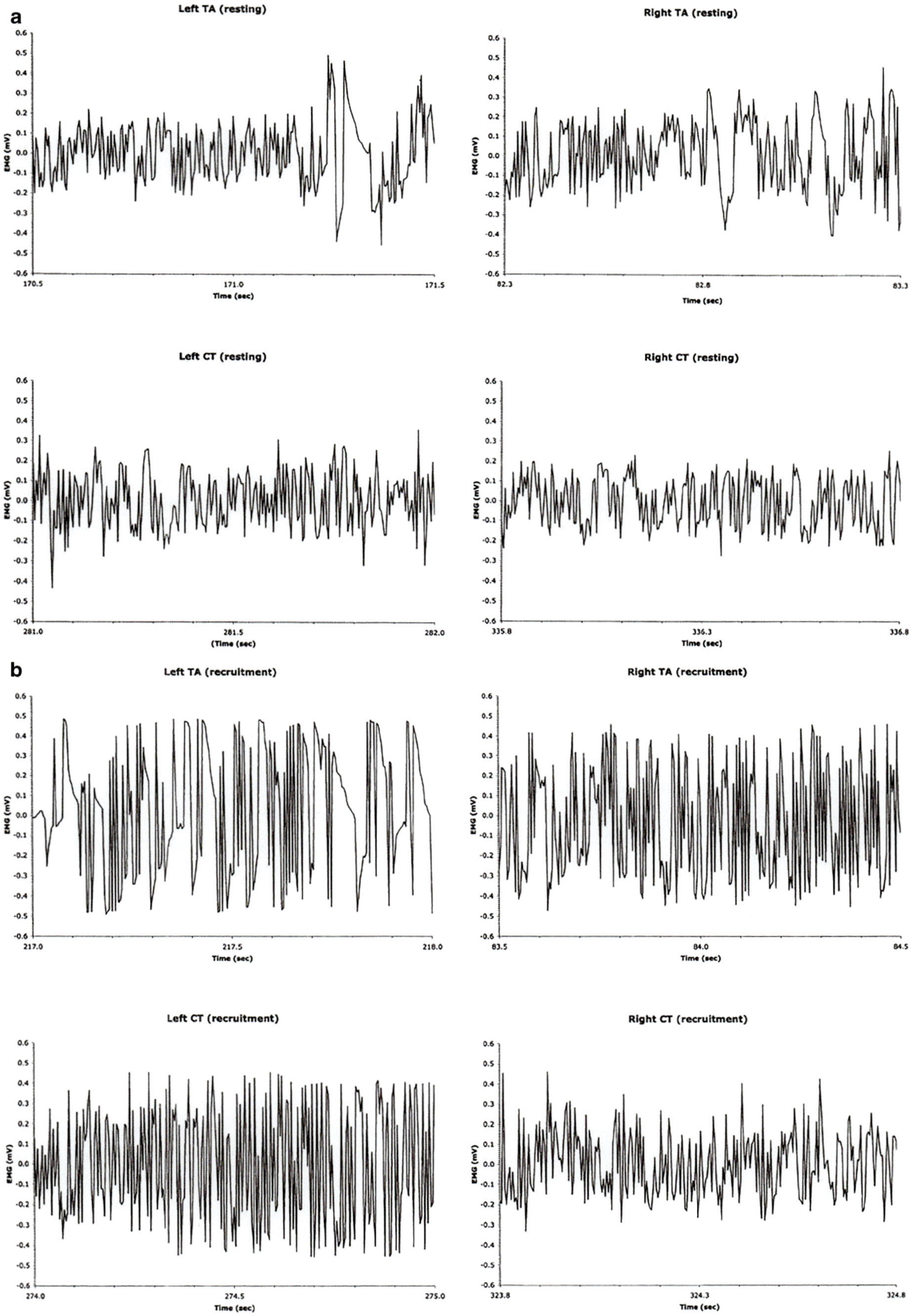

Fig. 12.2 EMG results in laryngeal transplant patient at 3 years. (**a**) EMG findings at rest, including bilateral thyroarytenoid muscles (TA) and cricothyroid (CT) muscles. (**b**) EMG findings during sustained/ee/ phonation (TA) and raising and lowering of pitch (CT). Upon volitional movement, the left TA and CT muscles demonstrated moderately reduced recruitment patterns, whereas the right muscle groups showed mild reductions in recruitment. All four muscles demonstrated increased numbers of polyphasic motor unit potentials of mildly increased duration and normal amplitude, firing at moderate to rapid rates

and objective measures of phonation including pitch, jitter, intensity, and maximal phonation time were within the normal range at 36 months posttransplant. As a vocation, the patient became a motivational speaker. He stated his quality of life improved "immeasurably" subsequent to the transplantation.

There were few postoperative complications. The patient experienced three early episodes of tracheobronchitis which were successfully treated with oral amoxicillin clavulanate. At 16 weeks posttransplant, the patient inadvertently stopped his trimethoprim sulfamethoxazole and developed *Pneumocystis carinii* pneumonia, which cleared rapidly with intravenous antibiotics. The patient presented with a decrease in voice quality 15 months posttransplant and was diagnosed with acute rejection. His larynx and voice returned to normal after being treated with three daily doses of methylprednisolone (1 g/day). A second episode of rejection occurred about 5 years later due to laboratory error in tacrolimus values measuring levels falsely high. As a result the patient's medication became below therapeutic levels. Laryngeal edema was observed during the acute rejection episode, but returned to normal once medication levels returned to the therapeutic range.

12.3 The Unpublished Colombian Experience

Dr. Luis Fernando Tintinago from Colombia has performed several laryngeal, tracheal, and esophageal transplantations starting in 2002 (personal communication). Tintinago and his team had performed a total of 21 transplants in total, including 5 laryngeal transplants (as defined by transplanting the entire larynx with reinnervation and partial hypopharynx), 10 laryngotracheal (partial laryngeal and partial tracheal without reinnervation), 4 tracheal, and 2 larynx, hypopharynx, and esophageal. Due to a variety of factors including heterogeneous outcomes and waning governmental support for transplant recipients, the program closed in 2012. Publication of the lessons and results has yet to be forthcoming, but his lessons learned from this voluminous and extensive experience have been captured in videotaped presentations:

Examples of Achieving Tolerance in Transplantation: The Colombian Experience.

http://webcast1.ccf.org/viewerportal/ccfe/video.vp?programId=esc_program:126814

Larynx, Trachea, and Esophageal Transplantation: Two Decades of Lessons Learned.

http://webcast1.ccf.org/viewerportal/ccfe/video.vp?programId=esc_program:126815

12.4 Second Published Human Composite Laryngeal Transplant

A second reported laryngeal transplant was performed in the USA in 2012 [13]. The patient was a 51-year-old woman with acquired laryngotracheal stenosis who was tracheotomy tube dependent and is fully described in Chap. 15. The main factor which lead to the consideration of laryngeal transplant was the presence of a previous kidney-pancreas transplant for her diabetic chronic kidney disease, obviating the need for additional immunosuppression for her laryngeal transplant.

12.4.1 Third Published Human Composite Laryngeal Transplant

The third reported larynx transplant was performed as part of a composite allograft in Poland in 2015 [14]. This patient was a 34-year-old man on immunosuppression for a renal transplant and was later treated for acute myeloid leukemia. He developed a T3N1 squamous cell laryngeal cancer and underwent a total laryngectomy with postoperative radiation in 2009. His cancer treatment course was complicated by pharyngeal necrosis and a large pharyngeal fistula. At the time of transplantation, the patient was disease free from leukemia for 12 years and laryngeal cancer for 6 years.

12.4.2 Surgical Details

Donor Graft: Larynx, 8 cm of trachea, pharynx with esophagus, thyroid and four parathyroid glands, hyoid bone with anterior bellies of digastric muscles, sternohyoid muscles, and anterior cervical wall skin paddle.

Arterial Anastomoses: End-to-end anastomoses between the donor superior thyroid arteries and the recipient left facial and right lingual arteries.

Venous Anastomoses: End-to-side anastomoses between the donor bilateral internal jugular veins with recipient internal jugular veins. In addition, the donor anterior cervical veins were anastomosed with the recipient external jugular veins.

Neural Anastomoses: End-to-side anastomoses of the donor superior laryngeal nerves to the recipient sublingual nerves and the donor recurrent laryngeal nerves were anastomosed end-to-side of the recipient left phrenic and right vagus nerves.

Induction immunosuppression consisted of antithymocyte globulin for 10 days, tacrolimus, mycophenolate mofetil, and methylprednisolone. During the maintenance phase, tacrolimus was administered to maintain the plasma concentration between 7 and 10 ng/mL. Mycophenolate mofetil was continued at a reduced dose of 1.5 g per day. Methylprednisolone was reduced to 4 mg per day.

No immediate postoperative complications were reported. An episode of cytomegalovirus reactivation was successfully treated with ganciclovir. A digestive tract contracture was treated endoscopically without the need for a repeat procedure within the 6 postoperative months.

Good functional results have been reported. The tracheostomy and gastric feeding tube were removed 10 days after surgery. Initial voicing occurred 2 weeks postoperatively. Per last report approximately 2 years after the transplant, the patient's vocal folds were functioning and he can communicate well. He is eating without difficulty and breathing without a tracheostomy. The transplanted thyroid and parathyroid glands are fully functional.

12.5 Immunosuppression Reduction

The primary limitation of laryngeal transplantation, and transplantation in general, is immunosuppression. The ability to significantly reduce or remove the need for immunosuppression would help to prevent associated complications and help to facilitate transplantation in cancer patients, thereby greatly expanding the potential candidate pool. Many innovative studies have been performed and are currently underway with this as the primary goal. The results of these studies may impact not only laryngeal transplantation but also both traditional and other vascular composite allograft transplants.

A variety of animal models have been developed to lessen the necessary immunosuppression for laryngeal transplantation including dog [1–3], mouse [15, 16], and pig [17]. These all offer complementary information forming the basis on which to build further understanding into laryngeal transplantation. The two authors' work has focused on the rat and mouse models since they are well-established transplant models, significant information is known about their immune systems, and are relatively inexpensive. Our model places the transplanted organ in tandem with the native larynx (Fig. 12.3a–c). An arteriovenous shunt is created with arterial inflow through one superior thyroid artery and venous outflow through the contralateral superior thyroid artery. Revisions to the rat model and a revised grading scale of rejection were published in 2002 [18]. The mouse model

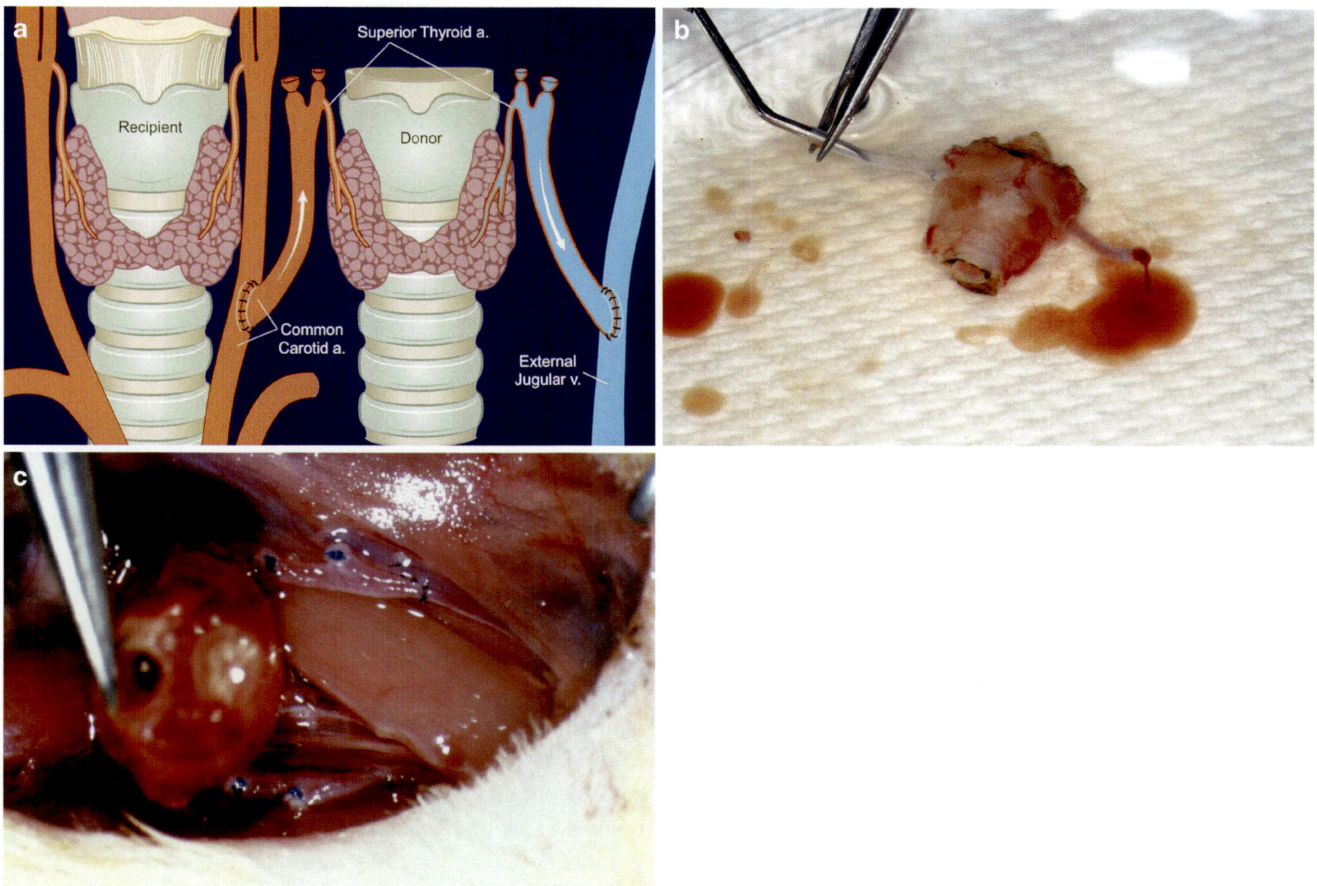

Fig. 12.3 (**a**–**c**) Mouse and rat laryngeal transplantation diagram. Arterial inflow is achieved through the donor common carotid artery anastomosed to recipient common carotid artery. Direct graft inflow and outflow is based on superior thyroid artery pedicled via the external carotid artery. Venous outflow continues through the donor contralateral common carotid artery anastomosed to recipient internal jugular vein. (**a**) (Reprinted with permission, Cleveland Clinic Center for Medical Art & Photography© 2015. All Rights Reserved)

[16] and a mouse rejection grading scale [19] were published later. With more than 3000 transplants, these models have shown overall nearly 100% survivability and a greater than 90% graft evaluability. Furthermore, performing a total parathyroidectomy on the recipient during transplantation can utilize the production of parathormone from the rat transplanted larynx as a marker of graft viability rather than having to sacrifice the animal for histologic evaluation [20]. This has allowed for a new generation of studies examining the ability to "pulse" immunosuppressives and "salvage" the organ if parathormone levels decrease.

Haug et al. [21] performed an interesting study that helped to develop the minimum level of CSA required to obtain optimum graft survival when used as the sole agent for immunosuppression. They correlated the laryngeal rejection grade, cyclosporine A (CSA) concentration, and CSA intramuscular dosing. This was a blinded study looking at different dosages for CSA monotherapy. CSA was dosed at 1.0, 2.5, 5.0, 7.5, or 10 mg/kg/day. Significantly different average CSA concentrations were achieved among each group of five transplanted rats. Rejection grading within the top three doses of CSA were not significantly different. However, significant pathologic allograft rejection correlated with CSA concentrations below 250 ng/mL.

A study in rats performed by Lorenz et al. [22] investigated the ability to decrease the overall amount of CSA by adding prednisone to the regimen. In a multi-arm study containing 220 transplantations, multiple doses of both cyclosporine and prednisone were administered. The transplanted organs were evaluated at both 15 days and 30 days posttransplantation. The addition of 1.0 mg/kg/day of prednisone allowed CSA doses to be reduced to 2.0 mg/kg and still demonstrate no significant rejection at 30 days posttransplantation. Although the combination of low-dose CSA and prednisone significantly improved graft survival when compared to CSA alone at the equivalent dose, prednisone monotherapy demonstrated rates of rejection similar to no immunosuppression at all.

Additional studies further demonstrated that combination therapy with other immunosuppressives would also allow for decreased levels while maintaining graft viability [23, 24]. A study by Nelson et al. [23] conducted experiments between tacrolimus (FK506) alone at varying levels, and tacrolimus combined with mycophenolate mofetil at varying levels. Groups were examined at either 15 or 30 days posttransplantation. As expected, increasing levels of tacrolimus demonstrated increasing efficacy of immunosuppression. However, low-dose tacrolimus in combination with mycophenolate mofetil achieved comparable results.

Akst et al. [24] elicited the exciting finding that tolerance of the transplanted organ can be induced with a very low dose of combined immunosuppressants. They treated transplanted rats with tacrolimus and mouse anti-rat alpha beta T-cell receptor monoclonal antibodies (αβ-TCR) for only 7 days following the transplant. All grafts demonstrated viability at 100 days. Skin grafting, mixed lymphocyte reaction, and flow cytometry revealed that tolerance was neither donor specific nor related to prolonged depletion of T-cell populations.

12.6 Immunosuppression in the Cancer Patient

The studies mentioned above demonstrate the possibility of inducing tolerance with very low doses of immunosuppression. However, that degree of immunosuppression is still prohibitive in cancer patients, which represent the vast majority of laryngeal transplantation candidates. It may be allowable to transplant patients with large benign or low-grade malignant laryngeal tumors, those with no sign of recurrent cancer after 5 years, or those with laryngeal cancer who are already on a post-transplant immunosuppression regimen.

Ultimately, the largest group of patients who stand to benefit are those presenting with locally advanced laryngeal cancer. There are approximately 12,000 new cases of advanced laryngeal cancer per year in the United States [25]. To date, two transplants have been performed for locally advanced head and neck cancer reconstruction—the non-revascularized partial laryngeal transplant in 1969 [4] and a tongue transplant in 2003. Unfortunately, both patients rapidly succumbed to recurrent disease. There are two primary areas of immunosuppression investigation that are promising for possible transplantation in malignancy. The first is to add an antineoplastic agent to the immunosuppression regimen. The second is to directly modify immune cells to maintain immunocompetence while accepting the transplant. The second will be discussed later in the chapter.

One intriguing immunosuppressive option for transplantation in cancer patients is Everolimus (SDZ-RAD) [26], which is a derivative of rapamycin and belongs to the mTOR (mammalian target of rapamycin) class of immunosuppressants. It blocks the translation of mRNA in critical cell cycle regulatory proteins, thereby inhibiting proliferation of intimal cells, lymphocytes, and tumor cells. Everolimus has shown both immunosuppressive and antitumor properties. The antitumor properties have been demonstrated in several animal and human tumor cell lines, including squamous cell carcinoma [27–29], which is the predominant laryngeal cancer type. In addition, it has been shown to inhibit the development of posttransplant lymphoproliferative disorders [30]. Findings from our laryngeal transplant models have provided support for the use of everolimus as an effective immunosuppressive and antineoplastic agent in laryngeal transplantation [29, 31].

An interesting study by Khariwala et al. used a mouse squamous cell carcinoma cell-line to determine the effect of everolimus on the growth of both intradermal tumors and pulmonary metastases [29]. Tumor inhibition occurred in both the intradermal primary tumors and pulmonary metastasis models studied (Fig. 12.4a–d). The authors concluded that everolimus provides potent tumor inhibition in animals inoculated with squamous cell cancer cells by decreasing local spread of disease as well as distant metastases.

Everolimus was then studied as a single agent immunosuppressive in the mouse transplantation model [32]. Everolimus at a dose of 1 mg/kg/day was given to transplanted mice and followed for 15, 30, and 60 days. The study showed that everolimus monotherapy successfully prevented laryngeal allograft rejection up to the study endpoint (60 days posttransplantation) (Fig. 12.5). Flow cytometry showed a blunted cytotoxic T-cell response, differentiation favoring regulatory T-cells, and decreased number and function of dendritic cells. This is a favorable environment for transplantation.

Once Everolimus demonstrated efficacy for both immunosuppression and antineoplastic activity, the feasibility of

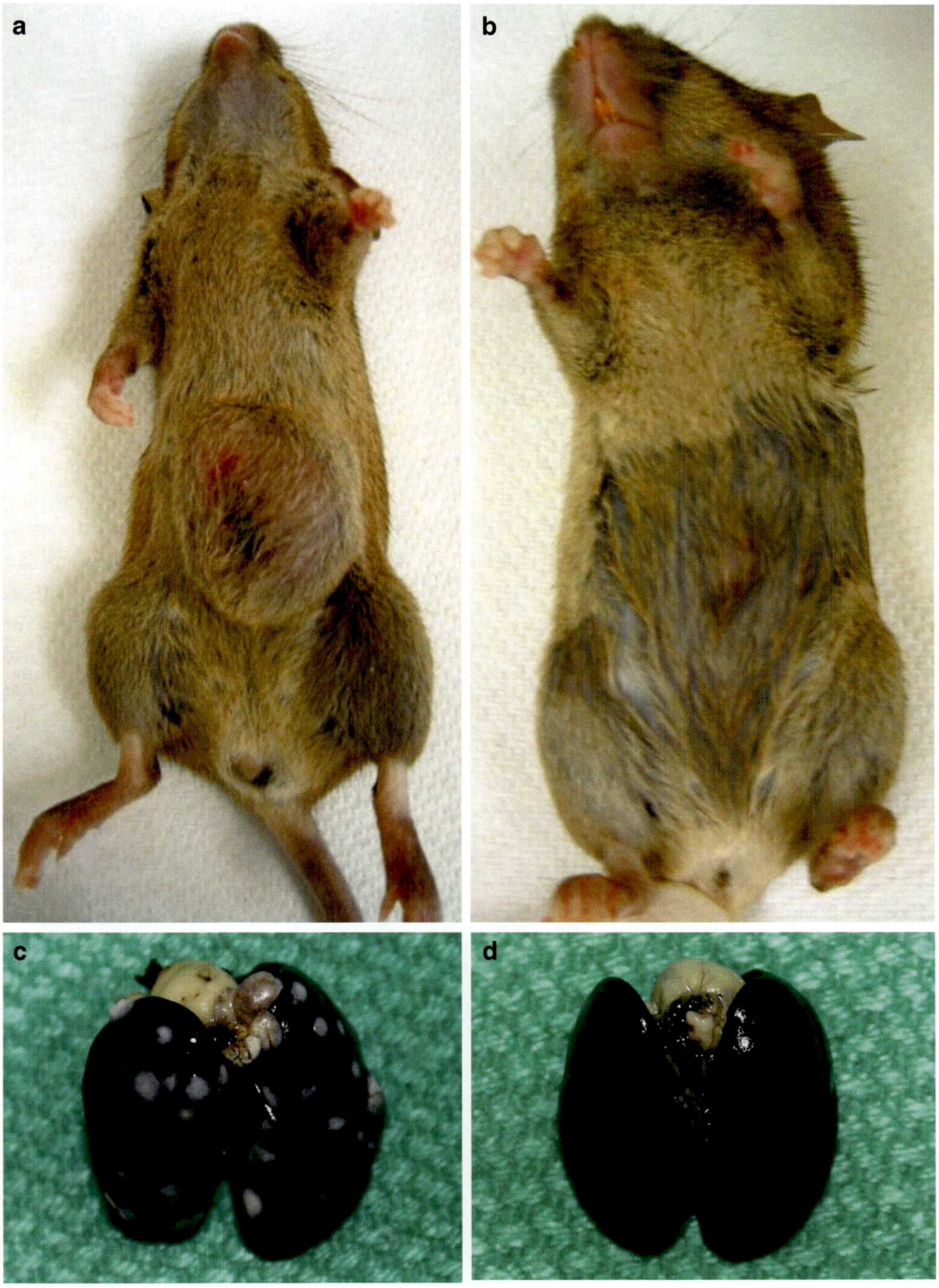

Fig. 12.4 Results of everolimus therapy in mouse squamous cell carcinoma. (**a**) Intradermal tumor in untreated animal. (**b**) Intradermal tumor in treated animal. (**c**) Pulmonary metastasis in untreated animal. (**d**) Pulmonary metastasis in treated animal

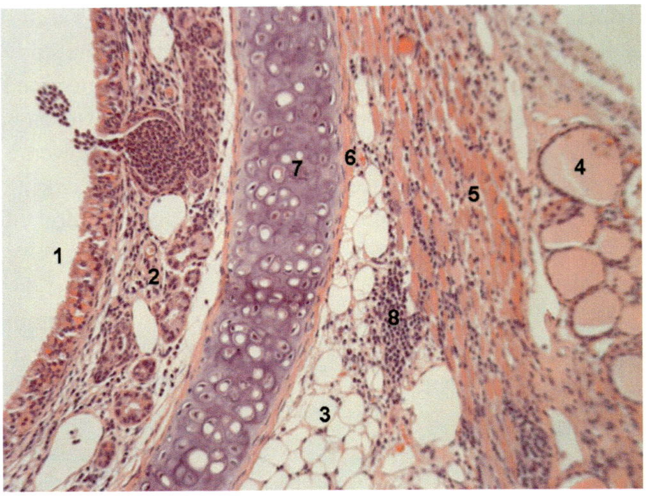

Fig. 12.5 Preservation of transplanted larynx with everolimus monotherapy. Hematoxylin-eosinophil analysis of laryngeal allograft at 60 days posttransplant. Note moderate lymphocytic infiltration with normal structures including ciliated epithelium (*1*) epithelium; (*2*) minor salivary glands; (*3*) fat; (*4*) thyroid gland; (*5*) muscle; (*6*) perichondrium; (*7*) cartilage; (*8*) lymphocytic infiltration

using it as a combination therapy (Everolimus and αβ-TCR) in a pulsed-dose regimen to reduce the total amount of immunosuppression and induce tolerance was investigated [31]. This study had the remarkable finding that tolerance can be achieved via a pulsed-dose combination therapy for 10 months with just a total of 15 days of immunosuppression. The promising immunosuppressive and antitumor profile of everolimus continues to suggest a prominent role for this agent in the future of laryngeal transplantation, and may 1 day serve to enable transplantation in the setting of malignancy.

12.7 Immunomodulation

An ideal immunosuppression regimen would be metabolically inert and induce donor-specific tolerance while leaving the remainder of the recipient's immune system functional. Directly altering immune cells through immunomodulation holds the promise of making that a reality. This concept was supported by Genden et al. [33] when they demonstrated that a single injection of UV-B irradiated donor splenocytes was sufficient to prevent rejection in a rat tracheal graft model.

Several studies have been performed to better understand the immunological environment of the larynx and trachea in an effort to further investigate immunomodulation as a viable immunosuppressive regimen for laryngeal transplantation. A dense, organized network of immunologically active cells has been identified in both pig and human laryngeal mucosa [34, 35]. The morphology of the cells in these early studies was suggestive of dendritic cells and was more closely analyzed by Friedman et al. [36] in the rat model. Rat larynges were stained for dendritic cells and enumerated by a combination of immunofluorescence, confocal microscopy, and imaging software. This revealed that the vast majority of dendritic cells were located in epithelium and subepithelium when compared to other laryngeal subsites. The epithelium was 11 times more highly populated than the subepithelium. A study by Govindaraj et al. [37] supports the importance of tracheal epithelium in the rejection process. Their studies of mouse tracheal grafts showed that replacement of the epithelium by host epithelial cells prevents rejection after withdrawal of immunosuppression.

The vastly increased density of dendritic cells in the epithelium coupled with the knowledge of the important role the epithelium has in graft rejection suggested an important role of dendritic cells in transplant tolerance. Dendritic cells are the primary antigen-presenting cells in the body and are known to have a significant role in determining graft rejection or survival. In the immature state (lack of a T-cell costimulatory molecule), they work to induce tolerance through T-cell anergy and apoptosis. Once maturation occurs through the presentation of a T-cell costimulatory molecule, dendritic cells facilitate rejection.

Lott et al. [38] were able to modify dendritic cells to resist maturation through the addition of nuclear factor kappa B (NF-κB) decoy oligodeoxyribonucleotides. Fortifying dendritic cells with NF-κB results in the suppression of costimulatory molecule expression causing resistance to maturation even after contact with activated allogenic T-cells, lipopolysaccharide [39], and antigen [40]. In their study, a single injection of immature dendritic cells (iDC) were injected into mice 7 days before transplantation. iDC-treated mice had significantly less rejection at all time points compared to non-immunosuppressed mice. Flow cytometry showed inhibition of cytotoxic T-cell infiltration and expansion of regulatory T-cells at the allograft site. The authors postulated that iDC immunotherapy may facilitate graft tolerance as a monotherapy or favorably affect concurrent immunosuppressive dose sequencing.

12.8 Reinnervation Research in Laryngeal Transplantation

Another major obstacle in laryngeal transplantation is the inability to restore functional reinnervation of the vocal fold musculature. Mass reinnervation of both the abductor and adductor muscle groups by the recurrent laryngeal nerve prevents net movement of the vocal folds. This process, called synkinesis, prevents proper glottic functionality. Similar to bilateral vocal fold paralysis, the patient is left with the option of having a permanent tracheostomy or a breathy voice following a laser cordotomy. The first transplanted patient rated his voice quality as "excellent" and was reluctant to undergo either lateralization of the true vocal fold or cordotomy in order to achieve closure of his tracheostomy due to the concern that such procedures would lessen his voice quality. In their 2010 transplant experience, Farwell et al. attempted to achieve some volitional movement on their recipient's left side, anastomosing the adductor branch of the RLN to the ansa cervicalis system, and the RLN truck end-to-side into the recipient's phrenic nerve [13]. By 18 months postoperatively, the authors described the glottis opening as limited and the patient continued to be tracheotomy tube dependent.

Return of volitional movement of the vocal folds is critical to the wide acceptance of laryngeal transplantation. To date, complete success has been elusive. Part of this difficulty is the complex anatomy of the recurrent laryngeal nerve. Stavroulaki and Birchall [41] reviewed the anatomy of the laryngeal nerves in humans, dogs, cats, and pigs. This review demonstrated that nerve specification is more complicated than the dogma suggests. The anterior recurrent laryngeal nerve is responsible for adductor function and the posterior recurrent laryngeal nerve controls abductor function. However, many branches of the anterior and posterior nerves exit and areas of cross-innervation abound that make reinnervation much less straightforward.

The primary goal of laryngeal reinnervation is to establish vocal fold abduction during inspiration. Therefore, the primary target of reinnervation is the posterior cricoarytenoid (PCA) muscle, which is the only laryngeal muscle that abducts the vocal fold. Given that vocal fold abduction must be timed with inspiration, the phrenic nerve is an attractive option for establishing function given that it is a motor nerve active during inspiration. Baldissera et al. [42] were able to selectively innervate the bilateral PCA muscles using a single branch of the phrenic nerve in a cat model. Some function was achieved bilaterally. An important consideration in selecting the phrenic nerve is the potential for diaphragmatic paralysis with an adverse effect on respiration. Animal studies have shown that using the first root of the phrenic nerve for reinnervation can preserve diaphragmatic innervation [43, 44].

Perhaps the most promising techniques described to date include those of Marie et al. [45, 46] who have developed a bilateral selective reinnervation schema. In this procedure, both PCA muscles are reinnervated with one right upper phrenic nerve root using an interposition free nerve graft. The adductors are reinnervated with the thyrohyoid branches of the hypoglossal nerve. In a preliminary report of the first 12 patients [46], four of six evaluable patients had decreased dyspnea. Three of six patients achieved active arytenoid abduction. All patients were decannulated. One of them did require an arytenoidectomy.

Zealear et al. [47] have been studying the placement of a laryngeal pacing device and have shown promising results. They performed a human clinical trial for electrically stimulated abduction of the PCA during thyroplasty using an external stimulation device. Seven patients (six women and one man, mean age 60 years) were implanted with an Itrel II device. All patients had a tracheotomy prior to this study. Two of the seven procedures resulted in long-term reanimation of the larynx. One of the patients was lost to follow-up after 4 years. The result of the other patient was maintained for more than 6 years. During that time, there was a slight shift of the electrode position and anode corrosion. The patient needed periodic injections of botulinum toxin to antagonize the adductors [48]. These results were promising but not ideal. The authors are currently working to overcome difficulties in the translation of the technology to humans and problems with electrode corrosion.

Ultimately what is requisite for laryngeal innervation in the context of transplantation is to consistently achieve a glottic aperture on abduction of 14–16 mm. The two episodes of rejection experienced by the first patient were associated with a sudden alteration in voice quality followed shortly thereafter by the onset of significant edema. Without attaining the aforementioned aperture, the airway could be seriously compromised during an episode of acute rejection.

Although most studies to date have focused on restoration of glottic motor function, sensory function of the transplanted larynx is also important to the success of the transplant. An interesting study performed by Blumin et al. [49] evaluated reinnervation of the transplanted dog larynx. In this randomized, controlled study, 10 dogs had their superior laryngeal nerves transected. Five of the dogs had the nerves reanastomosed. All dogs were tested for laryngospasm in response to hydrochloric acid stimulation both preoperatively and 6 months postoperatively. None of the dogs regained normal laryngospastic responses. However, the reanastomosed dogs exhibited protective EMG activity and coughing. The control group exhibited no response. In the first human laryngeal transplant patient, the supraglottis and vocal folds were sensitive to touch at 3 months postoperatively, initiating a severe cough. Stimulation through the stoma on the right side of the upper trachea elicited a sensation of touch without cough. Stimulation of the left side was not sensed.

12.9 Explantation

At 14.5 years after the first composite larynx transplant, explantation was necessary [50] (Fig. 12.6). Over the prior 5 years, a subtle but progressive contracture of the larynx could be noted in retrospect on sequential videos, suggesting

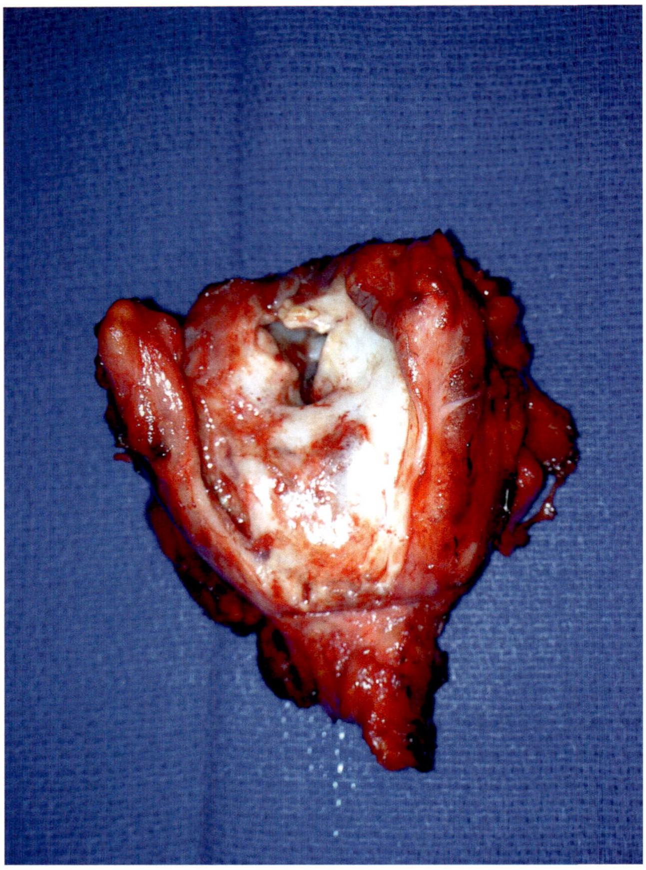

Fig. 12.6 Explanted larynx. Fourteen years after his transplant, the recipient and the senior author determined that the day had come for explantation. A fibrotic and shrunken organ was removed, with free-flap reconstruction of the pharyngeal defect and voice restoration with TEP speech. (See post-explantation video)

chronic rejection. Clinically, over the last year prior to explantation, the patient experienced increased aspiration with fluids, a decrease in voice quality, and persistent pain. Sensory testing revealed a dramatic reduction in sensation compared to prior testing. The thyroid function, which for 3 years posttransplant was found to be 80% donor derivation and 20% recipient, reverted to 100% recipient just prior to explant. The patient, on his own, decreased his steroid dose to help with the aspiration. The subsequent increased laryngeal swelling initially helped decrease the aspiration but was insufficient in the long-term. Attempted vocal fold augmentation by injection was unsuccessful. The decision was made to explant the larynx. Following extirpation, the pharyngeal remnant was augmented with a free flap. The histology of the excised larynx showed ulceration, acute and chronic inflammation, and dense fibrosis.

Upon careful examination of the explanted composite transplant, a small 3–4 mm HPV-associated oropharyngeal squamous cell carcinoma was identified at the margin of the pharyngeal mucosa. Given the size and early stage of disease, this was treated subsequently with endoscopic resection alone and is without evidence of disease now, 7 years into follow-up without adjuvant treatment. The relationship of HPV and immunosuppression in the context of the etiology of his cancer remains an open question. Our patient considers his experience worthwhile for multiple reasons (see Videos 12.1 and 12.2). Some of which include the ability to have a human voice with pitch control, sense of smell, and an overall feeling of well-being. Today he communicates via TEP speech. He has recently stated that, if given the opportunity, he would opt for another transplant.

12.10 Conclusion

Total laryngeal transplantation is a reality. With it, comes the potential of restored laryngeal function for many patients who have had to suffer the hardships and embarrassment of life without human voicing capability. There is still much to be learned and improved upon from the first transplant and the few that have followed.

With all of the research currently underway in transplantation medicine, the day is likely not too far away when many of the questions highlighted in this chapter will be answered. The immune system will be modified to allow for donor-specific tolerance while keeping immunosurveillance intact; or immunosuppression may be completely bypassed through other techniques. Glottic function might be restored through selective reinnervation or laryngeal pacing. Once these are a reality, laryngeal transplantation will be able to benefit the many people who have undergone a laryngectomy for malignancy. At that time, thousands of people will regain their voices, and their identities.

References

1. Boles R. Surgical replantation of the larynx in dogs: a progress report. Laryngoscope. 1966;76:1057–67.
2. Ogura JH, Kawasald M, Takenouchi S, et al. Replantation and transplantation of the canine larynx. Ann Otol Rhinol Laryngol. 1966;75:295–312.
3. Silver CE, Liebert PS, Som ML. Autologous transplantation of the canine larynx. Arch Otolaryngol. 1967;86:95–102.
4. Kluyskens P, Ringoir S. Follow-up of a human larynx transplantation. Laryngoscope. 1970;80:1244–50.
5. Genden EM, Urken ML. Laryngeal and tracheal transplantation: ethical limitations. Mt Sinai J Med. 2003;70:163–5.
6. Lott DG, Manz R, Koch C, Lorenz RR. Aggressive behavior of non-melanotic skin cancers in solid organ transplant recipients. Transplantation. 2010;90:683–7.
7. Potter CP, Birchall MA. Laryngectomees' views of laryngeal transplantation. Transpl Int. 1998;11:433–8.
8. Strome M, Wu J, Strome S, Brodsky G. A comparison of preservation techniques in a vascularized rat laryngeal transplant model. Laryngoscope. 1994;104:666–8.

9. Strome S, Brodsky G, Darrell J, Wu J, Strome M. Histopathologic correlates of acute laryngeal allograft rejection in a rat model. Ann Otol Rhinol Laryngol. 1992;101:156–60.
10. Strome M, Strome S, Darrell J, Wu J, Brodsky G. The effects of cyclosporin a on transplanted rat allografts. Laryngoscope. 1993;103:394–8.
11. Strome M, Stein J, Esclamado R, Hicks D, Lorenz RR, Braun W, Yetman R, Eliachar I, Mayes J. Laryngeal transplantation: a case report and 40-month follow-up. N Engl J Med. 2001;344:1676–9.
12. Lorenz RR, Hicks DM, Shields RW Jr, Fritz MA, Strome M. Laryngeal nerve function after total laryngeal transplantation. Otolaryngol Head Neck Surg. 2004;131:1016–8.
13. Farwell DG, Birchall MA, Macchiarini P, Luu QC, de Mattos AM, Gallay BJ, Perez RV, Grow MP, Ramsamooj R, Salgado MD, Brodie HA, Belafsky PC. Laryngotracheal transplantation: technical modifications and functional outcomes. Laryngoscope. 2013;123(10):2502–8.
14. Grajek M, Maciejewski A, Giebel S, Krakowczyk Ł, Ulczok R, Szymczyk C, Wierzgon J, Szumniak R, Dobrut M, Oleś K, Drozdowski P, Walczak D, Szpak-Ulczok S, Poltorak S. First complex allotransplantation of neck organs: larynx, trachea, pharynx, esophagus, thyroid, parathyroid glands, and anterior cervical wall. Ann Surg. 2017;266(2):e19–24.
15. Genden EM, Iskander A, Bromberg JS, Mayer L. The kinetics and pattern of tracheal allograft reepithelialization. Am J Respir Cell Mol Biol. 2003;28:673–83.
16. Shipchandler TZ, Lott DG, Lorenz RR, Friedman AD, Dan O, Strome M. New mouse model for studying laryngeal transplantation. Ann Otol Rhinol Laryngol. 2009;118:465–8.
17. Birchall MA, Bailey M, Barker EY, Rothkotter HJ, Otto K, Macchiarini P. Model for experimental revascularized laryngeal allotransplantation. Br J Surg. 2002;89:1470–5.
18. Lorenz RR, Dan O, Fritz MA, Strome M. Rat laryngeal transplant model: technical advancements and a redefined rejection grading system. Ann Otol Rhinol Laryngol. 2002;111:1120–7.
19. Lott DG, Shipchandler TZ, Dan O, Lorenz RR, Strome MA. New mouse laryngeal transplantation rejection grading system. Laryngoscope. 2010;120(1):39–43.
20. Nelson M, Dan O, Strome M. Evaluation of parathyroid hormone as a functional biological marker of rat laryngeal transplant rejection. Laryngoscope. 2003;113:1483–6.
21. Haug M 3rd, Dan O, Wimberley S, Fritz M, Lorenz RR, Strome M. Cyclosporine dose, serum trough levels, and allograft preservation in a rat model of laryngeal transplantation. Ann Otol Rhinol Laryngol. 2003;112:506–10.
22. Lorenz RR, Dan O, Fritz MA, Nelson M, Strome M. Immunosuppressive effect of irradiation in the murine laryngeal transplantation model: a controlled trial. Ann Otol Rhinol Laryngol. 2003;112:712–5.
23. Nelson M, Fritz M, Dan O, Worley S, Strome M. Tacrolimus and mycophenolate mofetil provide effective immunosuppression in rat laryngeal transplantation. Laryngoscope. 2003;113:1308–13.
24. Akst LM, Siemionow M, Dan O, Izycki D, Strome M. Induction of tolerance in a rat model of laryngeal transplantation. Transplantation. 2003;76:1763–70.
25. https://seer.cancer.gov/statfacts/html/laryn.html.
26. Sedrani R, Cottens S, Kallen J, Schuler W. Chemical modification of rapamycin: the discovery of SDZ RAD. Transplant Proc. 1998;30:2192–4.
27. Mabuchi S, Altomare DA, Cheung M, Zhang L, Poulikakos PI, Hensley HH, Schilder RJ, Ozols RF, Testa JR. RAD001 inhibits human ovarian cancer cell proliferation, enhances cisplatin-induced apoptosis, and prolongs survival in an ovarian cancer model. Clin Cancer Res. 2007;13:4261–70.
28. Fernández A, Marcén R, Pascual J, Galeano C, Ocaña J, Arellano EM, Alfaro C, Villafruela JJ, Burgos FJ, Ortuño J. Conversion from calcineurin inhibitors to everolimus in kidney transplant recipients with malignant neoplasia. Transplant Proc. 2006;38:2453–5.
29. Khariwala SS, Kjaergaard J, Lorenz R, Van Lente F, Shu S, Strome M. Everolimus (RAD) inhibits in vivo growth of murine squamous cell carcinoma (SCC VII). Laryngoscope. 2006;116:814–20.
30. Boulay A, Zumstein-Mecker S, Stephan C, Beuvink I, Zilbermann F, Haller R, Tobler S, Heusser C, O'Reilly T, Stolz B, Marti A, Thomas G, Lane HA. Antitumor efficacy of intermittent treatment schedules with the rapamycin derivative RAD001 correlates with prolonged inactivation of ribosomal protein S6 kinase 1 in peripheral blood mononuclear cells. Cancer Res. 2004;64:252–61.
31. Lott DG, Russell JO, Khariwala SS, Dan O, Strome M. Ten-month laryngeal allograft survival using pulsed Everolimus and anti-αβ TCR antibody immunosuppression. Ann Otol Rhinol Laryngol. 2011;120:131–6.
32. Lott DG, Dan O, Lu L, Strome M. Long-term laryngeal allograft survival using low-dose everolimus. Oto-HNS. 2010;142:72–8.
33. Genden EM, Mackinnon SE, Yu S, Hunter DA, Flye MW. Portal venous ultraviolet B-irradiated donor alloantigen prevents rejection in circumferential rat tracheal allografts. Otolaryngol Head Neck Surg. 2001;124:481–8.
34. Gorti GK, Birchall MA, Haverson K, Macchiarini P, Bailey M. A preclinical model for laryngeal transplantation: anatomy and mucosal immunology of the porcine larynx. Transplantation. 1999;68:1638–42.
35. Rees LE, Ayoub O, Haverson K, Birchall MA, Bailey M. Differential major histocompatibility complex class II locus expression on human laryngeal epithelium. Clin Exp Immunol. 2003;134:497–502.
36. Friedman AD, Dan O, Drazba JA, Lorenz RR, Strome M. Quantitative analysis of OX62-positive dendritic cell distribution in the rat laryngeal complex. Ann Otol Rhinol Laryngol. 2007;116(6):449–56.
37. Govindaraj S, Gordon R, Genden EM. Effect of fibrin matrix and vascular endothelial growth factor on reepithelialization of orthotopic murine tracheal transplants. Ann Otol Rhinol Laryngol. 2004;113:797–804.
38. Lott DG, Dan O, Lu L, Strome M. Decoy NF-kappaB fortified immature dendritic cells maintain laryngeal allograft integrity and provide enhancement of regulatory T-cells. Laryngoscope. 2010;120(1):44–52.
39. Xu MQ, Suo YP, Gong JP, Zhang MM, Yan LN. Prolongation of liver allograft survival by dendritic cells modified with NF-kB decoy oligodeoxynucleotides. World J Gastroenterol. 2004;10:2361–8.
40. Tiao MM, Lu L, Tao R, Wang L, Fung JJ, Qian S. Prolongation of cardiac allograft survival by systemic administration of immature recipient dendritic cells deficient in NFkB activity. Ann Surg. 2005;241:497–505.
41. Stavroulaki P, Birchall M. Comparative study of the laryngeal innervation in humans and animal employed in laryngeal transplantation research. J Laryngol Otol. 2001;115:257–66.
42. Baldissera F, Cantarella G, Marini G, Ottaviani F, Tredici G. Recovery of inspiratory abduction of the paralyzed vocal cords after bilateral reinnervation of the cricoarytenoid muscles by one single branch of the phrenic nerve. Laryngoscope. 1989;99:1286–92.
43. Marie JP, Tardif C, Lerosey Y, Gibon JF, Hellot MF, Tadié M, Andrieu-Guitrancourt J, Dehesdin D, Pasquis P. Selective resection of the phrenic nerve roots in rabbits: part II: respiratory effects. Respir Physiol. 1997;109:139–48.
44. Marie JP, Lacoume Y, Laquerrière A, Tardif C, Fallu J, Bonmarchand G, Verin E. Diaphragmatic effects of selective resection of the

upper phrenic nerve root in dogs. Respir Physiol Neurobiol. 2006;154:419–30.
45. Marie J, Lacoume Y, Magnier P, et al. Selective bilateral motor reinnervation of the canine larynx. Laryngorhinootologie. 2000;79:S188–9.
46. Marie JP. Nerve reconstruction. In: Remacle M, Eckel HE, editors. Surgery of larynx and trachea. Heidelberg: Springer; 2010. p. 279–94.
47. Zealear DL, Billante CR, Courey MS, Netterville JL, Paniello RC, Sanders I, Herzon GD, Goding GS, Mann W, Ejnell H, Habets AM, Testerman R, Van de Heyning P. Reanimation of the paralyzed human larynx with an implantable electrical stimulation device. Laryngoscope. 2003;113:1149–56.
48. Mueller AH. Laryngeal pacing for bilateral vocal fold immobility. Curr Opin Otolaryngol Head Neck Surg. 2011;19:439–43.
49. Blumin JH, Ye M, Berke GS, Blackwell KE. Recovery of laryngeal sensation after superior laryngeal nerve anastomosis. Laryngoscope. 1999;109:1637–41.
50. Lorenz RR, Strome M. Total laryngeal transplant explanted: 14 years of lessons learned. Otolaryngol Head Neck Surg. 2014;150:509–11.

Laryngotracheal Transplant

13

John E. Hanks and D. Gregory Farwell

13.1 Introduction

The following questions will be addressed in the following section of this chapter:

When did the program start?
How were the transplants funded?
Is the program still active?
How many patients have you screened?
How many patients were approved and how many are on the waiting list?
Is there any obstacle to the expansion of the program?

13.1.1 University of California-Davis (UCD) Laryngeal Transplantation Program

The University of California-Davis (UCD) laryngeal transplantation program began in 2008 in evaluation of a single operative candidate. Internal institutional funding was secured in order to fund the procedure and the patient's perioperative care. Two years of rigorous patient screening, counseling, medical clearance, and human cadaveric and live animal preparatory dissections followed prior to successful performance of the human laryngotracheal transplant by surgeons Gregory Farwell, M.D. and Peter Belafsky, M.D. at UCD in 2010 [1]. In addition to the selected patient, one other patient has been seriously screened for the procedure but was ultimately deemed not to be an ideal candidate. The UCD laryngeal transplant program remains active for judiciously selected, appropriately informed patients with qualifying lesions on a case-by-case basis as a potential adjunct to laryngectomy.

Including the aforementioned case, only three successful laryngotracheal transplants have been published with long-term follow-up. One transplant each has been performed at Cleveland Clinic in 1998 [2–6], UCD in 2010 [1, 7], and Maria Skłodowska-Curie Institute of Oncology (Cancer Center IMSC) in Poland in 2015 [8]. The first two successful transplants were performed for benign, posttraumatic laryngotracheal stenosis, and the third was performed to address numerous severe long-term wound and functional sequelae following remote laryngeal cancer treatment. The latter patient was disease-free for numerous years and was considered oncologically cured [8]. A variety of other cases have been mentioned in the literature since 1969, but these cases lack thoroughly reported outcomes, lack publication altogether, and/or were rapidly unsuccessful [9, 10]. No single institution has rigorously published any series including more than a single transplant to date.

Perhaps the primary obstacle to programmatic expansion and to the global adoption of laryngeal transplantation is the rarity of patients meeting ideal indications for the procedure. Although terminal laryngotracheal dysfunction and laryngectomy, particularly secondary to malignancy [11], are relatively common, a myriad of issues prevent routine laryngeal transplantation including ethical constraints related to the larynx being a non-life-sustaining organ, immunosuppression-mediated risks such as recurrent or *de novo* malignancies, and the existence of well-established highly functional gold-standard alternatives that lack the risks of immunosuppression (i.e., total laryngectomy, tracheoesophageal speech, etc.). Moreover, while voice and swallowing outcomes have been generally remarkable in the three prior transplants [1, 2, 8], consistent re-establishment of natural, tracheostomy-free respiration without collater-

J. E. Hanks (✉)
Department of Otolaryngology Head and Neck Surgery, Boston University School of Medicine, VA Boston Healthcare System, Jamaica Plain, MA, USA
e-mail: john.hanks@va.gov

D. G. Farwell
Department of Otolaryngology Head and Neck Surgery, University of California-Davis Medical Center, Sacramento, CA, USA

Department of Otolaryngology-Head and Neck Surgery, University of Pennsylvania Health System, Philadelphia, PA, USA
e-mail: greg.farwell@pennmedicine.upenn.edu

© Springer Nature Switzerland AG 2023
R. Gurunian et al. (eds.), *Reconstructive Transplantation*, https://doi.org/10.1007/978-3-031-21520-9_13

ally compromising voice or swallowing remains a distinct challenge with contemporary RLN reinnervation techniques [11]. While the most recent Polish transplant patient remains tracheostomy-free at 2 years [8], posttransplant functional RLN reinnervation and glottic abductor outcomes have been inconsistent [1, 3, 5]. All of these hurdles have reinforced historically strict selection criteria [1, 6, 11].

All previously published successful laryngotracheal transplants are summarized in Table 13.1.

13.1.1.1 Patients

Donor: age, sex, cause of death An otherwise healthy 38 year old female sustained unrecoverable anoxic brain injury and was ultimately found to be an allele-matched donor within 2 weeks of initiating the donor search [1]. Preharvest intubation period was only 3 days, and laryngoscopy showcased normal laryngotracheal anatomy without evidence of intubation-related pathology [1].

Recipient Age, sex, defect, etiology, follow-up, complications (immediate, intermediate, and long-term), functional outcomes (please detail motor recovery, sensory recovery, and organ-specific function); immunological outcomes (episodes of acute rejection, evidence of chronic rejection)

The recipient was a 51-year-old medically complex female who presented in 2008 with 11 years of complete laryngotracheal stenosis anatomically spanning from the laryngeal ventricle to the second tracheal ring Fig. 13.1 [1]. Her pathology arose from multiple traumatic self-extubations during prolonged intubation and ICU admission for diabetic renal failure in 1999. In light of her end-stage chronic kidney disease and diabetes, she ultimately received a renal-pancreas transplant in 2006, for which she was chronically immunosuppressed with tacrolimus and leflunamide at the time of our initial evaluation [1]. She failed repeated endoscopic airway interventions, and traditional means to re-establish laryngeal function and patency were felt to be expended [1]. At presentation, she was inexorably aphonic and tracheostomy-dependent, as her endoscopic exam showcased no anatomic communication between the trachea with the upper aerodigestive tract, which was confirmed with three-dimensional computed tomography. Residual laryngeal muscle function and deglutition were comprehensively assessed via laryngeal electromyography (EMG), esophageal manometry, pH probing, and video fluoroscopic swallow evaluation, and both laryngeal myometry and swallowing function were intact. Despite the preclusion of normal laryngeal respiration and vocalization by the patient's terminal laryngotracheal stenosis, bilateral thyroarytenoid muscle contractions were demonstrated with attempts at phonation, which confirmed intact bilateral RLN conduction [1]. Three-dimensional computed tomography (CT) of the UCD laryngeal transplant patient's complete airway stenosis from laryngeal ventricle to second tracheal ring (Fig. 13.1). Her candidacy for laryngotracheal transplantation was ultimately considered with the guidance of a global multidisciplinary expert panel.

To address the possibility of an unsuccessful transplant, the patient was thoroughly counseled preoperatively and prepared psychologically regarding the potential need for standard total laryngectomy in either the immediate or delayed setting [1]. Likewise, a surgical contingency for graft failure was planned for recipient site preparation, maintaining sufficient native distal trachea to formalize a stoma if needed. Moreover, the patient was also counseled regarding the possibility for patched or tubed pharyngeal reconstruction with a fasciocutaneous flap, jejunal flap, gasto-omental flap, or gastric pull-up procedure if the native and/or transplanted pharyngeal mucosa was deemed unsalvageable.

Complications (immediate, intermediate and long-term) With 10 years of clinical follow-up in the UCD patient, only minor, transient complications have been noted to-date. In light of the donor's cytomegalovirus immunoglobulin M (IgM) and IgG positivity, empiric ganciclovir was initiated in the perioperative period. No active CMV infection has since clinically manifested. Notably, intraoperatively the graft tracheal mucosa displayed evidence of mild tracheitis, which was covered with perioperative prophylactic antibiotics without subsequent issue. Otherwise, there were no notable intraoperative complications.

The patient required prolonged central venous access postoperatively due to repeated, difficult prior venipuncture secondary to dialysis and resultant poor venous access. Unfortunately, she sustained a femoral central line infection, and she acquired pneumonia postoperatively. Both infections were effectively treated with intravenous antibiotics. She sustained two episodes of mucosal candidiasis, which were successfully treated with antifungals. Moreover, she required a brief hospitalization at 2 months posttransplant secondary to diarrhea and resultant dehydration. An episode of tacrolimus-related toxicity was also observed. She has otherwise done very well [1, 7].

Functional Outcomes (motor recovery, sensory recovery, and organ-specific function) The UCD patient's tracheostomy balloon was uninflated on POD 10, and she was first able to vocalize on POD 14. By 3 months, normal bilateral adductor response was detected via laryngopharyngeal sensory testing, although glottic motion was restricted and primarily paradoxical at that time. Supraglottic edema, centered primarily at the bilateral aryepiglottic folds and epiglottis, was intermittently noted until postoperative week 8 but resolved thereafter. Endoscopic exam of the laryngeal transplant is shown at posttransplant week 9 in Fig. 13.2.

Table 13.1 Summary of published successful laryngotracheal transplants

Patient	Age/sex recipient (R) and donor (D) [cause of death]	Clinical history and indications	Recipient clinical deficit	Anatomic components of transplant	Vascular anastomoses, recipient (R) and donor (D)
Cleveland Clinic, 1998 [2, 3, 5–7, 11]	R: 40-year-old male D: 40-year-old male [ruptured cerebral aneurysm]	– Otherwise healthy – Irreparable laryngopharyngeal stenosis secondary to remote crush injury in motorcycle crash, refractory to repeated prior repairs	– Shortened, stenotic larynx – Immobile glottis – Traumatically segmented cricoid cartilage – Severely stenotic pharynx and esophagus – Pharyngolaryngeal fistula	– Larynx – Five tracheal rings – 75% pharynx – Thyroid – Four parathyroids	– Bilateral (D)/(R) superior thyroid arteries – Distal (D) internal jugular vein oversewn, proximal (D) right internal jugular vein: (R) right common facial vein – (D) middle thyroid vein: (R) internal jugular vein
	Neurorrhaphies	Preoperative recipient immunosuppression status	Rejection episodes	Complications	Follow-up, outcomes
	See Table 13.2 for comprehensive sensorimotor details and outcomes	Naïve	Y, acute and chronic (15 months, 5 years, 9 years)	– Cyclosporine-mediated renal dysfunction – Steroid-induced bone mineral density reduction – Oropharyngeal thrush – Tracheobronchitis – *Pneumocystis carinii* pneumonia – Progressive laryngeal dysfunction secondary to rejection, bilateral pharyngeal pain – Clinically occult HPV/p16-positive oropharyngeal squamous cell carcinoma noted in explant specimen	– First successful human laryngeal transplant – Laryngeal allograft explanted at year 14 – Return to OR for definitive excision of early stage HPV/p16-positive oropharyngeal squamous cell carcinoma. Remains disease free – Patient expresses desire to undergo second transplant if possible
Patient	Age/sex recipient (R) and donor (D) [cause of death]	Clinical history and indications	Recipient clinical deficit	Anatomic components of transplant	Vascular anastomoses, recipient (R) and donor (D)
University of California, Davis, 2010 [1, 7]	R: 51-year-old female D: 38-year-old female [anoxic brain injury]	– Complete laryngotracheal stenosis secondary to multiple traumatic self extubations while in ICU for end-stage diabetic renal failure – Refractory to repeated endoscopic airway interventions	– Complete laryngotracheal stenosis from laryngeal ventricle to second tracheal ring – Fused glottis with bilaterally immobile cricoarytenoid joints – Permanent tracheostomy dependence – Preserved preoperative bilateral thyroarytenoid muscle contraction on EMG – Maintained preoperative swallow function	– larynx – 8 tracheal rings – Pharynx – Esophagus – Thyroid – Parathyroids – Bilateral SLNs – Bilateral RLNs – Great vessels	– (D) right superior thyroid artery: (R) right superior thyroid artery – (D) right inferior thyroid artery: (R) right transverse cervical artery – (D) left inferior thyroid artery: (R) left transverse cervical artery – (D) right brachiocephalic vein: (R) right inferior jugular vein [end to side] – (D) left superior thyroid vein: (R) left jugular vein [end to side]
	Neurorrhaphies	Preoperative recipient immunosuppression status	Rejection episodes	Complications	Follow-up, outcomes
	See Table 13.2 for comprehensive sensorimotor details and outcomes	Previously chronically immunosuppressed with tacrolimus and leflunamide for renal-pancreas transplant	None	– Bacterial lung, central line, and tracheal infections – Mucosal candidiasis – Diarrhea	10 years

(continued)

Table 13.1 (continued)

Patient	Age/sex recipient (R) and donor (D) [cause of death]	Clinical history and indications	Recipient clinical deficit	Anatomic components of transplant	Vascular anastomoses, recipient (R) and donor (D)
Patient	Age/sex recipient (R) and donor (D) [cause of death]	Clinical history and indications	Recipient clinical deficit	Anatomic components of transplant	Vascular anastomoses, recipient (R) and donor (D)
IMSC Poland 2015 [8]	R: 34-year-old male D: Not reported [unknown]	– Numerous severe posttreatment wound complications related to prior T3N1M0 laryngeal cancer treatment (radiation followed by laryngectomy) – Successful jejunal-free flap, underwent three other failed traditional reconstructive attempts – History also notable for acute myeloid leukemia and IgA nephropathy – Remained disease free for 6 years from laryngeal cancer and 12 years from AML at time of laryngeal transplant	– Alaryngeal – Large pharyngocutaneous fistula – Permanent gastrostomy tube dependence – Severe neck soft tissue fibrosis – Marked psychosocial sequelae – Hypothyroid and hypoparathyroid – Functional outcome and quality of life deemed inadequate despite alimentary restoration with jejunal flap	– Larynx – Trachea (8 cm) – Pharynx – Esophagus – Large anterior neck soft tissue and skin paddle (>200 cm^2) – Bilateral anterior bellies of digastic muscles, bilateral sternothyroid muscles – Thyroid – Four parathyroid glands	– (D) right superior thyroid artery: (R) right lingual artery – (D) left superior thyroid artery: (R) left facial artery – Bilateral (D) inferior thyroid arteries: Bilateral (R) inferior thyroid arteries – Bilateral (D) internal jugular veins: Bilateral (R) internal jugular veins [end-to-side] – Bilateral (D) anterior cervical veins: (R) bilateral external jugular veins [venous coupler]
	Neurorrhaphies	Preoperative recipient immunosuppression status	Rejection episodes	Complications	Follow-up, outcomes
	See Table 13.2 for comprehensive sensorimotor details and outcomes	Previously chronically immunosuppressed for renal transplant	None	– "Digestive tract contracture"	– First successful transplant following laryngeal malignancy – 2 years follow-up – Remains tracheostomy free – Favorable aesthetic results – Thyroid and parathyroid supplementation weaned entirely

By 5 months postoperatively, her endoscopic evaluation continued to demonstrate bilateral median resting vocal fold position and minimal, largely paradoxical motion. Ten units of Botulinum toxin A was injected into the bilateral false vocal folds to antagonize the adductor musculature, thereby intending to promote selective reinnervation of abductor musculature. Regretfully, this resulted in drastic lateralization of the vocal folds and substantially diminished vocal tone and volume in addition to increasing her propensity to aspirate. Consequently, no further intralaryngeal botulinum toxin A injections were performed, and baseline tone, minimal coordinated movement, and median positioning returned 2 months later and have persisted thereafter [1]. Nonetheless, the temporary adductor paralysis in response to Botox injection confirmed the presence of baseline adductor tone, and thus reinnervation had taken place by 5 months.

At 18 months, endoscopic evaluation demonstrated bilateral vocal fold tone and bulk with a restricted glottic airway. The right vocal fold remained entirely immobile, while the left vocal fold demonstrated only synkinetic motion and minimal abduction. Also at that time, acoustic and vocal range assessments were performed. For an adult female, her posttransplant vocal fundamental frequency was slightly below normal, and vocal range was within normal range. Her

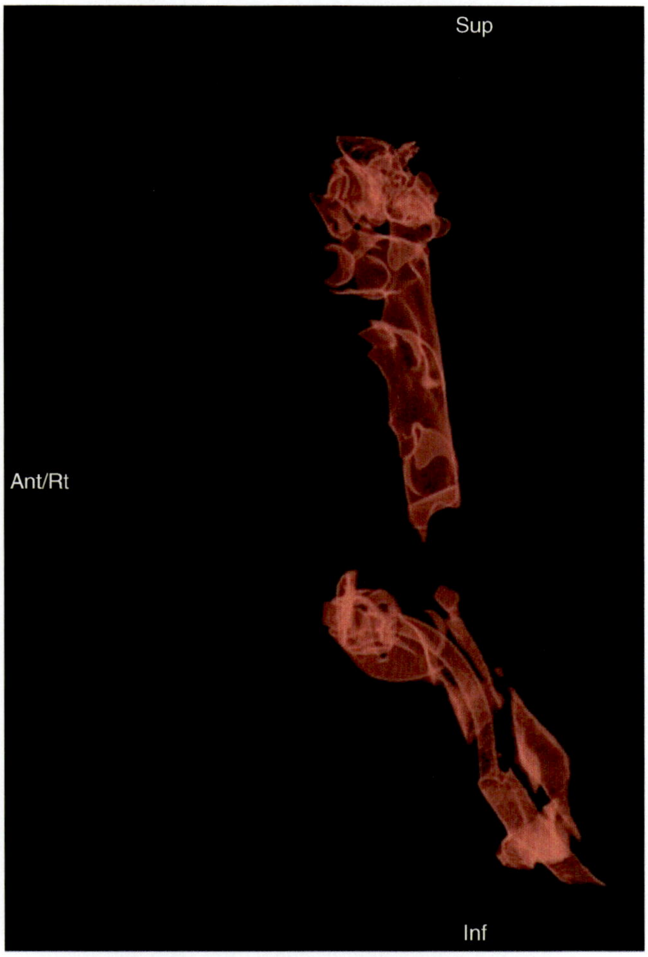

Fig. 13.1 Three-dimensional computed tomography (CT) of the UC Davis laryngeal transplant patient's complete airway stenosis from laryngeal ventricle to second tracheal ring. (Adapted with permission from Laryngoscope, 123:2502–2508, 2013).

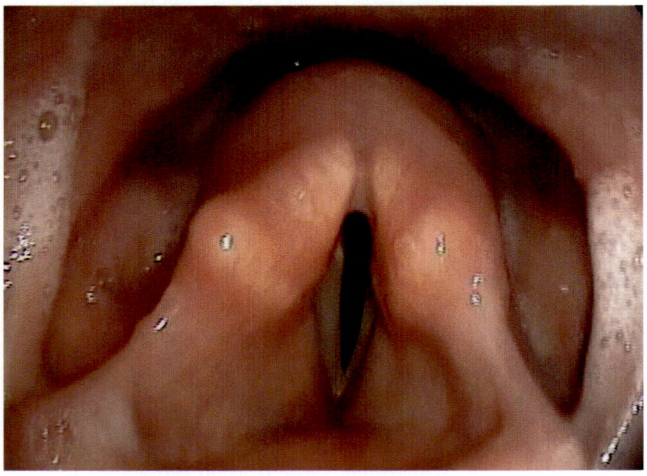

Fig. 13.2 Video laryngoscopy of the transplanted larynx posttransplant week 9. (Adapted with permission from Laryngoscope, 123:2502–2508, 2013)

median maximal phonation time was also within normal range for a healthy adult female, which lends further evidence to the competence of her transplanted glottis resultant of adductor tone provided by RLN reinnervation.

The consequent glottic airway restriction has disallowed decannulation, but the caliber of the trachea and subglottic airways remain widely patent and without evidence of restenosis [1, 7].

To preemptively address oropharyngeal secretions and to minimize perioperative aspiration risk, 20 units of Botulinum toxin A was injected into the bilateral parotid and submandibular glands 2 weeks preoperatively. The patient also underwent percutaneous endoscopic gastrojejunal tube placement 3 months preceding her transplant [1] in anticipation of potentially prolonged NPO status. Owing to postoperative pharyngeal anastomotic stenosis, the patient experienced a protracted return of swallow function relative to the other two published laryngeal transplant cases [2, 8]. At 2 months evidence of pooled pharyngeal secretions prompted repeated salivary Botox injection. Subsequently, at 5 months the mild pharyngeal anastomotic stricture was detected, and she tolerated a clear liquid diet without aspiration after successful endoscopic balloon dilation of the stenotic area to 20 mm.

Following intensive daily dysphagia therapy as an inpatient, she was transitioned to a rigorous three-times-daily home dysphagia therapy regimen administered via tablet computer application. At 7 months she was cleared for pureed diet. She required repeated endoscopic dilation at 9 months prior to being cleared for regular diet 11 months. Finally, her gastrojejunal feeding tube was discontinued at 13 months, and she has tolerated a general diet well without aspiration thereafter [1, 7].

Immunological outcomes (episodes of acute rejection, evidence of chronic rejection) The immunologic tolerance toward the patient's transplanted kidney and pancreas afforded by her pre-existing chronic tacrolimus and leflunamide regimen helped inform the selection of an appropriate laryngotracheal donor with an acceptable HLA antigen profile, including minor antigen mismatching [1]. Ultimately, functional and anatomic matching were weighed ahead of exact HLA matching between donor and recipient.

There have been no clinical, histological, or serological evidence of acute or chronic episodes of transplant rejection in our patient. Likewise, no interventions or adjustments to the immunosuppression regimen have been necessary [1]. This was evidenced by serial laryngeal biopsies at 6 hours, 1 day, 14 days, 30 days, and 137 days postoperatively, which all demonstrated normal laryngeal mucosal histology. Serologically, no anti-donor-HLA antibodies were detectable at 6 months postoperatively [1], which suggests that no detectable immune response had been mounted against the transplanted organ.

13.1.1.2 Surgical Technique

(Details of donor and recipient operation, ischemia time, use of preservation solutions, location of donor and recipient procedures, technical details of importance for success of surgery, and unique aspects of the approach used in our center)

Over the course of 18 hours, procurement of the donor larynx, liver, and kidneys was concurrently performed with laryngectomy and preparation of the recipient surgical bed in adjacent operating rooms at UCD Hospital [1].

The donor larynx, trachea, esophagus, thyroid, parathyroids, bilateral SLNs, bilateral RLNs, and great vessels were procured as a unit [1]. The cranial aspects of the great vessels, including the internal jugular veins, the common and external carotid arteries were isolated from lateral to medial taking care to preserve the laryngotracheal and thyroidal feeding vessels. Furthermore, the bilateral SLNs were isolated at their take-off from the vagus nerves. The strap muscles were excised.

A median sternotomy was performed in order to provide access for harvest of the intrathoracic RLNs, brachiocephalic veins, distal superior vena cava, and the subclavian arteries, which were eventually harvested medially at their take-off from the aorta and laterally with inclusion of the thyrocervical trunk. The laryngotracheal arterial supply was noted to be dominant on the right. Once pertinent structures were completely isolated and otherwise ready for harvest, the ascending and descending aorta, the post-scalenic subclavian arteries, and post-bifurcation carotid arteries were simultaneously cross-clamped in preparation of exsanguination of the isolated laryngotracheal specimen. The graft was flushed with 3 L of University of Wisconsin Perfusate (DuPont, Wilmington, DE) via ascending aortic cannulation until the thyroid and laryngeal mucosa were visibly pale. The distal trachea and esophagus were divided with surgical stapler in order to establish a temporary watertight closure, and the graft was removed allowing further preparation of the organ and feeding vessels under sterile iced University of Wisconsin solution bath. The esophagus was posteriorly split in a longitudinal fashion and stripped of mucosa, while the esophageal musculature was left intact to maintain additional blood supply to the membranous trachea. The common brachiocephalic venous trunk was truncated from the superior vena cava and prepared for anastomosis. The graft adductor and abductor branches of the left recurrent laryngeal nerve were preserved and isolated.

Recipient narrow field laryngectomy also included removal of the prior tracheostomy site and cricopharyngeal myotomy. Transplant inset began with microvascular re-anastomosis. The recipient right transverse cervical artery was anastomosed to the graft inferior thyroid artery, and transplant right brachiocephalic vein was sewn end-to-side to the host's right internal jugular vein, after which successful reperfusion of the entire graft was confirmed following 300 min total ischemic time. Subsequently, additional arterial anastomoses were performed between the donor and recipient right superior thyroid arteries and between the donor left inferior thyroid artery and the host left transverse cervical artery. The left superior thyroid artery was not utilized given its small 1 mm diameter. Further end-to-side venous anastomosis was performed between the graft left superior thyroid vein and the host left internal jugular vein. Epineural end-to-end neurorrhaphies were performed between the transplanted and recipient bilateral superior SLNs and the right RLNs. An attempt at selective left glottic reinnervation was made. In order to solicit abductor function synchronized with respiration, selective end-to-side neurorrhaphy of the abductor branch of the graft left recurrent laryngeal nerve innervating the left posterior cricoarytenoid muscle was performed to the host phrenic nerve. The transplanted left RLN adductor fibers were anastomosed to the ipsilateral host *ansa cervicalis* nerve trunk end-to-end to sustain adductor muscle tone and bulk [1].

Finally, soft tissue inset began with trimming to size of the transplant and recipient pharyngeal mucosa before inset. A tension-free distal tracheal reconstruction was accomplished incorporating a new tracheostomy site and insetting eight donor tracheal rings via parachute technique posteriorly and by interrupted technique laterally. The transplanted thyroid cartilage was suspended to the host hyoid with 2–0 polypropylene sutures. Delayed closure of the neck soft tissues and skin on postoperative day 1 was elected in order to allow donor tissue edema to subside and was ultimately performed successfully in tension-free fashion on postoperative day 1 [1] (Fig. 13.3).

Immunosuppression protocol (induction, maintenance and variations; treatment of rejection) No universal standard of care for immunosuppression for composite tissue allografts has been published to date [8], but the UCD patient had been chronically immunosuppressed for 4 years prior to surgery with tacrolimus and leflunamide in light of her prior kidney-pancreas transplant [1]. Leflunamide was initially selected due to the patient's BK polyoma virus positivity, aimed at preventing BK polyoma virus nephropathy [1].

Post-laryngeal transplant induction immunosuppression intravenous rabbit anti-thymocyte globulin was titrated to a cumulative dose of 5 mg/kg with does including 75 mg on postoperative days (POD) 1 and 2 and 50 mg on POD 3. 250 mg IV methylprednisolone was administered on POD 0,

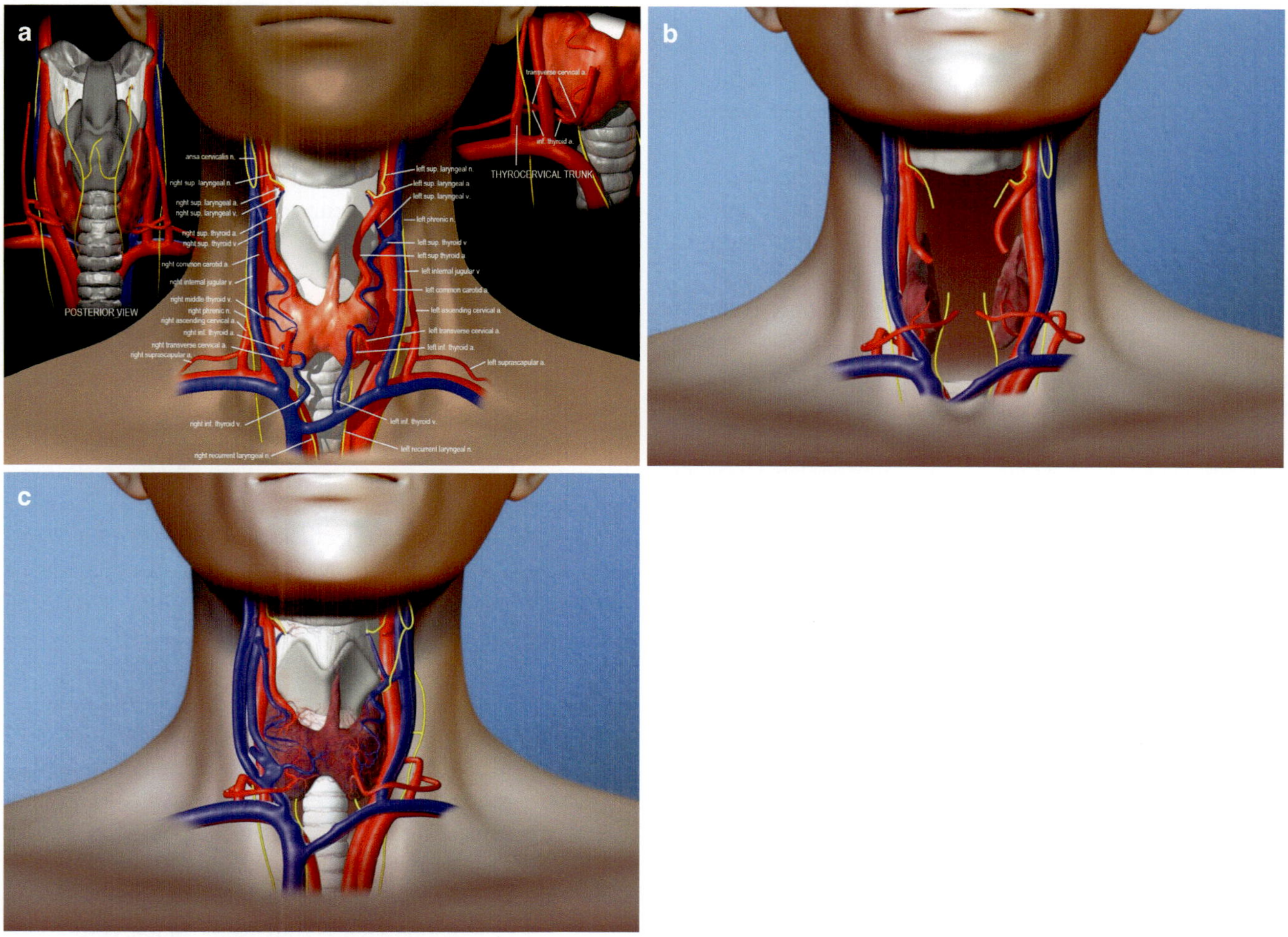

Fig. 13.3 . (**a**) Harvested laryngotracheal transplant. (**b**) Recipient surgical bed after narrow field laryngectomy. (**c**) Transplant after inset with microvascular anastomoses and neurorrhaphies. (Figure 3A previously unpublished. Figs. 3B and 3C adapted with permission from Laryngoscope, 123:2502–2508, 2013)

and 500 mg IV methylprednisolone was administered on PODs 2, 3, and 4. However, maintenance corticosteroids were deferred given UCD's institutional success with kidney transplant immunosuppression induced with rabbit antithymocyte globulin followed by maintenance regimens without chronic steroids. Accordingly, the patient had been previously successfully tapered off of corticosteroids for the maintenance of her kidney–pancreas transplant.

500 mg mycophenolate IV was administered BID from PODs 1 through 6 and was transitioned to 750 mg IV from PODs 7 through 14. Mycophenolate was ultimately stopped on POD 15 in favor of restarting 20 mg Leflunamide per day due to recidivistic BK viremia. Tacrolimus was resumed on POD 4 with titration to goal trough levels from 8 to 10 ng/mL for 3 post-operative months. Subsequently, the tacrolimus dose was transitioned over the next 3 months to final maintenance levels of 5–7 ng/mL [1].

No interventions or adjustments to the immunosuppression regimen for acute or chronic rejection events have been required to date [1].

Monitoring protocol (biopsy, blood work, general health monitoring) Rigorous posttransplantation monitoring protocols were developed by the UCD team, informed by our own experience in addition to the previously published protocols offered by the Cleveland Clinic team. The UCD protocol included evaluation of the immunosuppression regimen's efficacy, sensorimotor functional recovery, vocal and swallowing performance, gross exam findings, histologic findings, and serologic antibody profiles.

The efficacy of the immunosuppressive regimen in the prevention of acute and chronic organ rejection was monitored with serial biopsies and pathologic analysis at 6 hours, 1 day, 14 days, 30 days, and 137 days postoperatively to histologically assess for acute or chronic transplant rejection.

Routine awake endoscopic evaluation was performed daily via flexible videolaryngoscopy from POD 1–8 and subsequently on day 10, day 14, day 20, 3 months, 5 months, 7 months, 9 months, and 18 months to evaluate airway and pharyngeal patency, glottic tone and motor recovery, secretion handling, and signs of gross mucosal evidence of rejection. Throughout her course she continued rigorous dysphagia therapy and assessments, and multiple endoscopic pharyngeal dilations starting at 5 months were performed as appropriate based upon endoscopic or fluoroscopic diagnosis of stenosis and/or patient symptomatology.

Laryngopharyngeal sensory testing was performed at 3 months to assess for the return of the bilateral adductor response in response to tactile stimuli, which signals whether successful SLN reinnervation has taken place.

Additionally, the patient's serum anti-donor-HLA (or donor-specific-HLA) antibody level was evaluated at 6 months postoperatively [1]. While present in some patients prior to transplant following blood transfusion, pregnancy, or by unknown circumstances, the presence of anti-donor-HLA antibodies indicates that humoral immunity has been triggered in the host against the transplant [12]. Therefore, if absent preoperatively, newly present posttransplant anti-donor-HLA antibodies serve as a marker for transplant rejection [12].

Vocal acoustic testing was performed at 18 months assessing vocal intensity, range, fundamental frequency, noise-to-harmonic ratio, and median maximal phonation time was also within normal range for a healthy adult female, which lends further evidence to the competence of her transplanted glottis resulting from adductor tone provided by RLN reinnervation.

Preoperatively, laryngeal EMG was performed to ensure that despite gross glottic immobility that the patient's native RLN and SLN circuitry remained intact. Additionally, while not performed to-date in the UCD patient postoperatively, postoperative laryngeal EMG was employed at 4 years postoperatively in the Cleveland Clinic patient and represents another potentially useful monitoring tool to assess the status of RLN reinnervation and glottic motor activity. Neurophysiologic data from LEMG can aid in determining the quality, time course, and pattern of RLN and SLN reinnervation. Particularly as new reinnervation techniques and technologies are developed, these findings can be correlated with the clinical scenario to determine the efficacy of the strategy and may help inform adjunctive procedures. For instance, the use of laryngeal EMG may be employed adjunctively with endoscopic findings to inform the optimal location, dosing, and time course for botox injections or other antagonists such as vincristine or myelin-associated glycoprotein to encourage selective reinnervation [13, 14]. The UCD and Cleveland Clinic patients shared similar clinical glottic motor outcomes despite having utilized different reinnervation techniques [1, 5].

In the Cleveland Clinic patient, volitional contraction of the bilateral cricothyroid muscles was demonstrated with postoperative laryngeal EMG, affording excellent pitch control. However, while bilateral thyroarytenoid electrophysiologic signals were detected on EMG, the functional outcome of motor reinnervation of the right RLN was seemingly limited. Only baseline adductor tone was present without coordinated volitional abduction of either thyroarytenoid muscle, leaving the vocal folds in the midline position. From an electrophysiologic standpoint, the right vocal fold EMG tracings were only marginally better than the left, which notably had not undergone RLN microneurorrhaphy because it could not be located intraoperatively [5].

13.1.2 Rejection

To date, no evidence of rejection has been noted on biopsy, exam, or with serologic evaluation in the UCD patient [1]. Lorenz and Strome described the symptomatic, histologic, and gross examination manifestations of the only recorded case of acute or chronic rejection following laryngeal transplant, which began approximately 10 years postoperatively, ultimately culminating in explantation of the Cleveland Clinic patient's graft [3].

Rehabilitation protocol (timeline and details) A postlaryngeal transplant rehabilitation program should revolve around restoration of the three cardinal laryngeal functions: airway protection, respiration, and speech. Our patient's airway has not been adequate to consider decannulation due to lack of coordinated bilateral arytenoid abduction, and she functions well with a tracheostomy. She has declined procedures to facilitate decannulation such as cord lateralization, cordotomy, or arytenoidectomy in order to maintain her voice quality.

Having attained early functional postoperative voicing and having declined procedures aimed at tracheostomy decannulation, postoperative swallowing has been the centerpiece of the patient's rehabilitation regimen. Rapid return of both laryngopharyngeal sensation and motor activity was noted at 2 months and 3 months, respectively. While discrete, coordinated glottic adduction and abduction was ultimately unsuccessful resulting in near-median bilateral resting vocal fold position, the early return of sensation and muscular tone is felt to have been crucially beneficial in airway protection during swallow. She did not have persistent aspiration events in the postoperative period or beyond. As an inpatient, she underwent daily face-to-face swallowing therapy with a licensed speech language pathologist. This rigorous regimen was continued at home with three-times-daily dysphagia therapy sessions under the guidance of iSwallow, a digital smartphone application designed by the UCD dysphagia team with detailed text and pictographical instruction and automated reminders to complete a variety of desired exercises as directed by the supervising provider. Her return of swallow function was protracted and complicated by ongoing recurrent pharyngeal anastomotic stricture requiring serial endoscopic dilations. Her preexisting diabetes and diabetic neuropathy may have also complicated her swallowing recovery and pharyngeal stenosis by facilitating uncoordinated pharyngeal swallowing. However, she was ultimately successful with this regimen with advancement to a regular diet by 11 months, removal of her gastrojejunal feeding tube at 13 months, and complete resolution of her dysphagia symptoms at 18 months [1]. She has since been managed with repeated endoscopic dilations but maintains good swallowing function.

Unique problems or challenges encountered (E.g. *amputation or removal of the transplant, re-transplantation, malignancy, death).*

13.1.3 Laryngeal Anatomical Complexity and Associated Challenges in Autologous Rehabilitation of End-Stage Laryngeal Dysfunction or Laryngotracheal Stenoses

An inherent reality faced by otolaryngologists caring for end-stage laryngeal dysfunction or laryngotracheal stenoses is that these pathologies are notoriously challenging to address. The larynx is arguably the most complicated articulating human organ, integrating its densely innervated, highly dynamic, mechanically complex, paired human motor system with infinitesimally delicate bilateral sensory input [11, 15]. This successful relationship is crucial to maintaining three principal laryngeal functions including respiration, airway protection, and voice production [15], but the larynx's complexity also makes rehabilitation following loss of function exceedingly difficult.

Laryngeal sensorimotor function, which is governed by coordination of the recurrent laryngeal and superior laryngeal branches of the bilateral vagus nerves [16], is particularly difficult to re-establish when lost. The multifaceted, bilateral interplay is crucial and chiefly complementary, yet the restoration of laryngeal functions is complicated by the complexity of RLN neuromuscular activity required to fulfill these functions.

Therefore, recreating all native laryngeal functions with high fidelity via traditional autologous reconstructive methods or via substitution with alaryngeal speech techniques remains an elusive challenge. Unfortunately, the RLN's role simultaneously governing both arytenoid adduction and abduction undermines successful regeneration because axons instead often regenerate in uncoordinated, synkinetic fashion where both adductors and abductors activate concurrently, thereby yielding a dysfunctional minimally mobile glottis [16].

Additionally, even if idealized glottic neuroregeneration were realized, the intricate biomechanical properties of laryngeal tissues represent additional currently insurmountable barriers to *de novo* laryngeal bioengineering. Current regenerative techniques have failed to recreate the fluidity and interplay between the various layers of the vocal folds, most importantly the superficial lamina propria, required to achieve advanced acoustic tasks, which are easily corrupted by the presence of scar tissue or other unnatural substances [17]. Despite continued advances in post-laryngectomy speech rehabilitation [18–20] as well as the continual emergence of autogenous and biologically engineered laryngotracheal reconstructive techniques [21–24], no alternative to laryngeal transplantation has faithfully restored natural-sounding voice in anatomically and/or functionally alaryngeal patients [6, 11].

Pharyngeal and laryngeal sensation is crucial for swallowing and airway protection, and the SLN is particularly impactful in this role by providing supraglottic sensory innervation via its internal branch [25]. Supraglottic sensory stimulation signals elevation of the larynx and glottic closure during swallow. It further serves as the primary defense against aspiration by soliciting cough and glottic adduction in response to offending stimuli [25]. Moreover, subglottic sensation is supplied by the RLN [11], while glottic sensation is likely mediated by both the RLN and SLN [25]. In both animal models and in previously published human laryngeal transplants, laryngeal sensation has been effectively restored following primary SLN and RLN neurorrhaphies [1, 5, 11]. While only unilateral RLN repair could be performed in the Cleveland Clinic patient because the recipient's left RLN could not be identified among the extensive scarring, there was no resultant clinically apparent effect on swallowing or aspiration in this patient [2].

Motor input to the larynx plays an integral role in all three laryngeal functions: vocal fold adduction plays a key role in phonation and airway protection while abduction facilitates respiration [25]. To this end, there are five sets of paired laryngeal muscles, including the laryngeal adductors (thyroarytenoid, interarytenoid, lateral cricoarytenoid), laryngeal abductors (posterior cricoarytenoid), and the cricothyroid muscles, which rotate the larynx about the cricothyroid joint to lengthen the vocal folds and modulate vocal pitch [16, 26]. All intrinsic laryngeal muscles including competing laryngeal adductor and abductor muscles obtain predominant motor innervation by interlaryngeal branches of the RLN aside from the cricothyroid muscle, which is supplied by the external branch of SLN [16]. There is currently no known reinnervation technique to address Sunderland III [27] or greater neural injury that guarantees reunion of regenerating damaged axons with their embryologically intended motor units [11]. Therefore, such injuries frequently preclude restoration of physiologic motion [15] and instead predispose synkinetic, unorganized glottic electrical and motor activity without purposeful adduction or abduction [15]. This mechanism frequently leaves the vocal fold(s) in the paramedian position. If bilaterally paralyzed, as by definition in the postoperative laryngeal transplant, the resting paramedian position is serviceable but limited for phonation and airway protection. Conversely, the lack of meaningful coordinated vocal fold abduction compromises the resting glottic airway and frequently requires tracheostomy or adjunctive procedures (e.g., cordotomy, arytenoidectomy, lateralization, etc.) to improve glottic patency [11].

On the other hand, the cricothyroid muscle represents SLN's singular motor target, and thereby deleterious, synkinetic reinnervation of this muscle following primary neurorrhaphy is thought to be avoided. Therefore, pitch modulation via reinnervated cricothyroid muscle activity following bilateral SLN neurorrhaphy is excellent [5], and "normal"-sounding voice has been reported even the absence of functional RLN recovery [5, 7]. Successful SLN motor and sensory reconstitution is currently considered the primary driver of vocal recovery and protection against aspiration in laryngeal transplant [11].

Alternative methods aimed to improve spontaneous coordinated glottic motion after complete transection have been described, such as phrenic nerve or phrenic nerve root, hypoglossal nerve, and ansa cervicalis transfers. These procedures inherently require sacrifice of a different motor nerve other than RLN, whose original target organ then experiences its own loss of function [15]. Moreover, using traditional nonselective reinnervation techniques, results have shown that when supplied to the intrinsic laryngeal muscles, reinnervation using these techniques provide bulk and tone with mass movement rather than sufficiently restoring the intricate fine movements required for high-level dynamic speech [11].

An emerging field within laryngeal reinnervation has been the expansion and refinement of selective laryngeal reinnervation techniques, in which intralaryngeal nerve branches are isolated to target reinnervation of a single muscle, thereby mitigating the risk of synkinesis. A particular goal is to isolate the reinnervating neural input to the PCA in order to allay its tendency to receive synkinetic adductor reinnervation. To replace input from the complex multifunctional motor neurons supplied by the damaged RLN, this technique frequently instead couples the repaired PCA branch to the uniformly composed phrenic nerve in order to synchronize arytenoid abduction with inspiration [28]. An undoubted risk of this technique is resultant diaphragmatic paralysis, which may prove especially deleterious to respiratory reserve if the procedure does not successfully improve glottic competency [28]. However, animal models showcase the sacrifice of only upper phrenic cervical roots (i.e., C3 in humans) typically preserves adequate diaphragmatic excursion [29, 30]. Regardless, the sectioning of the entire unilateral phrenic nerve has been shown to manifest minimal adverse clinical effects in a patient with otherwise intact pulmonary function [31]. In bilateral vocal fold paralysis, Marie et al. described selective use of the bilateral *ansa hypoglossi* to reinnervate the bilateral RLN adductor branches and the bilateral RLN abductor branches reinnervated with a unilateral upper root of the phrenic nerve (C3) via direct neurorrhaphy to the ipsilateral and retrocricoid cable nerve graft to the contralateral side [28]. Preliminary data showed four of six patients experienced improved dyspnea, three of six demonstrated spontaneous arytenoid abduction with respiration, and all six were successfully decannulated using this technique, including one following arytenoidectomy [28].

Addressing concern for the anatomic complexity of PCA innervation, which frequently receives additional synkinetic input from the interarytenoid branch of RLN, and the resultant challenge of isolating abductor branches, Kwak et al. described a refinement to this technique [32]. Kwak describes additional sectioning of the RLN between the interarytenoid branch and the PCA branch and inserting the interarytenoid branch into the PCA to facilitate abduction. This technique requires at least 5 mm separation between the branches, and if the PCA branch is obscured by the thyroid cartilage, as is the case in over half of patients, they described creation of a cartilaginous window to expose it and to facilitate the surgery [32]. No human cases of this technique have been published, however. Regardless of the complexity of PCA innervation, numerous studies have shown the efficacy of selective reinnervation in animals, and feasibility has been shown in human cadavers [28, 32].

An alternative to PCA reinnervation methods requiring the sacrifice of non-RLN source motor axons was introduced by Zealear and Dedo in 1977 via the concept of an implanted electrical laryngeal pacemaker [33]. Over the next four decades, various animal and human studies affirmed the feasibility of laryngeal pacing via either direct PCA muscular stimulation or RLN abductor nerve branch stimulation, allowing coordination of PCA pacing to contractile thoracic diaphragm EMG signals via minimally invasive techniques [34]. However, technical limitations arose from electrode corrosion and durability against the mechanical forces exerted by laryngeal motion and elevation. Further, there were concerns regarding the safety and reliability of off-label use of a spinal stimulating device employed in the first randomized human laryngeal pacemaker trial in 1995. Moreover, further study also elucidated that direct muscular stimulation was suboptimal compared to residual RLN branch stimulation due to the relatively high current required for direct muscular pacing, the associated risk of muscle and tissue damage, and the increased tendency for electrode corrosion [34]. Fortuitously, the presence of synkinetic reinnervation also better facilitates successful laryngeal pacing and relies upon lower stimulation currents than completely paralyzed larynges. Therefore, an additional benefit of low current abductor nerve fiber pacing is that it is perhaps best employed in the delayed setting after the laryngeal neurodegenerative process has already declared itself. Moreover, this provides the opportunity to first perform immediate selective or non-selective reinnervation techniques, reserving either unilateral or bilateral laryngeal pacing as a fallback option should abduction not be achieved with the immediate reinnervation methods. Most recently, Mueller [34–36] has published feasibility data from the first prospective human trial examining a device specifically designed for laryngeal pacing. The device was successfully implanted in eight of nine patients, and seven completed the study duration of 6 months. Two patients who were tracheostomy dependent prior to implantation were decannulated, and all patients demonstrated increased peak expiratory flow without compromising voice or swallowing outcomes [35, 36]. Further study is needed to validate this preclinical data, but these promising results may represent an additional option for restoring spontaneous arytenoid abduction in laryngeal transplantation in the future.

Long-term neurophysiologic outcomes are available for the first transplant, while clinical and endoscopic data are available for the second and third transplants [1–3, 5–8, 11]. While EMG signals demonstrated that reinnervation had taken place in the first laryngeal transplant patient, the functional benefit of the repaired right RLN was seemingly limited. Only baseline adductor tone was present without coordinated volitional abduction of either posterior cricoarytenoid muscle, leaving the vocal folds in the midline position. Unfortunately, from an electrophysiologic standpoint, the right vocal fold EMG tracings were only marginally better than the left, which had notably not even undergone RLN neurorrhaphy [5]. Differing from the Cleveland Clinic patient, in addition to right primary donor-to-recipient RLN neurorrhaphy, the UCD patient underwent attempts at more selective reinnervation on the left including end-to-end neurorrhaphy of *ansa cervicalis* to the RLN adductor fibers and end-to-side neurorrhaphy of RLN abductor fibers to the phrenic nerve [1]. Regardless of the varied techniques, both the Cleveland Clinic and UCD patients' functional clinical outcomes were similar including relatively good speech and swallow but lacking coordinated volitional glottic adduction and abduction [1, 5].

Consequent to the limited electrophysiologic and functional improvement with long-term follow-up following RLN neurorrhaphy, restoring volitional glottic abduction has been cited as the greatest remaining hurdle to laryngeal transplantation's widespread adoption [11]. In order to maintain favorable vocal outcomes achieved by both patients and in light of the laryngeal edema experienced during the Cleveland Clinic patient's episodes of transplant rejection, pursuit of tracheostomy decannulation was deferred in both the Cleveland Clinic and UCD patients [1, 3, 7]. Amazingly, with 2 years of follow-up the Polish group reports that the third patient's transplanted glottis showcases at least partial bilateral glottic abduction with respiration and the patient has remained tracheostomy free. This outcome is especially remarkable given that their technique described only nonspecific end-to-side neurorrhaphies of the donor RLN stumps to the recipient vagus and phrenic nerves [8]. Prior reported outcomes have suggested that nonspecific reinnervation strategies would only provide tone, synkinetic activity, and bulk motion that is only marginally better than spontaneous reinnervation seen in the absence of any attempted neurorrhaphy [7, 11, 15]. Posttransplant laryngeal EMG data of the Polish patient has not been published, but this patient's reported clinical outcome is extremely promising [8]. Long-term follow-up is required to verify the durability of these findings, and further research must be done to consistently emulate this outcome. A full summary of airway, vocal, and swallowing outcomes in the three laryngeal transplants is presented in Table 13.2.

13.1.3.1 Lessons Learned

What are the strengths of your program?

The complexity of this procedure and the challenges of the recovery of function serve as reminders of the necessity of a team approach to these cases. Certainly, skill in complex laryngopharyngeal and microvascular surgery are critical. Coordination of organ procurement and need for mediastinal access argue for involvement of a thoracic or transplant surgeon with appropriate skills. Given UCD's longstanding and high-volume transplant program, the immunosuppression regimen was carefully implemented by physicians with great experience and skill.

It is impossible to emphasize the importance and necessity of speech and language pathology support. Relearning to speak and swallow after this procedure requires the engagement and expertise of dedicated and talented specialists in this critical rehabilitation area. Fortunately, the UCD group has a longstanding dedicated group of experts in speech and language pathology who were critical to our patient's successful outcome.

What did you change over time?

Due to the fact that there has been only a single procedure performed at each institution, it is challenging to discuss programmatic changes at length. However, in the time elapsed since the Cleveland Clinic program began in 1987 [2], there has been significant evolution of the field of laryngeal transplantation and composite tissue transplants including changes in the ethical paradigm, surgical indications, will-

Table 13.2 Summary of airway, vocal, and swallowing outcomes in the three published laryngeal transplants

Patient	Neurorrhaphies performed, recipient (R) and donor (D)	Laryngeal EMG findings	Sensory recovery	Endoscopic laryngeal findings at latest follow-up	Clinical speech and swallow outcomes	Tracheostomy present as of latest publication (Y/N)
Cleveland Clinic [2, 3, 5–7, 11]	– (D) bilateral SLN: (D) bilateral SLN – (D) right RLN: (R) right RLN – Unable to locate left (R) RLN due to post-traumatic fibrosis, (D) left RLN situated "free field" in adjacent neck musculature	– SLN reinnervation: Volitional bilateral cricothyroid contraction – RLN reinnervation: Electrophysiologic signals present in bilateral thyroarytenoid muscles – Baseline adductor tone present without coordinated activity – Right vocal fold EMG signals only marginally better than unrepaired left RLN	Successful reinnervation of the bilateral SLNs and right RLN distributions	– Vocal folds in the midline position – Bulk motion only – No coordinated or volitional vocal fold abduction	– "Normal" sounding voice – Excellent pitch control – Gastrostomy tube removed at 14 weeks	Y, "self-sustaining" permanently formalized tracheostomy in place prior to explantation, narrow field laryngectomy at year 14
UCD [1, 7]	– (D) bilateral SLN: (R) bilateral SLN – (D) right RLN: (R) Right RLN – Adductor branch (D) Left RLN: (R) left ansa cervicalis nerve – Abductor fibers (D) left RLN: (R) left phrenic nerve [end to side]	Not reported	Normal bilateral adductor response via laryngopharyngeal sensory testing at 3 months	– Baseline bilateral VF tone – Synkinetic bilateral VF motor activity – Right VF immobile, left VF abduction limited – Median bilateral VF positioning – Glottic airway restricted – Tracheal and subglottic airways patent – Return of pharyngeal motor activity, epiglottic inversion	– Maximal phonation time within normal range – For adult females: Vocal fundamental frequency slightly below normal, vocal range within normal range – Protracted return of swallow function due to stenosis at pharyngeal anastomosis, successfully managed with endoscopic dilation – Cleared for regular diet 11 months, Gastrojejunal feeding tube discontinued 13 months – Currently swallows normally, with intermittent ongoing endoscopic dilations – No aspiration	Y
Polish [8]	– (D) right RLN: (R) right vagus nerve [end-to-side] – (D) left RLN: (R) left phrenic [end-to-side] – (D) bilateral SLN:(R) bilateral lingual nerves [end-to-side]	Not reported	Not reported	– Functioning vocal folds with documented adduction and abduction – Breathing comfortably via mouth and nose	– Intelligible speech – Unrestricted diet – Mild pharyngoesophageal stenosis, managed successfully via endoscopic techniques – No aspiration	N, decannulated POD #10

ingness of surgeons to pursue transplantation in patients with malignant history, and surgical technical advances. Additionally, given the UCD patient's experience with the pharyngeal stenosis, necessitating multiple dilations over time, additional pharynx would be incorporated into the transplant in future patients.

13.1.4 Shift in the Transplant Surgery Ethical Paradigm

For instance, the transplant surgery ethical paradigm has experienced a major shift in which not only are vital, life-prolonging organs being transplanted but now composite tissue transplants of organs are being performed with the primary goal of improving quality of life [37]. Thus, composite tissue allografts encompassing the face, hands, penis, uterus, abdominal wall, larynx, and other traditionally non-canonical transplanted organs are gaining traction and performed with increased frequency [37].

Prior to Strome's work, laryngeal transplantation faced similarly intense ethical and logistical challenges due to the larynx representing a "non-vital" organ [11]. Indeed, laryngectomy has long been the gold standard to address malignancies and end-stage laryngotracheal dysfunction, and it is backed by 150 years of excellent functional and oncologic outcomes dating back to Billroth in 1873 [4, 38]. Perhaps most notably, laryngectomy lacks the risk of initiating immunosuppression in the naïve patient. Likewise, the potential for highly intelligible tracheoesophageal speech following total laryngectomy in motivated patients [18, 19] may also disincentivize exposing patients to the risk and costliness of laryngeal transplantation.

Notwithstanding the fact that an intact larynx is not mandated for survival, the psychosocial effects of total laryngectomy are immense and well-studied. The effects of laryngectomy on patients' lives are far-reaching and omnipresent, potentially including speech and swallowing difficulties, loss of smell, sinonasal congestion, depression, and anxiety [39]. Laryngectomy has also been linked to diminished mutual sexual function and intimacy between couples [40]. The classic 1981 study by McNeil examined the attitudes of laypersons toward laryngeal cancer, laryngectomy, and the perceived effects of loss of natural speech on function and quality of life [39]. Thirty-seven healthy fireman and executives were interviewed and given a passage describing the functional consequences and survival outcomes of total laryngectomy versus available non-surgical alternatives (i.e., primary radiation or "experimental chemotherapy") for locally advanced laryngeal cancer at the time [39]. After listening to recorded speech samples, 20% of the respondents noted that if faced with laryngeal cancer that they would forgo laryngectomy with artificial speech options. Instead they favored natural speech preservation with primary radiation even when informed that 3-year survival was up to 30% worse for non-surgical therapies at the time [39]. Those surveyed stated an average willingness to forgo 14% of expected lifespan in order to avoid loss of natural speech accompanying laryngectomy [39]. Importantly, this study demonstrates that despite the larynx's non-vital status, some human subjects express that laryngeal preservation provides value that outweighs threatened mortality. In addition, one may postulate that a similar attitude may be expressed toward the risks of initiating immunosuppression to facilitate a laryngeal transplant if the alternative is laryngectomy without transplantation. A variety of studies have been conducted to survey patients and healthcare providers regarding the risks of composite tissue allotransplantation and initiating immunosuppression [41–44]. Perhaps not surprisingly, Jo et al. reported that when surveyed regarding the acceptable risks associated with laryngeal allotransplantation, patients who were already taking immunosuppressive medications (90.6%) are most willing to accept the risks of immunosuppression for the purpose of laryngeal transplantation, followed very closely by the general population (88%). Conversely, patients having already undergone laryngectomy (55.9%) were least likely to accept the risks followed by physicians (63%).

Likewise, although no significant difference was shown, immunosuppressed patients and the general public also tended to trade the highest percentage of life expectancy to obtain a laryngeal transplant relative to laryngectomy patients and physicians. Finally, solid organ transplant recipients and the general public each reported higher expected quality-of-life improvements provided by a laryngeal transplant than laryngectomy patients and physicians. Therefore, those most familiar with post-laryngectomy aesthetic and functional outcomes (physicians and laryngectomy patients) were most reticent to the risks of initiating immunosuppression and transplant rejection and were less optimistic that it would provide a meaningful and worthwhile improvement on quality of life and function. On the other hand, the willingness of kidney transplant patients to undertake the risks of laryngeal transplantation and their collective optimism regarding its positive effects on quality of life are likely attributable to their prior experience with renal transplantation [45]. For physicians, the combination of familiarity with immunosuppression risks, post-laryngectomy voice and swallow function, and perhaps a more comprehensive assessment of the potential risk–benefit ratio following laryngeal transplant may have yielded a more cautious and less optimistic outlook. Therefore, careful assessment of preexisting patient quality of life and function in addition to patient functional and aesthetic goals and expectations are crucial considerations prior to recommending laryngeal transplantation.

A logical compromise for some providers was to consider CTA in only idealized patients, including those already on chronic immunosuppression for a prior transplant for whom no additional non-surgical risk was levied. Interestingly, with the first ever laryngeal transplant in 1998, Strome and colleagues were early adopters of the emerging ethical paradigm by selecting a patient that required de novo initiation of immunosuppressive medications [2]. This patient did well with immunosuppression, although he sustained a variety of minor related adverse events. The patient sustained one episode of cyclosporine-mediated renal dysfunction and hypertension 6 months postoperatively, which resolved upon optimization of his antihypertensive regimen and cyclosporine dose. Additional side effects included oropharyngeal thrush, *Pneumocystis carinii* pneumonia, tracheobronchitis, and steroid-related bone mineral density diminution [3]. Importantly, he developed an occult HPV/p16-positive oropharyngeal squamous cell carcinoma, which later compelled return to the operating room for definitive excision. However, this cancer's relationship to the *de novo* administration of immunosuppression will never be known with certainty given its HPV-positivity and the patient's high-risk status as a young, otherwise healthy non-smoker. As of his most recent follow-up, he remained cancer-free and sustained no untoward effects of weaning the immunosuppression [3].

13.1.5 Evolving Indications for Laryngeal Transplantation and Attitudes Toward Laryngeal Transplant and Malignancy

No strict inclusion criteria or guidelines for laryngotracheal transplant have been universally proposed or published. However, in the authors' experience and with review of the limited literature, ideal laryngotracheal transplant candidates likely include previously immunosuppressed patients with nonmalignant, noninflammatory/autoimmune end-stage laryngotracheal stenosis not otherwise amenable to traditional endoscopic or open airway procedures [1]. Patients with bulky benign laryngotracheal tumors leading to irreversible dysfunction and/or those requiring laryngectomy have also been proposed as ideal laryngotracheal transplant candidates [6]. Real-time transplantation performed concurrently with benign laryngotracheal tumor extirpation is an additional theoretical consideration, assuming adequate margins can be confirmed.

Other considerations include patient smoking status, pulmonary function, history of head and neck malignancy, and prior surgical treatment and/or radiation of the neck.

While prior laryngeal transplant patients have enjoyed adequate swallowing function without significant aspiration, this risk should be considered strongly when assessing patient candidacy. Therefore, patients with poor baseline pulmonary status such as those with COPD and limited pulmonary reserve should be considered poor candidates. This is informed by the increased risk of pulmonary complications and prolonged hospital stays seen in supracricoid laryngectomy patients with COPD, smoking history, and FEV1/FVC <59% [46].

For many surgeons and patients, the dangers of immunosuppression are sufficiently prohibitive to cause reticence toward the initiation of chronic immunosuppression to facilitate nonessential, non-life-sustaining laryngeal transplant in an immunosuppressive-naive patient [47]. Therefore, a patient who has previously been committed to lifelong immunosuppression for another indication (i.e., solid organ transplantation) helps justify laryngotracheal transplantation in qualifying patients [47]. However, as discussed, the ethics and safety of composite tissue allografting is gaining traction in immunocompetent patients [41–44].

In a patient whose end-stage laryngotracheal disease arises from autoimmune etiology, the potential for recidivistic inflammatory laryngotracheal stenosis (e.g., idiopathic/autoimmune subglottic stenosis) may also give surgeons pause prior to considering laryngeal transplantation in such cases. While the immunosuppression regimen would potentially aid both the prevention of autoimmunity and graft rejection, various studies have noted recurrent autoimmune hepatitis following liver transplantation in 16–43% of cases [48]. Laryngotracheal transplantation and inflammatory laryngotracheal stenosis are each sufficiently rare that the study of recurrent stenosis following transplant is improbable, and no laryngeal transplant has been attempted in this setting to our knowledge.

Another critical consideration in laryngeal transplantation is the patient's oncologic history and history of prior cancer treatments. Real-time laryngeal transplantation following laryngectomy for active malignancy or radiotherapy-related laryngeal dysfunction and has long-represented an alluring goal but faced historical reticence due to the risk of cancer recurrence [10] and the development of de novo cancers [49]. Both risks are heightened by transplant-mandated lifelong immunosuppression, with as high as five-fold cancer risk compared to immunocompetent hosts [50]. In fact, the earliest apparent laryngeal transplantation attempt took place concurrently with total laryngectomy for bilateral glottic squamous cell carcinoma in 1969 [10], although no revascularization or reinnervation attempts were made [51]. The graft was expeditiously explanted after the patient sustained rapid peristomal disease progression within 8 months of the initial operation prior to eventually succumbing to this recurrence [10, 51]. Skepticism has since been expressed that the failed outcome likely stemmed from an oncologically substandard initial resection rather than an immunosuppression-mediated recurrence [51]. Nonetheless, this poor outcome led the authors of the 1970 publication to discourage laryngeal transplant in the context of malignancy, calling it "unjustifiable" prior to further study on cancer immunobiology [10]. In kind, the consideration of malignancy as a contraindication to laryngeal transplantation persisted for decades despite rejection of the concept within the field of solid organ transplantation, which enjoyed successful long-term survival outcomes in liver transplantation following resection for malignancy [51].

Unfortunately, the first published human lingual composite tissue transplant also died of rapid disease recurrence in 2003 [11, 52, 53]. Rapid recurrence and death of both patients in the last 50 years having undergone immediate head and neck CTAs in the context of active locally advanced malignancy [10, 11, 52] may have reinforced concerns within the head and neck oncology community.

Nonetheless, the fact remains that over 13,000 cases in the US and over 150,000 global cases of locally advanced laryngeal malignancy were diagnosed yearly in the United States yearly as of 2017, which easily represents the largest source of potential subjects [11, 54]. While malignant history is certainly an important consideration, the disease-free interval is another pivotal consideration for patients whose head and neck cancer has been treated. Consequently, support for pursuing laryngeal transplant following malignancy has gained momentum in patients with greater than 5 years of disease-free survival and are considered oncologically cured [6].

The Cleveland Clinic and Polish laryngeal transplants each offer significant insight into the challenges and ethical dilemmas faced associated with laryngeal transplant in the context of prior malignancy and the development of *de novo* malignancies. The Cleveland Clinic patient's initial transplant was performed to address benign posttraumatic stenosis, and the explanted laryngeal specimen was otherwise cancer-free. However, an incidental clinically occult focus of HPV/p16-positive oropharyngeal squamous cell carcinoma was excised at the margin of the specimen and the native tonsil, which later compelled return to the operating room for definitive excision. The unexpected presence of occult malignancy highlights the potential risks of initiating immunosuppression medications in a naïve patient for a non-life-sustaining transplant. Viral mediated malignancies, such as those related to high-risk HPV strains, herpes viruses, and EBV, are at generally increased prevalence in immunosuppressed patients such as in solid organ transplantation [55]. However, the HPV-positivity of the oropharyngeal lesion in an otherwise healthy non-smoking young male obscures any direct causal link to immunosuppression due to the generally increased incidence of HPV-mediated oropharyngeal cancer in his demographic even in the absence of immunosuppression [56].

Strome and colleagues note that the timing of the explant serendipitously led to the early detection and removal of this lesion [3]. Regardless, the development of an upper aerodigestive tract malignancy in the first laryngeal transplant highlights the need for caution, patient counseling, and strict surveillance of high-risk organ systems (i.e., the upper aerodigestive tract, skin, vulva/cervix, anus, liver, and for hematologic malignancies such as Non-Hodgkin Lymphoma and Kaposi's Sarcoma) [55].

The most recent reported transplant performed in Poland also adds crucial experience to the literature, since it represented the first successful laryngotracheal transplant performed in a patient having previously completed treatment for laryngeal cancer. This case is also noteworthy for his treatment having included therapeutic radiotherapy to the neck. A 34-year-old chronically immunosuppressed kidney transplant recipient and previous acute myeloid leukemia patient underwent definitive chemotherapy and radiation for T3N1M0 laryngeal squamous cell carcinoma followed by salvage laryngectomy. Thankfully, by 2015 the patient remained disease-free from both leukemia (12 years) and laryngeal cancer (6 years). However, the patient's long-term quality of life was severely limited secondary to numerous severe postoperative complications, including pharyngeal necrosis, large pharyngocutaneous fistula, permanent gastrostomy tube dependence, severe neck scarring, and marked psychosocial sequelae. Three initial attempts at traditional reconstructive measures failed, although jejunal free flap was ultimately successful in restoration of alimentary function [8]. Nonetheless, the patient's functional outcome and quality of life remained inadequate. Given the nature and extensiveness of the postoperative wound sequalae, laryngotracheal transplantation was eventually pursued, entailing an extensive composite laryngotracheal allograft with a large anterior neck soft tissue component, thyroid, and parathyroid glands. When it was performed in 2015, this became the first successful documented transplant performed following a head and neck malignancy [8]. To re-establish supraglottic and glottic sensory and laryngeal motor innervation, end-to-side neurorrhaphies were performed between the bilateral graft SLNs to the recipient "sublingual" nerves, and ipsilateral graft RLNs were anastomosed to the right vagus and left phrenic nerves. Moreover, with 2 years of follow-up, the patient remarkably possessed an adequately functioning transplanted glottis such that he remained tracheostomy-free, demonstrated intelligible speech, and swallowed an unrestricted diet without aspiration [8].

Real-time laryngeal transplantation in the setting of laryngeal malignancy represents a highly attractive but elusive strategy that has not been widely adopted for myriad reasons elaborated previously. Concurrent laryngectomy and laryngeal transplant is also potentially complicated by the frequent need for adjuvant radiation required for locoregionally advanced laryngeal malignancies, which although unstudied could theoretically harm the transplant or potentiate wound complications. Stereotactic radiation appears to be safe following radiation for hepatic malignancies, but its role in hepatic malignant recurrences is not clear [57]. Therefore, radiation to a laryngeal transplant may theoretically increase the risk of delayed secondary graft malignancy synergistically with immunosuppression. If the patient sustains severe wound complications related to the transplant, radiation therapy may also require delay, which has been shown to worsen survival outcomes in head and neck cancers [58].

Consequently, delay of the transplant until oncologic clearance is strongly favored prior to consideration for laryngeal transplant in patients with a head and neck cancer history. Likewise, posttreatment transplantation also gives rise to its own distinct technical and functional challenges, due to the fact that dissecting and isolating native SLN and RLN stubs in a previously operated and/or radiated surgical field characterized by postoperative and/or radiation-mediated fibrosis may prove exceedingly difficult. For instance, the Polish team performed only end-to-side RLN and SLN neurorrhaphies 6 years after radiation and laryngectomy [8], and Strome's team was also unable to locate the recipient left RLN due to extensive trauma-related fibrosis [2].

Notwithstanding, the vast majority of irreversible laryngeal dysfunction arises consequent to malignancy or associated treatments, and laryngotracheal transplantation, as a means to rehabilitate patients in this setting, remains an intriguing possibility for surgeons and patients. It remains to be seen whether immediate transplant in the setting of laryngeal cancer is a viable option. Therefore, Strome and colleagues have sought alternative immunosuppressive regimens to mitigate the risk of recurrence or de novo malignancies [49] by exploring drugs with concurrent antitumor and immunosuppressive mechanisms. Both sirolimus [6] and everolimus [49] have been explored as an addition to immunosuppressive regimens for patients with malignancies, due to dual anti-cell cycle tumor suppressive activity and anti-calcineurin immune inhibitory properties. Rapamycin-based immunosuppressives in place of tacrolimus in standard regimens demonstrated promising results in a combination rat allograft-tumor model [49], and this has been corroborated in renal transplant literature [6].

Evolving Surgical Techniques and Lessons Learned Regarding What to Avoid (What will you not repeat in the future?) Since Strome and colleagues' first groundbreaking laryngeal transplant in 1998, significant technical advancements have been made in laryngeal transplantation and RLN and SLN reinnervation. Farwell and colleagues UCD transplant in 2010 [1] became the first to include a long segment (8 cm) of trachea, to preserve the transplanted pharyngoesophageal muscular blood supply from inferior thyroid arteries to the membranous tracheal wall, and to attempt unilateral selective PCA muscle and adductor muscle reinnervation. This reinnervation technique was modified from the previously published technique described by Marie [28], but in order to avoid diaphragmatic paralysis, end-to-side neurorrhaphy was performed between the RLN abductor fibers to phrenic while end-to-end anastomosis was performed between the adductor fibers and *ansa cervicalis*. Unfortunately, the UCD patient remains tracheostomy-dependent due to robust adductor tone and bulk without meaningful arytenoid abduction [1], and the Cleveland Clinic patient also showcased similar results until explantation after not having undergone selective reinnervation [3]. In future transplants, consideration of Marie's bilateral end-to-end selective upper phrenic root reinnervation to PCA branches [59] and/or Kwak's sectioning and transposition of interarytenoid nerve branches [32] may improve chances of success of either unilateral or bilateral selective reinnervation, may restore glottic airway patency with respiration, and may ultimately facilitate decannulation. Moreover, either real-time or delayed implantation of laryngeal pacing devices may help deliver similar outcomes [60, 61]. Both the Cleveland Clinic and UCD patients chose to remain tracheostomy dependent and to defer procedures such as cord lateralization, cordotomy, or arytenoidectomy in order to maintain voice quality [1, 3]. These procedures remain options for patients with chronic bilateral vocal fold paralysis to aid in decannulation. However, significant caution should be taken prior to the decannulation of laryngeal transplant patients due to the risk of airway edema that may accompany acute and chronic transplant rejection episodes, which may occur at any point after transplantation [3].

The UCD transplant demonstrated that anastomosis of a single inferior thyroid artery supplied adequate arterial perfusion to the entire graft intraoperatively, but preservation of the cervical muscular esophagus theoretically improved perfusion to the graft, particularly to the long tracheal segment. The redundant inferior thyroid artery blood supply via the transplant's demucosalized pharyngoesophageal musculature safeguarded the graft from ischemic damage in the event of an arterial thrombosis. Moreover, this technical advancement may be crucial in undertaking complete tracheal transplantation in the future [1, 62]. While trimming of the mucosa was initially intended to prevent pooling of secretions and associated aspiration risk, an unexpected outcome associated with this pharyngeal inset may have been the development of pharyngeal stenosis due to an anastomotic stricture in this patient. While the patient sustained protracted dysphagia, which was potentially worsened by her diabetic neuropathy, the pathology was managed entirely with two rounds of endoscopic dilations. She was advanced to a general diet by 11 months and her gastrojejunal feeding tube was removed by 13 months [1]. It is possible that insetting the redundant graft mucosa rather than trimming it may have improved this course by reducing the chance for clinically significant stenosis.

Significant surgical technical advances were also performed in the Polish transplant patient also notably differed from prior patients due to the prior surgical excision of all native parathyroid tissue during laryngectomy and the need for a large composite soft tissue component in light of the severe post-cancer treatment scarring and pharyngocutaneous fistula [8]. Post-operative thyroid scintigraphic scans and laboratory values demonstrated that thyroid and parathyroid function that had been absent preoperatively were restored. Therefore, this was the first transplant to confirm that thyroid and parathyroid function could be derived solely from transplanted organs [8], and as of 2017 no pharmacologic supplementation was required. The allograft was particularly unique due to its large anterior composite neck soft tissue and skin paddle over 200 cm^2. Due to a dense population of dendritic cell antigen presenting cells, allogenic skin is typically highly immunogenic and increased the complexity of the graft and the potential for organ rejection. The large skin paddle doubly improved monitoring capabilities via visual inspection. It also provided an easily accessible biopsy site for formal pathologic assessment, but this was deferred to-date due to the lack of evidence of clinical rejection episodes. The neck skin paddle remained completely integrated without evidence of acute or chronic rejection and with favorable aesthetic results as of the latest publication in 2017 [8].

13.1.6 Lessons Learned from Explantation of First Laryngeal Transplant

The clinical and histopathologic manifestations of acute and chronic rejection episodes experienced by the Cleveland Clinic patient in addition to evaluation of the post-explantation specimen are informative. The Cleveland Clinic patient remains the sole laryngeal transplant patient to have sustained documented acute and/or chronic episode of rejection.

The patient manifested his first episode of acute transplant rejection at 15 months, requiring high-dose prednisone and transition from cyclosporine to tacrolimus [3, 6]. This episode resolved 3 days thereafter. Perhaps attributable to a dip in the serum tacrolimus trough, he sustained an additional acute rejection episode at year 5, characterized by bilateral glottic and epiglottic edema and vocal degradation. Symptoms and concerning exam findings quickly resolved with up-titration of his tacrolimus dose and a course of IV solumedrol.

Ultimately, the first transplant was successful for many years with remarkable functional outcomes including speech and swallowing [3, 5]. However, approximately 10 years into his postoperative course, the patient gradually manifested the effects of "slowly progressive chronic rejection" beginning with unilateral and subsequently bilateral glottic edema and ultimately yielded a nonfunctional larynx [3, 6]. At year 12 the patient developed an unresolving ulcerated post-cricoid mucosal lesion characterized by acute inflammation and bacterial overgrowth on biopsy, which improved only with debridement and protracted IV antibiotics. Over the next 2 years, the authors note that in spite of adjustments to the immunosuppression regimen, after initial improvement the patient's voice quality and swallow function declined irreparably, which were highlighted by breathy voice, poor pitch control, and increasingly severe aspiration. Additionally, he began to suffer from bilateral radiating pharyngeal pain and otalgia, and the patient's long-term use of oral corticosteroids manifested as diminished bone mineral density [3, 6]. The patient elected for explantation 14 years after transplantation due to gradually progressive severe laryngeal dysfunction and pharyngeal pain [3]. He underwent laryngopharyngectomy with additional explantation of the donor thyroid. Parathyroid tissue was not identified in the explanted specimen. Concurrently, pharyngeal reconstruction was performed with an anterolateral thigh free flap. Interestingly, while its relationship to the immunosuppression regimen remains unclear, an incidental clinically occult focus of HPV/p16-positive squamous cell carcinoma was excised at the margin of the specimen and the native tonsil. The laryngeal specimen was otherwise cancer-free, but this malignant oropharyngeal focus later compelled return to the operating room for definitive excision. The explanted laryngotracheal allograft also allowed for the previously undescribed gross and histopathologic analysis of the characteristic of end-stage chronic rejection in this setting, including acute and chronic inflammation, chondritis, tissue atrophy, severe fibrosis, and microcirculatory occlusion.

Postoperatively, the patient underwent tracheoesophageal puncture for insertion of a speech prosthesis, and he became fluent with tracheoesophageal speech. The patient otherwise sustained only minor and/or transient adverse events related to his immunosuppression regimen, which was successfully ceased post-explantation without significant issue [3]. The patient emphatically noted that he did not regret the procedure and stated that he would undergo a second transplant if given the opportunity [3]. As the first laryngotracheal transplant, it stands as the longest surviving first-of-its-kind transplant of any organ system for which immunosuppression was initiated in a previously naïve patient [3, 6].

13.1.7 How Do You See the Future of VCA?

We anticipate that the field of vascularized composite tissue allotransplantation will continue its expanding trajectory, as prior ethical restraints surrounding non-vital organ transplants become increasingly normalized to patients, medical professionals, and the lay-public. Head and neck CTAs have at present consisted predominately of facial transplants, for which over 35 cases have been reported [63], but the acceptance of and indications for laryngeal transplantation also promises to expand with the continued advancement of surgical techniques and laryngeal neuromuscular rehabilitation strategies including selective reinnervation and pacing. Moreover, lessons learned from continually accruing follow-up in previously published laryngeal transplants will further inform management and avoid pitfalls in the future. Additionally, we anticipate that improved immunosuppression regimens with dual immunosuppressive and tumor suppressor mechanisms [49], combined with rigorous oncologic surveillance, will increase access of laryngeal and lingual CTAs to qualifying patients with adequate disease-free follow-up to be deemed oncologically cured of prior head and neck cancers. Once solutions are developed to re-establish the profoundly complex neural network provided by associated cranial nerves, including somatosensory, special sensory, autonomic, and motor interplay, the possibilities for organ transplantation within the head and neck are seemingly endless. Future directions for CTAs of the head and neck may include the globe, temporal bone, scalp, cranium, olfactory neuro-epithelium, and more. Moreover, as the risks of immunosuppression are diminished, it is possible that smaller isolated components of previously published larger CTAs may be pursued, including transplant of the parathyroid, thyroid, trachea, esophagus, nose, lymphatics, eyelids, and/or oral aperture.

References

1. Farwell DG, et al. Laryngotracheal transplantation: technical modifications and functional outcomes. Laryngoscope. 2013;123(10):2502–8.
2. Strome M, et al. Laryngeal transplantation and 40-month follow-up. N Engl J Med. 2001;344(22):1676–9.
3. Lorenz RR, Strome M. Total laryngeal transplant explanted: 14 years of lessons learned. Otolaryngol Head Neck Surg. 2014;150(4):509–11.
4. Strome M. Human laryngeal transplantation: considerations and implications. Microsurgery. 2000;20(8):372–4.
5. Lorenz RR, et al. Laryngeal nerve function after total laryngeal transplantation. Otolaryngol Head Neck Surg. 2004;131(6):1016–8.
6. Knott PD, et al. A 12-year perspective on the world's first total laryngeal transplant. Transplantation. 2011;91(7):804–5.
7. Krishnan G, et al. The current status of human laryngeal transplantation in 2017: a state of the field review. Laryngoscope. 2017;127(8):1861–8.
8. Grajek M, et al. First complex allotransplantation of neck organs: larynx, trachea, pharynx, esophagus, thyroid, parathyroid glands, and anterior cervical wall: a case report. Ann Surg. 2017;266(2):e19–24.
9. Duque E, et al. Management of larynx and trachea donors. Transplant Proc. 2007;39(7):2076–8.
10. Kluyskens P, Ringoir S. Follow-up of a human larynx transplantation. Laryngoscope. 1970;80(8):1244–50.
11. Birchall MA, et al. Laryngeal transplantation in 2005: a review. Am J Transplant. 2006;6(1):20–6.
12. McCaughan J, Xu Q, Tinckam K. Detecting donor-specific antibodies: the importance of sorting the wheat from the chaff. Hepatobiliary Surg Nutr. 2019;8(1):37–52.
13. Paniello RC, Park A. Effect on laryngeal adductor function of vincristine block of posterior cricoarytenoid muscle 3 to 5 months after recurrent laryngeal nerve injury. Ann Otol Rhinol Laryngol. 2015;124(6):484–9.
14. Ali SA, et al. Comparison of myelin-associated glycoprotein with vincristine for facial nerve inhibition after bilateral axotomy in a transgenic Thy1-Gfp rat model. JAMA Facial Plast Surg. 2019;21(5):426–33.
15. Kupfer RA, et al. Spontaneous laryngeal reinnervation following chronic recurrent laryngeal nerve injury. Laryngoscope. 2013;123(9):2216–27.
16. Singh JM, Kwartowitz G. Vocal fold paralysis unilateral. In: StatPearls. Treasure Island, FL: StatPearls; 2020.
17. McPhail MJ, Janus JR, Lott DG. Advances in regenerative medicine for otolaryngology/head and neck surgery. BMJ. 2020;369:m718.
18. Onofre F, et al. Effect of singing training on total laryngectomees wearing a tracheoesophageal voice prosthesis. Acta Cir Bras. 2013;28(2):119–25.
19. Mendelsohn M, Morris M, Gallagher R. Speaking proficiency after primary tracheoesophageal puncture. J Otolaryngol. 1993;22(6):435–7.
20. Rameau A. Pilot study for a novel and personalized voice restoration device for patients with laryngectomy. Head Neck. 2020;42(5):839–45.
21. Loos E, et al. Tracheal autotransplantation for functional reconstruction of extended hemilaryngectomy defects: a single-center experience in 30 patients. Ann Surg Oncol. 2016;23(5):1674–83.
22. Moser PT, et al. Creation of laryngeal grafts from primary human cells and decellularized laryngeal scaffolds. Tissue Eng Part A. 2020;26(9–10):543–55.
23. Wang Q, Chen R, Zhou S. Successful management of the supraclavicular artery island flap combined with a sternohyoid muscle flap for hypopharyngeal and laryngeal reconstruction. Medicine (Baltimore). 2019;98(41):e17499.
24. Gilbert RW, et al. Vertical partial laryngectomy with temporoparietal free flap reconstruction for recurrent laryngeal squamous cell carcinoma: technique and long-term outcomes. Arch Otolaryngol Head Neck Surg. 2012;138(5):484–91.
25. Erman AB, et al. Disorders of cranial nerves IX and X. Semin Neurol. 2009;29(1):85–92.
26. Hong KH, et al. Functional differences between the two bellies of the cricothyroid muscle. Otolaryngol Head Neck Surg. 1998;118(5):714–22.
27. Sunderland S. A classification of peripheral nerve injuries producing loss of function. Brain. 1951;74(4):491–516.
28. Marina MB, Marie JP, Birchall MA. Laryngeal reinnervation for bilateral vocal fold paralysis. Curr Opin Otolaryngol Head Neck Surg. 2011;19(6):434–8.
29. Marie JP, et al. Selective resection of the phrenic nerve roots in rabbits. part II: respiratory effects. Respir Physiol. 1997;109(2):139–48.
30. Marie JP, et al. Selective resection of the phrenic nerve roots in rabbits. Part I: cartography of the residual innervation. Respir Physiol. 1997;109(2):127–38.
31. Fackler CD, Perret GE, Bedell GN. Effect of unilateral phrenic nerve section on lung function. J Appl Physiol. 1967;23(6):923–6.
32. Kwak PE, et al. Selective reinnervation of the posterior cricoarytenoid and interarytenoid muscles: an anatomical study. Laryngoscope. 2010;120(3):463–7.
33. Zealear DL, Dedo HH. Control of paralysed axial muscles by electrical stimulation. Acta Otolaryngol. 1977;83(5–6):514–27.
34. Mueller AH, Pototschnig C. Recurrent laryngeal nerve stimulator. Otolaryngol Clin North Am. 2020;53(1):145–56.
35. Mueller AH, et al. Laryngeal pacing for bilateral vocal fold paralysis: voice and respiratory aspects. Laryngoscope. 2017;127(8):1838–44.

36. Mueller AH, et al. Laryngeal pacing via an implantable stimulator for the rehabilitation of subjects suffering from bilateral vocal fold paralysis: a prospective first-in-human study. Laryngoscope. 2016;126(8):1810–6.
37. Caplan A, Purves D. A quiet revolution in organ transplant ethics. J Med Ethics. 2017;43(11):797–800.
38. Karamanou M, et al. A historical overview of laryngeal carcinoma and the first total laryngectomies. J BUON. 2017;22(3):807–11.
39. McNeil BJ, Weichselbaum R, Pauker SG. Speech and survival: tradeoffs between quality and quantity of life in laryngeal cancer. N Engl J Med. 1981;305(17):982–7.
40. Gür H, et al. The effect of partial and total laryngectomy on couples' sexual functions in men with larynx cancer. Eur Arch Otorhinolaryngol. 2020;277:3397.
41. Brouha P, et al. Risk acceptance in composite-tissue allotransplantation reconstructive procedures. Microsurgery. 2006;26(3):144–9; discussion 149–50.
42. Barker JH, et al. Investigation of risk acceptance in facial transplantation. Plast Reconstr Surg. 2006;118(3):663–70.
43. Reynolds CC, et al. Risk acceptance in laryngeal transplantation. Laryngoscope. 2006;116(10):1770–5.
44. Majzoub RK, et al. Investigation of risk acceptance in hand transplantation. J Hand Surg. 2006;31(2):295–302.
45. Jo HK, et al. Risk acceptance and expectations of laryngeal allotransplantation. Arch Plast Surg. 2014;41(5):505–12.
46. Joo YH, et al. Factors that predict postoperative pulmonary complications after supracricoid partial laryngectomy. Arch Otolaryngol Head Neck Surg. 2009;135(11):1154–7.
47. Birchall M. Human laryngeal allograft: shift of emphasis in transplantation. Lancet. 1998;351(9102):539–40.
48. Faisal N, Renner EL. Recurrence of autoimmune liver diseases after liver transplantation. World J Hepatol. 2015;7(29):2896–905.
49. Shipchandler TZ, et al. Laryngeal transplantation in the setting of cancer: a rat model. Laryngoscope. 2008;118(12):2166–71.
50. Acuna SA. Etiology of increased cancer incidence after solid organ transplantation. Transplant Rev (Orlando). 2018;32(4):218–24.
51. Strome M, Strome S. Laryngeal transplantation: a program for investigating new parameters. J Voice. 1994;8(1):92–4.
52. Kermer C, Watzinger F, Oeckher M. Tongue transplantation: 10-month follow-up. Transplantation. 2008;85(4):654–5.
53. Birchall M. Tongue transplantation. Lancet. 2004;363(9422):1663.
54. Hamilton NJI, Birchall MA. Tissue-engineered larynx: future applications in laryngeal cancer. Curr Otorhinolaryngol Rep. 2017;5(1):42–8.
55. Cangemi M, et al. Dissecting the multiplicity of immune effects of immunosuppressive drugs to better predict the risk of de novo malignancies in solid organ transplant patients. Front Oncol. 2019;9:160.
56. Rahimi S. HPV-related squamous cell carcinoma of oropharynx: a review. J Clin Pathol. 2020;73:624.
57. Au KP, et al. Initial experience with stereotactic body radiotherapy for intrahepatic hepatocellular carcinoma recurrence after liver transplantation. World J Clin Cases. 2020;8(13):2758–68.
58. Goel AN, et al. The impact of treatment package time on survival in surgically managed head and neck cancer in the United States. Oral Oncol. 2019;88:39–48.
59. Marie JP, et al. Selective reinnervation of the abductor and adductor muscles of the canine larynx after recurrent nerve paralysis. Ann Otol Rhinol Laryngol. 1989;98(7 Pt 1):530–6.
60. Zealear DL, et al. Reanimation of the paralyzed human larynx with an implantable electrical stimulation device. Laryngoscope. 2003;113(7):1149–56.
61. Mueller AH. Laryngeal pacing for bilateral vocal fold immobility. Curr Opin Otolaryngol Head Neck Surg. 2011;19(6):439–43.
62. Salmeron J, et al. Tracheal transplantation: superior and inferior thyroid artery perfusion territory. Laryngoscope. 1998;108(6):849–53.
63. Tasigiorgos S, et al. Face transplantation-current status and future developments. Transpl Int. 2018;31(7):677–88.

Part IV

Upper Extremity Transplantation

Hand and Upper Extremity Transplantation

14

Alexander de Heinrich, Marina Ninkovic, Zvjezdana Milacak, and Milomir Ninkovic

14.1 Introduction

Traumatic arm amputations can be treated with replantation or surgical shaping of an adequate stump with or without subsequent prosthetic fitting. The superior reconstructive option for an amputated extremity is always replantation when possible. However, in the last 25 years modern immunosuppressive therapy has opened new horizons in composite tissue allotransplantation, opening possibilities for facial and extremity allotransplantation as one reconstructive option.

The main goal of treating amputees is to obtain a usefully functioning, sensate, and surviving allotransplant of the upper extremity. In the emerging field of allotransplantation, experience and knowledge in the field of reconstructive microsurgery are the key to the successful use of this technique. In 1962 Malt and McKhann are credited with performing the first successful reconstruction of an amputated arm, and Komatsu and Tamai presented the first successful digital replantation in 1968 [1, 2].

A. de Heinrich (✉) · M. Ninkovic
Department of Plastic, Reconstructive, Hand and Burn Surgery, Munich Clinic Bogenhausen, Academic Teaching Hospital Technical University Munich, Munich, Germany

Department of Surgery, University Hospital for Visceral, Transplant and Thoracic Surgery, Medical University of Innsbruck, Innsbruck, Austria

Office of Plastic and Reconstructive Surgery, Munich, Germany
e-mail: Alexander.deHeinrich@muenchen-klinik.de; Milomir.Ninkovic@muenchen-klinik.de

M. Ninkovic · Z. Milacak
Department of Plastic, Reconstructive, Hand and Burn Surgery, Munich Clinic Bogenhausen, Academic Teaching Hospital Technical University Munich, Munich, Germany

Department of Surgery, University Hospital for Visceral, Transplant and Thoracic Surgery, Medical University of Innsbruck, Innsbruck, Austria
e-mail: Marina.Ninkovic@i-med.ac.at; Zvjezdana.Milacak@muenchen-klinik.de

The first unilateral hand transplantation was performed in 1964 in Ecuador [3], but the extremity was rejected 3 weeks postoperatively and had to be removed. It was not until 1978 that the immunosuppressant drug cyclosporine (calcineurin inhibitor) was developed. The first unilateral hand transplantation, using a modern immunosuppressive therapeutic regimen was performed in Lyon, France, in 1998 [4]. It had to be re-amputated on an outpatient basis after 1.5 years in London.

The program started 1998 in Innsbruck, Austria and moved with the transfer of Prof. Ninkovic to Munich, Germany in November 2003. During this time more than 100 patients were screened, which of three were approved and successfully operated on. The transplants always were covered fully by insurance.

The program is still active defying local bureaucracy. In 2003, we still had the approval by the state government. At that time, composite tissue transplantation was categorized as organ transplantation. When the government changed the status to tissue transplantation, which requires a humane laboratory. Due to lack of the latter on our premises, our license for transplantation was revoked putting our program on hold. Now, with our new and very promising candidate, we are fighting once more to regain authorization for composite tissue allotransplantation, which would also allow expansion of the program.

In 2000, both hands were transplanted for the first time in Lyon; this was followed by the first bilateral hand transplantation in Innsbruck in March of the same year [5]. From 1999 to 2021, 120 hands were transplanted, either isolated or in combination with a face or lower extremity transplant in approximately 81 patients [6].

Since then, an increasing number of replantation surgeries have been performed around the world with a boosting survival rate of amputated parts. Justifiably, the focus of surgeons has turned to function, by far the most important consideration in hand surgery, due to increasing experience [7, 8].

Initial survival in the case of transplants depends on the perfectly functioning microvascular anastomosis as well as

© Springer Nature Switzerland AG 2023

R. Gurunian et al. (eds.), *Reconstructive Transplantation*, https://doi.org/10.1007/978-3-031-21520-9_14

immediate postoperative care, but the final function and acceptability depend on carefully selected patients, precise matching, the correct surgical procedure, the proper reconstruction of bones, muscles, tendons, nerves, and soft tissues, as well as long-lasting patient-tailored rehabilitation program. Hence, vascularized composite allotransplantation requires a highly trained and full-range hand surgeon with high skills and experience in microsurgery to be able to predict outcomes of allotransplants as well as knowledge of immunosuppressive therapy. To maintain a high degree of viability and maximum functional efficiency, a single surgeon working alone is unlikely to achieve the same high success rate in allotransplantation as a team. A well-coordinated team includes a plastic surgeon, an orthopedist/trauma surgeon, a transplant surgeon, a psychiatrist/psychologist, and a specialist in physical medicine and rehabilitation. Additionally, also other specialists like anesthesiologists, neurologists, immunologists, radiologists, and internists are involved in treatment of these patients.

14.2 Indications and Patient Selection

The recruited patients are healthy and mentally stable, aged 18 years and older, approved for allotransplantation only after a thorough preoperative assessment, including their own as well as their family's anamnesis, the course of events resulting in the injury, pre-existing trauma, or medical conditions. Patients under the age of 18 years should only be considered if they are undergoing immunosuppressive therapy in connection with other organ transplants. The main objective in vascularized composite allotransplantation is the functional and esthetic restoration. Its consequences (risks and benefits), autonomy and adherence to future medications (e.g., immunosuppression), and a rehabilitation program are prerequisites for passing [9].

Apart from this, the patient must be placed in a healthy social environment, be of adequate intelligence, highly motivated, and endure a high tolerance for frustration to actively participate in the tedious process of rehabilitation, both mentally and physically [10–12].

Obviously, Guillotine amputees of both hands at level of wrist and distal forearm are ideal candidates. However, most hands are amputated more proximally due to the most common injury mechanisms. These include explosion, crush, electrical, or avulsion injuries that increase the difficulty of reconstructive surgery and decrease the percentage of functional viability. Particularly after electrical accidents, electricity causes fibrosis in particular of the nerves [13], leading to an increase in phantom pain, a decrease in surface sensitivity, and a delay in reinnervation of the intrinsic muscular system [10].

In addition, after very proximal muscle damage, no resting function remains, and the high proximal nerve damage makes nerve recovery questionable. Therefore, the patient should be fully aware of the possible complications and side effects and would only be eligible in the event of unsatisfactory myoelectric prosthetic alternatives. Developments in new prosthetic treatment are very promising and must be considered as a better alternative in high proximal upper extremity amputation compared to extremity allotransplantation. Providing an indication for extremity allotransplantation, we must take all benefits and risks of immunosuppressive therapy into consideration and find the optimal solution accordingly.

Patients with unilateral hand amputation as well as blindness are still questionable [14]. The question in increasing unilateral amputees is whether loss of the dominant hand with retained awareness of the missing extremity (painless phantom representation) an indication for transplantation is [15], or whether a one-handed human is capable of doing facing everyday life with skill. In our opinion unilateral hand amputation is not yet indicated for allotransplantation. There are many reasons for that. First, side effects of immunosuppressive therapy are higher than their benefit; second, hand matching after allotransplantation is very difficult to achieve and is psychologically unacceptable for the patient which will constantly compare his healthy hand to the transplanted one [16].

Bilateral hand transplantation in blind patients is more demanding for the rehabilitation initially without tactile sensation or optical control, but ultimately improve quality of life by recovering sensory qualities in new hands compared to non-sensory prostheses [17].

14.3 Patient Expectations

In our current time and state of mind, quality of life is of increasing importance and therefore the possibilities in adapting medicine in order to meet patients' wishes and expectations. Life without hands is equal to a massive loss, both physically and mentally, and hindrance in day-to-day life, and many patients refuse their myoelectric prosthesis since they do not impart sensitivity. Hence, an amputees' wish for "new" hands, and with them adequate function, sensitivity, and restoration of self-perception are understandable [18, 19].

The expectations of an amputee must be realistic with regard to function and sensitivity, and therefore, the possibility of failure of surgery, rejection, or re-amputation be addressed quite plainly [20].

The candidate must be willing and eager to undergo a lengthy and strenuous rehabilitation program (e.g., cognitive training, physiotherapy, hand therapy, electrotherapy) and must be aware that lifelong immunosuppressive therapy including all side effects, that might harm his health, will be necessary [11].

Due to a patients' injury history, hope for restoration of self-image and function of the hand might surpass the fear of all unpleasant consequences. In order to bring a patients' expectations in order with the surgical procedure, the tedious rehabilitation, and all possible consequences, the decision for transplantation must be taken by the patient, his closest relatives, and the team of attending physicians, (plastic-hand surgeon, orthopedic-trauma and transplantation surgeon, anesthetist, specialist for physical medicine and rehabilitation, psychiatrist) [10].

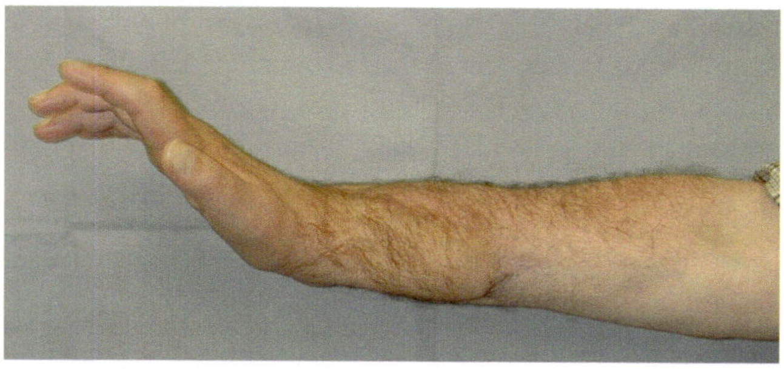

Fig. 14.1 Two years post hand allotransplantation. Notice exceptional integration of the distally based Z-flap of the transplant covering the radial part of the forearm. No sign of circular scar strangulation. (The operation was performed in March 2000, Medical University of Innsbruck, Innsbruck, Austria)

14.4 Surgical Technique

Allotransplantation has to be performed simultaneously by two teams in adjacent operating theaters, one operating on the donor and the other on the recipient [21–23].

Only perfectly coordinated simultaneous surgeries can guarantee minimal ischemia time according to the required transplantation time as well as the quantity of tissue needed and harvested for optimal functional and esthetic results. Ideally, excessive lengths of all donor structures are connected with the recipient tissue in a tension-free manner. That especially applies to the neurovascular structures. For optimal identification of the individual neurovascular structures, tendons, and muscles, both teams must operate in an anemic field, thus using a tourniquet.

Depending on the type of surgery, the number of teams may vary. In case of a bilateral hand transplantation, the ideal number of simultaneously working teams would be four to enhance chances of an optimal outcome [4, 21–24].

14.4.1 Incising the Skin

Depending on the level of amputation, skin incisions in both donor and recipient should be chosen extensively for adequate exposure of the neurovascular structures of the forearm. The section should be planned in a manner adequate for closing with z-plasties and shall never be placed directly above nerves or vessels, as swelling may prevent direct closure.

The recipients' stump can be incised above the midpalmar and the middorsal compartment allowing access to the bone and main neurovascular structures, maintaining ideal blood supply to the skin flaps, one being fed by the radial artery, the other by the ulnar. Alternatively, choosing radio-ulnar skin incisions can raise a dorsal and a palmar skin flap. For closure around the extremities, incisions on the transplanted hand or forearm have to be planned accordingly, allowing aligning skin flaps as z-plasties. Hence, if team A decides to incise in a mid-palmar and middorsal fashion on the stump, team B needs to make radio-ulnar incisions in order to enable transposition as a z-plasty. Closure in a circumferential zigzag manner is crucial to avoid constrictive circular scarring, since postoperative edema can cause remarkable reduction of available skin (Fig. 14.1).

14.4.2 Dissecting and Identifying the Neurovascular Structures and Tendon-Muscle Units

Beginning in the subcutaneous level, dissection and identification continue downward to the surface of the bone. All available vessels and nerves are easily visible at this point and are marked by using different types of sutures or plates for muscle-tendon units. In our habit, we tag each vessel with two equally long and every nerve with single-ended sutures. Microvascular clamps have proven not suitable for tagging, as they tend to slip off during subsequent manipulation and can be the cause of damage to the intima or might be forgotten in situ. Marking of each individual structure will prove to be helpful and above all timesaving when working in a bloody operating field at a later stage. After transplantation, tissues are bloodstained and the neurovascular structures are prone to be retracted into an amorphous mass of soft tissue, inducing pure frustration to the surgeon. We see no necessity in marking tendons in the transplant as they are easily identified during transplantation.

All available and functioning muscle-tendon units have to be identified and prepared for transfer according to the muscle-tendon injuries and scarring to the stump, thereby following the principles of tendon transfer in the upper extremity.

14.4.3 Hemostasis

After all available structures have been identified, prepared, and tagged, the tourniquet is released and exact hemostasis is performed in both donor and recipient sites. When accurate blood flow is restored (approximately 20 min later) at the distal flap levels of the stump and donors' fingertips, the tourniquet can be reapplied for osteotomy and final amputation of the transplant. At last, the closure of the donor site is performed in a way to later fit custom-made esthetic prosthesis.

14.4.4 Transplantation

After accurate preparation of all structures and hemostasis of the transplant are complete, the transplant is perfused with 500 mL of UW solution (University of Wisconsin solution) via the brachial artery and then can be taken off. Depending on the type of injury (clean cut, explosion, crush, or avulsion) and level of amputation (wrist or forearm), the sequence of transplantation varies slightly.

The usual sequence is the following:

- Osteosynthesis.
- Vessel anastomosis.
- Muscle-tendon suture/transfer.
- Definite vessel anastomosis.
- Nerve suture.
- Soft tissue closure.
- Dressing.

14.4.4.1 Osteosynthesis

The preferred technique of osteosynthesis is firm internal fixation since it encourages early union and joints are not immobilized promoting early functional exercising. The periosteum must be preserved while preparing and shortening the bone in order to enhance bone healing and prevent tendon adhesions. In case of bone fixation with plates, the periosteum should be sutured, usually using a 5–0 absorbable stich.

Key to all osteosynthesis is correct bone length, alignment, rotation, and angulation since subsequent re-osteotomy would cause unnecessary procedures and delayed healing.

14.4.4.2 Vessel Anastomosis

Following bone fixation, the ulnar, being the dominant hand artery, and radial arteries are prepared under microscopic vision and one of them anastomosed in an end-to-end fashion. In our preference, the ulnar artery is the first to be repaired and the clamps opened in order to have blood circulation of the transplant. Meanwhile the cephalic vein is anastomosed with the advantage of early revascularization with minimal ischemia time and easier identification of the dominant superficial veins. We found it useful to anastomose a temporary superficial vein (basilic vein) to reduce bleeding from the transplant. Moreover, venous drainage from the bulk muscle freely entering the circulation might cause considerable danger of uncontrolled acidosis resulting in reduced local perfusion. Therefore, some bleeding from the transplanted hand should occur before opening the re-anastomosed cephalic vein. We have found it beneficial providing the patients with intravenous sodium bicarbonate prior to opening of the venous anastomosis.

Early revascularization has the advantage of complete tendon-muscle repair without time pressure. Furthermore, short ischemia time is prerequisite for optimal functional recovery of all structures, especially muscles.

14.4.4.3 Muscle-Tendon Suture/Transfer

Extensor tendon repair should follow osteosynthesis and primary revascularization for gaining stability. Various suture techniques can be applied to different levels of amputation. In general, a series of interrupted figure-of-eight synthetic nonabsorbable sutures have proven sufficient. In cases of severe avulsion injuries of the recipient site with missing extensor muscles, the standard techniques of tendon transfer (i.e., pronator muscle for wrist joint extensors or flexor carpi radialis or flexor carpi ulnaris for extensor digitorum) are useful for improvement in function. To obtain adequate balance between the extensors and the flexors, it is essential to always keep the wrist extensor under sufficient tension, at least at 45°.

The flexor tendons are sutured using different techniques depending on the level of amputation, particular care given to an accurate repair for best chances of a good functional result. Stability and strength of the core suture are key for the desired early functional exercising. In case of missing flexor muscles due to explosion or avulsion injuries, several possibilities for functional tendon transfer must be taken into account.

In tendon transfer, it is crucial to always consider the synergistic muscle function among flexors and extensors and maintaining a straight direction of tendon transfer to achieve optimal functional recovery.

Adjoining tendon sutures should be placed at different proximal/distal levels in order to prevent scarring and thus adhesions (Fig. 14.2). From a top view the suture lines would be arranged in a zigzag fashion leaving a minimum of 1.5–2 cm in between each one of them. This is achieved by using different lengths of proximal/distal tendon stumps.

Once all sutures have been performed, testing of correct tension between flexor and extensor tendons is essential, restoring a natural palmar cascade from small to index finger. The tension is easily tested by passively moving the wrist checking for correct balance between flexion and extension [25] (Fig. 14.3).

Complete palmar flexion of the fingers should be achieved with the wrist in dorsiflexion and full metacarpi-phalangeal extension (not hyperextension!) with the wrist in volar flexion. Performing these two tests, we can manage exact tendon balance between digital flexors and extensors [25].

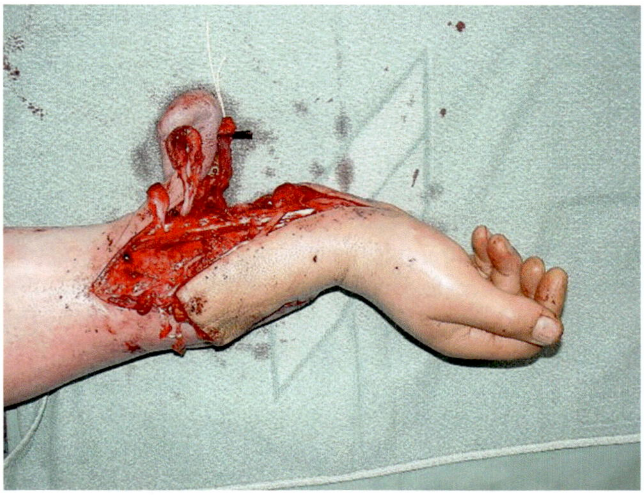

Fig. 14.2 Intraoperative view showing the position of the wrist joint and the normal digital cascade as well as the insertion of the Z-plasty flap. (The operation was performed in March 2000, Medical University of Innsbruck, Innsbruck, Austria)

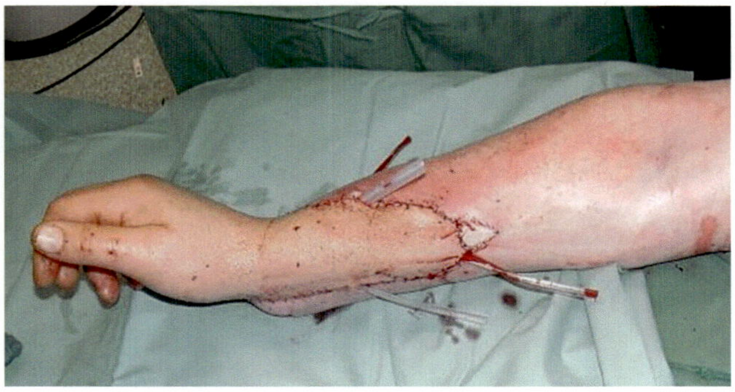

Fig. 14.3 View at the end of surgery showing great integration of the Z-plasty flap with excellent wrist joint position presenting natural balance between extensor and flexor tendons. Notice the small split thickness skin graft to avoid any tension on the suture line. (The operation was performed in March 2000, Medical University of Innsbruck, Innsbruck, Austria)

14.4.4.4 Definite Vessel Anastomosis

When optimal flexor-extensor balance is restored, final vessel repair is obtained. Primary objective is adequate vessel length preventing kinking or excess tension, in which case vessel stumps cannot be approximated by a single 9–0 nylon suture or with a double microvascular clamp. Anastomosing vessels under excessive tension with traction or oversized sutures will lead to leakage and, when uncorrected, eventually to transplant failure. Therefore, appropriate vessel length is prerequisite for a functioning anastomosis.

First, the second main artery (radial artery) is anastomosed followed by at least one vena comitantes. Then the excess length of the primary repaired ulnar artery is corrected and reanastomosed. For optimal drainage one or two deep veins (venae comitantes) have to be anastomosed as well as all other superficial veins of suitable caliber. So, if both main arteries of the hand are repaired, a minimum of four to six adequate veins (profound comitantes & superficial) must be anastomosed to guarantee maximum outflow [25].

14.4.4.5 Nerve Suture

The main forearm/hand nerves, the median, ulnar, and radial (or superficial radial nerve, depending on the amputation level) are approached and identified from the intact side of the nerve proximal of the neuroma. They are individually prepared and isolated under the microscope and separated from fibrotic tissue and the neuroma by sharp dissection. Then, far proximal to the neuroma (in particular after electric or avulsion trauma) the nerve is trimmed to its normal fascicular tissue using a no. 11 blade. The fascicles are aligned without distortion, strangulation or surplus and sutured in a tension free manner. A10–0 monofilament nylon is recommended for nerve suture; however, a larger size suture can be applied when more force is needed for accurate coaptation. The technique of nerve repair is left to the surgeon. Our preference is the suture of groups of fascicles on major forearm nerves and either fascicular or epineural repair on smaller nerves. The emphasis is less on the technique (fascicular or epineural) but on its correct execution regarding the fascicles upon completion of suturing. The number of sutures used in fascicular repair depends on the way the fascicles relate to each other after placement of each stitch (one, two or maybe three). The fewer sutures are used, the less fibrous tissue is evoked obstructing axonal sprouting and maturation.

14.4.4.6 Soft Tissue Closure

After meticulous hemostasis, the skin is loosely adapted using the skin flaps in the z-plasties in a manner as indicated above. Appling this technique is prerequisite for avoiding edema and compression with consecutive circular scar contracture. In any case, the most special attention is given to the fingertips. Any change of color, duskiness, or accelerated refill after blanching on the digital pulp must be immediately corrected by releasing tension at the corresponding skin suture.

14.4.4.7 Dressing

The suture lines are covered longitudinally (never circumferential!) with paraffin strips, followed by an excessive layer of fluffed dry gauze. Then, a plastic sponge 1–3 cm thick is wrapped around the transplanted limb extending the fingertips leaving a longitudinal gap on one side, held in place by an elastic gauze. At last a rigid splint is applied (longitudinally!) incorporating the flexed elbow with a sling beyond the length of the fingertips, from which it is suspended. Once again, the digital pulp is checked for any obstruction caused by the dressing, and finally, the splint is raised above elbow level with the sling.

14.4.5 Postoperative Care

14.4.5.1 Observation

Circulation Checks

Initially, circulation checks are performed at hourly intervals. Color, pulp turgor, capillary refill, and warmth are very useful aids in monitoring of the transplanted hands. The color of the nail bed and return of the blood after blanching must be controlled continuously.

A perfect response is accomplished with pink skin color, with refill comparable to that in an adjacent non-transplanted area.

Digital pulse monitoring, oxygen probe, and temperature monitoring using a thermocouple are also very useful tools.

14.4.5.2 Medication

Heparin is given to maintain prothrombin time at approximately 50s. It can be replaced 1 week postoperatively by oral acetylsalicylic acid (100 mg/day), which can be maintained for a long period of time [25].

14.5 Outcomes of Hand Transplantation

Hand and upper extremity transplantations are becoming more common. The goal of postoperative rehabilitation is to improve function, quality of life, and self-esteem of transplant patients [26] (Figs. 14.4, 14.5, 14.6, and 14.7).

There is currently no standardized assessment protocol to evaluate the posttransplant outcomes; the majority of the transplantation centers has developed its own [27–29].

The International Registry on Hand and Composite Tissue Transplantation (IRHCTT) [30, 31] has prospectively collected information on the most cases since 2002. Considering all other reported cases together, more than 100 known transplantations of hand/upper extremities have been performed in over 80 patients worldwide since 1998. Overall, a 22.4% total transplant loss rate has been described [6].

This has to be carefully interpreted because not all countries that perform upper extremity transplantations have the same medical standard with different peri-hospital care systems. Considering only the Western World (USA, Europe, Australia) and taking out all combined heterogeneous multi-

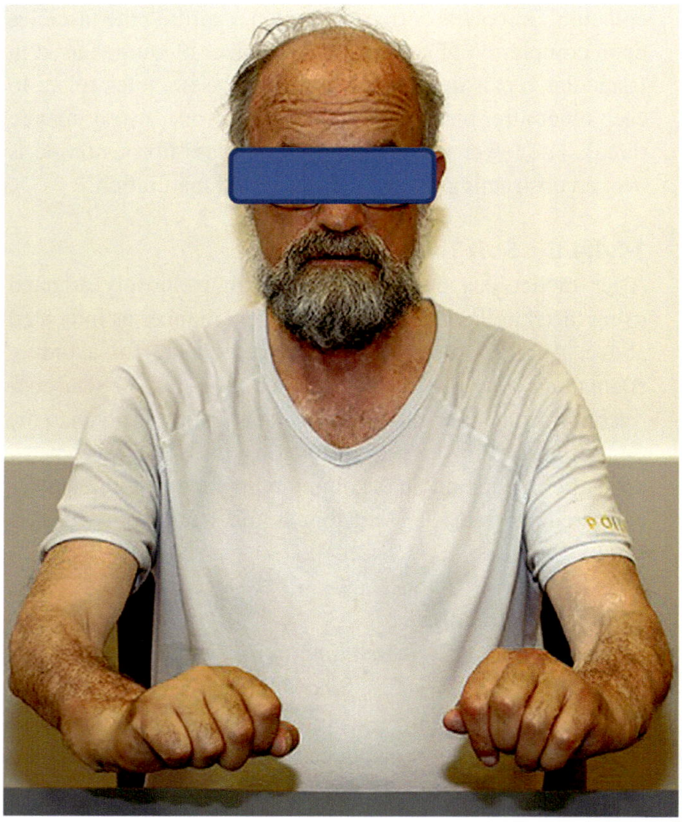
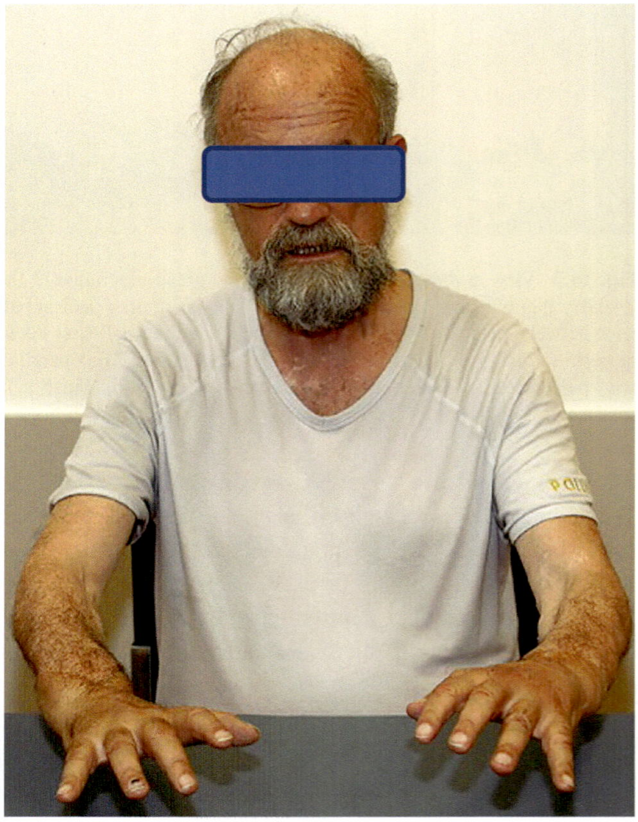

Figs. 14.4 and 14.5 Functional result 20 years after allotransplantation. Note full flexion and extension of the finger. (The operation was performed in March 2000, Medical University of Innsbruck, Innsbruck, Austria)

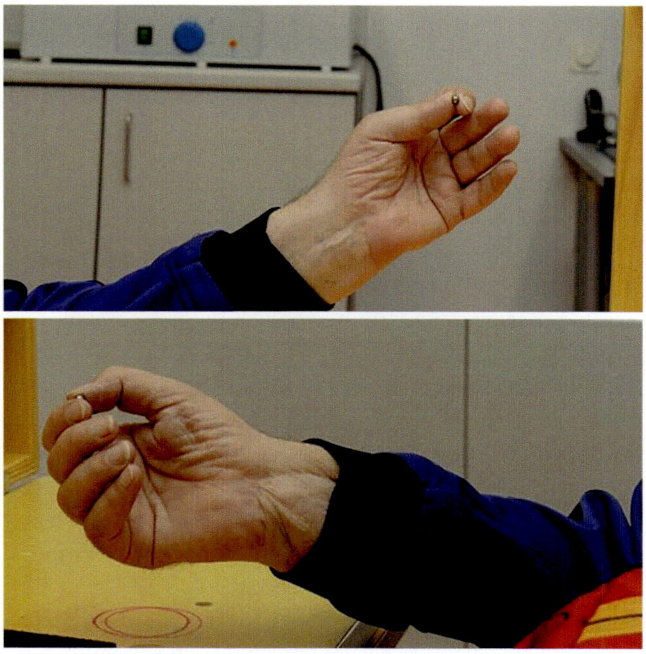

Figs. 14.6 and 14.7 Functional result 20 years after allotransplantation. Note holding of small pieces with pinch grief with left and right hand. (The operation was performed in March 2000, Medical University of Innsbruck, Innsbruck, Austria)

site transplantations (four cases), an overall graft survival rate of over 90% per limb transplanted and a 0% mortality rate in patients (50 cases) undergoing *isolated* unilateral or bilateral upper limb transplantation has been reported [6].

Functional outcomes are difficult to compare internationally since different assessment methods and scores are used by each transplantation team. Different existing score systems are being applied (i.e., the Hand Transplantation Score System from International Registry on Hand and Composite Tissue Transplantation, the Chen score for limb replantation, the Carroll score, DASH and Action Research Arm Test—ARAT [32]), but until now the Hand Transplantation Score System is the most specific established score system which takes almost all levels of upper limb transplantation into consideration. Mobility, dexterity, and strength have also been reported inconsistently. However, a significant functional improvement has been described in the majority of all transplanted patients in the posttransplant time. According to Petruzzo et al. the extrinsic and intrinsic functions recover over variable time frames depending on the level of amputation (usually 9–15 months postoperatively, confirmed by EMG if possible) [31].

Almost all patients seem to acquire at least protective sensation. Petruzzo et al. also showed that about 90% develop tactile sensibility and over 80% develop discriminative sensation [31].

In order to demonstrate sensory recovery, the Semmes-Weinstein Monofilaments test, the two-point discrimination and the modified Highet scale [33] were frequently used.

Even with the difficulties of comparison, most patients were able to perform activities of daily living and returning to an occupation. Seventy-five percent of hand-transplant recipients report improvements in quality of life [31].

In general, Shores et al. stated that patients with distal forearm transplants could expect the best absolute function, with some expectation of limited intrinsic recovery, some discriminative sensation, faster functional recovery, and more specific sensory/motor recovery. Patients undergoing mid-forearm and proximal forearm transplantation can expect limited to no intrinsic recovery, protective sensation, and possibly some discriminative sensation, weaker overall grip strength, but still substantial functional improvement from baseline [6].

Interestingly, the reported data, related to transplants above the elbow, show very encouraging results concerning the capacity of functional improvement with partially similar range of motion, better strength in replants, and better sensibility in the transplant patient [34–36]. This might be due to the greater potential of improvement since preoperative disability is typically higher than in candidate patients for extremity transplant at a more distal level.

14.6 Upper Extremity Amputations and Prosthetics

The indications for upper-extremity replantation are far from timeless, evolving with patients' needs, surgeons' skill, and technology. However, common to all cases is the critical need to identify the goal of reconstruction, which should be individually targeted to the patient's occupation, hobbies, health, and socioeconomic status. Function must remain the predominate goal, requiring restoration of skeletal stability, joint mobility, power, and sensibility. Although indications are relative to each patient, most would agree that the absolute indications for replantation are thumb amputations, multiple finger amputations, and any upper-extremity amputation in a child. The risks of a replantation procedure and the extent of the necessary postoperative treatment should reasonably relate to the expected benefit.

Upper limb prosthetics may be needed for a variety of reasons, including disease, accidents, and congenital defects. A congenital defect can create the need for a limb prosthesis when the newborn is born with a missing or damaged limb. Industrial, vehicular, and war-related accidents are the leading cause of amputations in developing areas, such as large portions of Africa. In more developed areas, such as North

America and Europe, disease is the leading cause of amputations. Cancer, infection, and circulatory disease are the leading diseases that may lead to amputation.

Despite recent significant advances in technology and medicine, the number of patients who undergo amputation of body parts for various reasons continues to increase. Assistive devices such as prosthetic arms can enable limited activities in upper limb amputees and improve their quality of life.

The limitation of daily life activities due to disability has a significant correlation with depression of the disabled. Social isolation is a serious consequence of amputation because amputees often significantly decrease social activities and avoid meeting new people. Therefore, to lower depression and relieve social isolation in people with disabilities, the development of assistive devices that enable physical activity can play a role.

Beekman and Axtell argued that amputees believe that assistive devices not only enable limited activities due to disability but also improve the quality of life, thereby lowering social isolation.

14.7 Activities of Daily Living

Disabled people have limited activities of daily living (ADL), such as bathing, dressing, and toilet use. Furthermore, instrumental activities of daily living (IADL) such as housework, hobbies, and social activities are also subject to restrictions. The daily life performance test is used to evaluate people's ability to move the body for tasks required for living, and the most used test method measures the ability to perform daily life movements. ADL is categorized into physical ADL, which includes the most basic physical activities performed in daily life, IADL, which comprise activities that are required for living such as cleaning, washing, using transportation, preparing meals, and using the phone. Such limitations and the inability to perform ADL and IADL increase depression and further deteriorate the quality of life of persons with disabilities. The level of daily life movements and instrumental daily life movements led to a lower degree of depression. Thus, disabled individuals continuously require the help of others in performing daily life movements, and if people cannot independently perform daily life movements for a long time, they may easily get depressed. This can, in turn, act as factors that negatively affect rehabilitation and treatment [37].

Consequently, active physical activities of persons with disabilities expand their talents, prove their abilities, eventually improving their quality of life. Winnick argued that the physically or psychologically limited range of activities and variables such as environment or dependence limit participation, resulting in poor physical activity participation by the disabled. It has been reported that the physical activity participation rate of people with physical disabilities is lower than that of nondisabled individuals because most of the physical activities performed by people with disabilities are passively performed [38].

14.8 Definition

In medicine, a prosthesis (plural: prostheses; from Ancient Greek *prosthesis*, "addition, application, attachment") or prosthetic implant is an artificial device that replaces a missing body part, which may be lost through trauma, disease, or a condition present at birth (congenital disorder). Prostheses are intended to restore the normal functions of the missing body part. Amputee rehabilitation is primarily coordinated by a physiatrist as part of an inter-disciplinary team consisting of physiatrists, prosthetists, nurses, physical therapists, and occupational therapists. Prostheses can be created by hand or with computer-aided design (CAD), a software interface that helps creators design and analyze the creation with computer-generated 2D and 3D graphics as well as analysis and optimization tools [39].

14.9 Types and Functions of the Upper Limb Prosthetic

In recent years, several upper-limb prosthetic devices have been proposed. Available cutting-edge prosthetic devices can be classified considering different criteria [31].

- DEKAs (DARPAs) Luke Arm.

  The Luke Arm is the latest upper arm prosthesis developed by **D**efense **A**dvanced **R**esearch **P**rojects **A**gency (DARPA), designed by Dean Kamen. Its advanced dexterity makes the Luke Arm better than the prosthetics currently on the market. In addition, high quality electronics and software allow for fine control of the arm, which will allow amputees to perform complex tasks such as plucking chocolate covered coffee beans one by one, picking up a power drill, unlocking doors, or shaking hands. The Luke Arm is modular-based, adjustable to be used by anyone with any level of amputation distal to the shoulder, elbow, or forearm.
- Proto 2.

  Proto 2 was launched as one of the phases of a 4-year DAPRA-program creating a prosthetic arm with better imitation of natural arm movement. It is built with 100 sensors that connect the natural neural signals of the body to the mechanical prosthetic arm, creating a sensory feedback loop. Thus, the prosthetic arm gives feedback in real time of the patients' interactions with objects. The user should get a feel for where the arm is in space, which object it is touching, whether that object is smooth or rough, with which force the hand is holding it, and what temperature the object has.

- Transhumeral and Elbow Prosthetic Devices.

  These are worn by amputees with elbow disarticulation or transhumeral amputations.
- Gas-Actuated Transhumeral Prosthesis.

  This is an anthropomorphic nine degree-of-actuation prosthesis arm for transhumeral amputees. The arm utilizes a monopropellant, hydrogen peroxide as a gas generator to power nine pneumatic type actuators that drive elbow, wrist, and a 17DoF compliant hand. The design makes the arm compact and integrated in elbow and wrist joints are sensors for position and force. The prosthesis is expected to approach the dexterity of an anatomical arm and is projected to deliver half of the force and power output of an average human arm. The usage of the gas-type actuators let the arm achieve better volumetric and gravimetric power density.
- Saga University Prosthetic Arm.

  The robotic prosthetic arm developed by Saga University targets to mimic the human anatomy as closely as possible. Emphasizing on forearm motion, it focuses to pronation/supination with introduction of two shafts acting as the ulnar and radial bones of the human arm.
- MSUM elbow–2.

  This prosthetic is mainly capable of providing elbow flexion and extension. In the design, gears are tied with linkages increasing the mechanical efficiency of the hand by over 80%. The prosthetic could also be integrated with other mechanisms to develop a transhumeral or shoulder prosthetic.
- Transradial and Hand Prosthetic Devices.

  There are three state-of-the-art transradial and hand prostheses worn by amputees with wrist disarticulation or transradial amputation:
  - Touch Bionics i-Limb.

    Touch Bionics i-Limb was the first commercially available prosthetic device with five individually powered digits. Its inclusion of a thumb that works like the human thumb, let the hand achieve different positions, enables important grip configurations, many of which have not been available to amputees before. The articulating fingers are able to close tightly around objects. Furthermore, built-in stall detection locks each individual finger in its position until the patient voluntarily triggers an open signal via muscle signal.
  - Under-actuated Hand Prosthesis.

    Nasser et al. proposed this hand to overcome the drawbacks of commercially available hand prostheses. Each finger is fully independent from the other and adaptable to grasp any object of any geometry. The system is capable of providing safe and reliable grasping without the need for feedback sensors, multiple servos, or any type of data processing.
  - FLUIDHAND III.

    FLUIDHAND is a prosthesis with enhanced functionality, enabled security, and adaptive grasping as well as esthetic appealing design. The combination of flexible fluidic actuators and soft passive elements reduces the required grasping force for a wide range of objects. Further, the enhanced actuator system allows high grasping forces if necessary. Two myoelectrodes in the socket together with the developed controller board and software enable quick selection of the most important grasping patterns. Vibrotactile force feedback and wireless programming as well as control options complete the characteristics of the FLUIDHAND III.

With hands, a person interacts directly with the external environment and loss of hand use has a direct impact on life situations. A prosthetic hand is a representative assistive device for people who underwent an upper limb amputation and compensates for hand function. In general, prosthetic hands refer to cosmetic hands designed only for esthetic purposes. Furthermore, body-powered hands have been developed to perform grasping movements by using the shoulder movements.

The electric-powered prosthetic hand, which was proposed to solve the problems of body-driven prostheses, was first introduced in 1954 announced as an industrial robot with versatility for repetitive work. The battery for the electric-powered prosthetic hand, which is shaped like a regular hand, was used to generate motive power. The motor-driven prosthetic arm is used as a control signal for hand movements such as grip or wrist rotation by recognizing the myoelectric signal detected from the residual muscle of the cut area, leading to the proposal of a myoelectric hand prosthesis. This muscle anterior prosthesis controller compares the mean absolute value of the muscle potential signal generated by the voluntary contraction of the user's residual muscle with a preset threshold value to determine the user's intention.

The most representative commercialized myoelectric prosthesis is the System ElectroHand (OttoBock Co., Duderstadt, Germany) and Utah ProControl (Utah Arm Co., Salt Lake City, UT, USA) [37, 39–41].

14.10 Upper Extremity Prostheses Controls and Components

Prostheses can serve a cosmetic (passive) role or a functional role, or both. The components of upper extremity prostheses consist of a socket, a suspension component, a terminal device, and an interposing joint (if applicable). Functional prostheses are further divided into two categories, body-powered (cable-controlled) or externally powered (myoelectric).

The mechanism of control is often the focal point in the prescription of a prosthetic unit.

Cable-controlled prostheses enable an amputee to harness residual body movements to generate controlled movement and force of a terminal device. Cable-operated prostheses boast improved sensory feedback through the harness system and are notably durable, but they possess a limited range of motion and limited prehensile strength [31].

An externally powered prosthesis uses electric power and can be controlled by several distinct methods: myoelectric, switch, or servo control. Myoelectric prostheses use the electric signals of residual muscle contractions to direct the movement and force of a terminal device. If the residual limb possesses measurable EMG signals, myoelectric control is considered a functionally viable option and is often used for forearm amputees. Because a prosthesis lacks sensory feedback and there are limitations with grip strength, users often prefer to pick up an object with the native hand and transfer it to the prosthetic hand. In the absence of a useable myoelectric signal, the prosthetic can be directed by switch control, a mechanism in which small switches are turned on and off by residual digits or bony prominences to operate the terminal device.

Furthermore, for higher-level amputees (e.g., transhumeral amputees) who possess limited myoelectric inputs, switch control can be coupled with limited myoelectric control (hybrid control). For instance, switch control can be used for elbow positioning as EMG signals control hand and wrist orientation. As expected, the binary (on/off) nature of switch control has functional limitations. Servo control attempts to mitigate these limitations by permitting the amputee to control the speed of the prosthetic component by one of two techniques: varying the force applied to the switch (force-activated servo) or varying the degree of movement of a harness system (position servo) [37].

Standard myoelectric control systems use either a dual-site system, in which paired electrodes can use forearm flexion and extension to control terminal device pronation and supination, or a single-site system, in which a single electrode placed on a given muscle belly elicits two opposing movements, depending on the strength of the EMG signal. Although the movements of these binary systems are restricted, a recent study demonstrated that distinct finger movements, including independent digit flexion and lateral pinch grip, can be replicated by a terminal device through control of eight bipolar electrodes on select forearm flexors and extensors of a forearm amputee [37].

The electrodes must have good soft tissue covering (skin and subcutaneous tissue) to withstand the contraction inside the socket. For transhumeral amputees who lack the distal muscle contractions needed for such control, targeted muscle reinnervation can be used. Targeted muscle reinnervation is a surgical technique that transfers residual arm nerves (i.e., median, or ulnar nerves) to alternative muscle sites (i.e., pectoralis major muscle) that are no longer biomechanically functional. These sites can then produce surface EMG signals used for myoelectric control of a terminal device.

Along with a comfortable socket and suspension system, an amputee's choice of a terminal device is integral to successful interaction with the environment. Terminal devices can be passive, primarily serving an esthetic function, or they can be active. There are several terminal devices that can be used for specialized activities, as well as more traditional, multiple-purpose terminal devices [42].

Active terminal devices are further divided into two categories: a hook terminal device (or other specialized purpose) or a prosthetic hand. Terminal devices can be designed to serve distinct functions and are considered adaptive in such cases. Although current devices enable flexion/extension and pronation/supination movements, researchers are continually refining current prostheses [43].

14.11 Indications and Appropriate Prescription

Successful rehabilitation of an upper extremity amputee and prosthetic success have been linked to distinct factors, some of which are within the control of the rehabilitations team.

Unfortunately, rejection rates of upper extremity prostheses are common and can approach 38% for more proximal amputations.

Forearm-level amputations are associated with the greatest acceptance rate, followed by transhumeral amputations, and finally by shoulder disarticulations. These acceptance rates can partially be explained by literature that links rejection and abandonment of upper extremity prostheses to increased prosthetic weight, socket discomfort, and associated pain, as well as decreased sensory feedback and lack of functionality.

To ensure an optimal prosthetic adoption, an amputee should be fit for a prosthesis within 30 days of amputation. The duration of this period is subject to changes in residuum volume due to edema, limb sensitivity, maintenance of the range of motion, and the amputee's mental status. It is imperative that the healthcare team attend to these variables to expedite the amputee's rehabilitation. The duration of this period is subject to own techniques to assist in the daily activities of life [44].

Literature research of the available level III literature indicates that replantation of the traumatically amputated arm leads to good functional outcomes and higher patient satisfaction rates than prosthetic fitting, regardless of the objectively measured functional outcome. In clinical practice this could mean that if technically possible, replantation could be the preferred option of treatment. That being said, careful patient selection and surgical common sense remain the most important parameters in choosing replantation over revision surgery and prosthetic fitting.

Upper extremity amputations are devastating and will profoundly impact the life of the affected patient. A successful amputation and reconstruction can decrease the extent of the loss. Surgical goals include removing the damaged or diseased limb, minimizing long-term complications, and preparing a limb stump that can be fitted for a prosthetic. Following surgery begins the long rehabilitation process in which the most comfortable and functional prosthetic is determined for the individual. During this process, the rehabilitation team adopts the responsibility to adequately match the patient's physiological and psychological needs to an appropriate device and make consequential strides in enabling the patient to function independently. With advancing technology, new prosthetic options will continue to be developed, thus helping to ameliorate the substantial loss associated with an upper extremity amputation.

14.12 Lessons Learned

In the future, improvements in immunosuppressive therapy may make hand transplantation a less controversial issue from an ethical standpoint.

Our expertise and experience are strengths and the technical requirements have been resolved over the years, reducing ischemia times through improvements in organization, resulting in improvement of functional long-term outcomes. Donor selection with respect to anatomical features and gender identity must become more stringent, and the age difference between donor and recipient should by no means be too great. Patients with unilateral hand amputation are not suitable for vascularized composite allotransplantation. From the beginning, the recipient must be assured of lifelong drug therapy.

The risks of life-long immunosuppressive therapy and the late effects caused by it must be reduced. By inducing donor-specific tolerance, the risk would decrease compared to the benefit of transplantation. Only innovations in immunomodulatory therapy will allow vascularized composite allotransplantation to be offered as a routine procedure in the future. Until then, the indications for this should be stricter and should only be given at selected centers; furthermore, long-term results, disadvantages, complications as well as side effects should be openly presented.

14.13 Conclusion

Motor function after hand allotransplantation is clearly superior to that of a myoelectric prosthesis; in particular, compound movements as well as fine motor control of movements are easier for the patient. Of particular importance for both patients is the regaining of bodily integrity, which had not been imparted to them by the prostheses. As a result, the ability for social interaction as well as intimate contacts has improved significantly. Overall, patients are highly satisfied with both the functional and cosmetic results. Our findings show that motor function after hand allotransplantation is slightly better than that after forearm transplantation. The achieved function after hand transplantation is >60% of a normal hand. Together with the very good sensitivity without cold intolerance, the achieved function enables patients to perform numerous activities that they could not manage with the prostheses. Not only can they perform more complex movements in everyday life, such as buttoning shirts or picking up small coins from a flat surface, but self-confidence and thus interaction with the environment improve significantly.

References

1. Malt AR, McKhann FC. Replantation of severed arms. JAMA. 1964;189:716.
2. Komatsu S, Tamai S. Successful replantation of a completely cut-off thumb. Plast Reconstr Surg. 1968;43:375.
3. Gilbert R. Transplant is successful with a cadaver forearm. Med Trib Med News. 1964;5:20–3.
4. Dubernard JM, Owen E, Herzberg G, Lanzetta M, Martin X, Kapila H, et al. Human hand allograft report on first 6 months. Lancet. 1999;17:1315–20.
5. Piza H. Händetransplantation in Innsbruck. Wien Klin Wochenschr. 2000;112:563–5.
6. Shores JT, Brandacher G, Lee WPA. Hand and upper extremity transplantation: an update of outcomes in the worldwide experience. Plast Reconstr Surg. 2015;135:351–360e.
7. Chow AJ, Bilos JZ, Chunprapaph B, et al. Forearm replantation-long-term functional result. Ann Plast Surg. 1983;10:15.
8. Kleinert EH, Jablon M, Tsai T. An overview of replantation and results of 347 replantants in 245 patients. J Trauma. 1980:20:390.
9. Petruzzo P, Revillard JP, Kanitakis J, et al. First human double hand transplantation: efficacy of a conventional immunosuppressive protocol. Clin Transpl. 2003;17(5):455–60.
10. Piza-Katzer H, Wechselberger G, Estermann D, Gabl M, Arora R, Hussl H. Ten years of hand transplantation experiment or routine? Handchir Mikrochir Plast Chir. 2009;41(4):210–6. Epub 2009 Aug 17. https://doi.org/10.1055/s-0029-1225628.
11. Kumnig M, Massey EK, Parker LS. Why quality-of-life data collection and use should be standardized when evaluating candidates for hand transplantation. AMA J Ethics. 2019;21(11):E974–9. PMID: 31742546. https://doi.org/10.1001/amajethics.2019.974.
12. Kumnig M, Jowsey SG, DiMartini AF. Psychological aspects of hand transplantation. Curr Opin Organ Transplant. 2014;19(2):188–95. PMID: 24503494. https://doi.org/10.1097/MOT.0000000000000047.

13. Li QF, Zang DS, Guan WX. Functional evaluation of electrical-injury nerve using somatosensory evoked potential technique. Zhongguo Xiu Fu Chong Jian Wai Ke Za Zhi. 2000;14:332–5.
14. Lúcio MJ, Horta R. Hand transplantation-risks and benefits. J Hand Microsurg. 2020;13(4):207–15PMID: 34776710. https://doi.org/10.1055/s-0040-1715427.eCollection.2021.
15. Lanzetta M, Nolli R, Borgonovo A, et al. Hand transplantation: ethics, immunosuppression and indications. J Hand Surg Br. 2001;26:511.
16. Cooney CM, Siotos C, Aston JW, Bello RJ, Seal SM, Cooney DS, Shores JT, Brandacher G, Lee WPA. The ethics of hand transplantation: a systemic review. J Hand Surg Am. 2018;43(1):84.e1–84.e15. Epub 2017 Oct 4. https://doi.org/10.1016/j.jhsa.2017.08.004.
17. Carty MJ, Bueno E, Lehmann LS, Pomahac B. A position paper in support of hand transplantation in the blind. Plast Reconstr Surg. 2011;128(5):510e–5e. https://doi.org/10.1097/PRS.0b013e31822b62e7.
18. Jones NF. Concerns about human hand transplantation in the 21st century. J Hand Surg. 2002;27:771–87.
19. Kverno HD, Gorantla VS, Gonzalez RN, et al. Hand transplantation a future clinical option? Acta Orthop. 2005;76:14–27.
20. Maizoub RK, Cunningham FG, Maldonado C, et al. Investigation of risk acceptance in hand transplantation. J Hand Surg. 2006;31A:296–302.
21. Piza-Katzer H, Ninkovic M, Pechlaner S, Gabl M, Ninkovic M, Hussl H. Double hand transplantation functional outcome after 18 months. J Hand Surg. 2002;27B:385–90.
22. Piza-Katzer H, Hussl H, Ninkovic M, Pechlaner S, Gabl M, Ninkovic M, Schneeberger S, Margreiter R. Beidseitige handtransplantation. Handchir Mikrochir Plast Chir. 2002;34:75–83.
23. Margreiter R, Brandacher G, Ninkovic M, Steurer W, Kreczy A, Schneeberger S. A double-hand transplant can be worth the effort. Transplantation. 2002;74:85–90.
24. Jones JW, Gruber SA, Barker JH, Breidenbach WC. Successful hand transplantation. One-year follow up. N Engl J Med. 2000;7:468–72.
25. Ninkovic M. Technical and surgical details of hand transplantation. In: Lanzetta M, Dubernand JM, Petruzzo P, editors. Hand transplantation. New York: Springer Italia; 2007. p. 197–203. ISBN: 978–88–470-0373-6 (Print) 978–88–470-0374-3.
26. Ninkovic M, Weissenbacher A, Gabl M, et al. Functional outcome after hand and forearm transplantation: what can be achieved? Hand Clin. 2011;27(4):455–65, viii-ix.
27. Bueno E, Benjamin MJ, Sisk G, Sampson CE, Carty M, Pribaz JJ, Pomahac B, Talbot SG. Rehabilitation following hand transplantation. Hand (N Y). 2014;9(1):9–15. https://doi.org/10.1007/s11552-013-9568-8.
28. Tombak K, Özkan Ö, Uysal H, Özkan Ö. An individualized physiotherapy and rehabilitation program for bilateral hand transplantations. Ann Plast Surg. 2021;86(2):217–22. https://doi.org/10.1097/SAP.0000000000002668.
29. Severance G, Walsh L. Rehabilitation after bilateral hand transplantation in the quadrimembral patient: review and recommendations. Tech Hand Up Extrem Surg. 2013;17(4):215–20. https://doi.org/10.1097/BTH.0000000000000024.
30. International registry on hand and composite tissue transplantation (IRHCTT). http://www.handregistry.com. Accessed 29 Aug 2015.
31. Petruzzo P, Lanzetta M, Dubernard JM, et al. The international registry on hand and composite tissue transplantation. Transplantation. 2010;90(12):1590–4.
32. Ninković M, Weissenbacher A, Pratschke J, Schneeberger S. Assessing the outcome of hand and forearm allotransplantation using the action research arm test. Am J Phys Med Rehabil. 2015;94(3):211–21. https://doi.org/10.1097/PHM.0000000000000151.
33. Dellon AL, Curtis RM, Edgerton MT. Reeducation of sensation in the hand after nerve injury and repair. Plast Reconstr Surg. 1974;53:297–305.
34. Schneeberger S, Landin L, Jableki J, et al. Achievements and challenges in composite tissue allotransplantation. Transpl Int. 2011;24:760–9.
35. Jablecki J, Kaczmarzyk L, Domanasiewicz A, et al. Result of arm-level upper-limb transplantation in two recipients at 19- and 30-month follow-up. Ann Transplant. 2012;17:126–32.
36. Cavadas PC, Ibanez J, Thione A, Alfaro L. Bilateral transhumeral arm transplantation: result at 2 years. Am J Transplant. 2011;11:1085–90.
37. Ju N, Lee K-H, Kim M-O, Choi Y. A user-driven approach to prosthetic upper limb development in Korea. Healthcare (Basel). 2021;9:839. https://doi.org/10.3390/healthcare9070839.
38. Yamamoto M, Chung KC, Sterbenz J, et al. Cross-sectional international multicenter study on quality of life and reasons for abandonment of upper limb prostheses. Plast Reconstr Surg Glob Open. 2019;7:e2205.
39. Wright TW, Hagen AD, Wood MB, Rochester MN. Prosthetic usage in major upper extremity amputations. J Hand Surg. 1995;20A:619–22.
40. Bieringer S, Sibbel B. Exoskelettale prothesen der oberen extremität. Orthopädie Unfallchirurgie Up2date. 2012;7:367–94.
41. Behrend C, Wayne Reizner BS, Marchessault JA, Hammert WC. Update on advances in upper extremity prosthetics. J Hand Surg. 2011;36A:1711–7.
42. Maat B, Smit G, Plettenburg D, Breedveld P. Passive prosthetic hands and tools: a literature review. Prosthet Orthot Int. 2018;42:66.
43. Aman M, Sporer ME, Gstoettner C, Prahm C, Hofer C, Mayr W, Farina D, Aszmann OC. Bionic hand as artificial organ: current status and future perspectives. Artif Organs. 2019;43(2):109–18. https://doi.org/10.1111/aor.13422.
44. Tintle SM, Baechler MF, Nanos GP 3rd, Forsberg JA, Potter BK. Traumatic and trauma-related amputations: part II: upper extremity and future directions. J Bone Jt Surg. 2010;92A:2934–45.

Hand Transplantation Program at Amrita Institute of Medical Sciences, Kochi, India: Technical Considerations (Part 1)

15

Mohit Sharma, Abhijeet Wakure, Devajyoti Guin, and G. Srilekha Reddy

15.1 Introduction

The Indian subcontinent, owing to its huge population, has a large burden of hand injuries. Despite the rapidly improving healthcare infrastructure and increased number of people accessing high-quality health care, there is a progressive accumulation of a patient pool with severely debilitating hand injuries, especially the bilateral upper limb amputees. High-end prostheses and reconstructive transplantation are the two options for such patients to enable them achieve reasonable hand function. The advantage of a prosthesis is rapid rehabilitation with minimal side effects. However, this is offset by the high cost of advanced prosthesis, need for replacement every 5–7 years, absent sensations, and hence no tactile feedback which fails to restore body image. An additional significant problem is that current prostheses are poorly compatible with water. This is especially important in the Indian context, where handling water is an essential part of living. As a result of these problems, most of our patients in India are reluctant to use prosthesis and wish for more permanent solution. The other option in such a situation is bilateral upper extremity allotransplantation, which has been one of the most important advances in plastic and reconstructive surgery over the last two decades. The presence of sensations in the transplanted hands [1] apart from varying degrees of motor recovery makes it superior to prosthesis. Till date at least 178 upper extremity transplantations have been done (ISVCA 2019 Proceedings).

In the Indian subcontinent, Amrita Institute of Medical Sciences, Kochi, Kerala started the first upper limb vascularized composite allotransplantation programme in January 2015, and since then, we have performed eight bilateral upper limb transplants. Figures 15.1, 15.2, 15.3, 15.4 and 15.5 show the pre-operative photos of our patients. We have trained plastic and reconstructive surgeons from other centres in India, who wish to make this complex procedure available to a wider section of the population, and now there are three more active VCA programmes at Chennai, Puducherry and Mumbai. Our programme is picking up pace because of greater public awareness regarding the limb donation and active efforts of transplant coordinators. We have screened more than 300 patients with upper limb amputations and approved 32 bilateral upper limb amputees for transplantation and presently 24 patients are on the waiting list.

Although many unilateral hand transplantations have been done worldwide, there is always an ethical dilemma while performing single hand transplantation, as it subjects the patient to life-long immunosuppression. The unilateral upper limb amputee is not as dependent on others for his or her daily activities as is the bilateral upper limb amputee. In case of the bilateral upper limb amputee, the risk–benefit ratio is more favourable for performing transplantation, as the person is severely incapacitated by loss of both upper limbs [2]. This is the reason why we have confined our transplant programme to bilateral amputees alone.

Our inclusion and exclusion criteria for donor as well as recipients is given in Table 15.1 [3]. This chapter discusses the donor and patient characteristics of all cases in our series. It also discusses surgical techniques of the transplants and the immediate post-operative outcomes. Immunosuppression, monitoring and rehabilitation protocols as well as long-term functional outcomes have been discussed in part 2 of this chapter.

M. Sharma (✉) D. Guin
Department of Plastic and Reconstructive Surgery, Amrita Hospital, Faridabad, Haryana, India
e-mail: mohitsharma@fbd.amrita.edu

A. Wakure
Department of Plastic and Reconstructive Surgery, VPS Lakeshore Hospital and Research center, Kochi, Kerala, India

G. Srilekha Reddy
Department of Plastic and Reconstructive Surgery, Amrita Institute of Medical Sciences, Kochi, Kerala, India

© Springer Nature Switzerland AG 2023
R. Gurunian et al. (eds.), *Reconstructive Transplantation*, https://doi.org/10.1007/978-3-031-21520-9_15

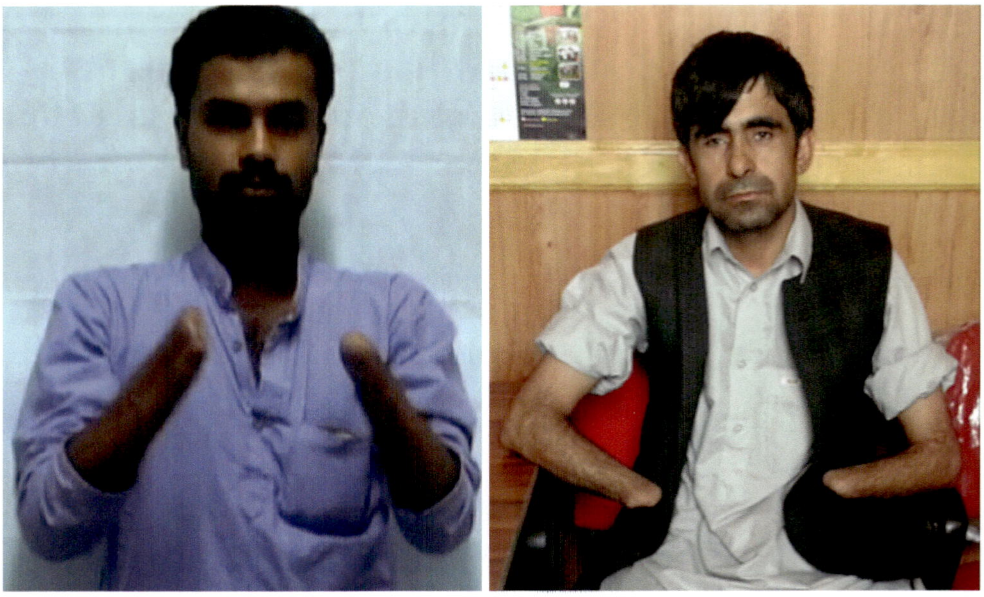

Fig. 15.1 Patient 1 (left) and patient 2 (right)

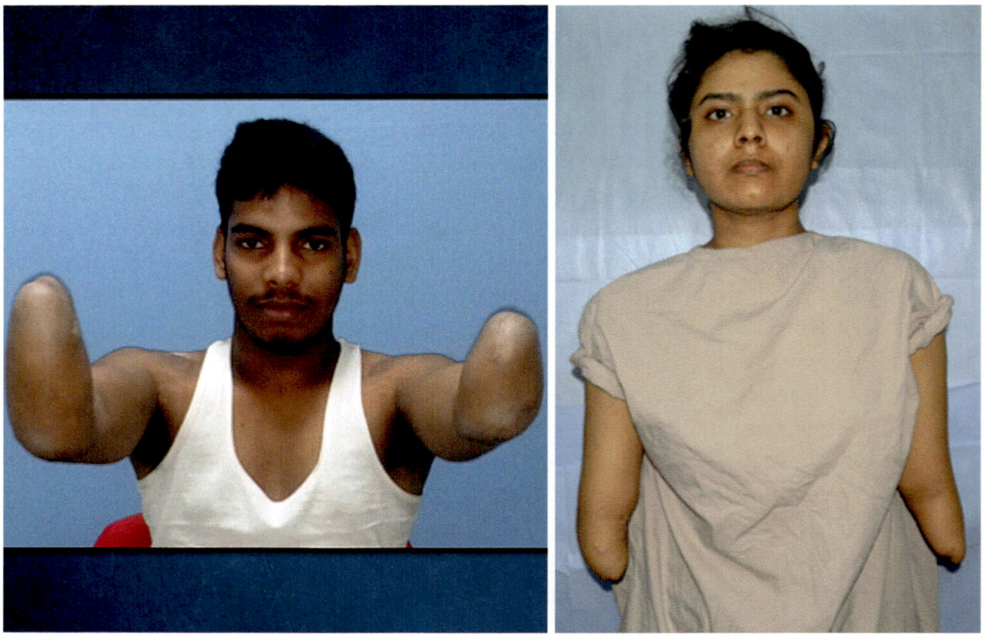

Fig. 15.2 Patient 3 (left) and patient 4 (right)

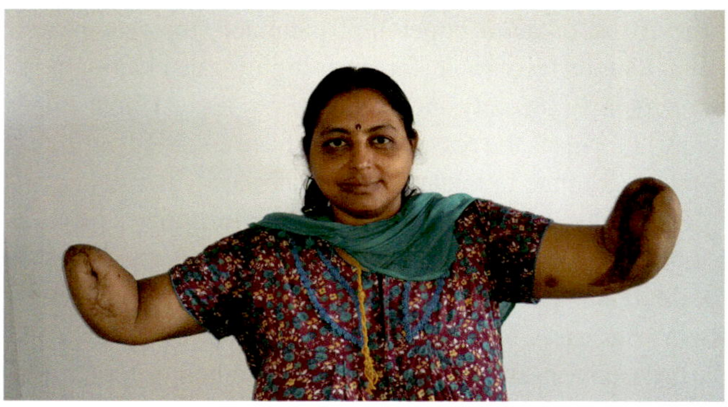

Fig. 15.3 Patient 5

15.2 Case Series

The pre-operative evaluations of all the recipients and donors are summarized in Table 15.2. The surgical details of all patients and their hands including ischemia times are provided in Table 15.3. The donor and recipient characteristics are described as follows.

Case 1

Donor: The donor was a 24-year-old male who was brain dead due to motor accident-related traumatic brain injury. The donor was admitted in the same institute as the recipient.

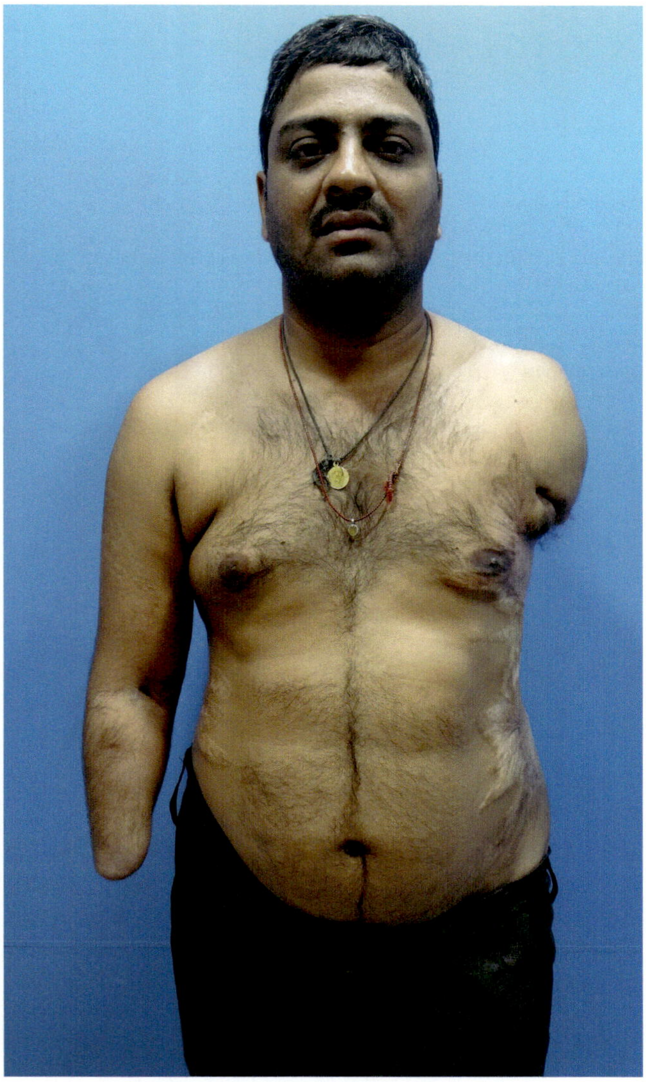

Fig. 15.4 Patient 6

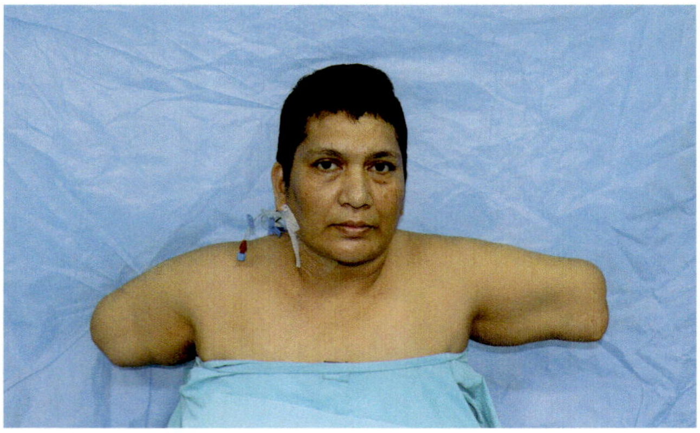

Fig. 15.5 Patient 7

Graft procurement and recipient surgery happened in adjacent operating rooms. Both hand grafts were normal.

Recipient: The recipient was a 30-year-old male. He had lost his hands in a train accident 1.5 years before the surgery. He was thrown off a running train by antisocial elements. Both the hands were amputated at the distal forearm level. The transplantation was done at distal forearm level. The right hand had all motor and sensory stumps intact. The left hand had only the motor stumps available of tendons of palmaris longus (PL), flexor digitorum superficialis (FDS), brachioradialis (BR), abductor pollicis longus (APL), and extensor digitorum communis (EDC). Hence, tendon transfers were done for this patient as described—PL to APL; FDS (1) to FPL (flexor pollicis longus); FDS (2, 3, and 4), to FDP (flexor digitorum profundus) (1, 2, 3, 4); APL to ECRB (extensor carpi radialis brevis); EDC to EDC; BR to EPL (extensor pollicis longus). His right-hand graft had an acute skin flap necrosis within 12 h of surgery and was managed by debridement and free anterolateral flap cover on post-operative day 2. Subsequently there were no surgery-related short-term or long-term complications. He has the longest follow-up of 5 years and 8 months.

Case 2

Donor: The donor was a 52-year-old male who was brain dead due to motor accident-related traumatic brain injury. The donor was admitted in the same institute as the recipient. Graft procurement and recipient surgery happened in adjacent operating rooms. Both hand grafts were normal.

Recipient: The recipient was a 31-year-old male. He had lost his hands in an explosion while attempting to defuse a mine during army operations in Afghanistan 2.5 years before the surgery. Both the hands were amputated at the distal forearm level. Both the hands had all motor and sensory stumps intact. The transplantation was done at distal forearm level. Immediate post-operative period was uneventful. He has the longest follow-up of 5 years. He died 5 years after his transplant in a terrorist attack in Afghanistan.

Case 3

Donor: The donor was a 29-year-old male who was brain dead due to traumatic head injury sustained in a road traffic accident. The donor was admitted in an institute 30 km away. Graft procurement was done in the donor's institute and was transferred to our institute for preparation and transplantation. Both hand grafts were normal.

Recipient: The recipient was a 24-year-old male. He had lost his hands due to electrocution 1.5 years before the surgery. Both the hands were amputated at the mid-forearm

Table 15.1 Inclusion and exclusion criteria

Donor		Recipient	
Inclusion criteria	Exclusion criteria	Inclusion criteria	Exclusion criteria
Essential			
Documented brain death	Age < 18 years or > 60 years	Age 18–60 years	Unilateral hand amputee with no major functional impairment
Hemodynamic stability	Congenital/traumatic upper extremity deformities	Bilateral upper limb amputee	Brachial plexus injuries
Blood group matching	Connective tissue disorders	Psychologically stable to manage the transplant post-operatively	Congenital or syndromic hand deformities
Favorable lymphocyte crossmatch	Peripheral neuropathy	Financial stability	Pediatric traumatic amputees
	Cancer	Social and family support	Severe medical co-morbidities including malignancy
	Non-correctible acute traumatic injuries		Non-correctable acute traumatic injuries
	HIV, hepatitis B or hepatitis C infection/carrier		HIV, hepatitis B, hepatitis C
Desirable			
Same gender			
Same race			
Body habitus			
Skin tone			
Negative CMV/EBV screening			

level. All structures at this level were intact. He had transplantation done at proximal forearm level. Immediate post-operative period was uneventful. He has the longest follow-up of 4 years and 4 months.

Case 4

Donor: The donor was a 20-year-old male who was brain dead due to traumatic brain injury. The donor was admitted in an institute 35 km away. Graft procurement was done in the donor's institute and was transferred to our institute for preparation and transplantation. The donor radial arteries were cannulated for arterial lines.

Recipient: The recipient was a 19-year-old female who had lost her hands in a road traffic accident 1 year back. Both the hands were amputated at the proximal forearm level. All structures at this level were intact. She underwent a supracondylar level upper limb transplantation. Due to cannulation of radial artery, the radial arterial pulse was not flowing at the right side in the post-operative period. Hence she was started on intravenous prostaglandin E1 infusion. After 24 h the radial artery pulsations returned back to normal. After that the post-operative period was uneventful. She has had a longest follow-up period of 3 years and 2 months.

Case 5

Donor: The donor was a 29-year-old male who was brain dead due to traumatic brain injury. The donor was admitted in the same institute as the recipient. Graft procurement and recipient surgery happened in adjacent operating rooms. Both hand grafts were normal.

Recipient: The recipient was a 46-year-old diabetic female. She had lost her hands due to electrocution 2 years back. Both the hands were amputated at the mid forearm level. All structures at this level were intact. She had transplantation done at proximal forearm level. Immediate post-operative period was uneventful. Her longest follow-up is for 2 years and 5 months.

Case 6

Donor: The donor was a 65-year-old female who was brain dead after a massive stroke. She was admitted in an institution in another city which was more than 500 km away. Radial artery cannulation had been done on the right side. Grafts were harvested by the surgical team and were flown down to the parent institution by air. Logistical problems caused delay in transfer of the grafts hence the delay in ischemia time (given in the Table 15.3). On arrival to the parent institute, both grafts were perfused with cardiopulmonary bypass machine with human blood, and as the grafts were being perfused, graft preparation was done. Blood was recirculated back through the cardiopulmonary bypass machine while monitoring metabolic parameters. Transplantation proceeded once recipient and donor preparation was completed.

Recipient: The recipient was a 35-year-old male who had lost his hands due to electrical burns 10 years back. The left hand was amputated at the proximal arm level, and the right hand was amputated at the mid forearm level. Transplants were done at the proximal arm level for the left side and at the proximal forearm level for the right side. Due to differ-

Table 15.2 Donor and recipient characteristics

Cases	Case 1		Case 2		Case 3		Case 4		Case 5		Case 6		Case 7		Case 8	
Donor/recipient	Donor	Recipient	Donor	Recipient	Donor	Recipient	Donor	Recipient	Donor	Recipient	Donor	Recipient	Donor	Recipient	Donor	Recipient
Age	24	30	52	31	24	21	20	19	29	46	65	35	39	52	27	23
Sex	Male	Male	Male	Male	Male	Male	Male	Female	Male	Female	Female	Male	Male	Female	Male	Male
Type of trauma	Road traffic accident	Train accident	Road traffic accident	Land mine explosion	Road traffic accident	Electrical burns	Road traffic accident	Road traffic accident	Road traffic accident	Electrical burns	Cerebro-vascular accident	Electrical burns	Cerebro-vascular accident	Assault	Road traffic accident	Blast injury
Nationality	Indian	Indian	Indian	Afghan	Indian	Indian	Indian	Indian	Indian	Indian	Indian	Indian	Indian	Malaysian	Indian	Yemen
Blood type	A+	A+	O+	O+	B+	B+	A+	A+	B+	B+	B+	B+	O+	O+	O+	O+
Cytomegalovirus	Positive	Not done	Not done	Negative	Not done	Negative	Negative	Positive	Not done	Negative	Not done	Negative	Negative	Negative	Negative	Negative
Rubella	Not done	Not done	Not done	Not done	Not done	Negative	Positive	Positive	Not done	Negative	Not done	Negative	Negative	Negative	Negative	Negative
Toxoplasmosis	Not done	Not done	Not done	Not done	Not done	Negative	Negative	Negative	Not done	Negative	Not done	Negative	Negative	Negative	Negative	Negative
Epstein-Barr virus	Not done	Not done	Not done	Not done	Not done	Negative	Positive	Positive	Not done	negative	Not done	Negative	Negative	Positive	Negative	Negative
Lymphocyte cross-match	Favourable (<10%)		Favourable (<10%)		Favourable (<10%)		Favourable (<10%)		Favourable (<10%)		Favourable (<10%)		Favourable (<10%)		Favourable (<10%)	
Panel reactive antibody	Not done		Not done		Negative for class 1 and 2		Negative for class 1 and 2		Negative for class 1 and 2		Negative for class 1 and 2		Negative for class 1 and 2		Negative for class 1 and 2	
Human leucocyte antigen	Complete mismatch (0/6)		Complete mismatch (0/6)		Only done for recipient		Only done for recipient		Only done for recipient		Only done for recipient		Only done for recipient		Only done for recipient	
Donor specific antibody	Not done		Not done		Negative		Negative		Negative		Negative		Negative		Negative	

Table 15.3 Recipient surgical characteristics

	Patient 1		Patient 2		Patient 3		Patient 4		Patient 5		Patient 6		Patient 7		Patient 8	
	Left hand	Right hand	Left hand	Right hand	Left hand	Right hand	Left hand	Right hand	Left hand	Right hand	Left hand	Right hand	Left hand	Right hand	Left hand	Right hand
Date of surgery	1/13/2015		4/9/2015		5/25/2016		8/9/2017		4/3/2018		7/1/2019		7/18/2020		7/21/2020	
Time since amputation	1 and half years		2 and half years		1 and half years		1 year		2 years		10 years		6 years		3 years	
Warm ischemia time (min)	24	20	15	28	10	15	10	10	15	20	10	12	46	48	13	14
Cold ischemia time (min)	340	320	330	317	510	440	320	320	500	520	No perfusion	2040	280	320	542	403
Level of amputation	Distal forearm	Distal forearm	Distal forearm	Distal forearm	Mid forearm	Mid forearm	Proximal forearm	Proximal forearm	Mid forearm	Mid forearm	Proximal arm	Mid forearm	Mid arm	Mid arm	Mid forearm	Mid forearm
Level of transplantation	Distal forearm	Distal forearm	Distal forearm	Distal forearm	Proximal forearm	Proximal forearm	Supracondylar	Supracondylar	Proximal forearm	Proximal forearm	Proximal arm	Proximal forearm	Mid arm	Mid arm	Proximal forearm	Proximal forearm
Total time for surgery (h)	17		15		18		14		16		17		18		14	

ence in the sex and age of the recipient and donor, there was a gross mismatch between the donor and recipient upper limb. Ischemia times were also prolonged on both sides due to logistic issues of transport from different city (see Table 15.3).

On the left side, due to the size mismatch, vessel length fell short after osteo-synthesis and had to be bridged by using brachial artery vascular grafts harvested from the discarded portion of the donor right upper limb. The muscles of the arm and forearm did not perfuse despite vascular flow being established and hence a brachial artery to radial artery bypass graft was performed. There was adequate venous return but the muscles did not perfuse. After 24 h the graft was ischemic and gangrenous and was removed after tagging all structures in the native stump for future transplantation. This failure was attributed to a no flow phenomenon due to prolonged ischemia of large muscle mass.

On the right side, hand perfusion (as noted by peripheral pulses and signals on the pulse-oximeter from fingers) happened after 24 h. At 48 h gangrene of the tips of right index and thumb was noted. This could have been due to embolic shower from the radial artery cannulation site. Hence the patient lost the distal phalanx of the index finger and tip of thumb.

Case 7

Donor: The donor was a 39-year-old male who was brain dead due to haemorrhagic stroke secondary to accelerated hypertension. The donor was admitted in the same institute as the recipient. Graft procurement and recipient surgery happened in adjacent operating rooms. Both hand grafts were normal.

Recipient: The recipient was a 52-year-old female who had lost her hands due to assault by a sharp weapon 6 years back. Both the hands were amputated at the distal forearm level. She underwent a proximal forearm level transplantation.

During surgery, both brachial arteries thrombosed immediately after anastomosis. Hence the anastomosis was revised, and she was put on full dose of intravenous heparin. She developed a haematoma on the right side at the anastomotic site twice on the second post-operative day which were evacuated. She developed arterial bleed near the left humerus (recipient site) which again necessitated hematoma evacuation and control of the arterial bleeder. During this period she developed gram-negative sepsis. On the fifth post-operative day, she succumbed to gram-negative sepsis.

Case 8

Donor: The donor was a 27-year-old male who was brain dead due to road traffic accident. The donor was admitted in a hospital in a different city more than 200 km away. The grafts were harvested at the donor's institute and brought to our institute by aircraft. Graft preparation and recipient surgery happened in adjacent operating rooms. Both hand grafts were normal.

Recipient: The recipient was a 23-year-old male. He had lost his hands due to blast injury 3 years back. Both the hands were amputated at the mid-forearm level. He underwent a proximal forearm level transplantation on both sides. There were no immediate post-operative complications. He has had a follow-up of 2 months.

15.3 Surgical Technique

Surgical technique was standardized for all patients preoperatively and also tailored to the specific defects in the patient's amputation stumps. The warm and cold ischemia times have been mentioned in Table 15.3. All limbs were harvested in brain-dead donors before the harvest of other solid organs. We will describe the general technique according to the level of hand transplantation. Specific changes to the technique (according to the recipient limb characteristics) have been mentioned in the case series above.

15.3.1 Distal Forearm Level Hand Transplantation

15.3.1.1 Donor Hand Retrieval and Preparation

For distal forearm level transplantation, the donor upper limb was harvested through a fish-mouth incision given below the elbow. The brachial artery was cannulated for infusion after ligation proximally. Cephalic and basilic veins were identified and divided. The limbs were harvested by disarticulating through the elbow joint and perfusion was done with 1 L University of Wisconsin solution. The returning fluid velocity was noted in the superficial and deep veins to note the dominant venous system and prioritize the venous anastomosis. Wounds were closed and the prostheses attached to the amputated stumps. The limbs were placed in a tray with ice slush while avoiding direct contact with the skin and then were transferred for preparation.

Skin flaps were raised with excess length on the donor forearms through mid-axial incisions on the extensor and flexor aspect. Additional carpal tunnel release was done to avoid post-operative compression neuropathy. The skin flaps were raised preserving the skin perforators of the distal forearm on both the ulnar and radial aspects. The skin flaps raised on the donor and recipient limbs interdigitate to accommodate the post-operative oedema, to avoid constriction and scar contracture at the site of closure. The superficial veins and nerves were dissected off the skin flaps till some distance by incising the fascia over them. This step is important to ensure straight line anastomosis, avoid linking of the anasto-

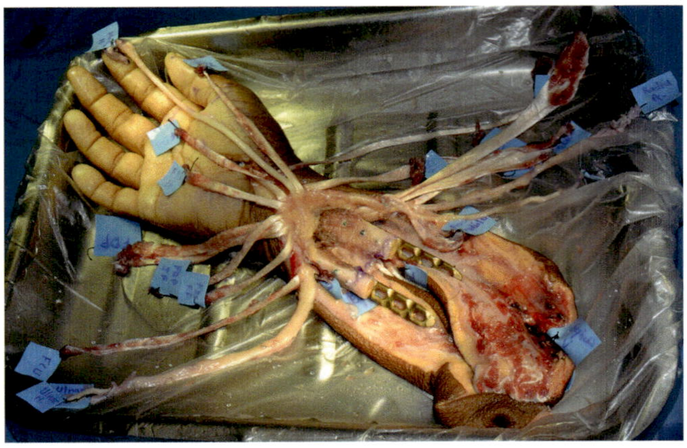

Fig. 15.6 Distal hand transplant—donor preparation

mosis and to be able to trim off excess skin flap as required. All the structures were dissected, identified and tagged at the ends. Most of the muscles were excised leaving behind only the tendinous part for repair. Aggressive periosteal stripping was avoided, and the bones were plated with 3.5 mm locking compression plates (Fig. 15.6).

15.3.1.2 Recipient Limb Preparation and Transplantation

Superficial veins were marked on the skin. Mid lateral incisions were given, and the skin flaps were raised on dorsal and volar aspects. The superficial veins and nerves were dissected off the skin for some distance by incising the fascia (for reasons described earlier). All the available musculotendinous units and neurovascular structures were identified, tagged and the missing structures noted. The final plan of anastomosis was made based on the availability of structures in the donor and recipient limbs. The sequence of repair was bone, one artery, one venae comitantes, one superficial vein, all extensor tendons, all flexor tendons, another artery, venae comitantes, superficial veins, all the nerves and skin.

Bone length was planned such that it would be maintained equal in both forearms appropriate to the patient's height. This is easily done by preoperatively measuring the bone length of an individual, who has a similar height with the recipient. Once this is done the existing bone length of the recipient is noted and the donor bone length could be extrapolated from that. At least 5 cm length was maintained in the donor bones to enable adequate plating. A 3.5 mm locking compression plate was used for osteosynthesis for each bone with three holes on each side of the bone (Fig. 15.7). In our programme, we have used both the volar and dorsal plating over the distal radius and ulna and have found no difference in the function.

Vascular anastomosis proceeded in the above-mentioned sequence using microsurgical techniques. Ulnar artery anastomosis was preferentially done earlier to avoid problems related to radial artery cannulation in the donor limbs. Tendons were reconstructed using Pulvertaft weave method. The tension in the extensor tendon repair was such that with wrist in 20° flexion, full extension of fingers was achieved. The tension in the Flexor tendon repair was such that normally graded cascade of finger flexion was achieved (Fig. 15.8). When the normal cascade is achieved, each finger is passively fully extended to ensure that there is no weakness in the repair [4]. Nerve repairs were done with epineural sutures after matching the nerve fascicles and was further reinforced with Fibrin tissue glue. Skin closure was achieved by inter-digitating the flaps on donor and recipient limbs as described earlier [5].

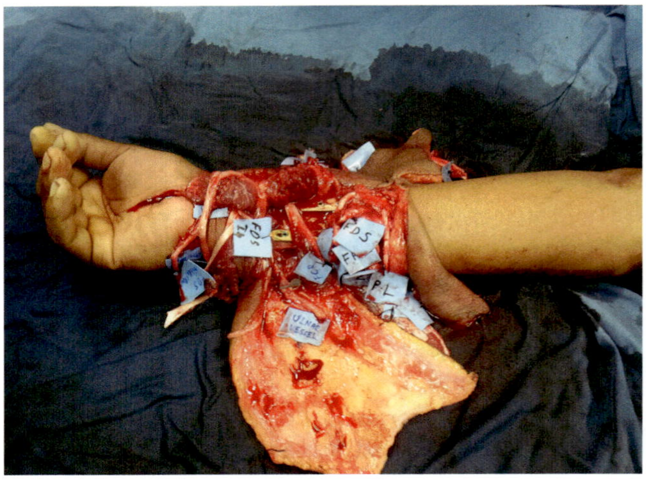

Fig. 15.7 Distal hand transplant after osteosynthesis

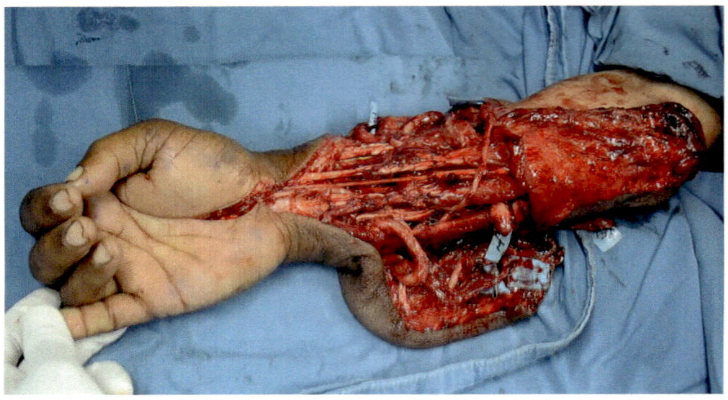

Fig. 15.8 Distal hand transplant after vascular and tendon repairs

15.3.2 Proximal Forearm Level Hand Transplantation

15.3.2.1 Donor Hand Retrieval and Preparation

Donor limbs were harvested by a circumferential incision at the mid-arm level. The superficial veins were clipped proximally, muscles and nerves were transected and humerus osteotomy was done at this level. Brachial artery was ligated proximally, divided and perfused with 1 L University of Wisconsin solution. The returning fluid velocity was noted in the superficial and deep veins to note the dominant venous system and prioritize the venous anastomosis. Wounds were closed and prostheses were attached to the amputated stumps. The limbs were placed in a tray with ice slush while avoiding direct contact with the skin and then were transferred to the bench for preparation.

Incisions were taken on mid-flexor and mid-extensor aspects from distal arm to mid-forearm level. Medial and lateral skin flaps were elevated so as to interdigitate with the volar and dorsal skin flaps of the recipient limb. Cephalic vein, basilic vein, medial antebrachial cutaneous nerve, and lateral antebrachial cutaneous nerve were dissected off the skin for some distance (allowing straight line closure, avoiding kink and allowing trimming of skin flaps as necessary). Ulnar nerve was dissected from proximal to distal until the origin of the branch to the flexor carpi ulnaris. The median nerve was dissected until the origin of the branch to pronator teres. The radial nerve was dissected and branches to the brachioradialis, extensor carpi radialis longus, extensor carpi radialis brevis were identified, tagged and transected at their origin from the radial nerve. The superficial and deep branches of the radial nerve were separately tagged. The brachial artery and vena comitantes were freed up to the division of radial and ulnar vessels. The flexor and extensor origins were detached from their origins along with the periosteum of medial and lateral epicondyles. This provides strong tissue for holding sutures while fixing them to the recipient bone. All structures were tagged to ensure easy identification during repair.

All muscles, nerves and vessels were gently mobilized en bloc by elevation in the sub-periosteal plane over the radius and ulna. After detaching the common flexor and extensor origin, an incision was given at the ulnar border and subperiosteal dissection was done in the medial and lateral direction. This makes it easy to reflect the forearm muscle mass. All the muscles attached to radius and ulna were reflected distally, taking special care to preserve the deep branch of the radial nerve. Some portion of the interosseous membrane may be split proximally to prevent the damage to posterior interosseous vessels during the distal flipping of muscle mass. Muscles raised off the bone in this way get reattached to the bone after some time and function normally after re-innervation. In the proximal forearm level transplantation as the donor limb length is recreated, it is easy to ascertain the length of bone to be discarded.

The donor and recipient limbs were brought together in an elbow-flexed position, and both the olecranon processes were matched on a flat surface and the exact length of radius and ulna present in the recipient was marked and discarded in the donor (Fig. 15.9). Sub-periosteal elevation of muscles (described earlier) continues to a level such that three holes of the LCDCP (limited contact dynamic compression plate) can be accommodated beyond the point of osteotomy.

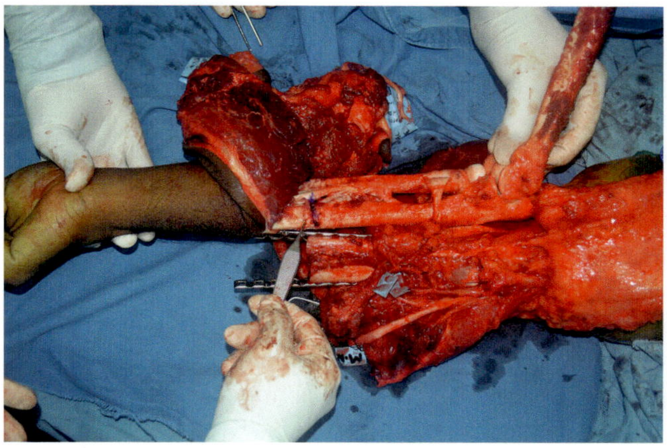

Fig. 15.9 Osteotomy site for proximal forearm hand transplantation

15.3.2.2 Recipient Limb Preparation and Transplantation

Volar and dorsal skin flaps were raised at subfascial level using mid lateral incisions. The superficial veins and nerves were dissected for some distance by incising the fascia (for reasons described earlier) and tagged. Native flexor and extensor muscle mass was left in situ. Median, ulnar and radial nerves were dissected till the most distal healthy nerve segment was seen; all neuromas were excised. Radial nerve branches to the ECRL, ECRB and BR were dissected and cut close to the point of muscle entry so that it could be later coapted to the donor ECRL, ECRB and BR branches. Superficial branch and deep branch were dissected separately for separate anastomosis. Ulnar nerve was transposed anteriorly to shorten recovery time and avoid stretch-induced neuropathy. The brachial artery and vena comitantes were dissected till the bifurcation of radial and ulnar arteries and divided here. The radius and ulna were exposed by reflecting the muscle mass. The upper limit of dissection was just distal to the radial tuberosity. The osteopenic bone was removed from the free ends, while the periosteum was reflected and preserved. Length was maintained adequate to accommodate three holes of LCDCP distal to the radial tuberosity. After contouring the plate according to the curvature of the radius and Ulna, it was fixed dorsolaterally on the radius, and it was fixed dorsomedially on the ulna. Contouring the plates is important to maintain normal anatomical gap between the radius and ulna thus facilitating normal supination and pronation on recovery of function. Close communication between the four teams preparing the donor and recipient limb bones is essential to maintain equal limb length on both sides.

Bicipital tuberosity was used as a guide for the correct orientation (it faces medially in full supination) at the time of osteosynthesis. Osteosynthesis was performed with screws traversing both the cortices, and the reflected periosteal flaps were kept back on the bone to facilitate union of the bones by promoting neo-osteogenesis. Brachial artery was anastomosed end to end using microsurgical technique followed by the dominant vein (which would have been noted earlier). The deep branch of radial nerve was anastomosed first because it becomes very difficult to anastomose the deep branch once the extensor origin is fixed as it gets buried within the extensor origin. Next, the common extensor origin was fixed to the lateral epicondyle with no. 1 polypropylene suture passed through holes drilled in the bone and multiple passes were made in the thick periosteum harvested along with the common origin.

The donor BR, ECRL and ECRB were overlapped over the partially debulked native BR, ECRL and ECRB respectively, and sutured with 3–0 polyglactin sutures. Thereafter the respective radial nerve branches were anastomosed to these muscle branches. The common flexor origin was fixed to the medial epicondyle in a similar fashion to the extensor origin. The median nerve, ulnar nerve, medial and lateral cutaneous nerves of the forearm were anastomosed to their counterparts in the donor limb using epineural sutures after matching their fascicles and this was reinforced by fibrin glue. The cephalic and basilic veins were repaired with microsurgical technique. Finally skin flaps were interdigitated and sutured together to accommodate the post-operative oedema, to avoid constriction and scar contracture at the site of closure (Fig. 15.10) [6].

15.3.3 Supra-Condylar Level Hand Transplantation

15.3.3.1 Donor Hand Retrieval and Preparation

The limbs were harvested using the same technique as described for the proximal forearm level transplantation.

Incisions were taken on mid-flexor and mid-extensor aspects from distal arm to mid-forearm level. Medial and lateral skin flaps were elevated to a short distance to interdigitate with the volar and dorsal skin flaps of the recipient limb. Cephalic vein, basilic vein, medial antebrachial cutaneous nerve and lateral antebrachial cutaneous nerve were dissected off the skin for some distance (allowing straight line anastomosis, avoiding kink and allowing trimming of skin flaps as necessary). The tendinous insertions of biceps brachii, brachialis and triceps were identified after removing all muscle mass. Brachial artery and its vena comitantes were dissected and freed for 2–3 cm in the distal arm. Radial nerve was dissected and branches to the ECRL, ECRB, BR, superficial branch and the posterior interosseous nerve were all prepared for separate anastomosis. Median nerve and ulnar nerve were dissected and prepared for anastomosis just proximal to the elbow. All structures were tagged to ensure easy identification during repair (Fig. 15.11).

15.3.3.2 Recipient Limb Preparation and Transplantation

Mid-lateral skin incisions were used to raise anterior and posterior skin flaps at subfascial level up to the mid-arm. Basilic vein, cephalic vein, medial and lateral antebrachial nerves were dissected for some distance after incising the fascia (for reasons described earlier). Radial, median and ulnar nerves were dissected from the arm from the stump till the distal arm level. The radial nerve branches were individually dissected from proximal to distal (branches to the muscles ECRL, ECRB and BR; the superficial branch and the deep branch). Presence of neuromas was noted, and healthy nerve was prepared for anastomosis. Biceps, triceps and brachialis muscles were dissected along with their tendinous insertions. The brachial artery and veins comitantes were dissected, and distal most healthy segment was mobilized for 2–3 cm. All structures were tagged to ensure easy identifica-

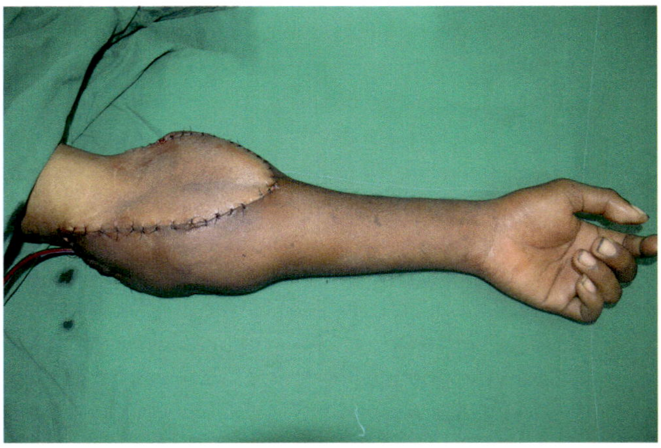

Fig. 15.10 Proximal forearm hand transplantation

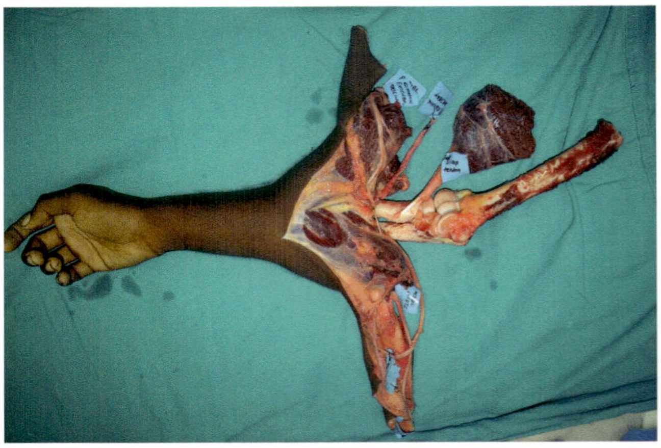

Fig. 15.11 Donor preparation for supracondylar hand transplant

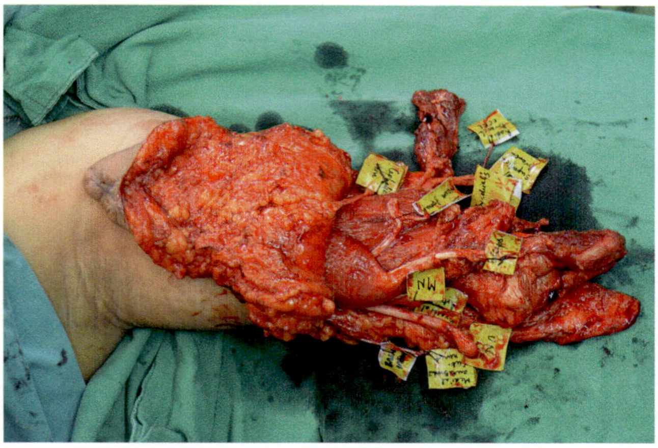

Fig. 15.12 Recipient dissection in supracondylar hand transplant

tion during repair (Fig. 15.12). Humerus was exposed circumferentially. A 4.5 mm LCDCP was used for osteo-synthesis. Osteotomy of the humerus was planned such that four holes of the LCDCP can be accommodated on either side of the osteotomy.

Length of the discarded lower end of the humerus was noted; and similar length was preserved on the lower end of the donor humerus (Fig. 15.13). Osteo-synthesis proceeded with 4.5 mm LCDCP with four holes on donor and recipient humerus each after aligning the plate along the lateral edge of the humerus shaft and along the lateral supra-condylar ridge (Fig. 15.14) [7]. This step ensures that at least one cortex is aligned properly since there is always a mismatch between the thickness of donor and recipient bones. The site of osteo-synthesis was covered with a 4 cm proximally based periosteal flap that was preserved while recipient limb preparation. The three muscles (biceps, brachialis and triceps) were then repaired using the Pulvertaft weave method keeping the elbow flexed at 90°. Excess tendon was used to reinforce the repair by folding onto itself. This was done before the vascular anastomosis to prevent disturbing the anastomosis later. Brachial artery and the dominant vein (noted earlier) were anastomosed next using microsurgical technique and the clamps were opened for limb perfusion. Brachioradialis muscle was sutured either to its counterpart or to the humerus directly depending upon availability. Other veins were anastomosed to their counterparts. The radial nerve branches were anastomosed individually; median and ulnar nerves were anastomosed by matching the fascicles. Finally, the medial and lateral antebrachial nerves were repaired. All nerve repairs were done with epineural sutures reinforced by fibrin tissue glue. Skin closure was achieved by inter-digitating the flaps on donor and recipient limbs as described earlier to accommodate the post-operative oedema, to avoid constriction and scar contracture at the site of closure (Fig. 15.15) [8].

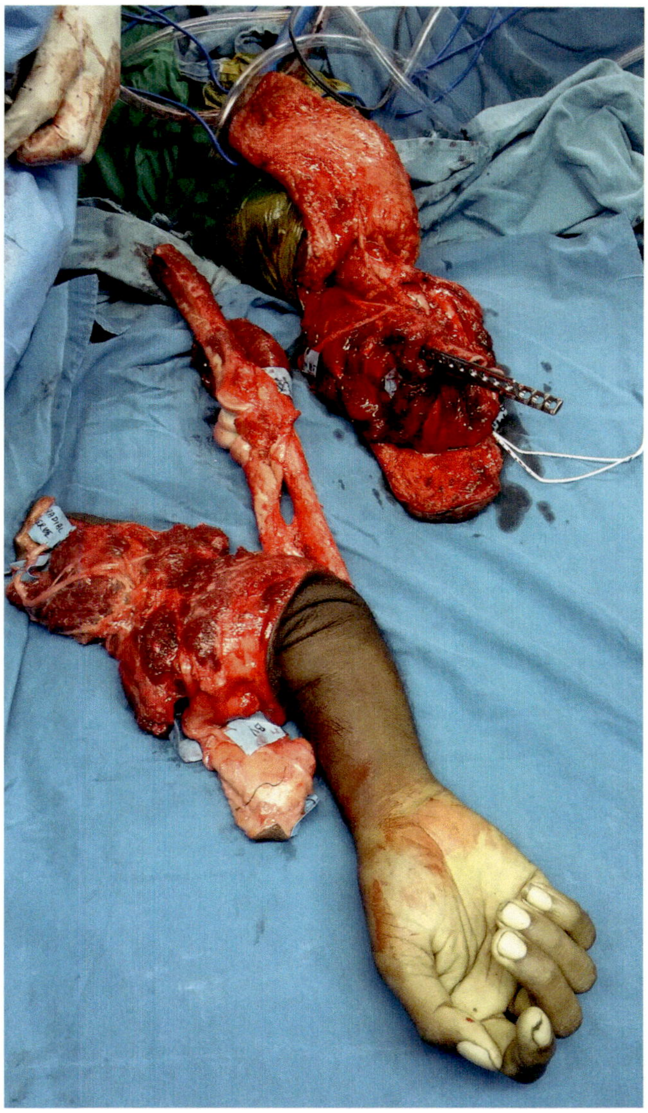

Fig. 15.13 Osteotomy site for supracondylar hand transplantation

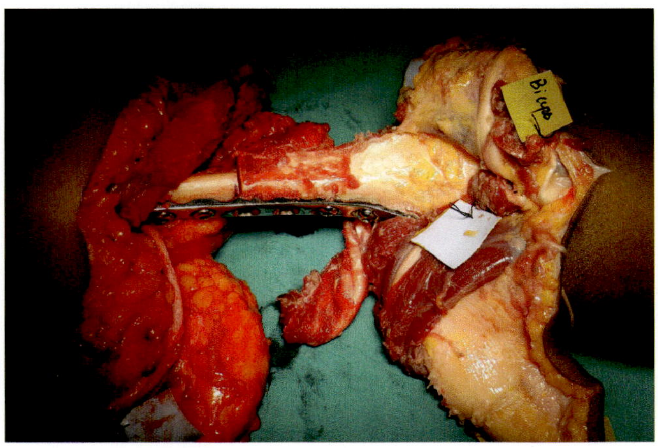

Fig. 15.14 Supracondylar hand transplant after osteosynthesis

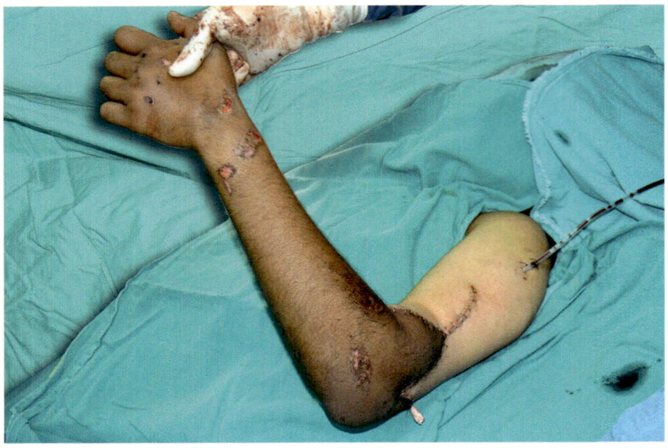

Fig. 15.15 Supracondylar hand transplant at the end of surgery

15.3.4 Mid-Arm Level

Mid-arm level hand transplant was performed similar to the supracondylar hand transplant described above. In this patient, although the bone was amputated at the mid arm level, adequate length of innervated muscle mass of biceps, brachialis and triceps was available for pulvertaft weave of the biceps brachialis and triceps tendons in the donor limb. The additional step was to harvest tendo-achilles from the donor to reinforce the tendon repairs of the major muscles.

15.4 Conclusion

Bilateral hand transplantation is a technically demanding surgery involving multiple teams and long operating hours. It is almost always undertaken as an emergency procedure whenever a donor is available. At the same time, every recipient would have peculiar defects in their amputation stump. It is therefore essential to have a surgical protocol ready for every level of amputation and also specific for every patient. Every member of the team needs to be thoroughly prepared with the surgical protocol for every patient. For successful execution of such complex procedures, the team also needs to perform mock cadaveric surgical dissections specific to the requirement of each amputation stump.

The chapter Part 1 has outlined our surgical plans and the reasoning behind the plans for different levels of upper limb allotransplantation. Part 2 will highlight the other important issues in upper limb allotransplantation, i.e. immunosuppression and rehabilitation. It also deals with the complications we encountered and the outcomes of our patients.

References

1. Landin L, Bonastre J, Casado-Sanchez C, et al. Outcomes with respect to disabilities of the upper limb after hand allograft transplantation: a systematic review. Transpl Int. 2012;25(4):424–32.
2. Petruzzo P, Lanzetta M, Dubernard JM, et al. The International Registry on hand and composite tissue transplantation. Transplantation. 2010;90(12):1590–4.
3. Iyer S, Sharma M, Kishore P, et al. First two bilateral hand transplantations in India (part 1): from vision to reality. Indian J Plast Surg. 2017;50(2):148–52.
4. Azari KK, Imbriglia JE, Goitz RJ, et al. Technical aspects of the recipient operation in hand transplantation. J Reconstr Microsurg. 2012;28(1):27–34.
5. Sharma M, Iyer S, Kishore P, et al. First two bilateral hand transplantations in India (part 2): technical details. Indian J Plast Surg. 2017;50(2):153–60.
6. Sharma M, Iyer S, Purushottaman K, et al. Indian subcontinent's first proximal forearm level double upper extremity transplantation. Indian J Plast Surg. 2019;52(3):277–84.
7. Shores JT, Higgins JP, Lee WP. Above-elbow (supracondylar) arm transplantation: clinical considerations and surgical technique. Tech Hand Up Extrem Surg. 2013;17(4):221–7.
8. Sharma M, Iyer S, Purushottaman K, et al. Indian subcontinent's first bilateral supracondylar level upper limb transplantation. Indian J Plast Surg. 2019;52(3):285–95.

Hand Transplantation Program at Amrita Institute of Medical Sciences, Kochi, India: Postsurgical Management, Outcomes, and Special Considerations (Part 2)

16

Mohit Sharma, Devajyoti Guin, Abhijeet Wakure, and G. Srilekha Reddy

"Faith is of no avail in absence of strength. Faith and strength, both are essential to accomplish any great work"

—***Sardar Vallabhbhai Patel***, *the Iron Man of India.*

The outcome of hand transplantation greatly depends on the dedicated and tenacious postoperative management and long-term follow-up. Several factors ranging from immediate to late postoperative management, immunosuppression therapy, regular monitoring and management of rejections, physiotherapy, and finally rehabilitation play equally important roles.

In this chapter, in addition to the above, we have discussed the unique problems and challenges we encountered at various stages of management of our first eight hand transplant recipients.

16.1 Immunosuppression

Immunosuppression was given as induction therapy, maintenance therapy, and for managing acute rejection.

16.1.1 Induction Therapy

Immediately after confirmation of a favorable lymphocyte cross-match of less than 10%, the recipient was started on an induction immune-suppression regimen (Table 16.1).

Table 16.1 Induction therapy regimen

Intraoperative (before vascular clamp release)	• Injection methylprednisolone IV 500 mg stat
Day 0 (immediate postoperative period)	• Injection thymoglobulin IV at 1.5 mg/kg stat • Injection methylprednisolone IV 250 mg stat • Capsule tacrolimus at 0.1 mg/kg in two divided doses (8 a.m. and 8 p.m.) • Tablet mycophenolate mofetil 1000 mg twice daily (8 am and 8 pm)
Day 1 onwards	• Injection thymoglobulin IV at 1.5 mg/kg × 3 days • Tablet prednisolone at 0.5 mg/kg/day × 5 days • Capsule tacrolimus at 0.1 mg/kg in two divided doses (8 a.m. and 8 p.m.) × 5 days • Tablet mycophenolate mofetil 1000 mg twice daily (8 am and 8 pm) × 5 days

M. Sharma (✉) · D. Guin
Department of Plastic and Reconstructive Surgery, Amrita Hospital, Faridabad, Haryana, India
e-mail: mohitsharma@fbd.amrita.edu

A. Wakure
Department of Plastic and Reconstructive Surgery, VPS Lakeshore Hospital and Research center, Kochi, Kerala, India

G. Srilekha Reddy
Department of Plastic and Reconstructive Surgery, Amrita Institute of Medical Sciences, Kochi, Kerala, India

© Springer Nature Switzerland AG 2023
R. Gurunian et al. (eds.), *Reconstructive Transplantation*, https://doi.org/10.1007/978-3-031-21520-9_16

16.1.2 Maintenance Therapy

Maintenance therapy with a triple-drug regimen was initiated after 5 days:

- Tablet prednisolone at 0.5 mg/kg/day.
- Capsule tacrolimus dose adjusted according to serum tacrolimus levels.
- Tablet mycophenolate mofetil 1000 mg twice daily (8 a.m. and 8 p.m.).

Some units prefer to wean their patients off the steroids at an early stage. Each unit performing CTA (composite tissue allotransplantation) has its protocols for immunosuppressive therapy, which usually mirrors the protocols used for solid-organ transplantation.

16.2 Monitoring Protocol

Monitoring was carried out by serial skin biopsies (using a 4 mm punch). Skin biopsies were carried out:

- Once a week for the first 3 months.
- Once in 2 weeks for the next 3 months.
- Once a month for the next 6 months.

In the eventuality of any suspicious lesions or skin changes, skin biopsy would be taken from the suspicious areas and assessed as per the Banff criteria [1] (Table 16.2).

Monitoring was carried out by skin biopsies using a 4-mm punch every week for the first 3 months, every 2 weeks for 6 months, and monthly thereafter up to 1 year. Any time after the first year, on suspicion of any rejection episode, skin biopsy was performed and the assessment was done using the Banff criteria. The presence of edema, skin blistering, scaling, erythema, hair weakness or loss, dermatitis, and papules of the allograft indicated possible graft rejection.

Systemic levels of tacrolimus were to be assayed weekly for the first 6 weeks; every alternate week for the next 6 weeks and then monthly. Tacrolimus assay was also repeated in the eventuality of suspicion of any rejection episodes. The target tacrolimus level was 5–10 ng/dL.

Table 16.2 Banff allograft rejection scale

Grade	Microscopic findings
Grade 0	None—rare inflammatory infiltrates
Grade 1	Mild—mild perivascular lymphocytic and eosinophilic infiltrates. No involvement of the overlying epidermis
Grade 2	Moderate—moderate to severe perivascular inflammation with or without mild epidermal and/or adnexal involvement
Grade 3	Severe—dense inflammation and epidermal involvement with epithelial apoptosis dyskeratosis and/or keratinolysis
Grade 4	Necrotising acute rejection—necrosis of single keratinocytes and focal dermal–epidermal separation

The common complications of immunosuppression were opportunistic infections. Other systemic complications included diabetes, hypertension, dyslipidemia, and chronic renal failure. There was also a definite risk of malignancies—lymphoma and skin carcinomas being the reported ones till date.

We, like most transplant programs, incorporated prophylactic antimicrobial therapy and surveillance for metabolic disorders and malignancies. The prophylactic antimicrobial therapy for *Cytomegalovirus* was Valganciclovir 900 mg/day for 6 months and for *Pneumocystis carinii* was Cotrimoxazole 400 mg/day for 6 months.

16.3 Rehabilitation Protocol

16.3.1 Distal-Level Transplants

The patients were given intense physical and occupational therapy for 5 h a day for 1 year. This was done in two sessions of 2.5 h each day. In the first 2 weeks, the aim was to prevent hand swelling, prevent joint stiffness, and promote tendon gliding. This was achieved by hand elevation and by passively extending the fingers with wrist flexion and by passively flexing the fingers with wrist extension. Controlled active motion of fingers and wrist was encouraged from the second postoperative day onwards. At other times, the hand was immobilized in a wrist extension splint.

Third week onwards, in addition to the above, activities of daily living like eating and drinking were begun gradually. The splint was changed to a dynamic splint during the day and a static splint during the night to maintain the hands in a functional position (Fig. 16.1a, b). The aim to be achieved by the end of the first month was a near-normal passive and active range of motion of the wrist and fingers. This was observed in both the patients.

In the second and third month, in addition to the above, passive stretching of the joints was started to prevent adhesion formation and joint stiffness. Full nonresistive use of the hands was permitted, and care was taken to protect the insensate hand from inadvertent injury.

Neuromuscular stimulation of the small muscles of the hand was started. Fourth month onwards, resistance training was started to improve the grip strength of the hands. At 6 months, attention was given to sensory re-education and fine motor coordination. Occupational rehabilitation was started at this time [2].

During the entire rehabilitation program, attention was given to functional rehabilitation of the hands. To ensure this, various activities were incorporated starting from simple ones like throwing and catching a ball, tearing bits of paper, opening and closing lids of bottles. Later on, this moved over to more complex ones like origami, playing the keyboard, sketching, and painting. These helped to make the rehabilitation process more interesting (Fig. 16.2) [3].

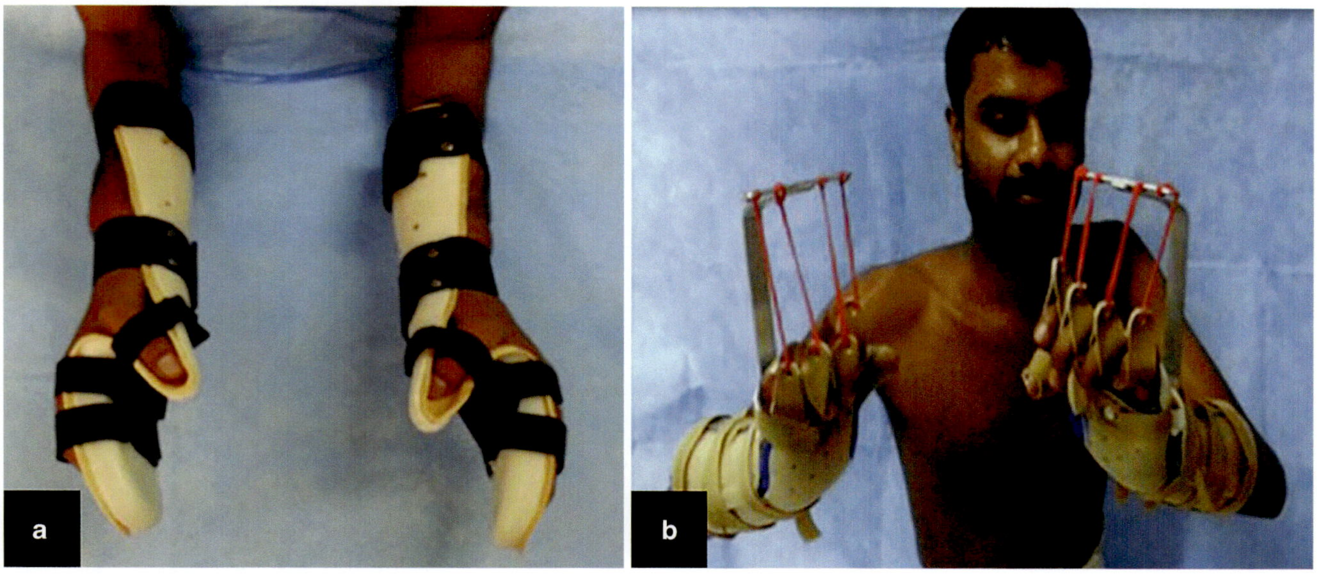

Fig. 16.1 (**a**) Static splint, (**b**) dynamic splint

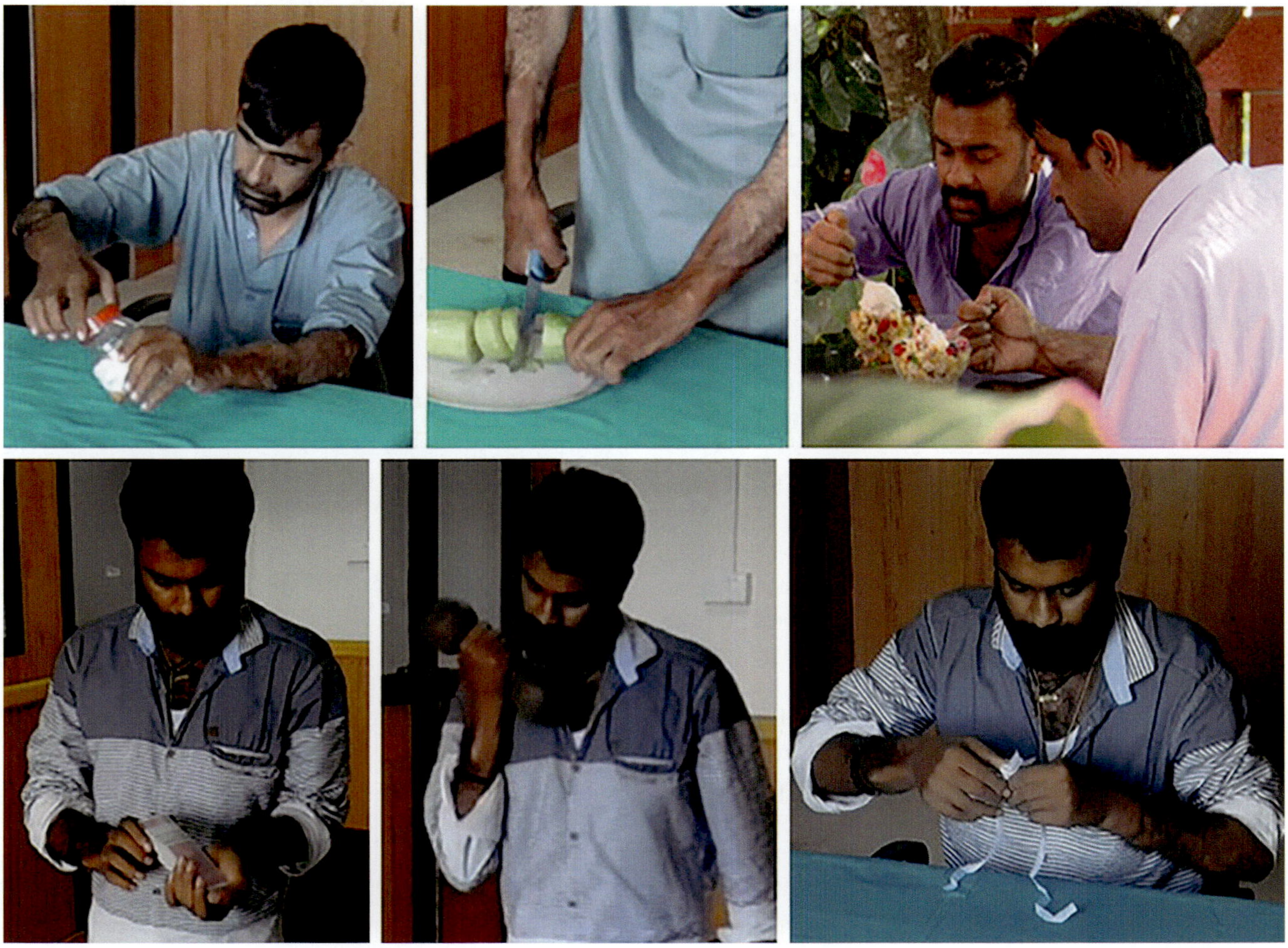

Fig. 16.2 Recipients 1 and 2 (bilateral distal forearm level transplant)—functional rehabilitation at 1 year

16.3.2 Proximal-Level Transplants

In these replants, the rehabilitation period was longer than in a distal-level transplant. The forearm and hand were flaccid in the postoperative period and usually, the first muscles to recover were the brachioradialis and long flexors at around 2–3 months.

The patient was mobilized early by third postoperative day, using a specially devised walker trolley with a supportive splint for hands.

Passive range of motion exercises was initiated in the second week with wrist flexion and extension. Active elbow mobilization began at 2–3 weeks. The limbs were maintained with wrist extension splints in a sling. In the second month, knuckle-bender splints are used to prevent clawing.

Galvanic stimulation, a square biphasic current of high strength that comes in intervals, was initiated for long flexors by the second month and long extensors by 4 months. Intrinsics were given stimulation at 6 months. Initially, the lowest strength that could initiate contraction was used. This current was delivered by placing a pen electrode over the muscle belly for not more than 30 seconds. All the relevant muscles were sequentially stimulated. In our experience recovery of intrinsic activity has been very good in the younger patients.

Active range of movement was encouraged after the second month. Once long flexors and extensors recovered, the rehabilitation was carried out with incorporation of activities of daily living (ADL).

As intrinsic recovery and active movements improved progressively, difficult tasks were incorporated into the physiotherapy as in the case of distal forearm transplants.

16.3.3 Supracondylar-Level Transplants

In supracondylar level transplants, the recipient biceps were anchored to the donor forearm, hence elbow flexion power was intact. The repair was allowed to heal for 2 weeks during which time the elbow and forearm were maintained in elevation with the wrist and hand splinted in the functional position. Ambulation was facilitated after postoperative day 3 with the help of a specialized walker to support the upper limbs. After 2 weeks active flexion and extension were allowed and passive stretching exercises were initiated. Resistive training and strengthening exercises were started after 3 months. Recovery of minimal flexor and extensor activity was anticipated by that time and rehabilitation followed similar principles as for the proximal forearm level transplants with the incorporation of galvanic stimulation, active range of motion exercises, ADLs, and occupational therapy [4].

16.4 Outcome Assessment

This was done every 6 months. The hand function was assessed by some definitive measurable parameters as follows:

1. The passive and active range of motion for the forearm (supination/pronation), wrist and fingers (flexion/extension).
2. Motor outcomes using the Kapandji score [4] for opposition (thenar intrinsic muscle and recovery), the grip dynamometer for strength, and the Medical research council (MRC) muscle power grading system [5] (Fig. 16.3).
3. Sensory recovery outcomes using the static 2-point discrimination (2PD), Semmes Weinstein monofilament (SWM) test [6] (Fig. 16.4), presence of pain and temperature, and assessment of stereognosis.

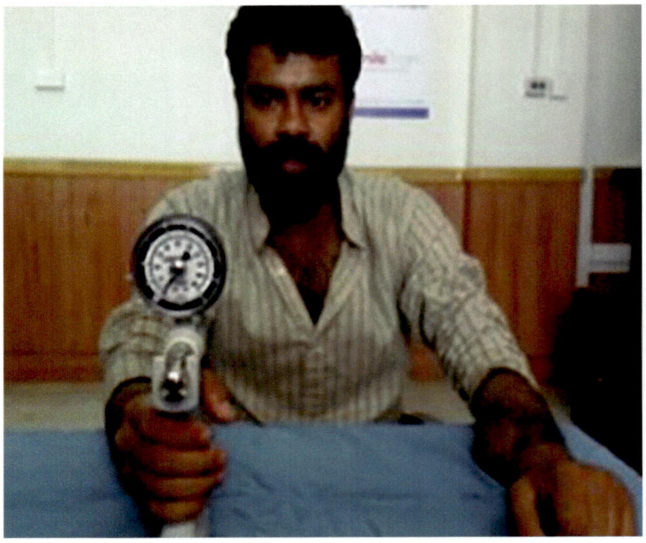

Fig. 16.3 Strength testing with a dynamometer at 1 year

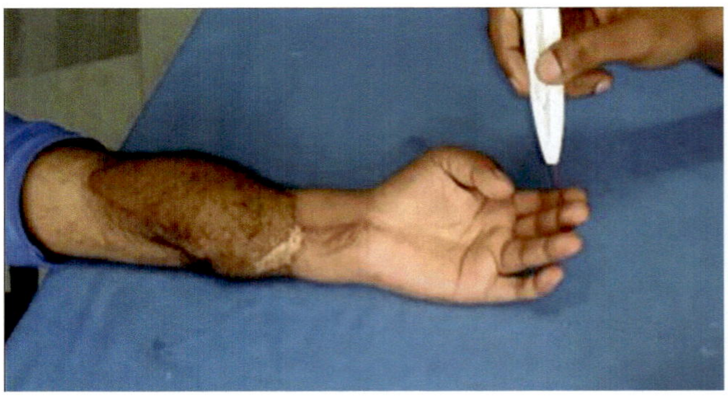

Fig. 16.4 Monofilament testing

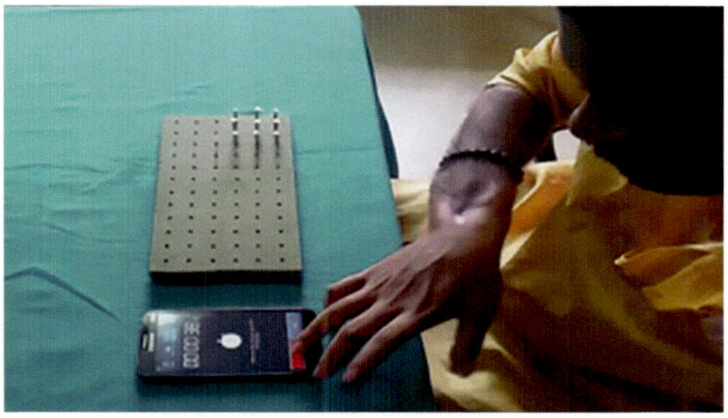

Fig. 16.5 Nine-hole peg test

4. Dexterity assessment test (Fig. 16.5).
5. The patient-reported outcome measures (PROMs) analyzed using the Disability of Arm Shoulder and Hand (DASH) score [7].
6. HTSS (hand transplantation score system) score [8] analysis at 1 year.

We used a questionnaire incorporating the above (Table 16.3). Besides, cortical reintegration of the transplanted hands was assessed by doing functional magnetic resonance imaging (MRI).

16.4.1 Functional Outcomes

The functional outcomes of our first six-hand transplant recipients have been discussed in detail in Table 16.4.

Functional MRI (fMRI) done as a part of the functional evaluation showed good cortical reintegration with right motor task showing activations in motor and premotor cortex of left frontal lobe and vice versa.

Reestablishment of lymphatic flow after transplant. Though no special consideration is given to surgically match lymphatic channels, we have not observed lymphedema following hand transplantation. On examination with ICG (Indocyanine green) lymphangiography and near-infrared imaging, all our hand transplant patients who completed 1-year posttransplant, it was found that axiality of flow is maintained, and lymphatic drainage is restored across the graft host interface (Fig. 16.6).

16.4.2 Immunological Outcomes

The transplant recipients are monitored closely and regularly to look for any rejection and when detected, are managed promptly. The details of the rejections in our first six recipients are mentioned in Table 16.5.

Table 16.3 Parameters used for functional assessment of transplanted upper limbs

1.	Range of motion										
a.	Passive										
PROM		Right					Left				
Elbow											
Forearm	Supination										
	Pronation										
Wrist	Flexion										
	Extension										
		Right					Left				
Hand		T	IF	MF	RF	LF	T	IF	MF	RF	LF
MCP											
PIP											
DIP		x					x				
b.	Active										
PROM		Right					Left				
Elbow											
Forearm	Supination										
	Pronation										
Wrist	Flexion										
	Extension										
		Right					Left				
Hand		T	IF	MF	RF	LF	T	IF	MF	RF	LF
MCP											
PIP											
DIP		x					x				

2. Strength

a. MRC

	Right	Left
Biceps		
Triceps		
BR		
ECRB/L		
FCR/		
FDS/P		
Intrinsic (ADM)		

(continued)

Table 16.3 (continued)

b. Dynamometer

	Right	Left
Grip		
Pinch		
Small		
Medium		
Large		

c. Kapandji score:

Left hand

Right hand

3. Sensation

	Right	Left
Pain		
Temperature (hot/cold)		
2-point discrimination	Dynamic-, mm Static—mm	Dynamic-, mm Static—mm
SWM[a]		
Stereognosis		

[a]Green=normal sensations; Blue=reduced tactile sensation; Purple=reduced protective sensation; Red=loss of protective sensation; Orange=deep pressure sensation only

4. Dexterity–9 Hole Peg test:

5. DASH score

Pre-op	1 Year	2 Year

6. HTSS:
(0-30=poor, 31-60=fair, 61-80=good, 81-100=excellent)

**Green* normal sensations, *Blue* reduced tactile sensation, *Purple* reduced protective sensation, *Red* loss of protective sensation, *Orange* deep pressure sensation only

SWM semmes weinstein monofilament, *DASH* disabilities of the arm, shoulder, and hand, *HTTS* hand transplantation score system, *MRC* medical research council for muscle strength

Table 16.4 Functional outcome for the first 6 recipients

	Motor	Sensory	DASH	HTSS
1 (at 5 years)	Passive and active ROM: good	Pain, temperature—very good	Preoperative: 91.7	Left: 74.5
	MRC grade: proximal 4–5 and distal 3–4 in both hands (ECRB weaker MRC 4 in left side)	Stereognosis achieved: large and small objects	1 year postoperative: 13.3	Right: 89
	Kapandji score: right 10, left 7	Mean static 2PD: 11 mm in both hands		
	Grip strength: right 20 kg, left 5 kg	SWM test: right hand—purple, left—red		

Table 16.4 (continued)

	Motor	Sensory	DASH	HTSS
2	Passive and active ROM: Good	Pain, temperature—very good	Preoperative: 86	Left: 81
(at 5 years)	MRC grade: proximal 4–5 and distal 3–4 in both hands	Stereognosis achieved: large and medium-sized objects	1 year postoperative: 9.1	Right: 84.5
	Kapandji score: right 4, left 3	Mean static 2PD: right 8 mm, left 6 mm		
	Grip strength: right 18 kg, left 10 kg	SWM test: purple in both hands		
3	Passive and active ROM: good	Pain, temperature—perceptible	Preoperative: 85	Left: 81
(at 1.5 year)	MRC grade: proximal 5 and distal 3–4 in both hands	Stereognosis not achieved	1 year postoperative: 6.6	Right: 82
	Kapandji score: right 4, left 3	Mean static 2PD: right 20 mm, left 18 mm		
	Grip strength: right 2.5 kg, left 5 kg	SWM test: right—purple left—purple		
4	Passive and active rom: good	Pain, temperature—very good	Preoperative: 69	Left:77
(at 2 years)	MRC grade: proximal 4–5 and distal 4 in both hands	Stereognosis achieved for small objects	1 year postoperative: 34	Right: 70.5
	Kapandji score: right 0, left 5	Mean static 2PD: right 4 mm, left 2 mm		
	Grip strength: right 5 kg, left 1 kg	SWM test: right—purple, left—purple		
5	Passive and active ROM: satisfactory	Pain, temperature—present	Preoperative: 90	Left: 60
(at 1 year)	MRC grade: proximal 4–5 and distal 3–4 in both hands	Stereognosis not achieved	1 year postoperative: 48	Right: 65
	Kapandji score: right 4, left 3	Mean static 2PD: right 18 mm, left 20 mm		
	Grip strength: right 4 kg, left 3 kg	SWM test: red in both hands		
6	Passive and active ROM: satisfactory	Pain, temperature—Present	Preoperative: 62.5	Left (explanted)
	MRC grade: proximal 5 and distal 4 in both hands	Stereognosis achieved: Nil	1 year postoperative: 40	Right: 51
	Kapandji score: 1	Mean static 2PD: right >5 cm, left >5 cm		
	Grip strength: right 0.5 kg, left 0.5 kg	SWM test: purple		

SWM semmes weinstein monofilament, *MRC* medical research council for muscle strength, *ROM* range of motion

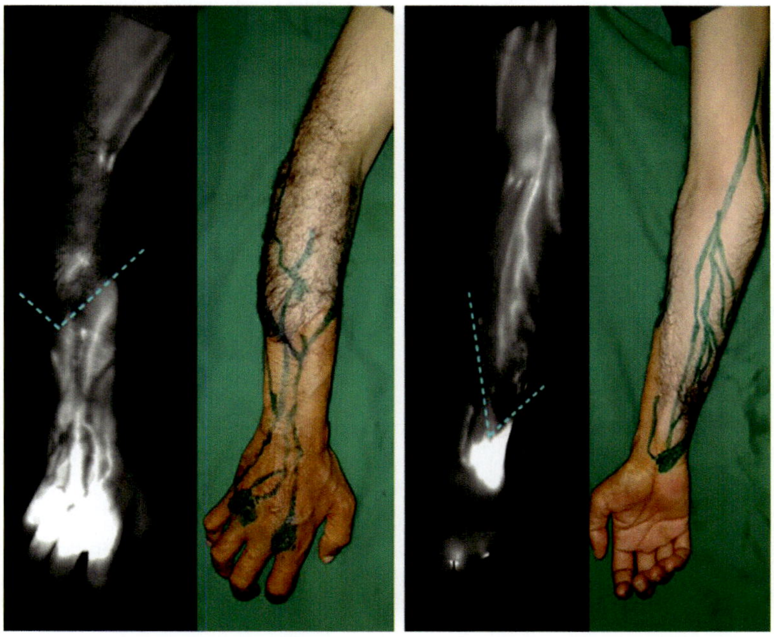

Fig. 16.6 Linear flow pattern noted on ICG lymphangiography and near-infrared imaging in recipient 2, 4 years postoperatively. Lymphatic flow traced in green

Table 16.5 Details of rejections in the first 6 recipients

Recipient	Rejection episode	Timing	Management	Tacrolimus level
1	Antibody-mediated rejection	2 weeks	Rituximab 2 × 500 mg	4.6
	Grade I ACR	4 weeks	Tapering of tacrolimus and oral steroid dosage	7.3
	Grade II ACR	4 months	Pulse therapy with methylprednisolone (500 mg × 3)	8.6
	Grade III ACR	8 months	Pulse therapy with methylprednisolone (500 mg × 2)	8.3
	Grade II ACR	9 months	Tapering of tacrolimus and oral steroid dosage	8.8
	Grade I–II ACR	10 months	Pulse therapy with methylprednisolone (250 mg × 3)	8.8
	Grade II ACR	13 months	Pulse therapy with methylprednisolone (250 mg × 3)	7.2
	Grade II–III ACR	14 months	Pulse therapy with methylprednisolone (250 mg × 3)	7.7
2	Grade I ACR	1 month	Pulse therapy with methylprednisolone (500 mg × 3)	8.9
	Grade II ACR	2 years 2 months	Pulse therapy with methylprednisolone (500 mg × 6)	10 [a]Episode possibly triggered due to reduction of tacrolimus dosage for an erroneously high serum tac level due to ongoing diarrhoea and hemoconcentration
	Grade II ACR	2 years 5 months	Pulse therapy with methylprednisolone (500 mg × 6)	
3	Moderate ACR	2 months	Pulse therapy with methylprednisolone (500 mg × 3)	14.4
	Insect bite/allergic reaction	3 months	Pulse therapy with methylprednisolone (500 mg × 3)	13.9
	Grade II ACR	4 months	Pulse therapy with methylprednisolone (500 mg × 3)	11
	Grade II ACR	6 months	Pulse therapy with methylprednisolone (500 mg × 3)	11
	Atypical chronic rejection (GvHD picture)	2 years and continuing	Inj ATG 50 mg in 500 mL dextrose IV over 6 h 3 cycles alternate days T sirolimus 1 mg 0–1–0	6.8–7.78
4	Grade II ACR	2 months	Pulse therapy with methylprednisolone (500 mg × 3)	12.17
	Grade II ACR	2.5 months	Pulse therapy with methylprednisolone (500 mg × 3)	11.99
	Grade II ACR	3 months	Pulse therapy with methylprednisolone (500 mg × 3)	14.52
	ACR	4 months	Resolved spontaneously	18.82
	Grade II ACR	6 months	Pulse therapy with methylprednisolone (500 mg × 4)	4.04
5	Nil			
6	Grade II ACR	2 months	Pulse therapy with methylprednisolone (250 mg × 3)	15
	Grade 1 ACR	4 months	Pulse therapy with methylprednisolone (250 mg × 3)	11.85
	Grade II ACR	6 months	Pulse therapy with methylprednisolone (250 mg × 3)	17.25
	Grade II TCMR	7 months	Pulse therapy with methylprednisolone (250 mg × 3)	13.38
	Grade I ACR	10 months	Pulse therapy with methylprednisolone (250 mg × 3)	9.7

[a]The patient was suffering fom diarrhoea and hence had dehydration and hemoconcentration when the Tacrolimus levels were checked. This caused the Tacrolimus levels to be erroneously reported as "high"

ACR acute cellular rejection, *TCMR* T-cell mediated rejection, *GvHD* graft versus host disease

16.5 Complications, Unique Problems, and Challenges Encountered

16.5.1 Recipient 1: Bilateral Distal Forearm Level Transplant

Postoperative: The ulnar skin flap of the left hand which had shown some intraoperative congestion started to show signs of significant congestion 12 h after surgery (Fig. 16.7). On account of the risk of infection and potential life-threatening sepsis in an already immune suppressed patient, it was immediately debrided (Fig. 16.8a) and covered with an end-to-side anterolateral thigh flap (Fig. 16.8b) under regional anesthesia as the patient was just recovering from a major procedure under general anesthesia.

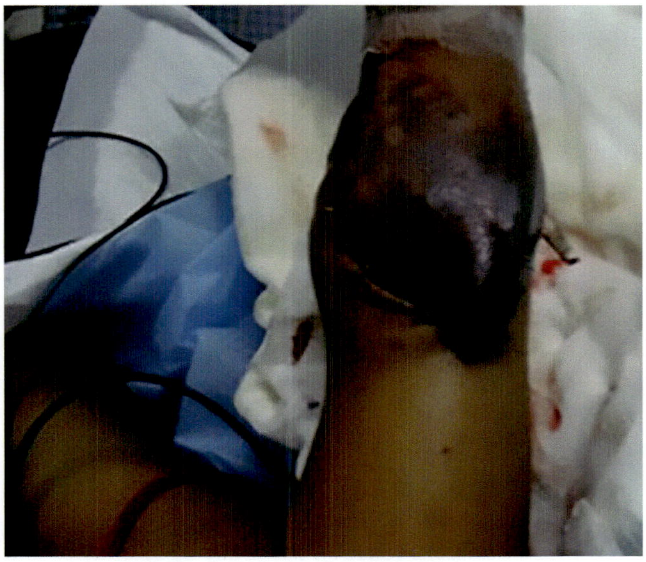

Fig. 16.7 Congestion of the ulnar skin flap of the left hand of recipient 1, 48 h postoperative

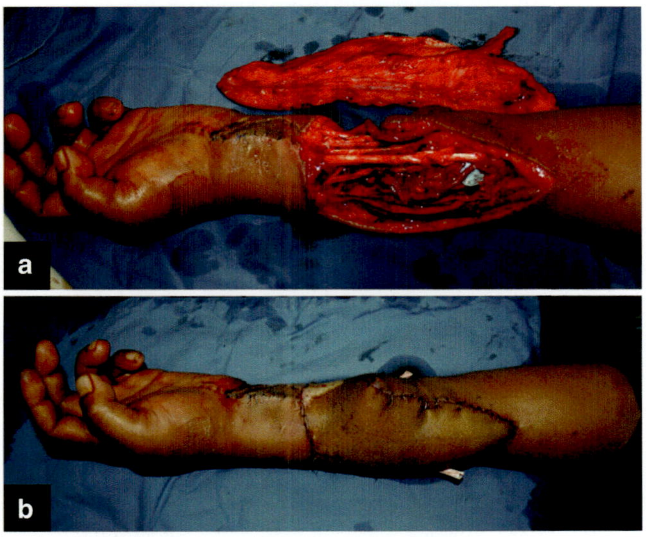

Fig. 16.8 (**a**) After debridement of the congested part. (**b**) Resurfacing the defect with an anterolateral thigh flap

16.5.2 Recipient 2: Bilateral Distal Forearm Level Transplant

Preoperative: Color matching of the skin was not ideal since he was from Afghanistan, and it was almost impossible to find the same racial and color match. We proceeded with the transplant as the recipient was not bothered about the disparity in the color.

On Follow-Up: Over 2 years the transplanted hand skin complexion became significantly lighter and matched that of the recipient skin (Fig. 16.9a, b). This phenomenon has been observed in all our transplant patients. Notably, all the donor grafts have been either a few shades darker than the recipient or of good color match. We have not had any recipients who received grafts of lighter or fairer complexion to establish that the transplanted hand skin eventually matches the recipient skin. Rather, till date, all the grafts have become lighter, adequate to match the recipient and never lighter than the recipient skin.

On serial histopathological examinations conducted either as protocol examination or when there was an episode of rejection, melanocyte pigment incontinence has been a consistent finding. It has been reported in inflammatory skin conditions where dyskeratosis led to scavenging of the affected epidermis by macrophages which also ingest melanosomes [9]. These get deposited in upper dermis and present as pigment incontinence.

Tacrolimus which is routinely used in maintenance immunosuppression is known to increase melanin production and facilitate melanocyte migration. It is currently used in vitiligo. However, in the context of VCA, it may have a role in melanocyte migration from the recipient skin across the interface [10].

Fourteen months following the transplant he developed weight loss of 10–12 kg over 4 months associated with a severe distaste for food and loose stools (3–4 episodes per day) for 2 months. An esophago-gastro-duodenoscopy and colonoscopy were performed which was unremarkable except for gastric inflammation. Duodenal biopsy showed chronic active duodenitis with giardiasis. Microscopy of stools showed ova of giardia. He received a 10-day course of metronidazole following which he recovered well.

During this period routine surveillance for serum tacrolimus levels was carried out and was found to be twice the required therapeutic level. The diarrhea caused severe hemoconcentration, and serum levels of tacrolimus were erroneously high. Dose adjustment was reconsidered after adequately hydrating the patient.

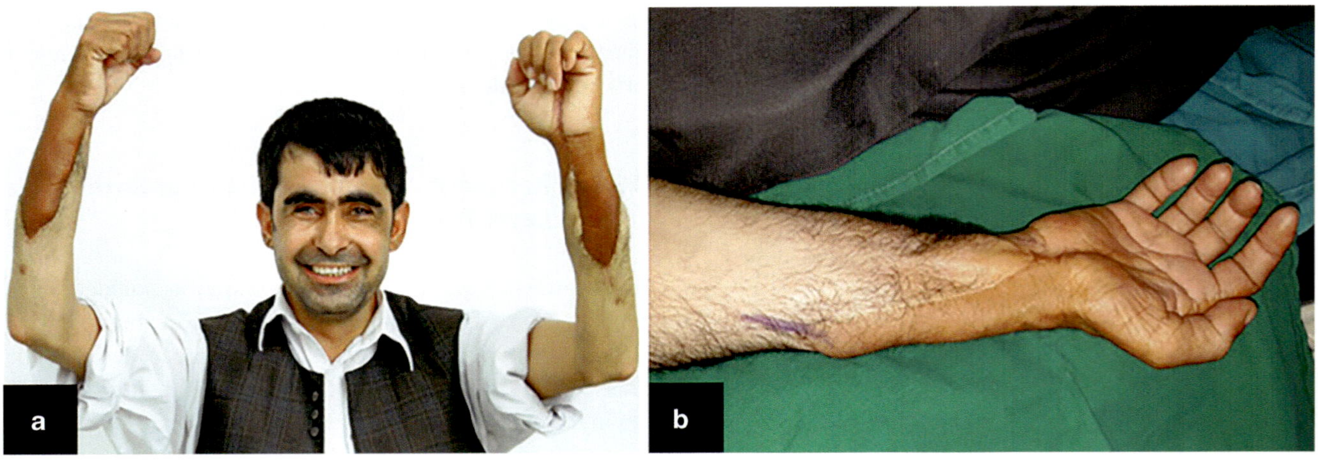

Fig. 16.9 (**a**) Notable color mismatch in the initial months posttransplant in recipient 2. (**b**) Significant lightening of skin of the transplanted hand 2 years posttransplant

16.5.3 Recipient 3: Bilateral Forearm Level Transplant

Operative: In this proximal forearm level transplant, only half or one-third of the muscle mass was present, which might not have given sufficient excursion to the digits if an end-to-end approximation was performed. Therefore, first, the recipient muscle groups were denervated by diligently dissecting out the radial, median, and ulnar nerves. Thereafter, some of the denervated recipient muscle bulk was discarded. This helped in accommodating the donor muscle overlap over the recipient muscles [11].

On Follow-Up: The transplant surgery and postoperative rehabilitation up to 1.5 years were uneventful with excellent functional recovery. In the first-year posttransplant, he developed four rejection episodes in the second, third, fourth, and sixth months, which were ACR (acute cellular rejection) grade II. He responded well to pulse steroid therapy and immunosuppressive treatment was titrated accordingly. Following this, he was asymptomatic with a stable course and recovery. At 1-year posttransplant his HTSS showed excellent function (right = 82, left = 81) and DASH score improved by 78.4 points (Fig. 16.10). He was employed and was reintegrated into a routine successfully.

However, after 1.5 years he was lost to follow-up for 4 months during which he had lapses in immunosuppression. He then presented to us with dystrophic nail changes. Under clinical suspicion of onychomycosis, he received empirical antifungal Itraconazole. Skin biopsies revealed a picture of chronic atypical cellular rejection which was CD8 T-cell predominant. He was treated with pulse steroid therapy, and a repeat biopsy 1 week later showed improvement. Four weeks later, he presented with gross edema, hyperpigmentation, and stiffness. Ultrasound of the forearm showed edema in deeper intermuscular planes. Muscle biopsy, skin biopsies from the graft and recipient skin were done. His histopathology resembled a graft versus host disease (GvHD) and it was diagnosed as a form of grade III chronic rejection [12]. Histopathology had no evidence of capillary thrombosis or ischemic changes. Rather, it was perivascular and periappendageal lymphoid proliferation with extension into the dermo-epidermal interface and epidermal tagging of lymphocytes.

He received ATG (three cycles on alternate days) along with pulse steroid therapy. Sirolimus, an mTOR inhibitor known for potent immunosuppressive and anti-fibrogenic activity, started to retard further fibrosis [13, 14].

Even after this, his function has gradually worsened and stiffness has become progressive despite adequate immunosuppression. Sensory and motor deterioration has been progressive and grafts have developed woody fibrosis and desquamation of palmar skin (Fig. 16.11).

16.5.4 Recipient 4: Bilateral Supracondylar Level Transplant

Preoperative: There was a gender mismatch (donor was a young male and the recipient was a young female) in this case. Though she had below elbow amputation, the stump was inadequate for plating; hence, a supracondylar transplant was planned [15].

Operative: Challenges faced intraoperatively were as follows:

1. A discrepancy in the vessel circumference.
2. A discrepancy in the size of the humerus, due to which only lateral surface was matched and osteosynthesis was performed using a single LCDCP (limited contact dynamic compression plate).

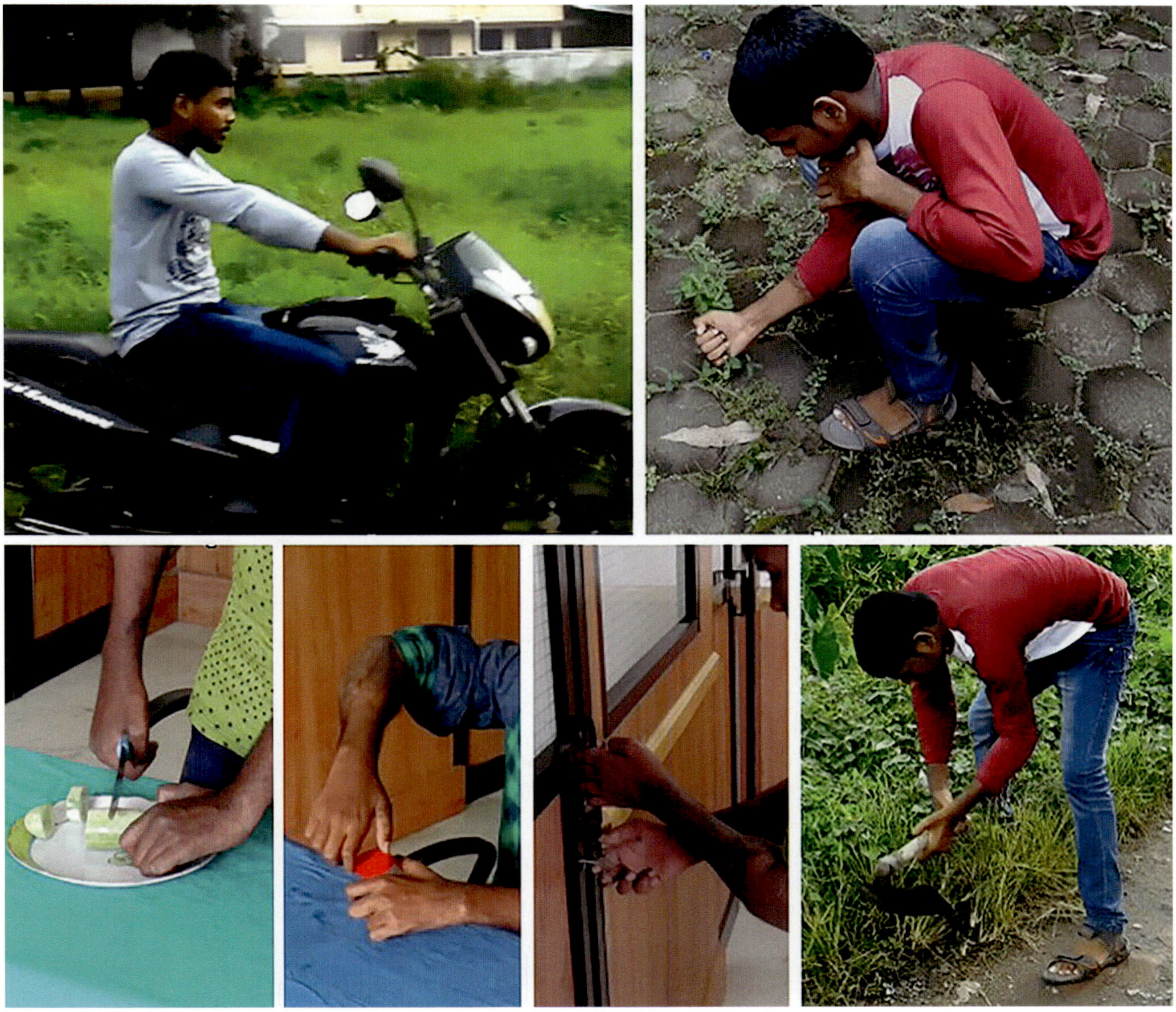

Fig. 16.10 Recipient 3 (bilateral proximal forearm) at 1-year postop he developed good recovery of gross and fine motor skills

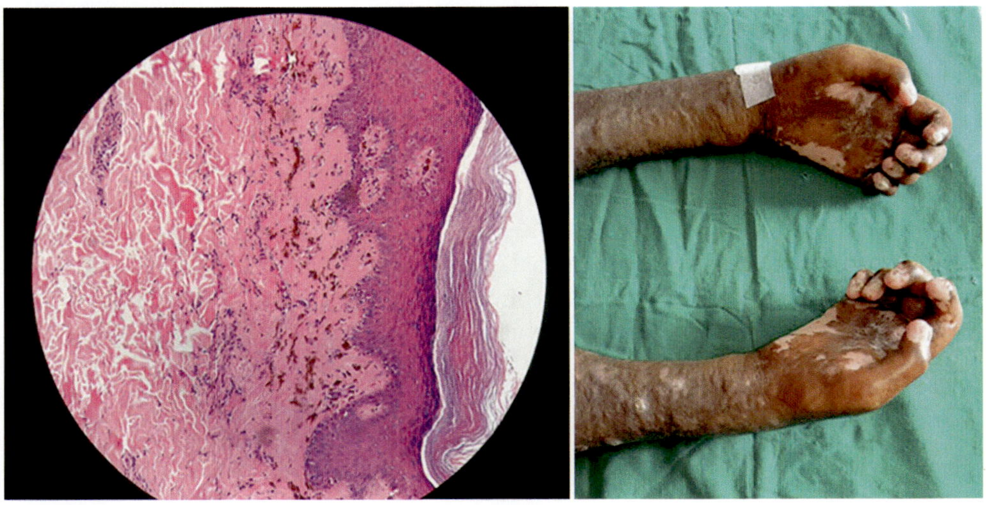

Fig. 16.11 Histopathology shows GvHD-like-features; the current clinical picture of recipient 3, with fibrosis, nail dystrophy, and flexion contractures

3. A large bulk of muscles was transplanted; hence, it was important to keep the ischemia time as short as possible.
4. Due to the presence of neuromas, the median nerve on the right side was resected at a level 10 cm higher than the left side and similarly, the scar and fibrosis at the site of the right radial nerve required excision 10 cm higher than the left-sided radial nerve that would eventually delay the return of function in the right upper limb.

Postoperative: The right limb of the donor had one radial arterial line placed when she was on a ventilator; as a result some intimal damage might have been there, resulting in a localized block in the flow of right radial artery, and for the initial 2 postoperative days the right hand was perfusing on the ulnar artery alone.

Prostaglandin E1 (PGE1) infusion was started intravenously with a concentration of 500 μg/50 mL normal saline diluted to 200 mL administered at the rate of 1 mL/min for 2 days postoperatively. The effective dose that was given was 2.5 μg/min; the maximum safe dose is up to 10 μg/min. By the third postoperative day, the radial pulse was detectable.

The use of PGE1 infusion has been described to be of benefit in patients with critical limb ischemia secondary to peripheral vascular occlusive disease. PGE1 agonist binds to the PGE receptors causing corporal smooth muscle relaxation that in turn leads to an increase in peripheral blood flow by vasodilation and inhibits platelet aggregation [16].

On Follow-Up: On the 70th-day posttransplantation, she had the first episode of rejection. This was followed by two more episodes of rejection each, weeks apart. All episodes were treated with pulse doses of methylprednisolone. Valganciclovir was temporarily discontinued because of leukopenia. The patient recovered from the episodes of rejection.

Four weeks after the last episode of rejection, she developed loose stools, which was initially treated with antibiotics. Symptoms recurred in a few weeks when gastroscopy and colonoscopy were done, which showed features of CMV (Cytomegalovirus) colitis (confirmed on biopsy). CMV DNA-PCR quantitative sent during the start of treatment showed 112,633 copies/mL. She was initially started on injectable Ganciclovir, and later oral (900 mg twice daily). At the end of 2 weeks of treatment, CMV DNA-PCR quantitative assessment showed a reduction in viral load (16,365 copies/mL). Because of severe leukopenia, MMF was temporarily stopped for a few days and restarted once her counts improved. For the next 2 months, she was free from symptoms and there was a further reduction in viral load.

Seven months posttransplant, she had abdominal pain, vomiting, and fever. CT abdomen showed focal thickening in the stomach, an endoscopic biopsy of which showed Monomorphic B cell type of posttransplant lymphoproliferative disease (PTLD). It was decided to significantly reduce immunosuppression. Only local application of steroid and tacrolimus creams was done. She received four cycles of Rituximab. It was spaced out 1 week apart with 600 mg given on the first and third weeks and 500 mg on second and fourth weeks. Repeat endoscopies showed healed ulcers, and she is disease-free till date. During this period she received topical Tacrolimus ointment application to the grafts to avoid high levels of Tacrolimus in the blood while maintaining adequate levels in the grafts to prevent rejection.

She is on two immunosuppressive agents only (Tacrolimus and Prednisolone), has no further episodes of rejection, and has good functional outcome at 3 years posttransplant (Figs. 16.12 and 16.13).

16.5.5 Recipient 5: Bilateral Proximal Forearm Level Transplant

Preoperative: Recipient was a 46-year-old female, a known hypothyroid with uncontrolled diabetes mellitus. The donor was a young male with a favorable lymphocyte cross match. Given her poor glycemic control, a steroid-based regimen was avoided. She received a two-drug regimen containing mycophenolate (1000 mg BD) and tacrolimus (6 mg BD) with weekly monitoring for plasma levels of tacrolimus.

Postoperative: She developed necrosis of donor skin flap on the left side, it was debrided and resurfaced with a split-thickness graft.

She underwent weekly protocol biopsies for the first month followed by monthly biopsies for the first 6 months and 6 monthly for the next 1 year. She has had no frank episodes of rejection, and her protocol biopsies were consistent with the same with only mild perivascular infiltrate and occasional eosinophils.

She however required insulin supplementation as her HbA1c was 11 g/dL at the time of transplant and with strict control, it improved. However, she continues to require injectable long-acting insulin.

On Follow-Up: Her functional recovery was compromised and the recovery of sensory and motor function was delayed (Fig. 16.14).

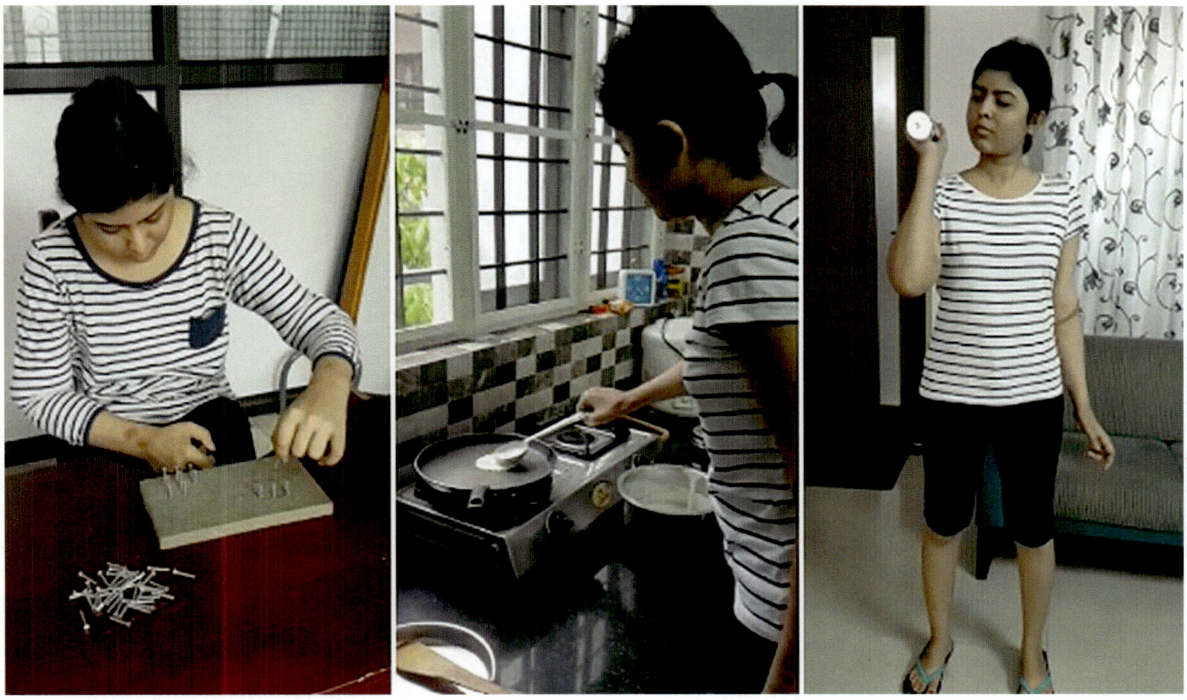

Fig. 16.12 Recipient 4 (bilateral supracondylar level transplant) at 1-year posttransplant with the recovery of gross motor function as anticipated and inadequate fine motor function improving

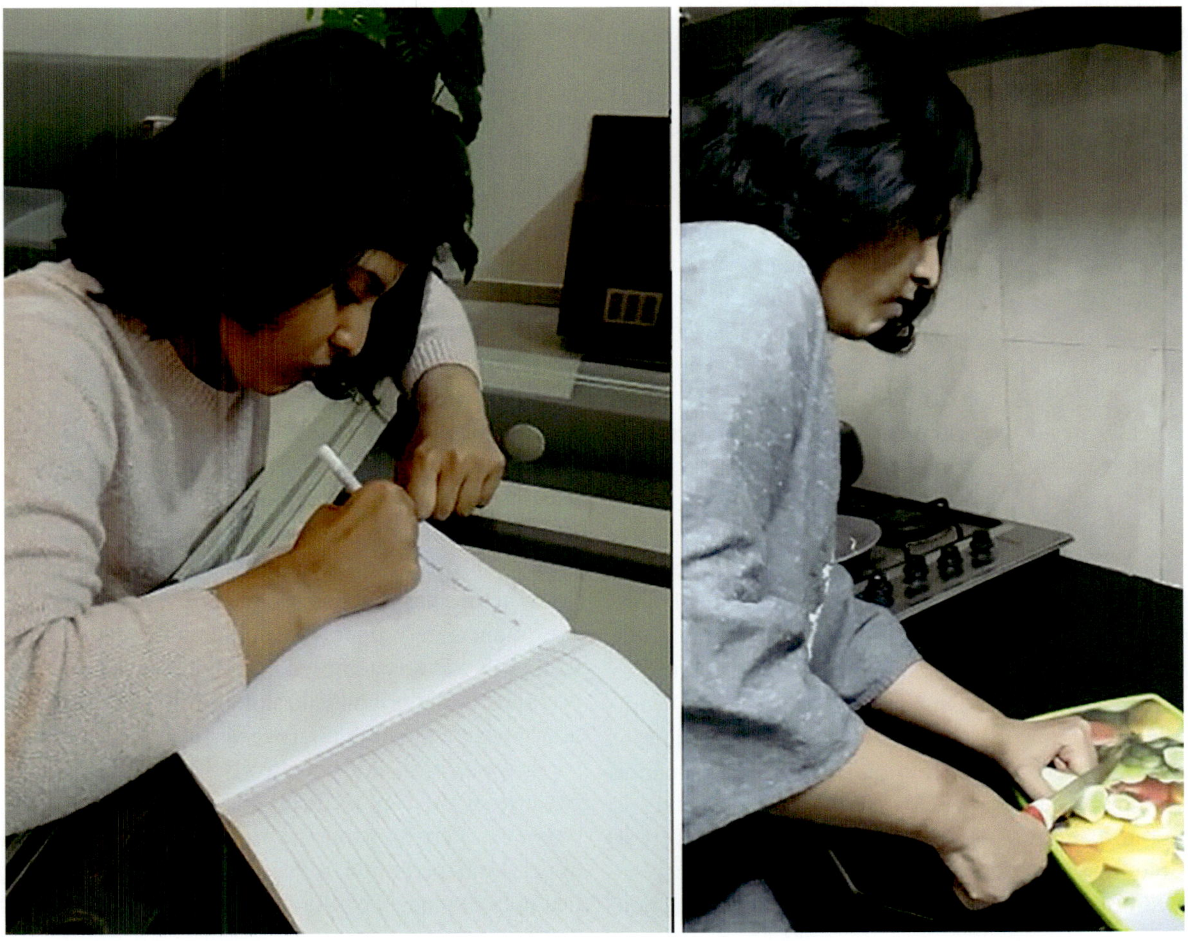

Fig. 16.13 Recipient 4 with good recovery of gross and fine motor function at 2 years posttransplant

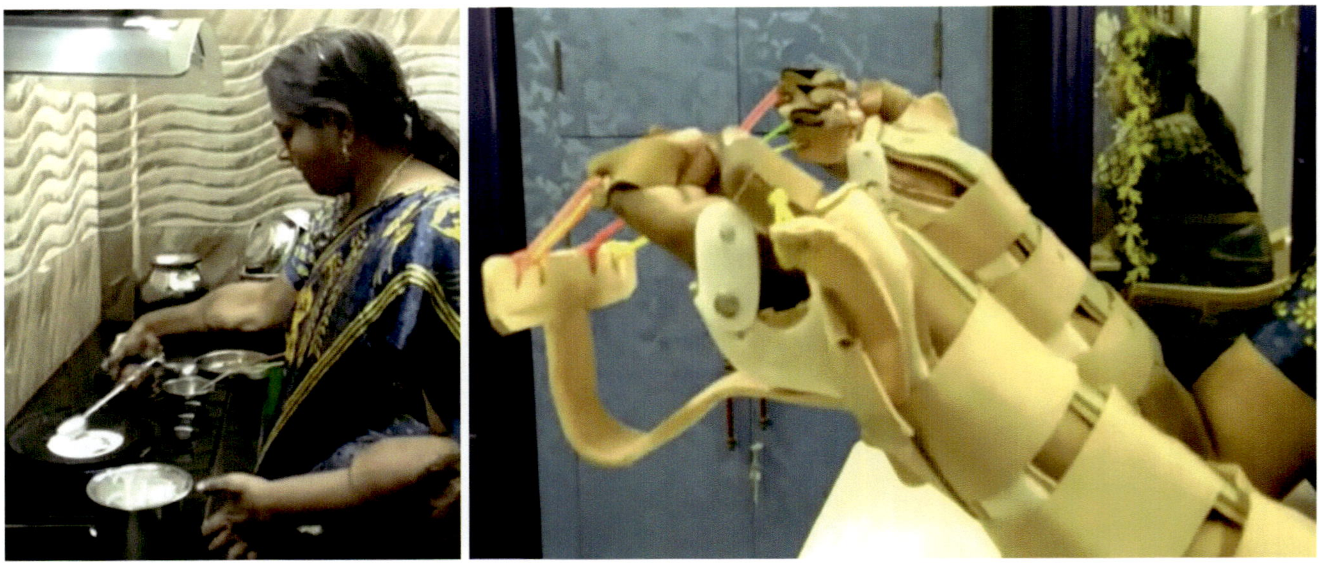

Fig. 16.14 Recipient 5 (bilateral proximal forearm level transplant) at 1-year posttransplant. Recovery of gross motor function was poor with weak flexors and weaker extensors. She required extension splints to perform ADLs for a longer time

16.5.6 Recipient 6: Right Proximal Forearm Level and Left Proximal Arm Level Transplant

Background and Operative: Recipient was a 36-year-old civilian who was working for the Indian navy and lost his hands in a tragic electrical accident. He sustained a proximal arm amputation on the left side and proximal forearm level amputation on the right side which greatly affected his quality of life. He presented to us 10 years following his injuries. He was listed in the organ recipient registry of the state, unfortunately during this period, the organ donation had come to a standstill for a couple of years due to various reasons. He waited for about 2.5 years staying near the campus in hope of getting a donor. This made us look at avenues of procuring hands from elsewhere.

We have had extensive discussions from various organ procurement teams in the country and reached a consensus to accept suitable donations from neighboring states where helicopter transport can be done with a time-lapse of 1–2 h. In case of any unforeseen delay, we planned on extracorporeal perfusion of the limbs for graft preparation as a means to reduce the ischemia time [17, 18]. Unfortunately the day we procured the hands the timing of procurement did not allow the heli-ambulance late in the night, and we had to resort to the transfer of hands by a commercial flight. This resulted in further delay. Ultimately 8 h had elapsed from the time of harvest and delivery of limbs to our center. This situation was also explained to the patient, and he insisted to proceed with the transplant procedure even accepting the grave risk of possible limb loss. As previously planned in this contingency, we used a cardiopulmonary bypass (CPB) machine for perfusion along with simultaneous preparation. The brachial artery and cephalic vein were cannulated, and graft dissection was performed in a big bowl to facilitate collection of blood spilt from the stump. This blood was reintroduced into the circulation of the CPB by intraoperative cell salvage. The positioning in a bowl and compromised field due to ongoing perfusion made dissection technically challenging. Despite this, we completed the dissection, osteosynthesis, and vascular anastomosis by 11 h.

The right limb remained cold but viable postoperatively. It took about 34 h and PGE1 infusion to regain full perfusion of the digits and a detectable waveform. Tips of thumb and index were found cyanosed, possibly secondary to radial artery cannulation of the donor in the previous institute. After reperfusion, the distal phalanx of index and tip of thumb remained dusky and progressed to gangrene over 2 weeks. Ultimately it resulted in the amputation of the index finger at distal phalanx level.

The donor was a very short-statured female, and despite harvest at a very proximal level for the left upper limb, there was a significant gap between the donor and recipient vessels. This was bridged with the discarded brachial artery from opposite limb. Following anastomosis, perfusion of forearm muscles was not satisfactory. A forearm fasciotomy was immediately done. An additional bridging saphenous vein graft was anastomosed to the side of the brachial artery proximal to the original anastomosis and to the donor radial artery in an attempt to improve perfusion.

Postoperative: Postoperatively PGE1 infusion was given because of the lack of distal pulse and waveform on pulse oximetry. Perfusion on the right side improved. The left upper limb perfusion remained poor postoperatively and had to be explanted on the morning of the second postoperative day.

He developed patchy necrosis of right forearm donor skin at the proximal aspect which was debrided and resurfaced with a skin graft.

Despite prolonged ischemia, the patient developed meaningful recovery, his DASH score improved from 62.5 to 40 at the end of 1 year.

His intrinsic recovery was poor and was further complicated by a shortened index finger. He adapted by developing a pinch grasp between thumb and middle finger. He writes comfortably by grasping a pen between middle and ring fingers (Fig. 16.15).

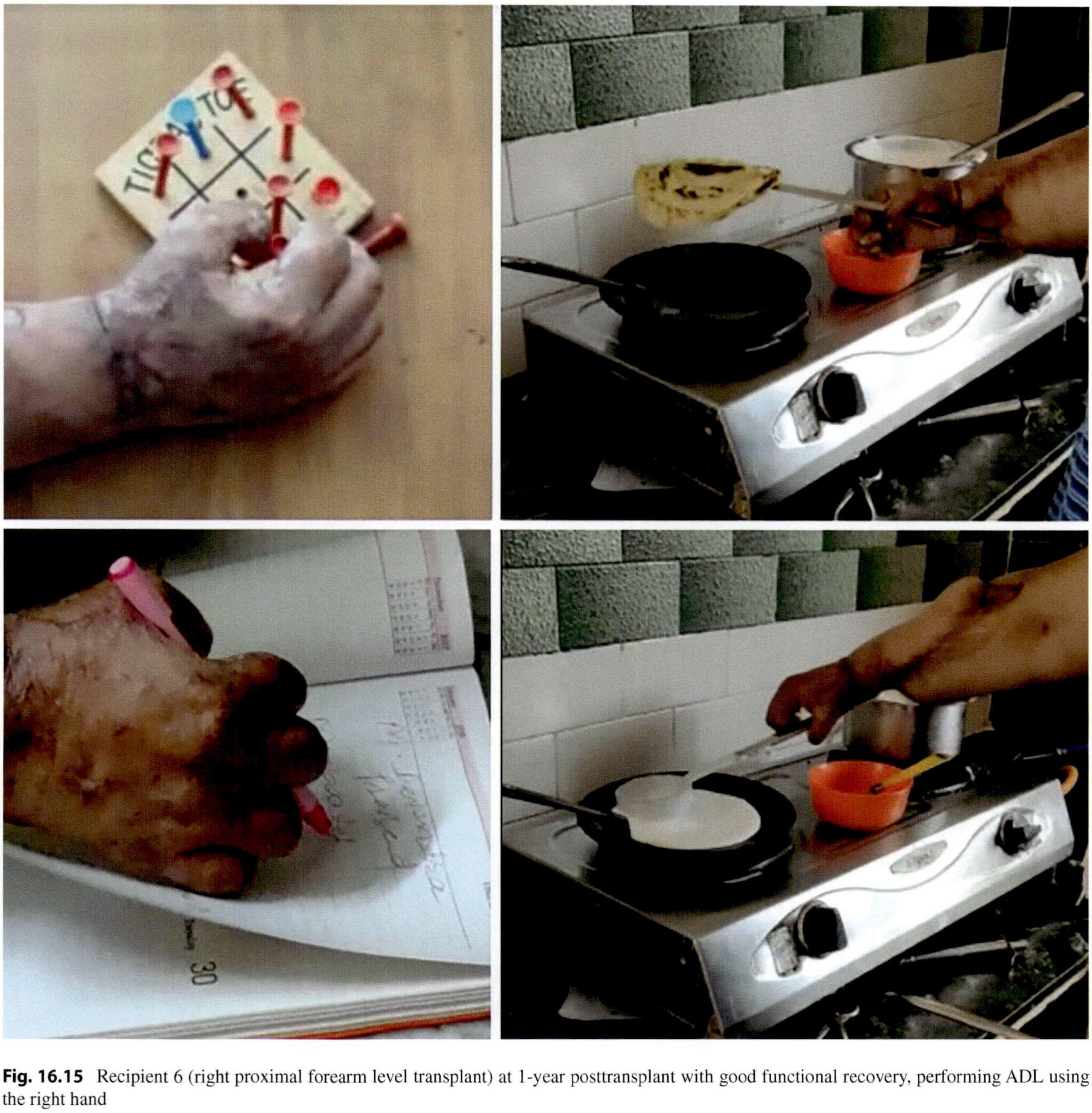

Fig. 16.15 Recipient 6 (right proximal forearm level transplant) at 1-year posttransplant with good functional recovery, performing ADL using the right hand

16.5.7 Recipient 7: Bilateral Mid-Arm Level Transplant

Preoperative: A 52-year-old Malaysian lady, quadruple amputee (bilateral upper limb above elbow and bilateral lower limb below knee) following an assault by husband, underwent bilateral upper limb transplant at the supracondylar level. The donor was a 39-year-old male, hypertensive who was declared brain dead following a hemorrhagic stroke.

Operative: There was thrombosis at both the brachial arterial anastomotic sites immediately after clamp removal and was successfully revised patient was heparinized intraoperatively and was converted to therapeutic low molecular weight heparin.

Postoperative: Therapeutic low molecular weight heparin was continued postoperatively because of the thrombotic episodes intraoperatively. The grafts showed satisfactory perfusion postoperatively; however, she developed hematomas in the right arm on postoperative day 1 and 3 which were promptly evacuated. On the left side, she developed active bleeding which required re-exploration on postoperative day 2.

She became febrile on the third day and antibiotic therapy was initiated. She had a continuous high-grade fever which was poorly responding to antipyretics. Procalcitonin was marginally elevated on second postoperative day (level = 2.2) and rapidly increased over the next 48 h (level = 87). Blood cultures did not show bacterial growth. Her respiratory and hemodynamic status deteriorated on postoperative day 4, and she required elective intubation and inotropic support.

The possibilities considered were gram-negative sepsis or cytokine storm syndrome. Along with broad-spectrum antibiotics, pan cytokine removal by CytoSorb® therapy was administered on postoperative day 4 and 5 with which hypotension and pyrexia improved transiently. However, she rapidly deteriorated on postoperative day 6 and succumbed.

16.5.8 Recipient 8: Bilateral Proximal Forearm Level Transplant

Background: The recipient, a 23-year-old male was bilateral below-elbow upper limb amputee following a blast injury and had corneal scarring. His vision was severely impaired and was a relative contraindication for the procedure. He underwent a corneal transplant in his left eye and regained meaningful vision. He underwent hand transplant 3 years following the blast injury.

Postoperatively: Proximal aspect of the donor skin flaps developed marginal necrosis which was revised.

16.6 The Future

Over the last 5 years, our team has acquired vast experience in the nascent field of vascularized composite allotransplantation (VCA). Our greatest strength has been a cohesive and dynamic team of reconstructive surgeons working together in a charitable tertiary care institute of excellence. An excellent cadaveric lab for surgical training and drills, a state-of-art animal lab with microvascular training facility, a transplant research facility along with our plastic and reconstructive surgery residents and post-doctoral fellows, a dedicated physiotherapy unit—all played an important part.

Over time, our team has acquired much better synchronization in executing such complex operations. However, since the ischemia time in VCA may be linked to the phenomena of chronic rejections [19], our main emphasis was on reducing the ischemia time. One of the advances in the field of transplantation has been in the field of oxygen delivery to the tissues. The French company Hemarina has developed Hemo2Life®, extracellular hemoglobin derived from the marine invertebrate *Arenicola marina*, which has shown promising results in preserving organs, as it has high oxygen affinity and can deliver it to tissues even at low temperatures [20]. As it could be easily mixed with the commercial tissue preservative solutions, this could protect against ischemia and allow the transfer of organs over long distances. We could take advantage of this development in our future hand transplants. Simultaneously, the advances in the field of organ decellularization and cell seeding might make organs available to us in future, without the need of immunosuppression.

In the field of rehabilitation, we have been actively working to develop a tool in which a 3D camera could sense the movement of a hand and project it onto a computer screen by which the range of motion can be instantaneously calculated. In future, this would be an excellent tool to record the progress of rehabilitation and improvement in hand functionality (Fig. 16.16).

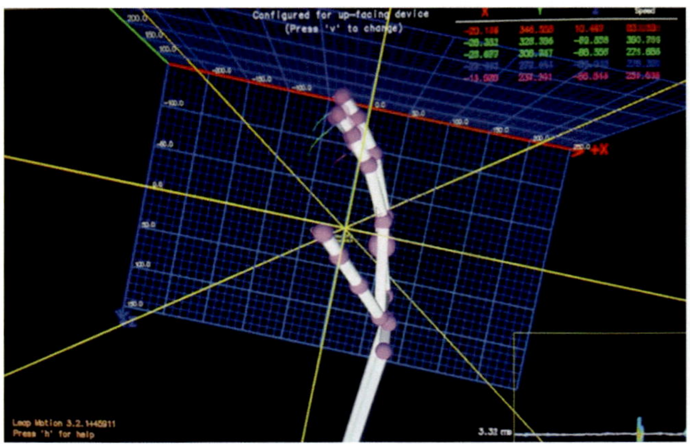

Fig. 16.16 Real-time projection of hand for measurement of range of movement

No prosthesis has come close to providing near-normal pain and temperature perception, stereognosis, sweating, and the mental freedom to jump in a swimming pool without a second thought. In a time trade-off study on quality of life done at our institute, we found that bilateral hand amputees are willing to trade-off a significant portion of their life years to obtain functional hands after transplantation, even taking all risks into account [21].

16.7 Conclusion

The field of transplantation is here to stay as we simultaneously work on achieving methodologies to create graft tolerance and better immunosuppression along with perfecting the existing surgical techniques.

Finally, what matters for the patient is normal body image, functionality and ability to live without the stigma of an amputee. With the progressive reduction in the cost of immunosuppression, the future of a large number of unfortunate upper limb amputees appears to be bright.

References

1. Cendales LC, Kanitakis J, Schneeberger S, Burns C, Ruiz P, Landin L, Remmelink M, Hewitt CW, Landgren T, Lyons B, Drachenberg CB, Solez K, Kirk AD, Kleiner DE, Racusen L. The Banff 2007 working classification of skin-containing composite tissue allograft pathology. Am J Transplant. 2008;8(7):1396–400.
2. Bueno E, Benjamin MJ, Sisk G, Sampson CE, Carty M, Pribaz JJ, Pomahac B, Talbot SG. Rehabilitation following hand transplantation. Hand (N Y). 2014;9(1):9–15.
3. Sharma M, Iyer S, Kishore P, et al. First two bilateral hand transplantations in India (part 3): rehabilitation and immediate outcome. Indian J Plast Surg. 2017;50(2):161–7.
4. Kapandji A. Cotation clinique de l'opposition et de la contre-opposition du pouce [clinical test of apposition and counter-apposition of the thumb]. Ann Chir Main. 1986;5(1):67–73.
5. Medical Research Council. Aids to examination of the peripheral nervous system. Memorandum no. 45. London: Her Majesty's Stationary Office; 1976.
6. Bell-Krotoski J, Weinstein S, Weinstein C. Testing sensibility, including touch-pressure, two-point discrimination, point localization, and vibration. J Hand Ther. 1993;6(2):114–23.
7. Solway S, Beaton DE, McConnell S, Bombardier C. The DASH outcome measure user's manual. Toronto: Institute for Work & Health; 2002.
8. Lanzetta M, Petruzzo P. A comprehensive functional score system in hand transplantation. In: Lanzetta M, Dubernard JM, editors. Hand transplantation. Milan: Springer-Verlag; 2007. p. 355–62.
9. Masu S, Seiji M. Pigmentary incontinence in fixed drug eruptions. Histologic and electron microscopic findings. J Am Acad Dermatol. 1983;8(4):525–32.
10. Kang HY, Choi YM. FK506 increases pigmentation and migration of human melanocytes. Br J Dermatol. 2006;155(5):1037–40.
11. Sharma M, Iyer S, Purushottaman K, et al. Indian Subcontinent's first proximal forearm level double upper extremity transplantation. Indian J Plast Surg. 2019;52(3):277–84.
12. Gorantla V, Demetris A. Acute and chronic rejection in upper extremity transplantation: what have we learned? Hand Clin. 2011;27(4):481–93.
13. Yoshizaki A, Yanaba K, Yoshizaki A, et al. Treatment with rapamycin prevents fibrosis in tight-skin and bleomycin-induced mouse models of systemic sclerosis. Arthritis Rheum. 2010;62(8):2476–87.
14. Abouelnasr A, Roy J, Cohen S, Kiss T, Lachance S. Defining the role of sirolimus in the management of graft-versus-host disease: from prophylaxis to treatment. Biol Blood Marrow Transplant. 2013;19(1):12–21.
15. Sharma M, Iyer S, Kishore P, et al. Indian Subcontinent's first bilateral supracondylar level upper limb transplantation. Indian J Plast Surg. 2019;52(3):285–95.
16. Weiss T. Mechanisms of action of prostaglandin E1 in therapy of peripheral arterial occlusive diseases. Vasa. 2003;32(4):187–92.
17. Werner NL, Alghanem F, Rakestraw SL, et al. Ex situ perfusion of human limb allografts for 24 hours. Transplantation. 2017;101(3):e68–74.
18. Greaney PJ, Cordisco M, Rodriguez D, Newberger J, Legatt AD, Garfein ES. Use of an extracorporeal membrane oxygenation circuit as a bridge to salvage a major upper-extremity replant in a critically ill patient. J Reconstr Microsurg. 2010;26(8):517–22.
19. Qayumi AK, Nikbakht-sangari MN, Godin DV, et al. The relationship of ischemia-reperfusion injury of transplanted lung and the up-regulation of major histocompatibility complex II on host peripheral lymphocytes. J Thorac Cardiovasc Surg. 1998;115(5):978–89.
20. Kaminski J, Hannaert P, Kasil A, et al. Efficacy of the natural oxygen transporter HEMO life in cold preservation in a preclinical porcine model of donation after cardiac death. Transpl Int. 2019;32(9):985–96.
21. Harijee A, Thankappan K, Sharma M, et al. Estimation of health utility and quality adjusted life years in bilateral hand transplantation: a time trade-off study. Ann Plast Surg. 2020;86:345. Epub ahead of print. https://doi.org/10.1097/SAP.0000000000002544.

Hand Transplantation CM Kleinert Institute for Hand and Microsurgery Experience

17

Laxminarayan Bhandari and Tuna Özyürekoglu

17.1 The Beginning

One small step for man one giant leap for mankind—a famous Kleinert Kutz patient.

In more than a few ways hand transplantation and the lunar landing have similarities. Both were considered impossible, yet, both were achieved, celebrated, and reproduced world over. With the changing world, both are being debated and scrutinized. In Louisville, our experience ranged from as far as the moon and back. This journey of being the first to perform a successful hand transplantation as well as the largest series till date does put us in a unique vantage point. The scientific success, the patient triumph as well as tragedies and the endless debates make this an interesting chapter not only in hand surgery but also in modern medicine.

The first successful solid organ transplantation happened in 1954 [1]. It took another forty-four years for successful hand transplantation to be achieved. Hand transplant is unique compared to solid organs and even other composite tissue allotransplantations (CTA). Some of the factors unique to CTA over other solid organs are the fact that they improve quality of life and not necessarily add years to lifespan. Second, the concerns for causing harm by lifelong immunosuppression. Third, hand transplantation is performed in patients who are healthy and unlike solid organ transplantations do not have chronic medical conditions. While face and hands transplants both contribute to body image, the identity issues are less with hand transplantations. Transplanted hands can be amputated, if needed, an option seldom possible for face transplant.

The factors behind our group's consideration to work in the field of hand transplantations were mainly three-fold. First, the hand prosthetics were still in infancy. The functional outcome of a prosthetic device was considered poorer to hand replantation [2]. Advances in microvascular techniques and instrumentations led to consistent success in replantation surgeries at our institution. The outcomes of replantation were superior compared to prosthetics [2]. However, replantation was not possible when the amputated part was missing or beyond salvage. This kindled interest in allotransplantation. Second, when hand transplantation was still a concept, several components of CTA were being transplanted with good outcome. These included nerves [3], tendons [4], skin [5] bones and joints [6], vessels [7], and muscles [8]. Hand, being a combination of the above tissues was considered to be within reach. Third, advances in understanding the immunological basis of rejection led to development of multiple immunosuppression medications. The introduction of cyclosporin A (CsA) in 1983, tacrolimus (FK 506) in 1994, mycophenolate mofetil (MMF) in 1995, and sirolimus in 1999 heralded an era in transplantation, where long term immunosuppression could be managed with relatively low dose and lower risks [9].

These factors led our teams to conduct multiple preclinical experiments—three among them deserve a mention. The first one related to low dose CsA and MMF combination. Low dose CsA and MMF combination had showed promising results in rat hind limb allografts [10]. With an eye toward future clinical application, our group developed pig brachial artery based radial forearm osteomyocutaneous flap allograft model [11]. Only two of the ten pigs showed acute rejection. Three pigs showed no rejection and three showed stable mild

L. Bhandari
CM Kleinert Institute for Hand and Microsurgery, Louisville, KY, USA

Kleinert Kutz Hand Care Center, Louisville, KY, USA

Department of Surgery, University of Louisville, Louisville, KY, USA
e-mail: lbhandari@kleinertkutz.com

T. Özyürekoglu (✉)
CM Kleinert Institute for Hand and Microsurgery, Louisville, KY, USA

Kleinert Kutz Hand Care Center, Louisville, KY, USA

Department of Surgery, University of Louisville, Louisville, KY, USA

Department of Orthopedics, University of Louisville, Louisville, KY, USA
e-mail: tozyurekoglu@kleinertkutz.com

© Springer Nature Switzerland AG 2023
R. Gurunian et al. (eds.), *Reconstructive Transplantation*, https://doi.org/10.1007/978-3-031-21520-9_17

to moderate rejection. Two pigs died without any evidence of rejection. The second study evaluated FK506 and MMF combination in the same porcine model [12]. Five of the nine pigs survived 90 days without rejection. The other four died, three from pneumonia and one from gastric rupture. There were multiple complications noted—septic arthritis, toe abscesses, diarrhea, and decreased weight gain. Thus, combination oral FK506-MMF treatment provided a superior antirejection effect but more toxicity [12]. In the third study the "Louisville Pig" model was created to include the radial digit along with the radial forelimb osteomyocutaneous flap on brachial artery and cephalic vein. Since the previous model of radial forearm osteomyocutaneous flaps had not included joints, the current "Louisville Pig" model had the closest resemblance to human hand allograft [13].

As the preclinical models successfully demonstrated long term graft survival for composite tissue allotransplantation, the clinical trials seemed to be the next logical step. However, multiple barriers needed to be crossed before it could be a reality. In order to address these concerns, Louisville Hand Transplant team was constituted in June 1996. Dr. Warren Breidenbach organized a team of hand surgeons, plastic surgeons, and transplant surgeons along with psychiatrists, pathologists, hand therapists, and organ procurement team. As hand transplant was a novel treatment modality, multiple ethical questions needed to be addressed [14]. In order to address these concerns, a medical ethicist of national recognition was consulted. The ethics of introduction of innovative surgical procedure was guided by six criteria suggested by Dr. Francis Moore: (i) scientific background of the innovation; (ii) skill and experience of the team; (iii) ethical climate of the institution; (iv) open display; (v) public evaluation; and (vi) public and professional discussions. All these criteria were included in the Louisville program [14].

The proposed hand transplant trial was submitted for Institutional Review Board approval. To avoid institutional bias, an Independent Ethics Committee outside our institution was invited to review the protocol. Each candidate underwent a careful psychologic screening by a committee of psychologists, psychiatrists, and social workers. Each patient was asked to select a patient advocate. The patient advocate had a relationship with only the patient and advise him or her throughout the entire process. A thorough public and professional scrutiny was invited by advance announcements of the clinical trial.

The First International Symposium on Composite Tissue Allotransplantation held on November 1997 at Louisville could not have happened at a better time. With a goal to discuss the "scientific, clinical, and ethical barriers standing in the way of performing the first human hand transplant," eminent scholars from around the world deliberated on the feasibility of hand transplant [15]. International experts predicted that limb allotransplantation was not far from "becoming a clinical reality." As noted in the closing remarks, in the words of a few of the symposium speakers and others, it was time to "Just Do It" [15].

University of Louisville Institutional Review Board and Jefferson County Medical Society Ethics Board approved hand transplant clinical trial in July 1998 which opened the doors to patient recruitment and the preparations to make it a clinical reality for America's first and the world's longest surviving hand transplant.

17.2 Criteria and Protocols

As the Louisville Hand Transplant Team got the scientific, ethical clearance as well as support from global scholars, donor and recipient criteria were formulated [16]. Most of our selection criteria for donor and recipient mirrored similar criteria which were in practice for solid organ transplantation [1]. There were a few notable differences which would be detailed in the subsequent text. The proposed organ procurement as well as transplant surgery was designed. The postoperative monitoring, immunosuppression, and rehabilitation protocols were set up [1].

17.3 Donor Considerations

Selecting a donor for a hand transplantation had some notable differences compared to solid organs. In contrast to internal organs, the external appearance of hand is an important consideration in hand transplant [1]. Skin color, tone, hairiness, gender, and race were matched between the donor and recipient. Extremities with extensive or offensive tattoos were rejected. Donors with history of congenital anomaly, malignancy, traumatic deformity, connective tissue disorders, peripheral neuropathy were excluded.

17.4 Donor Procurement

Donor procurement was done in collaboration with the local organ procurement organization (OPO) [17]. When the local OPO received information about a case of probable brain death, the representatives were sent to approach the patient's family to attempt consent for donation. If consent was obtained, OPO performed donor evaluation in accordance with our criteria (Table 17.1) [1, 9, 17]. If the donor was a suitable candidate, the information was communicated to our transplant team. Once intimated, a team of two surgeons for unilateral limb and four surgeons for bilateral limb procurement, fully complemented with surgical technicians and the necessary surgical instrumentation was dispatched on a charter flight irrespective of geographic location [1, 9, 17, 18].

Table 17.1 Louisville donor criteria

Selection criteria • Brain dead • Aged 18–65 years • Matches the age, sex, skin tone of the recipient • Not on excessive vasopressors to maintain blood pressure
Exclusion criteria • Infections: Unresolved sepsis, HIV, active cytomegalovirus or Epstein–Barr virus, active tuberculosis, viral hepatitis (B or C) viral encephalitis • Malignancy • Current intravenous drug use • Tattoo (within past 6 months) • Any systemic or limb-related neuropathies, rheumatoid arthritis, and osteoarthritis
Additional role of OPO • The OPO should, in collaboration with the donor hospital's critical care team, maintain the hemodynamic stability, normothermia, optimal oxygenation, fluid and electrolyte balance, and infection prevention in the donor patient • Responsible for affirming the initial serologic testing for infections • Obtaining the posteroanterior and lateral radiographic scans of both upper extremities, including both elbow and wrist joints • The OPO is responsible for providing the limb packing materials, such as a proper sterile container that can store the limb with ice water at the desired temperature

OPO would work with the local critical care team to maintain the donor on ventilator and stabilize with fluids and medications. Any arterial/venous lines on the upper limbs would be removed. The limb would be prepared using 4% chlorhexidine gluconate scrub and kept in a non-dependent position. An above elbow tourniquet would be placed anticipating the arrival of the procurement team [1, 18].

Ideally, to lessen ischemia time to the hand, the hand procurement team performed the arm retrieval first, followed by procurement of the other organs. If the patient was unstable, the other transplantation teams began the dissection. However, before cross clamping the aorta and icing the patient, tourniquet would be inflated. Limb retrieval began with a sterile technique with inflated tourniquet and the limb was disarticulated at the elbow joint. Later the protocol was modified to include more graft and skin from the upper arm. In the last patient the tourniquet was placed high in the upper arm and the arms were harvested at mid-upper arm level. Anterior and posterior circumferential dissections were made sharply and large vessels were dissected and cut at the level of the incision. The bone was exposed, soft tissues were protected using Hohman retractors, and the bone was cut with a Gigli saw or an oscillating saw. The tourniquet was left in place to prevent blood loss. Skin staplers were used to hasten the closure. The total time for procurement of an upper extremity was, on average, less than 20 min. The harvested limb was wrapped in moist gauze and put in a sterile container maintaining temperature at 4–6 °C. Further dissection continued at the back table, dissecting the brachial artery and vein, which were subsequently cannulated and connected to a continuous irrigation of University of Wisconsin (UW) solution. The limb was packaged and stored at 4C to 6C and prepared for transport back to the transplant center. Upon procurement of the donor limb, the donor body was fitted with a cosmetic prosthesis to allow the family an open-casket funeral [1, 9, 17, 18].

17.5 Recipient Selection

Prospective patients contacted the transplant coordinator to express their interest [16]. After ruling out the exclusion criteria (Table 17.2), the transplant coordinator and the transplant nurse met with the patient for a comprehensive assessment (Table 17.3). The patient would also undergo extensive evaluation by the transplant psychiatrist, transplant psychologist, and transplant social worker (Table 17.4). The potential adverse effects of immunosuppressive medications were also discussed with the patients (Table 17.5). The nurse coordinator would then present the summary of the medical data/tests/assays collected to each member of the selection committee. The selection committee consisted of hand surgeons, transplant physician, transplant surgeon, transplant coordinator, hand therapists, immunologists, tissue typing director, psychiatrist, psychologist, social worker, and any other specialist (cardiology, etc.) as needed. Each member of the selection committee presents their concerns and recommendations. The final decision is made by the primary investigators of the clinical trial. To date, committee member opinions have been nearly unanimous either for or against listing a specific candidate for transplantation.

All the potential recipient candidates were required to have at least attempted prosthetic use prior to transplant. This served as an exit plan in case of graft failure. Additionally,

Table 17.2 Exclusion criteria for recipient

• Pediatric amputee—due to ethical issues regarding consent and the potentially increased risk of post-transplant lymphoproliferative disorder (PTLD)
• Congenital defect—As the patient may not have adequate cerebral representation
• Inappropriate amputation (digit only or above elbow)
• Not medically appropriate for transplant (i.e., heart disease or viral status)
• Insufficient financial resources/no insurance
• Insufficient social support
• Inability to travel and stay in Louisville for three months with support person
• Poor surgical candidate
• Patients with blindness were excluded as sight provides the only means of protecting the hand during and before protective sensation is achieved
• Unrealistic expectations does not comprehend the risks involved

Table 17.3 Hand transplant candidate screening evaluation

- History and physical exam, including height and weight
- Serum pregnancy test for all female subjects of childbearing potential
- Complete blood count, differential, reticulocyte count, platelet count, ABO blood type
- Panel reactive antibody
- Liver functions tests, PT.PTT with INR
- Serum electrolytes and kidney function panel, urinalysis, and creatinine clearance test
- Infectious disease studies: HIV antigen, HTLV I–II antibody, antibodies to HIV 1 and 2, hepatitis A and C virus, syphilis, hepatitis B core antibody, and hepatitis B surface antigen titers, cytomegalovirus, HSV, toxoplasmosis, and VZV (IgG and IgM when indicated)
- Pulmonary function test and chest X-ray
- Electrocardiogram and MUGA or echocardiogram
- Ultrasound of the gallbladder (if indicated)
- Dexascan (if indicated)
- Panorex of all teeth, sinus X-ray (if indicated).
- Ophthalmologic (eye) examination
- CT scans/MRI studies as indicated by medical history and physical examination
- PSA blood test and any other cancer screening tests as recommended by the American Cancer Society based on age of the recipient
- SF36 Health Survey
- DASH: Disabilities of the Arm, Shoulder, and Hand Instrument

Table 17.4 Hand transplant candidate psychosocial evaluation

Transplant psychiatrist	Transplant psychologist	Social worker
Social history	Clinical interview	History of amputation
Accident history	Behavioral observations	Family history including presence/ absence of abuse
Medical history	Bender-gestalt	Work history
Substance abuse history	Wechsler abbreviated scale of intelligence (WASI)	Presence/absence of substance abuse/ gambling
Psychiatric history	Geriatric depression scale (GDS)	Discussion of available social support
Mental status exam	Beck hopelessness scale (BHS)	Discussion of expectations of hand transplant
Support system	Beck anxiety inventory (BAI)	
History of medical compliance	Minnesota multiphasic personality inventory (MMPI-2)	
Emotional/ cognitive preparedness for Tx DSM-IV diagnosis	Derriford appearance scale (DAS 59)	
	Incomplete sentences blank (ISB)	
	Draw A person test (DAP)	

Table 17.5 Common side effects of immunosuppressants discussed with candidates

Drug	Risks that are Rare (0–5%)	Risks that are less common (6% - 50%)	Risks that are common (over 50%)
Campath 1H	Allergic reaction	Fevers, chills, nausea, vomiting, infections and bone marrow suppression. Lymphocyte counts are reduced for weeks or months	
Simulect	Allergic reactions	Increased infections, anemia, headaches	Nausea, vomiting diarrhea, dizziness
FK506 (Tacrolimus, Prograf)	Elevated potassium level in your blood. You may need to be on a potassium-restricted diet	Signs of kidney dysfunction, such as a decrease in urine output, or swelling of hands and feet Tremor or a slight shaking of the hands High blood pressure Elevated blood sugars Nausea/vomiting/diarrhea Burning or tingling sensation on the skin, especially on the fingers or toes	Nausea/vomiting/diarrhea
Cyclosporine	Breast enlargement in males, lymphomas (tumors of the lymph glands), convulsions, liver toxicity	Acne Flushing Decreased white blood cell count Sinusitis A burning or tingling Sensation of the skin especially of the fingers and toes Growth of excess hair on your body and thickening of the hairs	Stomach discomforts (cramping, nausea, and/ or vomiting) Diarrhea Tremor or a slight shaking of your hands High blood pressure Swollen or bleeding gums Headache Burning sensation in eye

Table 17.5 (continued)

Drug	Risks that are Rare (0–5%)	Risks that are less common (6% - 50%)	Risks that are common (over 50%)
		Signs of kidney dysfunction, such as a decrease in urine output, fever, or swelling of your hands and feet.	Excessive tear production
Prednisone or Solumedrol (side effect strongly related to dose and length of administration	Stomach pain, rapid weight gain, nausea, poor wound healing	Decreased or blurred vision; frequent urination: increased thirst, loss of bone density, cataract formation Emotional problems	acne, development of a round or moon-shaped face, weight gain, high blood pressure, thinning of the bones (osteoporosis), increased risk of diabetes, and an increased risk of infection
Antithymocyte Globulin	Chest pain Wheezing or shortness of breath Rash Tumors, with extended use	Nausea Vomiting Diarrhea Increased blood pressure Increased pulse	Headache Fever or chills
Mycophenolate Mofetil	Stomach bleeding Lymphomas (Tumors of the lymph glands)	Lowered white blood count	Increased risk of infection Headache Diarrhea Nausea Vomiting

serious potential hand transplant candidates were required to meet or have a phone call with one or more of our current hand transplant recipients. These interactions have provided data for the selection process as well [1, 16, 17].

17.6 Recipient Surgery

The recipient was notified immediately when the donor family's consent was obtained. The recipient was admitted to our hand transplant center and worked up for surgery. The patient was placed in a terminally cleaned room with a high efficiency particulate air filter. The nurse would perform an initial assessment of the patient including a psychosocial evaluation of the patient and the family [1, 17].

Once the limb was on way, the recipient was administered anesthesia, prepped, and kept ready. On arrival of the donor limb the recipient team started the surgery, working the distal stump and tagging vessels, nerves, and tendons. Another team (donor team) worked on the back table to prepare the donor limb for transplant. Flaps were planned on donor limb, trimming excess skin. Bones, tendons, and nerves were kept up to adequate length depending on their respective status in the recipient. Chilled Ringer's lactate was used to flush out the UW solution from the donor graft. Biopsy specimens were taken from the donor and recipient's dorsal and volar skin, muscle, bone, tendon, nerve, artery, and vein and a donor core bone marrow for baseline histological assessment.

The technical aspects of hand transplantation are the same as replantation except for a few differences. While tissue deficiencies are common in replantation, transplants have tissue excess. This allows for stronger Pulvertaft repair for tendons enabling early active motion. The nerves can be repaired tension free and vein grafts for vascular repairs are seldom needed. The surgical steps were as follows [1, 17] (Fig. 17.1).

The ulna was fixed by 6 or 7 holes, 3.5 mm dynamic compression plates on the ulnar volar surface followed by fixation of the radius ventrally or radially using a similar plate. As prolonged warm ischemia could potentiate inflammatory responses and acute rejection, bone fixation was immediately followed by arterial and a few concomitant vein anastomoses. The two main arteries and at least one or two veins were anastomosed. In patients #4 and #5 brachial artery was harvested and a single arterial anastomosis was achieved at the antecubital fossa. Early vein repair decreased the pressure in the vascular tree and the remaining large veins were clipped until the end of the procedure to minimize blood loss.

After the repair of the tendons, nerve repair followed. At this point, the decision for the need for tendon attachment, grafts, or transfers was made as appropriate. Primary tendon transfers may be needed depending on the status of the donor muscles. Finally, the remainder veins were anastomosed. Excess of skin allows for planning of adequate flaps to cover without any tension or pressure. The incision on donor and recipient was offset by 90 degrees, allowing for interdigitating flaps. Forearm was covered in non-adherent dressing and hand was immobilized in long arm splint in a functional position.

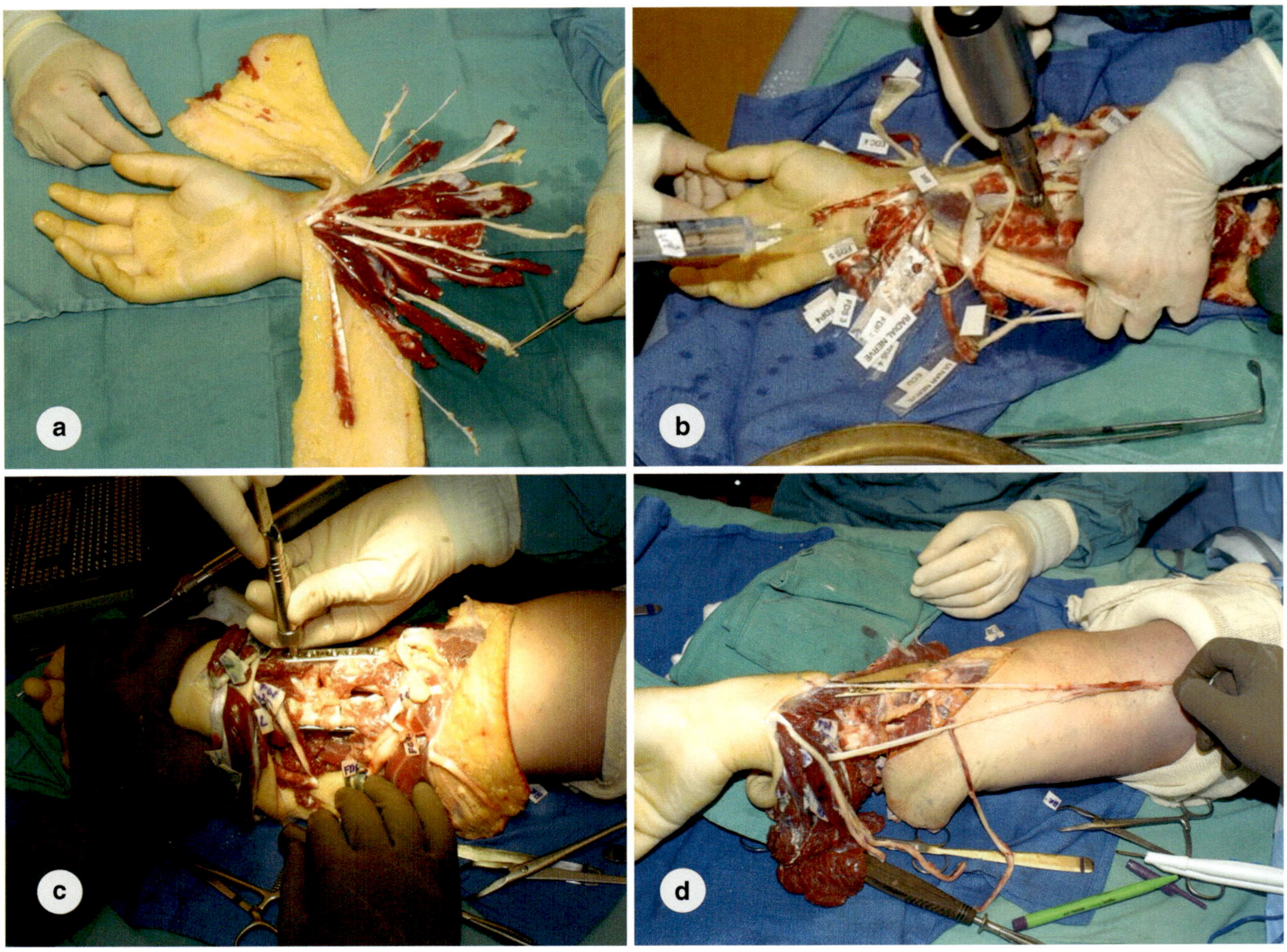

Fig. 17.1 Intraoperative pictures of recipient surgery. (**a**) The donor hand with all tendons, nerves, and vessels dissected out. (**b**) Osteotomy of donor and recipient bones done at appropriate levels. (**c**) Osteosynthesis with a 6-hole plate. (**d**) Donor and recipient tendons being prepared for Pulvertaft weave

The last two patients were included in an adipose derived stromal vascular fraction cell trial for studying tolerance induction. These patients underwent fat harvest after anesthesia was induced. About 60 ml of harvested fat tissue was centrifuged and processed in the operating room and the cell yield was standardized [19]. The specimens were checked for endotoxins and gram staining was performed. In our last patient who was a bilateral recipient a total of 70 million stromal vascular fraction SVF cells were injected in 30 aliquots on each side. In our ninth patient the cells were injected at the beginning of the transplant and in our tenth and last patient the cells were injected after the procedure was finished.

In order to keep the traffic in the operating room to a minimum, the surgery was telecasted live at an auditorium, where fellows, residents, and visitors could watch the procedure live.

17.7 Postoperative Care

Postoperatively, a continuous pulse oximeter device and a skin temperature device were placed on the transplanted limb and hourly monitoring was performed by an experienced nurse. The temperature in the recipient's room was maintained at 24 °C. The patient stays in an intensive care unit, and they were not allowed to consume caffeine, and smoking was prohibited. Pain control, nutrition, activity level, bowel and bladder function, and anti-embolic measures were continuously assessed by the nursing staff. The nurse also coordinated visits by the necessary personnel and family members to minimizing traffic in the room [17]. The initial braces are applied and therapy is begun when the patient is brought to a regular bed.

17.8 Immunosuppression

The first patient received Basiliximab (Simulect®, Novartis Pharmaceutical Corp, East Hanover, NJ), an interleukin-2 receptor chain blocking antibody as an inducting agent and tacrolimus (FK506; Prograf, Astellas, Deerfield, IL) along with MMF (CellCept, Roche, Nutley, NJ) and prednisone was used for maintenance immunosuppression [20]. For the second patient we used alemtuzumab (Campath 1H, Millennium Pharmaceutical Corp, Cambridge, MA), a monoclonal antibody that blocks the CD52 receptor as the induction immunosuppression. Maintenance was started with tacrolimus and MMF. A single dose of prednisone was given at surgery [21]. A similar alemtuzumab induction with tacrolimus and MMF with steroid avoidance was used for patients #3, #4, #5 and without steroid avoidance for patient #6. For patients #7, #8, #9, and #10, we used antithymocyte globulin (ATG) for induction and tacrolimus, MMF, and prednisone for maintenance [16, 20–23].

As our program evolved, we adapted different measures to reduce the immunosuppressive dose. Tacrolimus was reduced to tailor in such a way that minimal dose needed to keep patient off rejection. MMF was replaced with sirolimus (Rapamycin, Rapamune, Wyeth-Ayerst Labs, Philadelphia, PA) whenever possible. Additionally, patients were weaned off steroids as tolerated [22, 23].

Table 17.6 shows immunosuppression regimen given to our patients. The immunosuppression medications used for maintenance along with their target levels, dosing adjustments, and monitoring technique is listed in Table 17.7.

Table 17.6 Immunosuppression regimen given to patients

	Induction	Early maintenance	Currently on	Status of allograft
Patient #1 1999	Basiliximab	FK 506, MMF, prednisone	FK 506—2 mg Sirolimus—3 mg MMF—1440 mg Prednisone—None	Doing well
Patient #2 2001	Alemtuzumab	FK 506, MMF, single dose prednisone	FK 506—4 mg Sirolimus—3 mg MMF—None Prednisone—2.5 mg	Chronic rejection
Patient #3 2006	Alemtuzumab	FK 506, MMF, 506—None Sirolimus—2.5 mg MMF—1440 mg Prednisone—2.5 mg	Chronic rejection and deceased	Deceased
Patient #4 2008	Alemtuzumab	FK 506, MMF	Graft loss	Amputated
Patient #5 2008	Alemtuzumab	FK 506, MMF	FK 506—4 mg Sirolimus—5 mg MMF—1440 mg Prednisone—5 mg	Amputated
Patient #6 2010	Alemtuzumab	FK 506, MMF, prednisone	Deceased	Deceased
Patient #7 2011	ATG	FK 506, MMF, prednisone	FK 506—3 mg Sirolimus—3 mg MMF—None Prednisone—None	Doing well
Patient #8 2012	ATG	FK 506, MMF, prednisone	FK 506—3 mg Sirolimus—2 mg MMF—None Prednisone—None	Doing well
Patient #9 2014	ATG	FK 506, MMF, prednisone	Graft loss	Amputated
Patient #10 2016	ATG	FK 506, MMF, prednisone	FK 506—0.5 mg Sirolimus—1 mg MMF—None Prednisone—5 mg	Doing well

Table 17.7 Maintenance immunosuppressive medications monitoring and dose adjustment

Medication	Target level	Monitoring	Indication for dosage adjustment
Tacrolimus	Twelve-hour whole-blood trough concentration 10–15 ng/ml during months 1–6, then 5–10 ng/ml thereafter	Incstar ProTrac II enzyme-linked immunosorbent assay (Diasorin, Stillwater, MN)	If the 12 h trough is >20% above or below the target range
MMF	Trough plasma concentrations 3–5 ng/ml	EMIT 2000 assay [Dade Behring, Deerfield, IL]	If white cell count counts <4.0, MMF dose was reduced 50%, and at counts <2.5, MMF was discontinued
Methyl prednisone	At 2 mg/kg/day, which was decreased to 10 mg/day by month 3	Not monitored	
Sirolimus	4–12 ng/ml		

17.9 Antimicrobial Prophylaxis

Cephazolin was used for perioperative prophylaxis in all patients. Standard post-transplant prophylaxis included trimethoprim/ sulfamethoxazole, and nystatin swish and swallow. For prophylaxis against CMV, 5 mg of ganciclovir/kg (Cytovene, Hoffmann-La Roche, Nutley, NJ) was given intravenously every 12 h while the patient was hospitalized, followed by oral therapy (1000 mg t.i.d) until 3 months after transplantation.

17.10 Rehabilitation Protocol

The rehabilitation protocols were akin to the one for replantation [20]. We began early mobilization of the transplanted limbs within the first couple of days. After the first dressing change at 48–72 h, the patient was fitted with a dynamic crane-extension outrigger splint that mimics intrinsic function of the hand. With wrist in slight extension, the metacarpophalangeal joints were placed in 50–70 degree of flexion and the interphalangeal joints were held at in extension [16, 17]. The thumb was held in a balance between radial and palmar abduction. This splint reduced the force on the repaired fingers, minimizing risk of tendon rupture.

After the first month, the patient was transitioned into a hand-based anti-claw splint. Wrist and forearm range of motion were initiated at this time. Subsequently, other therapeutic modalities were added depending upon the level of healing and usage gained. At three months, a dynamic wrist extension splint was applied by connecting it to the anti-claw splint. This would strengthen the wrist flexors and extensors by allowing wrist flexion against resistance and assistive active extension. Light weights were also added to isolate and strengthen specific muscle groups such as the wrist flexor and extensors. Patient would alternate the use of this splint and the crane-extension outrigger splint. The anti-claw splint was worn at rest [16, 17].

17.11 Functional Assessment

Functional outcomes were assessed by a multitude of parameters. Grip strength was measured using a Jamar dynamometer and pinch strength (tip, three-jaw chuck, and key pinch) was measured using a pinchometer. Range of motion (ROM) including total active and passive ROM was measured according to the American Society for Surgery of the Hand (ASSH) guidelines. Tinel's sign was assessed until it advanced to the fingertips. Thereafter, Semmes-Weinstein monofilament testing, vibration, and static and moving 2-point discrimination were performed.

To assess integrated upper extremity and global hand function, Carroll test was performed. It is a measure of thirty-three tasks performed by the patient and scored by two independent observers leading to a possible maximum of 99 points. A score ≥ 85 is considered excellent, 75–84 is considered good, 51–74 is considered fair, and poor if <51 [24].

A summary of the current functional results of our patients is shown in Table 17.8.

Table 17.8 Current status of functional outcomes

Patient and duration	Carrol test	Grip strength	Sensation	ROM
Patient #1	61	7 lbs. on the transplanted left hand compared to 27 lbs. on the right	Two-point discrimination >15 mm but he can localize all fingertips He can detect hot, cold, and pain in the transplanted areas	Mild stiffness in the PIP joints (+3 to 73 deg. in long finger) but could make a near fist. Thumb had no active IP flexion
Patient #2	48	13 lbs. on transplanted left hand compared to 98 lbs. on the right	He could detect deep pressure sensation only with the 6.65 SW filaments	Worsening of the digit flexion. Unable to perform 2-point and 3-point pinch on the left
Patient #3	Deceased secondary to complications of squamous cell carcinoma 9 years post-transplant			
Patient #4	Transplanted hand amputated 9 months post-transplant			
Patient #5	Transplanted hand amputated 9 years post-transplant			
Patient #6	Deceased 9.5 years post-transplant			
Patient #7	73	40 lbs. on the transplanted left compared to 75 lbs. on the right	2PD > 15 mm in the thumb, small finger, and index finger. Unable to detect 2PD on ring and long finger He could detect S-W 4.56 (loss of protective sensation) with inconsistent touch localization	Full passive flexion and extension of the fingers and good ROM in thumb Palm to pulp 0 cm Thumb opposition 1.5 cm from small finger
Patient #8	79	25 lbs. on the transplanted right compared 116 lbs. on the left	2PD > 15 mm in all digits S-W test 3.61 (diminished light touch) in the thumb, index, and ring finger ulnarly	Full passive flexion and extension of all digits Thumb total active motion was 30 degrees. Active palm to pulp 2–3.5 cm
Patient #9	Transplanted hand amputated 5 days post-transplant			
Patient #10	60 (right) 10 (left)	17 lbs. on right 7 lbs. on left	Tinel's was still advancing at the tips but there was no response on the fingertips on Semmes-Weinstein or two-point discrimination testing	Right: Wrist—Was near normal Fingers—Full flexion but extension was limited clawing present Palm to pulp 0 cm Left: Wrist—Limited in flexion but good extension Fingers—Palm to pulp 1.0–3.4 cm

17.12 Immunological Monitoring

Skin was monitored in postoperative days 0, 5, 7, 10, 14, 21, and 30 and monthly thereafter. Any rash developed in the transplanted part was a concern for rejection. In case of maculopapular rash, edema, scaling, or blistering, skin biopsies were obtained. Additionally, all transplant recipients underwent skin biopsy during their annual evaluation. Skin biopsies were taken from the volar and dorsal surfaces of hand and forearm. Hand volume measurements were also used to check the edema in the transplanted hands. The family was taught on how to perform skin examination and hand volume measurements at home and report it back to the transplant team.

Presence of edema, erythema, escharification, and necrosis pointed toward acute rejection (AR). Scoring for acute rejection (AR) was accomplished using established criteria of acute skin ejection in VCA (Fig. 17.2); Grade 0: no or rare inflammatory cells, Grade I: mild perivascular infiltration without involvement of epidermis, Grade II: moderate perivascular inflammation with/without mild epidermal or adnexal involvement. No epidermal dyskeratosis or apoptosis, Grade III: dense inflammation and epidermal involvement with apoptosis, dyskeratosis, and/or keratinolysis, Grade IV: necrotizing acute rejection with frank necrosis of epidermis or other skin structures [25, 26].

Biopsies were also examined for evidence of chronic rejection (CR), such as intimal hyperplasia and subintimal foamy histiocytes in the vessels. Histologic evaluations of deep biopsies of skin and small arteries indicate some level of arteriopathy is present in all of our patients. Clinical diagnosis of graft versus host disease (GVHD) was done based on previously established criteria [27].

Monoclonal antibodies specific for host or donor class I or class II antigens and donor specific antibodies (DSA) were used to assess donor chimerism. The DSA antibody panel consisted of antibodies specific for T cells (CD3, CD4, CD8), B cells (CD19), NK cells (CD56), and myeloid markers (CD33, CD45).

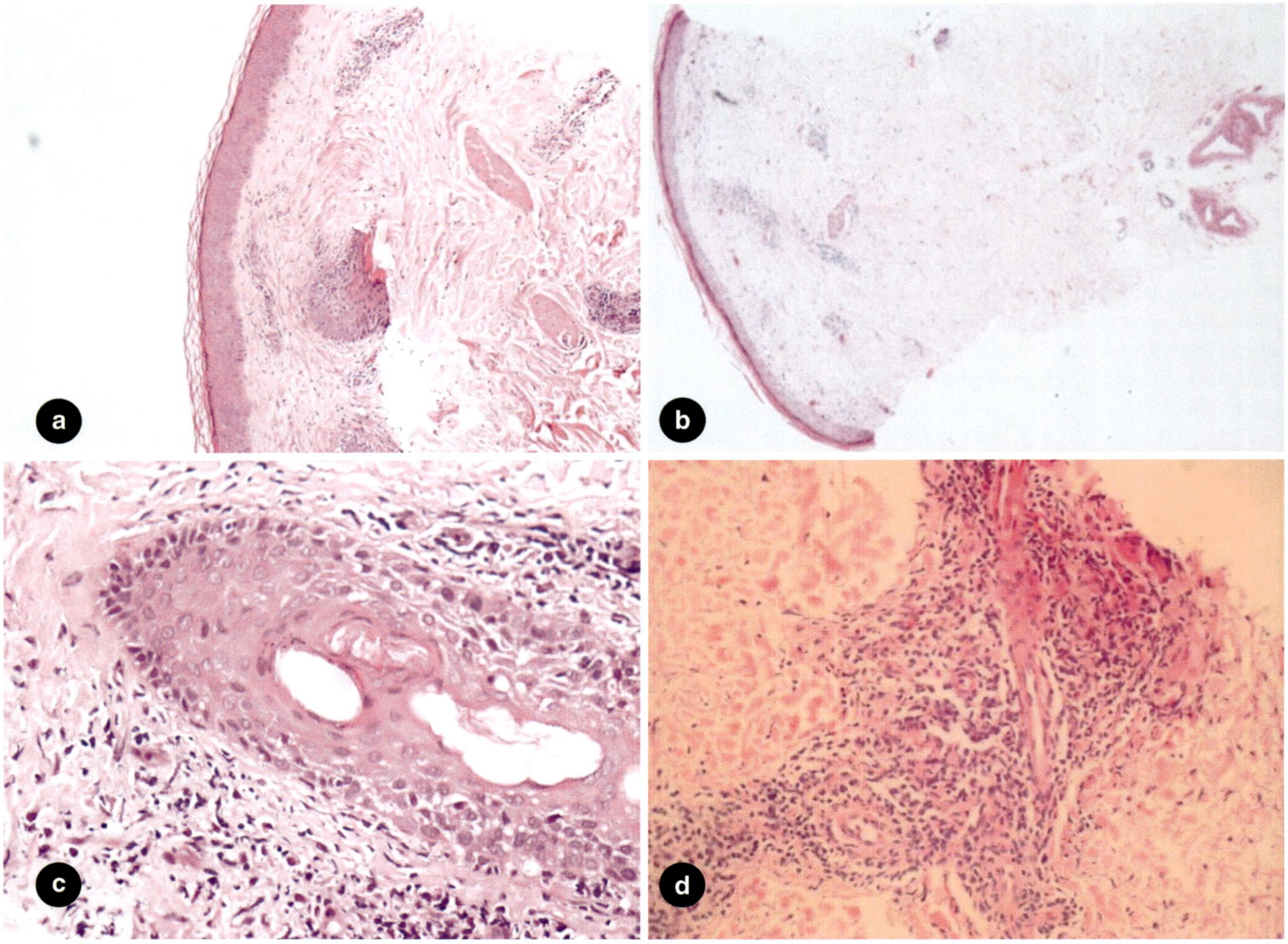

Fig. 17.2 Histopathology from skin demonstrating various grades of acute rejection (AR). (**a**) Grade I: mild perivascular infiltration without involvement of epidermis, (**b**) grade II: moderate perivascular inflammation with/without mild epidermal or adnexal involvement. No epidermal dyskeratosis or apoptosis, (**c**) higher magnification of grade II. (**d**) Grade III: dense inflammation and epidermal involvement with apoptosis, dyskeratosis, and/or keratinolysis

17.13 Monitoring Vasculopathy

The vasculopathy was monitored using CT angiogram and Duplex sonography. The CT angiogram was done with contrast injection to study the details about the arteries in cross sections as well as a 3D reconstruction. Any pathology or narrowing of the vessels was detected by the radiologist. B-mode duplex ultrasonography obtained the image of the vessels evaluated and the Doppler detected the velocity and the direction of blood flow.

Louisville program also imaged the blood vessels of hand transplant patients using a Vevo 2100® (VisualSonics, Toronto, ON, Canada) ultrasound biomicroscopy device which produces high-resolution images of the vessels. Ultrasound biomicroscopy (UBM) operates at 740 fps frequency frame rates and uses a solid-state array transducer that has 30-micron resolution. 20 MHz to 70 MHz probes are available. While the lower resolution probe (20 MHz) has a penetration to visualize most vessels, the higher resolution probes (70 MHz) produce the most detailed images, but reduced penetration [28]. The high-resolution imaging allows for measuring vessel wall thickness, the amount of blood flow through the artery and can provide early detection of vasculopathy in transplant patients. Our protocol reported in first six patients was using standardized measurements of the brachial artery at 3 cm distal to the antecubital crease, radial and ulnar arteries at 3 cm proximal to the wrist crease, palmar arch artery at mid-palm, and digital arteries at proximal phalanx of the ring finger and thumb. Our study determined the intimal hyperplasia and interstitial fibrosis which are standard features of chronic rejection can be detected earlier than conventional surveillance methods such as the radiological imaging or skin biopsies [28].

17.14 Tolerization of VCA with Adipose SVF

Louisville VCA program ran a clinical trial to test the therapeutic efficacy of freshly isolated, autologous stromal vascular fraction (SVF) cells in hand transplantation. This five-year project supported by AFIRM II grant aimed at induction of tolerance and prevention of rejection in hand transplantation. The stromal vascular fraction (SVF) contains a variety of immunomodulatory cell types that regulate immune homeostasis in adipose tissues [15, 16]. After harvesting adipose tissue under local or general anesthesia, the fat tissue is centrifuged to obtain the SVF cells [15]. Following centrifugation, three distinct layers are seen. The top layer consists of fat layer, the middle layer is the aqueous layer, and the bottom layer is the pellet that contains the stromal vascular fraction with immunomodulatory cell types. The SVF is harvested and administered within couple of hours without the need for enrichment or expansion.

We applied SVF cells in our last two transplant patients. One was at the beginning of the surgery and the other at the end of the surgery. In both instances endotoxin testing was done, and the patient's own cells were given in a standardized cell count dose. In our ninth transplant patient, 30 aliquots of SVF cells were injected at the thenar, hypothenar, and dorsal surface of the hand as well as volar and dorsal muscles of forearm (Fig. 17.3a, b). We were not able to observe the outcome because of early graft failure, but we had concerns that the cells got washed out with venous bleeding during the procedure. In the tenth patient, a total of 70 million cells were injected in both arms in 30 aliquots on the left and 40 aliquots on the right (Fig. 17.3c). This patient had no graft rejection. This was partly attributed to her old age as immune response gets weaker. However, the patient coincidentally had 6/6 match with the donor. We also used SVF cells during a rejection episode in the second patient. The temperature and swelling in the hand decreased the next day. Skin biopsy was not taken before the injections, and we had no comparison of before and after SVF application.

SVF cells and the related research are relatively new field. Adipose derived SVF cells' ability to regulate the immune response, inflammation, and wound healing wherever the response is needed, as the cells travel in the body, make the SVF cells an interesting topic for further research. Although our experience with adipose derived SVF cells is incidental only, these cells may be significant in achieving tolerance in transplant surgery [16].

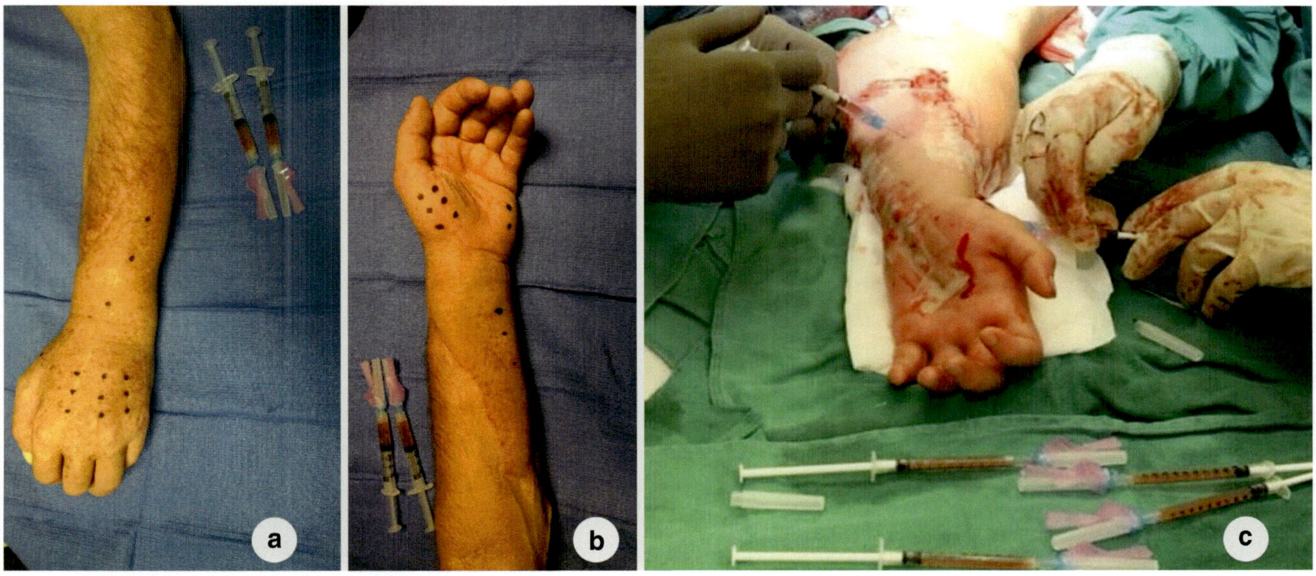

Fig. 17.3 Stromal vascular fraction injection to the transplanted hand. (**a** and **b**) 30 aliquots of SVF cells were injected at the thenar, hypothenar, and dorsal surface of the hand as well as volar and dorsal muscles of forearm in patient #9. (**c**) 30 aliquots on the left and 40 aliquots on the right injected in patient #10

17.15 Patient Profiles and Outcomes

17.15.1 Patient #1

Our first patient who received a hand transplant in January 1999 was also the first-hand transplant patient of the United States [23]. He was a 37-year-old male working as an administrator of a paramedic company. He had an amputation of his dominant left hand after a blast injury 14 years prior to his transplant in 1985. His past medical history was significant for type II diabetes with no secondary complications. He was a 20 pack year former smoker who quit three years earlier. He used an Otto Bock myoelectric prosthesis (Otto Bock, Inc., Minneapolis, USA) during work hours. He had passed all other medical or psychiatric evaluations [23].

He underwent a left-sided hand transplant on January 24, 1999. After bone fixation using plates and screws the tendon grafts from the lower extremity were needed to bridge the distal donor tendons to the recipient muscles. Skin grafting was needed to cover the defect on the forearm upon closure, which was excised later in the first year.

The immunosuppression was initiated using 20 mg of basiliximab, tacrolimus, MMF (1 g twice a day), and steroids. Tacrolimus levels were targeted to 15–20 ng/ml for the first 6 months. Steroids were tapered to maintenance dose of 10 mg of prednisone by the end of 3 months and 7.5 mg at the end of 6 months.

The patient developed CMV infection 3 months after the transplant and this was treated with Ganciclovir. He experienced 3 acute rejection episodes (one was grade 2 and two were grade 3) in the first year and these were successfully treated with methylprednisolone. After these episodes he had no other rejection.

His functional recovery was smooth after physical therapy. His Carroll score was 65 at 6 months and it improved to 72 between years 6 and 9. The score slightly decreased in the last 10 years and was 61 at his final full evaluation (Table 17.8). At 20 year follow-up, he had mild stiffness in the PIP joints (+3 to 73 deg. in long finger) but could make a near fist. Thumb had no active IP flexion. He had mild increase in volume of the hand but no edema or rashes were noted. His grip strength is 1/6th of the normal side and lateral pinch strength was 7 lbs. on the transplanted left hand compared to 27 lbs. on the right. His sensibility was difficult to assess as stimulation caused tingling throughout the hand and interfered with examination. Two-point discrimination was always >15 mm but he can localize all fingertips correctly and can detect hot, cold, and pain in the transplanted areas.

At his 20 year follow-up he was on tacrolimus 1 mg bid, sirolimus 3 mg daily. His skin biopsies showed grade 0 in dorsum of hand and grade 1 on his volar forearm. His diabetes was under control with long acting and fast acting insulin. He was on atorvastatin for hyperlipidemia, and losartan and amlodipine to treat high blood pressure and to help protect the kidneys from damage due to diabetes. His Doppler exam showed mild to moderate arterial disease in the left digital arteries. His class 1 and class 2 DSA were negative. At his annual exam at 20 years, he had decreased renal function with BUN 25 mg/dl, creatinine: 2.29 mg/dl, and GFR: 30 ml/min.

17.15.2 Patient #2

The second patient was a 36-year-old male who injured his nondominant left arm in a fireworks accident. He had a left mid-forearm level amputation. He had no medical problems, and he was not a smoker. He wore a cable hook prosthesis throughout day for 3 months and was able to perform all activities of daily living and work tasks including his hobby of motorcycle riding [22].

He underwent the transplant surgery on February 6, 2001 about 4–1/2 years after his injury. A mid-forearm level transplant was performed without any complications [22]. His induction was achieved with basiliximab, tacrolimus and prednisone but he developed diabetes due to high tacrolimus levels. Soon he was switched from tacrolimus to MMF and sirolimus to reduce the dose of tacrolimus. In the first year, the patient had 5 episodes of acute rejection which were treated with methylprednisolone [22]. At postoperative year 5, he developed another grade 3 acute rejection and was treated with a T cell depleting antithymocyte globulin (Thymoglobulin®). Another rejection episode happened 7 years after the transplant due to noncompliance with his medicines. He had class I donor antigen specific antibodies (DSA) that responded well to increased prednisone treatment. He developed osteonecrosis of the hips at years 2 and 6, most likely related to the course of years of acute rejection and its treatment, and underwent total hip arthroplasty.

His functional recovery improved gradually until the seventh year. His Carrol score was 50 at first year and 57 at the seventh year. On his last full evaluation at 18 years postoperatively, he had swelling on and off and he was using his isotoner edema glove. He was feeling his hand was tighter and harder to use. He reported no change in the functional use of the hand overall even when the swelling is down. On examination, his left hand showed rash and pitting edema up to the forearm. With the volume measurements left hand was 717 ml compared to 572 ml of the right hand and 52 ml more compared to the previous exam. There was worsening of the digit flexion and some improvement in extension possibly related to the dorsal edema. There was 5–35 degrees of decrease in the active and passive range of motion in the long, ring, and small fingers. His Carroll test score was 48. His grip strength was 13 lbs. and lateral pinch strength was 5.3 lbs. on the left compared to 98 lbs. and 21 lbs. on the right. He was unable to perform 2-point and 3-point pinch on the left. His sensibility at the fingertips was detecting deep pressure sensation only with the 6.65 S-W filaments.

At his 18th year annual visit, he was on sirolimus 5 mg daily, tacrolimus 2 mg two times daily, prednisone 2.5 mg daily. He was also taking metformin and glimepiride or type II diabetes, lisinopril, amlodipine, and terazosin for high blood pressure, simvastatin, aspirin, ranitidine, calcium, melatonin, multivitamins, and hydrocodone 5 mg daily. He was negative for class 1 and 2 DSA. His Doppler exam and CTA were normal. His biopsies revealed grade 2 acute rejection at dorsum of hand and forearm. He was started on prednisone taper. Three months later he developed ulceration on the ring finger, which was treated with doxycycline, trimethoprim/sulfamethoxazole, and later linezolid. There was another episode of swelling which was being treated with another round of prednisone taper.

17.15.3 Patient #3

Our third recipient was a 54-year-old male patient who lost his right dominant hand in industrial press accident in 1973. He was employed as a production and maintenance supervisor. He had a history of mitral valve prolapse and spontaneous pneumothorax and history or smoking which he quit five years ago. He was using a cable hook prosthesis which he wore full time at work and part time at home. His main goal in undergoing a hand transplant procedure was to be able to throw a football with his 10-year-old son [18].

He underwent a hand transplant surgery on November 2006. Induction was done with a single 30-mg dose of alemtuzumab and 3 doses of methylprednisolone in the perioperative period. Two drug regimen of tacrolimus and MMF was used for maintenance [18]. A severe neutropenia developed in the second month. Filgrastim was initiated and the prophylactic ganciclovir, trimethoprim/sulfamethoxazole, and MMF were halted. Two weeks later he developed CMV colitis and a grade 3 acute rejection of the transplanted hand. These complications were treated with intravenous ganciclovir, and topical tacrolimus and clobetasol.

During routine bloodwork 23 months after the transplant, an unusual B-cell clone and a monoclonal T cell clone were detected in the blood. After negative positron emission tomography and computed tomography but a positive bone marrow biopsy an initial diagnosis of post-transplant lymphoproliferative disorder (PTLD) was made. His tacrolimus was reduced and MMF was discontinued. After further monitoring of clinical status and review of histological specimens that were typical of a marginal zone lymphoma (MZL), and after identifying the B-cell clone in pretransplant frozen peripheral blood leukocyte specimens, the group decided that this is an MZL and not a PTLD. Unfortunately, after the immunosuppression was decreased due to the suspicion of PTLD the patient started a severe episode of rejection. This episode resolved when immunosuppression was restored.

His functional recovery was best at first year with a Carroll test score of 57. His sensibility testing showed >15 mm two-point discrimination but he had protective sensation in the fingers. His range of motion worsened in the hand over time and with chronic rejection. At his last full functional evaluation, he reported 2/10 to 7/10 pain at rest and 5/10 to 8/10 pain with use of his hand, on the VAS pain scale. He had hypersensitivity in the thenar eminence, fingertips, and dorsal web. He was feeling tingling in the fingers and palm with stimulation. He reported 10/10 hypersensitivity if any area of his hand was touched or exposed to cold air. He had similar hypersensitivity at his fingertips. Despite these complaints he still was using his hand as a stabilizer in bimanual task as long as he was wearing his cotton jersey glove. In winter months he wore a fleece mitt over the glove. We discussed amputation with him, and he felt he still could use his hand some to assist, and he had concerns about the level of amputation and the cost of a new prosthesis.

On year 11 evaluation he had widespread red and brownish mottled spots on the skin and contracted transplanted hand (Fig. 17.4a). He had adducted fingers with flexion contractures of the PIP joints. His TAM was 60 to 77 degrees in the fingers and 15 degrees in the thumb. His sensibility was intact for cold and hot and pain. S-W monofilament testing showed 6.65 on the thumb, 4.31 on the palm and the dorsal web, and no response in the fingers. He was unable to grip but he had a 2-point pinch of 2.5 lbs. in the IF and the thumb. His Carroll test was unchanged at 36 points compared to a year earlier.

In November of 2017, at year 8 post-transplant a whole-body PET/CT scan was performed as part of a routine study. This study showed he had a skin lesion in his back which was diagnosed as squamous cell carcinoma on biopsy. The skin lesion was excised, and the defect was covered with local flaps. In December of 2017, enlarged lymph nodes were observed in the left axillary region. Sentinel lymph node biopsy proved squamous cell carcinoma. He underwent a radiation treatment. He was hospitalized in his residential state and was investigated for any other source for the cancer. No other source was found. He passed away on December 3, 2018, in Detroit secondary to complications of cancer.

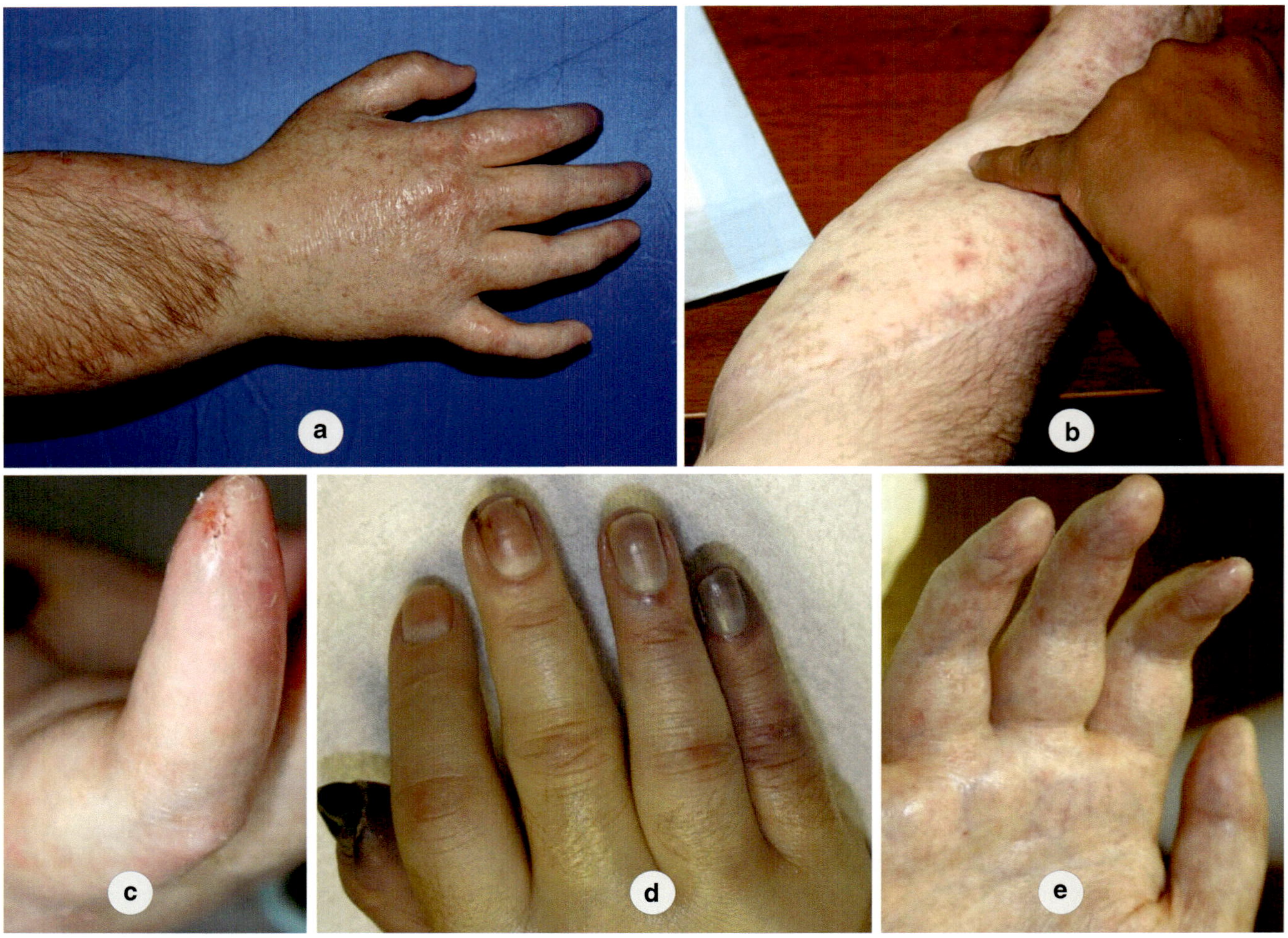

Fig. 17.4 Complications. (**a**) Acute rejection, (**b**) blanching rash suggestive of acute rejection, (**c**) loss of nail, (**d**) fingertip ischemia, (**e**) spider veins

17.15.4 Patient #4

The fourth patient of the program was a 32-year-old male who had an amputation at the distal third of his forearm after a grenade launcher had misfired two years earlier [29]. He was right-hand dominant and was using a cable prosthesis only when lifting weights. He was not using his myoelectric prosthesis or cable prosthesis routinely because he felt they slowed him with activities of daily living. He was feeling independent with ADLs at home and at work without any assistive devices. He used his stump for stabilizing objects. He had no health issues other than hypothyroidism.

A distal forearm level hand transplant was performed in July 2008. The bone was fixed with two plates and the radial and ulnar arteries were dissected up to the brachial artery and a single anastomosis was done at the antecubital level. Immunosuppression was induced using alemtuzumab, MMF, and a short course of steroid. He was maintained with tacrolimus and MMF shortly after bone healing. In his first year, three minor episodes of skin rash were treated successfully with topical tacrolimus and MMF [29].

Nine months following the transplant, he presented with bruising of the forearm and severe ischemia of the hand (Fig. 17.5a, b). During the exploration of the forearm thick scar was found around the vessels and the arteries were peeling from a bed of tubular scar. Despite the release of the arteries during exploration, circulation did not restore. Two days later a decision was made to amputate the transplanted hand [30]. In the histological specimens thickening of the vessel wall and intimal hyperplasia were discovered. Interestingly the skin biopsies before amputation were negative for rejection and he did not have DSA class I or class II antigens until several days after the amputation. While the intimal hyperplasia was likely related to an immune response, it was not clear if it was a result of humoral or cellular rejection, tissue response to ischemia, or of stripping of vessels during the surgery.

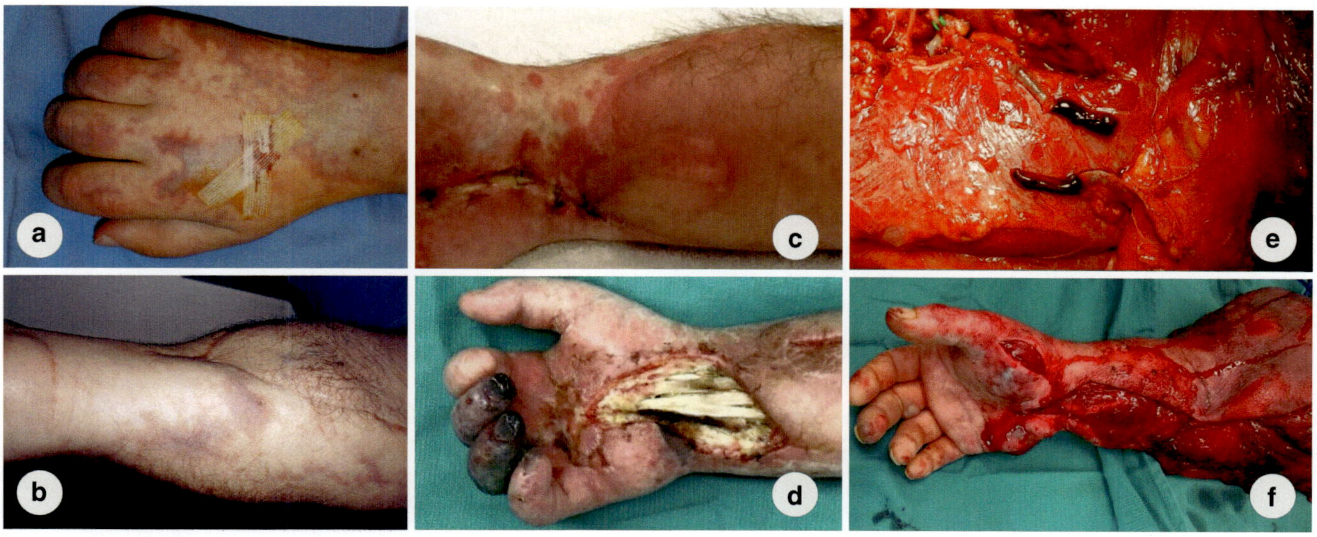

Fig. 17.5 Transplanted graft which was lost. (**a** and **b**) Nine months following the transplant, patient #4 presented with bruising of the forearm and severe ischemia of the hand. Despite surgical intervention, the graft was lost. (**c**) Patient #5 had a non-healing wound following carpal tunnel and Guyon's canal release. (**d**) Following debridement and negative pressure wound therapy, the fingers developed ischemia which ultimately led to amputation. (**e**) Third day after the transplantation, patient #9 developed cyanosis of his transplanted hand and intraoperatively, the veins were noted to be thrombosed. (**f**) Despite further fasciotomies the circulation declined, leading to amputation

17.15.5 Patient #5

Our fifth recipient was a 43-year-old male patient who lost his hand during an industrial injury when a furnace door crushed and burned his right hand two and a half years before the transplant [30]. He was using his prosthesis for mowing grass, driving, and during therapy exercises for about four hours a day. He had no significant medical problems. His hope in seeking hand transplantation was to return to employment at the same company in production and assembly of engine blocks.

He had a successful transplant on November 28, 2008 [30]. His induction was done using alemtuzumab, and he was on tacrolimus and MMF for maintenance. He had four episodes of grade II acute rejection in the first year. He was prophylactically switched back to standard sirolimus, mycophenolate mofetil (MMF), and prednisone at 7 months.

In November 2010, after driving 16 hours straight from our center to his hometown he started having chest pain and dyspnea. He was on medicine for hypertension, hypercholesterolemia, and depression. He was admitted and a pulmonary CT angiogram showed right pulmonary thromboembolism involving the distal right pulmonary artery extending into the right upper lobe. The patient was placed on heparin and the symptoms resolved. He was then discharged on warfarin. There were no other concerns with his treatment in the first six years other than slight decrease in renal function and increase in his hemoglobin A1c levels. He was maintained on tacrolimus, MMF, and 5 mg of prednisone. The patient underwent bariatric surgery at 3 and 5 years for weight control and tolerated the procedures well.

At year 6 postoperatively, he developed multiple macular rashes over his transplanted limb. Skin biopsy revealed modified Banff grade II rejection response. De novo Class II C1q and DSA were detected in the blood. He was converted back to sirolimus, MMF, and prednisolones for 18 months. His skin biopsy revealed similar changes with mild perivascular lymphocytic infiltrates suggesting Banff grade I mild acute cell mediated rejection.

He had initial improvement in his hand function. His Carroll score was 69 at two years. He had incomplete thumb abduction and lack of full pronation. At 5 years, his Carroll score increased to 76. However, his hand function decreased after multiple rejection episodes.

At late seventh year postoperative follow-up the patient had a recurrent rejection after performing CPR on a collapsed coworker. He was having swelling and stiffness of the hand. His skin biopsy revealed similar changes to the previous biopsy and the IHC staining revealed presence of C4D infiltrates along with the CD34 deposits across the graft capillaries. The patient was hospitalized and was treated with antithymocyte globulin (ATG) [1.5 mg/kg X 5 doses] and a steroid taper. Despite the symptomatic improvement the hand swelling did not turn to the preinjury level.

Early in the eighth year, the patient underwent a rotator cuff surgery on the native left shoulder and liposuction of his abdomen. Shortly after, he developed shooting pain in transplanted hand with swelling and rash, which responded to a prednisone taper.

At his last complete functional evaluation at 8 years and 9 months prior to his amputation, patient had a mottled, swollen, cool, and red to purplish hand. He was more sensitive to cold temperatures and had lost range of motion in the digits especially in the thumb. His hand volume was 597 ml on the left compared to 495 ml on the right. He had difficulty with thumb IP flexion and his thumb CMC extension was 0 degrees and abduction 25 degrees. Total active motion in the thumb was 53 degrees. His muscle testing showed grade 1 muscle strength in the APB and FPB muscles. His intrinsic muscles were 0 and the lumbricals were 3 +. His grip was 26 lbs. on the right compared to 83 lbs. on the left. His Carroll test score was 57. His S-W test showed no response in the thumb and ring fingers. Index finger showed loss of protective sensation, long and small fingers showed diminished protective sensation. He could detect hot, cold, and pain in the transplanted right hand.

The patient continued to complain of night pain, numbness, and hypersensitivity and a small wound on the small finger base ulnarly. This was treated with multiple and different doses of antibiotics. He had a nerve conduction and electromyography study that showed carpal tunnel and Guyon's canal syndromes. He responded well to steroid injection at carpal tunnel. His wound on contracted small finger resolved but his neuropathic pain continued. He also had a small abscess of the ulnar side of the forearm. He underwent a wide margin excision of the forearm abscess, a carpal tunnel release, and Guyon's canal release through a single incision. In this surgery plaques were observed on the median and ulnar nerves which turned out to be lymphocytic infiltration. In the postoperative two week follow-up the patient had wound dehiscence in the carpus (Fig. 17.5c). He underwent a reclosure of the wound after refreshing edges by his local surgeon. In one week follow-up, infection was seen. The patient underwent a debridement surgery and later severe infection was seen and was treated with a synovectomy and a vacuum assisted closure was applied. A day after the vacuum dressing application the circulation to the ulnar two fingers worsened. He had cold and purple discolored small and ring fingers (Fig. 17.5d). The patient was invited to Louisville and the options were discussed. An amputation was performed removing the transplanted hand and tissues.

17.15.6 Patient #6

Our sixth recipient was a 55-year-old right-hand dominant male chiropractor when he had a double hand transplant in 2010 [30]. He was injured four and a half years before transplant when he got trapped in his vehicle during a grassfire. He sustained second and third degree burns on 30% of his body including both of his hands and arms, face, and back. After his initial burn treatment, he underwent four surgeries on the right hand and one on the left hand. He was in good general health. He was taking escitalopram, oxycodone, zolpidem, flurazepam, hydroxyzine. His goal in seeking hand transplant was "to do all the things he could do before his accident."

He had bilateral post-burn scars with contractions. On the left-hand thick scarring was present on the dorsum causing limitation in flexion. On the right hand, scarring extended to the elbow. He had a radial artery flap done to cover the forearm. The scars on the wrist and palm were mobile and minimally tender. He had 2/10 hypersensitivity in most digits. Additionally, he had wounds on both thumbs, in the left first web space, and dorsally on the right thumb. He had normal sensibility on the left thumb, long, ring, and small fingers and diminished light touch in the left index finger. The right thumb, index finger, and long finger also had diminished light touch, whereas right long and ring fingers had lost protective sensation. The patient had hot, cold, and pain sensation on the left hand but no sensation on the right hand.

The patient received the nation's third double hand transplant after a 17.5-h surgery on August 24, 2010 [30]. His right and left hand were amputated while preserving his ulnar and median sensory and motor nerve branches individually till the palm level. The goal was to improve motor recovery. Radius and ulna were connected at the distal forearm level with 6-hole-plates. The radial and ulnar arteries were ligated at the distal forearm level. The donor hand radial artery and ulnar artery were prepped up to the brachial artery and the brachial artery was connected at the antecubital fossa level in an end-to-side manner. Two veins were connected at the elbow level. His flexor and extensor tendons were dissected and were connected at the distal forearm level to the corresponding tendons. The ulnar nerve repair was then performed at the Guyon's canal level connecting the motor branches and the sensory branches individually. The median nerve was connected as distal as possible at the common digital nerve level and at the recurrent nerve branch level. The radial nerve repair was performed at the wrist level.

The team had difficulty closing the right forearm especially proximally due to a deep burn scar. Skin graft was harvested from the right thigh to cover the forearm defect. The thumb circulation did not appear satisfactory initially; however, it pinked up with time. His induction was achieved with alemtuzumab without steroid avoidance and he was maintained with rapamycin, tacrolimus, and 10 mg of prednisone.

The right thumb and the right small finger had multiple ischemic episodes and were necrotic at the tip. Four months postoperatively, right thumb was amputated at the interphalangeal level and the flexor pollicis tendon was repaired to the proximal phalanx. The small finger was amputated at the distal interphalangeal level.

At about 4 months postoperatively he had some minor rash that responded well and quickly to topical clobetasol and tacrolimus creams. He had no swelling of the hands. He was using his anti-claw on the left consistently and was removing his right anti-claw undeservedly. He had new onset tremors on both arms that started 6 weeks earlier. This was attributed to the new medications of aripiprazole and bupropion he was recently started on.

At his 6-month and the last therapy evaluation at Kleinert Institute, he was reporting improved functionality in both hands. He described the right hand felt more natural to use. He revealed he could do new functional tasks such as eating independently, opening doorknobs, unzipping luggage, and more independence with bathing. He was having a disturbing ache and pain in the right thumb which woke him up regularly at night. ROM measurements showed he had excellent range of motion in both hands. He was able to do an active composite flexion and all fingertips touched the distal palmar crease except the right small finger. The distance from the thumb tip to the fifth digit distal palmar crease was 4.75 cm on the right and 3.8 cm on the left. His sensibility was improving with Tinel's detected at the fingertips, but SW microfilament tests showed loss of protective sensation. He was able to detect temperatures, was limited in detecting textures, and was unable to detect shapes.

This patient decided to follow up at University of Arizona and was taken off the protocol. He died on August 11, 2015, at age 60, nine and a half years after his accident and fighting depression [31].

17.15.7 Patient #7

Our seventh recipient was a 36-year-old right-hand dominant male who was a floor man at a steel fabrication plant. He had a crush injury with a steel splitter resulting in a partial amputation of the left hand. For years before his presentation to us he had revision amputation shortening the thumb and metacarpals, Leaving him with a short thumb and a metacarpal hand. He had injuries in the right hand at the same time as the left-hand injury, which were treated with right ring finger and right small finger PIP joint fusion. The patient was healthy and was on atorvastatin and paroxetine. He was given a prosthesis; however, he was wearing it only for cosmetic purposes and had no functional use of it.

He underwent a distal forearm level hand transplant following our usual surgical protocol. His immune suppression was achieved using antithymocyte globulin (ATG) for induction and tacrolimus, MMF, and weaning dose of prednisone for maintenance. As soon as the bone healed MMF was discontinued, and he was switched to rapamycin. He underwent a graft excision and closure after defatting the adjacent skin at two years post-transplant.

This patient had a smooth postoperative course, he was very responsive to physical therapy. He achieved Carroll score of 86 in his first year and maintained hand function over the course of his follow-up. At seven-year post-transplant he had symptoms of carpal tunnel syndrome that was treated conservatively, and he responded well to conservative treatment. His biopsy at 8 years was grade 0 on left forearm dorsum and grade 1 on left volar forearm. He had negative DSA class I and class II. He had positive DSA against HLA DQ8 antigens. His immunosuppression was maintained using tacrolimus 1 mg and rapamycin 3 mg daily.

At his last evaluation near 10 years postoperatively, he had no significant changes in his hand function, and he was using his hand regularly. The patient had full passive flexion and extension of the fingers and had good range of motion in the thumb (Fig. 17.6). His index, long, ring, and small fingers could touch the distal palmar crease and his thumb could oppose up to 1.5 cm away from the small fingertip. His grip strength was 40 lbs. on the left compared to 75 lbs. on

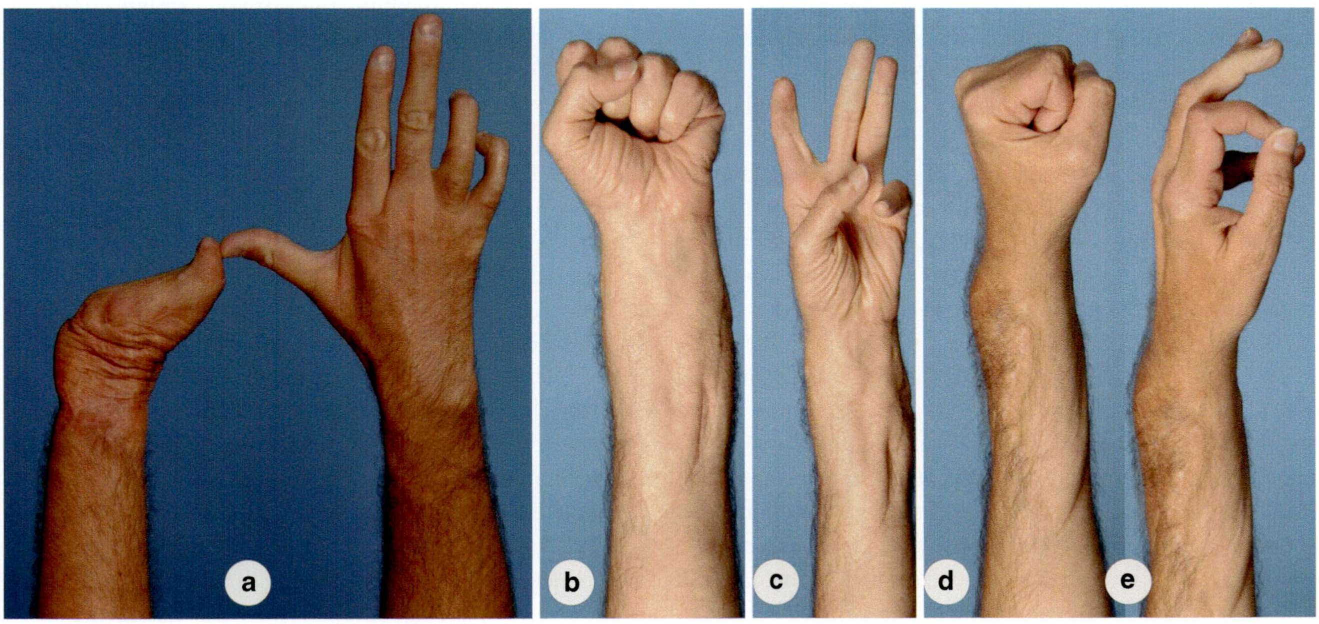

Fig. 17.6 (**a**) Pre-operative images of patient #7 showing partial amputation of left hand. (**b**–**e**) 10 years follow-up showing range of motion

the right. His two-point pinch strength was 3 lbs. on the left and 11 lbs. on the right, his lateral pinch was 5 on the left and 13 lbs. on the right.

On assessment of sensibility, he was unable to detect 2PD in the ring finger and long finger. His static 2PD was more than 15 mm in the thumb small finger and index finger. On Semmes-Weinstein monofilament testing patient was able to detect 4.56 (loss of protective sensation) at the tips of his left IF, RF, SF, but with inconsistent touch localization. In the thumb he was able to feel 4.31 (diminished protective sensation). He was able to complete Moberg test eyes open in 9.92 s on the left compared to 8.80 s; however, he was unable to perform this test eyes closed. He also was not able to identify objects with the left hand. His last measured Carroll score was 73 at 7 years postoperatively.

17.15.8 Patient #8

The eighth patient in our series was a 56-year-old male farmer who was previously right-hand dominant. A combined auger injury caused an amputation of his right forearm on November 2003, 9 years before his transplant. He received a myoelectric prosthesis in his first year, but he did not use it since it was slipping when he perspired and got in his way. He used a rocker knife to cut meat. His goal in seeking a hand transplant was to be able to play golf and use his right hand during activities of daily living from using a fork to tying his shoes. He had no medical problems.

His amputation was at distal third forearm level about 8 ¾ in. away from the olecranon. He was missing about 3 in. of his distal forearm compared to the opposite side. He had 45 degree supination and 70 degree pronation in the forearm. His existing volar muscles showed good contractility with electrical stimulation. He had a sensitive area on the volar and ulnar aspect on the stump with positive Tinel. This was considered as a painful neuroma of the ulnar nerve.

The patient underwent a successful hand transplant on February 2012. He had ulna and radius plating after release of the interosseous membrane. The surgical technique described above was followed without any significant event. His immunosuppression was achieved with ATG, and he was maintained on tacrolimus and MMF. He was later switched to rapamycin once healing of bones was confirmed.

He was doing well until he developed a rejection episode at year 6 after responding to a machinery fire in his farm. He was affected from the smoke and shortly after he developed swelling in his hand and arm, He was diagnosed with prostate cancer and received treatment including leuprolide injections. He was also having arthritic pain in the hips and shoulders treated with stretch and strengthening exercises.

On his seventh year postoperative evaluation, he had rash and slight edema on the transplanted arm. His DSA was negative for HLA class 1 and 2 antigens. His biopsy showed grade 1 rejection on the hand dorsum and grade 2 rejection on the dorsum of forearm. This was initially treated with topical clobetasol ointment and later by a short course three-day iv methylprednisolone followed by a prednisone taper. The rash and swelling responded well to this treatment but swelling returned without the rash. He was placed on prednisone taper and later prednisone 10 mg daily until the swelling subsided. He was kept on tacrolimus 1.5 mg bid, sirolimus 3 mg, and prednisone 5 mg daily.

His functional recovery was excellent. He reached a Carroll score of 64 at year 1 and improved to 79 at year 5. He was using both hands for bimanual tasks and his right hand was getting more skillful for one-handed tasks including using a regular knife and turning a key to start his car. He was still using his left hand for most tasks that required use of one hand.

He reported no changes in his hand function at his final evaluation at ninth year postoperatively. There were no rashes or swelling and he continued working on his farm under the set restrictions. He had limited shoulder ROM on both sides. He had full passive flexion and extension of all digits. His thumb total active motion was 30 degrees. He was able to oppose the thumb to the ring fingertip. His tip of the thumb to distal palmar crease measured 6 cm. During finger flexion his fingertip to distal palm crease distance stayed between 2 and 3.5 cm. He was able to detect hot, cold, and pain on his forearm. He could detect the point of a nail in palm and could differentiate between different textures at fingers. He can differentiate between a square and a round edge. His two-point discrimination was more than 15 ml in all digits. Semmes-Weinstein monofilament test showed improvement from 4.31 (diminished protective sensation) to 3.61 (diminished light touch) in the thumb, index, and ring finger ulnarly. His strength was 25 lbs. on the right compared 116 lbs. on the left. His pinch strength was 6 lbs. on the right compared to 17 lbs. on the left.

17.15.9 Patient #9

Our ninth patient was a 65-year-old male who was retired and was restoring classic and muscle cars and drag racing as a hobby. He had a motor vehicle accident on racetrack on July 20, 2012 while driving over 150 mph. He had bilateral forearm level injuries that were repaired on the left side and a below elbow amputation was done on the right side. The patient owned a hook prosthesis; however, he was able to use it on about 25% of his activities despite wearing it 75% of the time. He was able to open cabinet doors and push things onto shelves and garden. He had 14.6-centimeter amputation stump measured from the olecranon tip. He had contractions of the extensors and flexor tendons. He was not having phantom pain, but he had discomfort all the time. He slept through the night. His shooting pains were felt one or two times daily and no scar sensitivity was noted.

This patient was put on the transplant list and a donor was found. When the patient was invited for surgery, the patient did not feel comfortable and did not want to undergo a transplant. Later, he felt he was very disabled and was unable to do things, and he asked to be put on the transplant list again. This patient was also enrolled in the adipose derived stem cell therapy.

The patient underwent a transplant surgery on November 25, 2014. About 60 ml of fat graft was harvested to obtain standardized stromal vascular fraction (SVF) aliquots. The donor hand was injected with these cells at the beginning of the surgery. An exploration of the proximal forearm showed there were several muscles and tendons missing and the proximal muscles were not adequate for the repair. The ulna and radius were attached with 3.5 mm plates, then the brachial artery was repaired to the corresponding brachial artery in an end-to-side manner. The muscles of the donor forearm were repaired on the proximal forearm muscles. The nerve repairs were done at the elbow and proximal forearm level. Vein grafts were harvested from the donor hand dorsum and were used to bridge the gap at the elbow level. Immunosuppression was induced with ATG and MMF, tacrolimus, and prednisone.

On the third day after the transplantation, the color of the hand was slightly cyanotic, and a decision was made to explore the forearm. During the surgery we found the tissues were extremely edematous and two veins were thrombosed (Fig. 17.5e). The thrombosed veins were removed, and vein grafts were used to increase the venous drainage. Further fasciotomies were made in the hand to decrease the edema (Fig. 17.5f). The patient was placed on hyperbaric oxygen for the treatment of ischemia reperfusion injury. On postoperative day 5, the edema was significantly increased, and the circulation was decreased in the hand. A revision amputation was performed, and all the transplanted donor tissues were removed.

17.15.10 Patient #10

The last patient of the program was a 69-year-old female at the time of the transplant. Following systemic sepsis, she required bilateral below knee amputations, left mid-forearm level amputation, and right transmetacarpal amputation which also involved the thumb at the interphalangeal joint. She was living at home designed specifically for her physical needs. She used bilateral lower extremity prosthesis for walking. She needed assistance with activities of daily living including putting her prosthesis on. She had I-limb touch bionic prostheses for both arms, but she was having difficulty using them. They could not get wet, and they could not be around dirt or plants. She used a left body powered hook prosthesis when her myoelectric prosthesis was not working. Her goal in getting bilateral hand transplants was to be able to perform activities of daily living and possibly knitting again.

The right hand had thenar muscles available in the amputation stump and the left side had multiple muscles missing in the forearm. CT angiogram showed patent vessels on both sides. An MRI of the left forearm showed the available muscles and a surgical strategy for tendon transfers on the left side was considered. We also planned for stromal vascular fraction injection for this patient. A fluid resuscitation plan was made with anesthesia due to concerns regarding her total blood and fluid volume as she was a quadruple amputee. We proposed not to release both arm tourniquets at the same time but to stagger them by at least 20 min.

On September 17, 2016, a bilateral hand transplantation was performed in a 17-h long surgery. Fat graft harvest was performed first under general anesthesia and the harvested fat was processed in the operating room. Endotoxin screening and gram stating were performed. SVF cell yield was standardized, and the cells were kept on ice until the donor arms arrived. Four teams were formed, two exploring the recipient arms and two dissecting and preparing the donor arm.

The left side was addressed with two 7-hole 3.5 mm plate fixation and an end-to-side repair of the brachial artery. Two concomitant veins were immediately repaired, and the rest of the veins were clamped before the tourniquet was released. The tendon transfers were performed to compensate for the missing muscles. Pronator teres was transferred to extensor carpi radialis brevis, flexor carpi radialis was transferred to extensor digitorum, extensor carpi radialis longus was transferred to flexor digitorum profundus in reverse cascade. Brachioradialis was transferred to extensor pollicis longus and extensor carpi radialis brevis was lengthened and transferred to flexor pollicis longus. The nerves were repaired at the mid-forearm level and two more large veins were repaired.

The right hand was amputated at the distal forearm level during preparation and plate fixation was attained for both bones. The radial and ulnar arteries were repaired under the microscope. The nerves were connected at the wrist level. The tendons were repaired as in the previous transplants. Circulation to the right hand failed during the surgery; however, after washing the arterial system with continuous saline irrigation the clots were removed and the circulation was restored. After closure of the incisions, we injected arms with stromal vascular fraction cells in 30 aliquots. A total dose of 70 million SVF was injected, 30 million in the left hand and 40 million in the right hand.

Immunosuppression was inducted by ATG, and the patient was placed on tacrolimus, MMF, and prednisone.

Postoperatively, the patient showed delirium symptoms and her alertness and conscience levels were impaired. She was suspected of undiagnosed dementia. She became more responsive and cooperative when all pain medicines were stopped. Due to acute delirium, she required multiple braces and caused significant delays in her therapy.

Interestingly, this patient had no rejection episode during the entire follow-up: all biopsies were grade 0, DSA were negative. She had a six-antigen match with the donor with HLA typing. At her last follow-up she was on sirolimus 1 mg daily, and tacrolimus 0.75 mg extended release daily. She had recurrent urinary tract infections which were controlled with trimethoprim and solifenacin. She was on venlafaxine and gabapentin. She developed a lesion on her left malar area inferiorly which was reported as a basal cell carcinoma on shave biopsy. She also had a fall in her postoperative fourth year and was treated for a minimally displaced olecranon fracture and radial head fracture which healed well with a long arm cast.

On her third year full functional evaluation, she was ambulating without an assistive device during the day and was using a power chair at night. She had daily assistance from home health aides. She was using the right hand 90% of the time and the left hand 15% of the time for stabilizing objects. She could shower and wash her hair, make her bed, warm microwave meals, sweep the floor, and fold towels independently. She was unable to knit but was using her looms to make hats. She noted tremors in both hands that worsened with a busier day and impacted her ability to use her hands. She had multiple episodes of recurrent urinary tract infections and there was further decrease in her GFR after the last episode of kidney infection.

She had good skin color with soft and pliable scars. No rashes or areas of sensitivity were recorded. She had good shoulder and elbow function bilaterally. Her pronation and supination were full on the right and her pronation was limited on the left. Her right wrist motion was near normal. Left wrist was limited in flexion but had good extension. She had full flexion of the right-hand fingers but extension was limited. There was clawing of the fingers. She could touch the distal palmar crease with all right fingertips. She had no interossei or lumbrical contraction but had 2 + motor strength in the right abductor pollicis brevis. Her EPL was weak and other extrinsic muscles were about 4. Her grip strength was 17 lbs. on the right. Left hand was limited in her digital motion and the left wrist needed stabilization to neutral to have digital extension. She had 1.0 to 3.4 cm tip to palm distance in the digits on the left. There was no intrinsic muscle return on the left. Her extrinsic muscles were 2- to 3+ and grip strength was 7 lbs. at the second setting of the Jamar.

Her sensibility Testing showed Tinel's were still advancing at the tips but there was no response on the fingertips on Semmes-Weinstein or two-point discrimination testing. Carroll score was 60 on the right and 10 on the left. She was placed on night splinting to left upper extremity to address the tightening of the flexors of the fingers. Rejection episodes.

Acute rejection (AR): All of our patients had some episodes of AR (Fig. 17.4a, b) except patient #10. Skin biopsy were taken and grading was performed. Depending on the severity and patient specific factors, they were managed by prednisolone, ATG, MMF, sirolimus, intravenous ganciclovir, topical tacrolimus, clobetasol either alone or in combination. The details regarding individual AR and management are described earlier in patient profiles.

Chronic rejection: All patients had certain degree of graft vasculopathy, it was notably severe in patients #4 and #6 leading to loss of graft in patient #4 (Fig. 17.5a, b). In patients #2 and #3 loss of fingernails was also noted (Fig. 17.4c). Patient #6 had digital ischemia (Fig. 17.4d).

17.16 Complications

Complications could be divided into surgical complications, complications due to immunosuppression, and unrelated complications. Among surgical complications, acute graft loss due to ischemia reperfusion injury was noted in patient #9 (Fig. 17.5e, f). Patient #5 had pulmonary embolism. Thrombosis of ulnar artery was noted in patient #1. Other minor surgical complications were seroma (patients #1 and #3), delayed wound closure (patient #6), wound dehiscence, surgical site infection (patient #5) (Fig. 17.5c, d).

Immunosuppression produced a wide array of systemic complications. Infections such as CMV, MRSA, recurrent UTI were seen in patients #1, #3, #6, and #10. Renal dysfunction ranged from elevated creatinine levels (patients #3 and #5) to kidney failure (patient #1). Diabetes was noted in patients #2 and #3. Osteonecrosis of the hips was noted in patient #2 and neuropathy was noted in patients #3 and #5.

Two patients had malignancies. Patient #10 had basal cell carcinoma; patient #3 had a fatal squamous cell carcinoma. He also had a marginal zone lymphoma.

Other complications were excessive weight treated with bariatric surgery (patient #5), olecranon and radial head fracture (patient #10), spider veins (Fig. 17.4e).

17.17 Current Status of the Program

Louisville VCA program is created as a collaboration between two nonprofit organizations, a private practice, a private hospital, and a university. The core support was through multiple grants received from the Department of Defense and Jewish Hospital Foundation. This group of physicians led by Dr. Warren Breidenbach paved the way for the first transplant of the nation and was able to perform 10 hand transplants. The strength of this program comes from the expertise of physicians in hand surgery and from the training of all the physicians and researchers that went through this program. The group has the largest clinical experience and has faced multiple challenges successfully over time. Today we are celebrating 21 years since our first-hand transplant.

Unfortunately, there are multiple weaknesses as well. The most apparent one is the inadequacy of the grants, financial and administrative support to the program. The financial failure of the partnering private hospital system, dependency on grants for salaries of research personnel, lack of support from insurance industry, and the insufficient private donations to the institute forced the physicians to reevaluate the program. The funding issues, the number of complications, and the new developments in the field of prosthetic replacement of the hand were discussed. In December 2019, the hand surgeons of the program decided to suspend the hand transplant procedure and transfer the current patients to another well-sponsored program. The Louisville VCA program is now under the patronage of the University of Louisville Transplant Program and the group stays as a consult to the patients. No prospective patients are enrolled in the program.

Acknowledgments Louisville VCA program is a collaboration of Christine M. Kleinert Institute for Hand and Microsurgery, Kleinert Kutz Hand Care Center, Jewish Hospital, University of Louisville, and Cardiovascular Innovation Institute. There have been multiple changes to the program over the years. We would like to honor the contributors to the hand transplant program including the CMKI faculty Warren C. Breidenbach, Joseph E Kutz, Tsu-Min Tsai, Luis R. Scheker, Amit Gupta, Steve McCabe, Bill O'Neill, Martin Favetto, Russel Shatford, Margaret Napolitano, Huey Tien, Tuna Ozyurekoglu, Rodrigo Moreno, Michelle Palazzo, Scott Farner, Yorell Manon Matos, Elkin Galvis, Laxminarayan Bhandari, Rodrigo Banegas, CMKI therapists Anne Hodges, Ashley Emrich, Laurie Newsome, Jyoti Heipel, Greg Frey, COF, Brenda Blair RN, as well as dozens of CMKI hand surgery fellows who participated over the years including Linda Cendales, Vijay Gorantla, and many more research fellows. We would like to acknowledge the transplant surgeons and physicians Gordon R. Tobin, John H. Barker, Suzanne T. Ildstadt, Michael Marvin, Allan Ramirez, and Christopher M. Jones. We would also like to acknowledge the scientists who contributed to the program, namely Christina L Kaufman, Paula Chilton, Stuart Williams, and Jay Hoying.

References

1. Murray JE. The establishment of composite tissue allotransplantion as a clinical reality [internet]. In: Hewitt CW, Lee WPA, Gordon CR, editors. Transplantation of composite tissue allografts. Boston, MA: Springer; 2008. p. 3–12. https://doi.org/10.1007/978-0-387-74682-1_1.
2. Breidenbach WC, Tobin GR, Gorantla VS, Gonzalez RN, Granger DK. A position statement in support of hand transplantation. J Hand Surg Am. 2002;27(5):760–70.
3. Mackinnon SE, Hudson AR. Clinical application of peripheral nerve transplantation. Plast Reconstr Surg. 1992;90(4):695–9.
4. Guimberteau J-C, Baudet J, Panconi B, Boileau R, Potaux L. Human allotransplant of a digital flexion system vascularized on the ulnar pedicle: a preliminary report and 1-year follow-up of two cases. Plast Reconstr Surg. 1992;89:1135–47.
5. Wendt JR, Ulich TR, Ruzics EP, Hostetler JR. Indefinite survival of human skin allografts in patients with longterm immunosuppression. Ann Plast Surg. 1994;32:411–7.
6. Hofmann OG, Kirschner MH, Bühren V, Land W. Allogenic vascularized transplantation of a human femoral diaphysis under cyclosporin a immunosuppression. Transpl Int. 1995;8(5):418–9.
7. Carpenter JP, Tomaszewski JE. Immunosuppression for human saphenous vein allograft bypass surgery: a prospective randomized trial. J Vasc Surg. 1997;26(1):32–42.
8. Jones TR, Humphrey PA, Brennan DC. Transplantation of vascularized allogeneic skeletal muscle for scalp reconstruction in renal transplant patient. Transplant Proc. 1998;30(6):2746–53.
9. Kvernmo HD, Gorantla VS, Gonzalez RN, Breidenbach WC. Hand transplantation. Acta Orthop. 2005;76(1):14–27.
10. Benhaim P, Anthony JP, Ferreira L, Borsanyi J-P, Mathes SJ. Use of combination of low-dose cyclosporine and RS61443 in a rat hindlimb model of composite tissue allotransplantation. Transplantation. 1996;61(4):527–32.
11. Ustüner ET, Zdichavsky M, Ren X, et al. Long-term composite tissue allograft survival in a porcine model with cyclosporine/mycophenolate mofetil therapy. Transplantation. 1998;66(12):1581–7.
12. Jones JW Jr, Ustüner ET, Zdichavsky M, Edelstein J, Ren X, Maldonado C, Ray M, Jevans AW, Breidenbach WC, Gruber SA, Barker JH. Long-term survival of an extremity composite tissue allograft with FK506-mycophenolate mofetil therapy. Surgery. 1999;126(2):384–8.
13. Ustüner ET, Majzoub RK, Ren X, et al. Swine composite tissue allotransplant model for preclinical hand transplant studies. Microsurgery. 2000;20(8):400–6.
14. Tobin GR, Breidenbach WC, Klapheke MM, Bentley FR, Pidwell DJ, Simmons PD. Ethical considerations in the early composite tissue allograft experience: a review of the Louisville ethics program. Transplant Proc. 2005;37(2):1392–5.
15. Morris ME, Beare JE, Reed RM, Dale JR, LeBlanc AJ, Kaufman CL, Zheng H, Ng CK, Williams SK, Hoying JB. Systemically delivered adipose stromal vascular fraction cells disseminate to peripheral artery walls and reduce vasomotor tone through a CD11b+ cell-dependent mechanism. Stem Cells Transl Med. 2015;4(4):369–80.
16. Stivers KB, Beare JE, Chilton PM, Williams SK, Kaufman CL, Hoying JB. Adipose-derived cellular therapies in solid organ and vascularized-composite allotransplantation. Curr Opin Organ Transplant. 2017;22:490–8.
17. Gorantla V, Maldonado C, Frank J, Barker JH. Composite tissue allotransplantation (cta): current status and future insights. Eur J Trauma. 2001;27(6):267–74.
18. Ravindra KV, Buell JF, Kaufman CL, Blair B, Marvin M, Nagubandi R, Breidenbach WC. Hand transplantation in the United States: experience with 3 patients. Surgery. 2008;144(4):638–43.
19. Amirlak B, Gonzalez R, Gorantla V, Breidenbach WC 3rd, Tobin GR. Creating a hand transplant program. Clin Plast Surg. 2007;34(2):279–89.
20. Nseir I, Delaunay F, Latrobe C, Bonmarchand A, Coquerel-Beghin D, Auquit-Auckbur I. Use of adipose tissue and stromal vascular fraction in hand surgery. Orthop Traumatol Surg Res. 2017;103(6):927–32.
21. Banegas RN, Moreno R, Duggal A, Breidenbach WC. Surgical aspects of donor hand recovery for transplantation. J Reconstr Microsurg. 2012;28(01):21–6.

22. Breidenbach WC, Gonzales NR, Kaufman CL, Klapheke M, Tobin GR, Gorantla VS. Outcomes of the first 2 American hand transplants at 8 and 6 years posttransplant. J Hand Surg Am. 2008;33(7):1039–47.
23. Jones JW, Gruber SA, Barker JH, Breidenbach WC. Successful hand transplantation. One-year follow-up. Louisville hand transplant team. N Engl J Med. 2000;343(7):468–73.
24. Carroll S. A quantitative test of upper extremity function. J Chronic Dis. 1965;18:479–91.
25. Cendales LC, Kirk AD, Moresi JM, Ruiz P, Kleiner DE. Composite tissue allotransplantation: classification of clinical acute skin rejection. Transplantation. 2005;80:1676–80.
26. Starzl R, Brandacher G, Lee WP, Carbonell J, Zhang W, Schnider J, Gorantla V, Schneeberger S, Zheng XX. Review of the early diagnoses and assessment of rejection in vascularized composite allotransplantation. Clin Dev Immunol. 2013;2013:402980.
27. Granger DK, Briedenbach WC, Pidwell DJ, Jones JW, Baxter-Lowe LA, Kaufman CL. Lack of donor hyporesponsiveness and donor chimerism after clinical transplantation of the hand. Transplantation. 2002;74(11):1624–30.
28. Kaufman CL, Ouseph R, Blair B, Kutz JE, Tsai TM, Scheker LR, Tien HY, Moreno R, Ozyurekoglu T, Banegas R, Murphy E, Burns CB, Zaring R, Cook DF, Marvin MR. Graft vasculopathy in clinical hand transplantation. Am J Transplant. 2012;12(4):1004–16.
29. Kaufman CL, Blair B, Murphy E, Breidenbach WB. A new option for amputees: transplantation of the hand. J Rehabil Res Dev. 2009;46(3):395–404.
30. Kaufman CL, Breidenbach W. World experience after more than a decade of clinical hand transplantation: update from the Louisville hand transplant program. Hand Clin. 2011;27(4):417–21, vii-viii
31. Sonya Colberg, The Oklahoman. Published: Fri, August 21, 2015 12:00 AM Edmond chiropractor who received new hands dies at age 60 (oklahoman.com). Last accessed on 7/31/2021.

Hand Allotransplantation: The Penn Experience

18

Viviana M. Serra López, Zvi Steinberger, Erin L. Weber, Christine McAndrew, and L. Scott Levin

Abbreviations

DSA	Donor-specific antibodies
IV	Intravenous
LUE	Left upper extremity
OR	Operating room
RUE	Right upper extremity
VCA	Vascularized composite allograft

18.1 Introduction

The vascularized composite allograft (VCA) transplantation program at the University of Pennsylvania (Penn) was started in 2009. Dr. L. Scott Levin, the chair of Orthopaedic Surgery and professor of Surgery (Division of Plastic Surgery) and Dr. Abraham Shaked, director of the Penn Transplant Institute, worked closely with Gift of Life, local organ procurement organizations, and the United Network for Organ Sharing to establish the program. The first bilateral hand transplant was performed two years later on Patient #1, as described below.

To date, our program has completed a full screening of 25 patients and performed four bilateral hand transplants, two of which were international recipients. The transplants were hospital funded, with the exception of one, which was self-funded. The program is still actively screening patients, treating our current patients, and doing research. There is currently one patient on the waitlist.

V. M. Serra López · Z. Steinberger · E. L. Weber · C. McAndrew
L. S. Levin (✉)
Department of Surgery, Division of Plastic Surgery, Hospital of the University of Pennsylvania, Philadelphia, PA, USA
e-mail: viviana.serralopez@pennmedicine.upenn.edu; christine.mcandrew@pennmedicine.upenn.edu; scott.levin@pennmedicine.upenn.edu

The largest obstacle our VCA program faces moving forward is funding. The funding of this life enhancing transplant remains a challenge.

18.2 Protocols

During the development of the Penn Hand Transplant program, general protocols were developed to guide surgical technique, immunosuppressive regimens, post-operative monitoring, and rehabilitation. These protocols are outlined below, with any relevant adjustments highlighted during discussion of the individual patients.

18.2.1 Surgical Technique

The technique outlined here describes bilateral transplantation at the proximal forearm level. The procurement of donor limbs and the transplantation surgery are typically performed at different local hospitals. Donor arms are procured at the mid-humerus level. After ligation and transection of all structures, the brachial artery is perfused with University of Wisconsin cold storage solution until clear efflux is visualized from the brachial vein. Each arm is wrapped in blue towels, triple bagged, placed in a cooler, and transported to the site of transplantation. Once abdominal and thoracic teams have completed their respective organ procurements, a separate team obtains hemostasis at the donor sites, closes the skin, and ensures that upper extremity prosthetics are sent with the donor patient.

Four teams of surgeons, surgical technicians, and nurses perform the bilateral donor and recipient preparation simultaneously. On the recipient limbs, radial and ulnar incisions are made, allowing the elevation of dorsal and volar skin flaps. The brachial artery and vein, basilic and cephalic veins, cutaneous veins, radial, ulnar, and median nerves, and lateral and medial antebrachial cutaneous nerves are identified, dissected away from the residual bone and musculature, and

© Springer Nature Switzerland AG 2023

R. Gurunian et al. (eds.), *Reconstructive Transplantation*, https://doi.org/10.1007/978-3-031-21520-9_18

individually labeled with pre-made tags. The flexor/pronator mass and extensor wad are elevated from proximal to distal, taking care to maintain collateral ligaments at the elbow. Custom-made cutting guides, based on preoperative CT scans, are applied to the radius and ulna to facilitate osteotomy location. Six- or seven-hole locking compression plates are then pre-applied to the recipient with a single non-locking screw.

Donor extremities are prepared on separate back tables. Anterior and posterior incisions are made on the upper arm to create radial and ulnar skin flaps which are reflected distally. As with the recipient limbs, all neurovascular structures are identified and tagged (Fig. 18.1). The flexor/pronator origin and the extensor wad are elevated away from the epicondyles, such that the muscle remains attached to the skin. The radius and ulna are then exposed to allow placement of the cutting guides for osteotomies. Kirschner wires are used to maintain the relationship between radius and ulna and holes are pre-drilled for screw placement. The donor limbs are

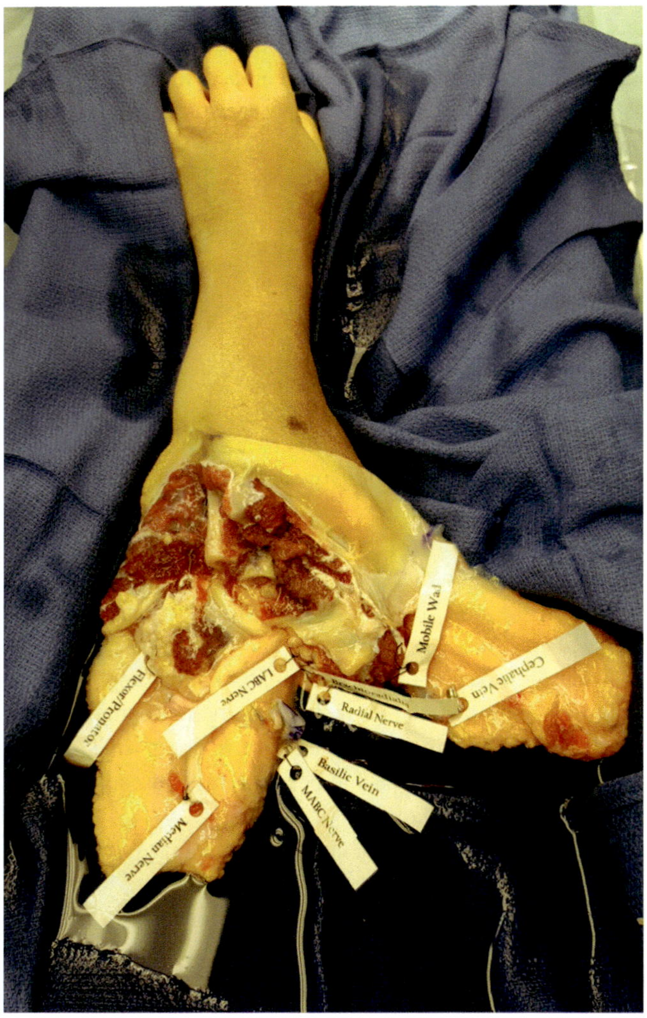

Fig. 18.1 Donor arm with custom-made tags identifying relevant structures in preparation for transplantation

then brought to the recipient limbs and osteosynthesis is performed. Unrestricted pronation and supination are confirmed before screw placement into the donor bone. The common flexor and extensor origins are affixed to the epicondyles with suture anchors. The brachial artery and vein are anastomosed and time-zero skin biopsies are taken immediately after anastomosis. The remaining structures are then repaired in the following order: median nerve, ulnar nerve, radial nerve, interdigitation of skin flaps, basilic vein, cephalic vein, median and lateral antebrachial cutaneous nerves. Skin is closed with excess to allow for serial biopsies and can be revised at a later date, if necessary. Cook Doppler probes are used to monitor arterial and venous anastomoses. Photographs are taken at the conclusion of the procedure for visual comparison of any changes during the post-operative period. A bulky dressing is placed.

18.2.2 Immunosuppression

A uniform immunosuppression protocol was designed for adult hand transplant recipients. The primary induction agent is rabbit antithymocyte globulin, referred to as thymoglobulin, with the first dose given in the operating room (OR) over a six hour period. Each patient should receive a total of 5 doses, as tolerated.

The primary calcineurin inhibitor used is tacrolimus. The starting dose is 0.15 mg/kg/day given orally in two divided doses 12 h apart within 24 h of the transplant. Target trough levels are 8–12 ng/mL for the first six months post-transplant, then 4–8 ng/mL if no rejection occurred within the first six months.

Mycophenolate mofetil is the antiproliferative agent of choice. Patients are administered 1000 mg orally every 12 h and the dose is adjusted based on adverse events. Routine level monitoring is not performed.

Corticosteroids are initially used in all transplant recipients and doses may be tapered or discontinued at the discretion of the clinician. Patients receive a methylprednisolone pulse in the OR, followed by a prednisone taper over the next 45 days.

18.2.3 Monitoring

To facilitate post-operative monitoring, patients are typically admitted to the hospital for four weeks after surgery. They are then discharged to either an acute rehabilitation facility or local housing in order to stay in the Philadelphia area for three additional months.

Punch biopsies are performed intraoperatively at day zero and weekly for the first six weeks after surgery. Three months post-operatively, biopsy frequency is decreased to once a month. During the second post-operative year, biopsies are performed quarterly and then yearly. Biopsies are typically 2 mm specimens, unless they are being collected to identify a cause of rejection, in which case they are 4 mm. Testing for donor-specific antibodies (DSA) is performed 14 days post-operatively, monthly for six months, then annually. In cases of rejection, DSA are also examined.

A diagnosis of rejection is based on the Banff 2007 classification of skin-containing composite tissue allografts [1]. Mild cellular rejection (Banff Grade 1) is treated with 500 mg of intravenous (IV) methylprednisolone daily for three days. One or more of the maintenance immunosuppression agents may also be increased and/or topical tacrolimus or topical steroids may be implemented at the discretion of the treating transplant clinician. For more severe episodes of rejection or episodes that do not respond to methylprednisolone, thymoglobulin is administered.

Patients require the input of many specialists in the immediate post-operative period and routine, long-term specialist visits may occur depending on their co-morbidities. All patients are followed closely by an infectious disease specialist for antibiotic prophylaxis. They are also evaluated by a psychologist in the immediate post-operative period, once in the first three months post-operatively and as necessary, thereafter. Other specialists are consulted as needed.

18.2.4 Rehabilitation

The post-operative rehabilitation protocol was developed specifically for patients undergoing hand transplants and is divided into six phases that build upon each other. Phase 1 begins during the first post-operative week. It consists of hand therapy for 1–3 h per day, focusing on splinting, range of motion (ROM), and cognitive retraining. Physical and occupational therapy are also included. Patients are fitted for resting splints (Fig. 18.2) and a crane outrigger splint to work on active digital flexion. They are not allowed to use their hands for any daily activities.

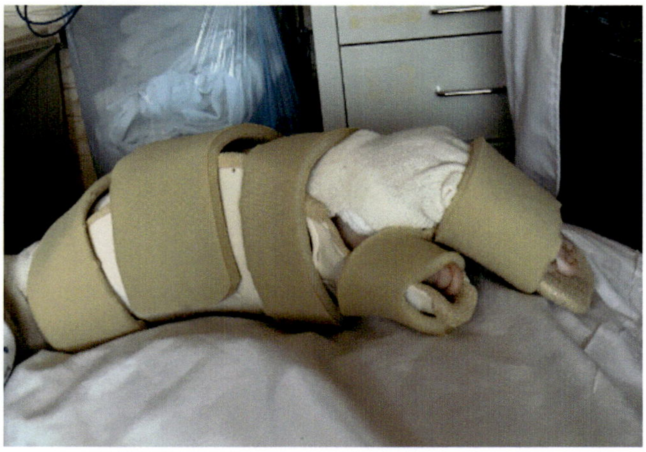

Fig. 18.2 Example of a left-sided custom-made resting splint

Phase 2 starts approximately three weeks post-operatively with the goal of progressing the patient to outpatient therapy. It includes initiation of an anticlaw splint for 15 min at a time three times daily, with increased use as tolerated. Hand exercises are progressed to protected digit ROM, active and passive wrist ROM, and active forearm and elbow ROM.

Phase 3 marks the beginning of motor and sensory development and occurs 1–3 months after surgery. As muscle function returns, tendon gliding and prehension and grab exercises are introduced. The patient is allowed to initiate light use of the hands. The therapists watch closely for sensory changes and educate the patient as these changes occur.

Phase 4 is the intermediate motor and sensory development phase, which occurs between 3 and 9 months post-operatively. At this time, arrangements are made to return patients back to their home base, including setup of local therapists with the goal of working 3 h per day. Light resistive use of the hand is added to the previous therapy protocols.

During Phase 5, referred to as the late motor and sensory development phase, patients use a hand-based intrinsic splint for light use of hand while continuing their initial splinting regimen at nighttime. Gross hand usage is increased as tolerated. Therapy goals are directed at preventing joint stiffness and motor strengthening. This leads into Phase 6, which is focused on return to work and activities of daily living.

18.3 Patients

Donor limbs are obtained through local and national organ procurement organizations. In addition to standard hematologic and immunologic matching, donor limbs are selected based on similarity to recipient gender, limb size, and skin tone. Per regulations of procurement agreements, we are unable to disclose any information about individual donors.

18.3.1 Patient #1—9/21/2011

Our first hand transplant recipient was a 28-year-old female who, four years prior, developed septic shock and multisystem organ failure following resection of her terminal ileum and colon for bowel obstruction arising from Crohn's disease. Due to a prolonged period of hypoperfusion leading to necrosis, the patient eventually underwent amputations of her bilateral upper and lower extremities. Once preoperative testing was completed, she was placed on the waiting list and, three months later, became the first patient to undergo bilateral hand transplantation through the Penn Hand Transplant Program.

Bilateral forearm transplantation was performed according to the surgical protocol detailed above. The time from the start of procurement until reperfusion was 5 h and 47 min for the right upper extremity (RUE) and 5 h and 12 min for the left upper extremity (LUE). After completion of the brachial artery and vein anastomoses, perfusion of the RUE was suboptimal, therefore an interposition vein graft was performed, using 3 cm of basilic vein. Her post-operative course was notable for the development of a right arm hematoma, which required evacuation and exploration in the OR eight days after transplantation. All anastomoses were verified to be intact and muscular bleeding was identified as the cause.

18.3.2 Functional Outcomes

Hand therapy followed the protocol outlined above. One month after the transplant, the patient was discharged to an acute rehabilitation facility, where she worked with occupational and physical therapists to achieve full pronation of the LUE, supination to 20° for the RUE, and 120° of elbow flexion. She practiced feeding and other light duty tasks. Four months after transplantation, she demonstrated signs of improvement in fine motor control such as picking up a cup and a set of keys. Nine months following surgery, she was able to feel temperature changes and continued to develop fine motor function. She eventually gained independence with the ability to drive and do housework. She has even participated in a competitive CrossFit event. At her most recent follow-up 8 years post-transplant, the patient demonstrated full strength and range of active elbow motion, though with some limits in supination. Wrist flexion and extension was within normal limits with 4 out of 5 digit motor strength bilaterally on the Oxford scale. The patient has limited right-hand active ROM due to extrinsic tightness and her left index finger rests in hyperextension. She is able to perform most activities of daily living; however, she continues to require assistance for fine motor skills, such as putting her hair into a ponytail, buttoning clothing, and tying shoelaces.

18.3.3 Immunologic Outcomes

The patient experienced an episode of Banff Grade 2 rejection four months after her transplant, which was treated successfully with a three-day course of intravenous steroids and topical tacrolimus. She also had five episodes of Banff Grade1 rejection, most recently eight years after their transplant, and one episode of Banff Grade 3 rejection nearly three years after their transplant. All of the episodes were successfully treated according to the previously described protocols. Currently, the patient's immunosuppression protocol consists of tacrolimus, sirolimus, and prednisone.

18.3.4 Other Outcomes and Challenges

In addition to routine follow-up with the surgical and transplant teams, the patient participated in routine follow-up with a psychiatrist for anxiety, a gastroenterologist for management of Crohn's disease, and an endocrinologist for management of diabetes mellitus associated with steroid use. The patient also experienced progression of her chronic kidney disease and is currently on the waitlist for a kidney transplant. Five years after transplantation, she developed left subclavian and innominate vein thrombosis which compromised outflow to her LUE. She subsequently underwent thrombectomy and angioplasty and was placed on chronic anticoagulation.

Five years after her bilateral upper extremity transplant, the patient moved to another state and faced difficulty continuing hand therapy sessions. As such, the patient required additional help and moved in with a family member after previously living independently. She also developed a painful cyst in her left lower extremity which prevented the use of her prosthetic and further limited her independence. The patient recently underwent excision of the left lower extremity bursa at the University of Pennsylvania to facilitate prosthesis use and was admitted to an acute rehabilitation facility, where she again received daily occupational and physical therapy. Prior to returning to her home state, arrangements were made to facilitate outpatient hand therapy and physical therapy.

18.3.5 Patient #2—7/7/2015

Our second upper extremity transplant patient was an 8-year-old male with bilateral upper and lower extremity amputations resulting from gastroenteritis complicated by staphylococcal sepsis at two years of age. He developed end stage renal disease and necrosis of bilateral hands and feet, necessitating distal transradial amputation of the right upper extremity, amputation at the radiocarpal joint of the left upper extremity, bilateral below-knee amputations, and a living related donor kidney transplant at 4 years of age. Given his quadruple amputee status and lifelong pre-existing need for immunosuppression, the patient was a candidate for bilateral distal forearm transplantation from a pediatric donor.

Transplants were performed at the distal forearm level and, thus, involved both radial and ulnar arterial anastomoses as well as multiple individual tendon transfers. Otherwise, the surgical procedure followed a similar sequence to that described above. Tourniquet time for the recipient was 1 h and 42 min for the LUE and 1 h and 56 min for the RUE. The patient's early surgical course was complicated by return to the operating room within one hour of transplantation for right upper extremity arterial thrombosis. The radial artery, ulnar artery, and multiple vein anastomoses were revised. The ulnar artery was found to be redundant and bent, with absence of flow distally; it was shortened and re-anastomosed with excellent outflow. The radial artery was found to have a proximal thrombosis in the forearm which was evacuated with a Fogarty catheter. The trajectory of the radial artery was then redirected to reduce tortuosity, achieving excellent outflow. A high amount of outflow volume was noted through the venae comitantes during artery revision and, thus, two additional venous anastomoses were performed. There were no further operative complications.

18.3.6 Functional Outcomes

Rehabilitation protocols largely followed the adult protocol described above, with additional emphasis on judgment in the absence of protective sensation and modification of splints and dressings to restrict picking and biting at the transplants. At two weeks post-operatively, goals for passive range of motion, edema control, and activation of extrinsic muscles were met. At four weeks post-operatively, the patient was transferred to a pediatric rehabilitation center and passive and active range of motion training was intensified. The patient was discharged home at six weeks post-operatively and resumed therapy through a local day hospital program, consisting of three hours of occupational therapy and one hour of physical therapy a day for five days per week, with schooling intermixed. He returned to his regular school ten months after limb transplantation and, at that time, continued with outpatient therapy. Most recently, he was attending occupational therapy once a week and has participated in intensive month-long therapy camps during summer breaks. Figure 18.3 shows the appearance of his bilateral hand transplants four years after their transplant.

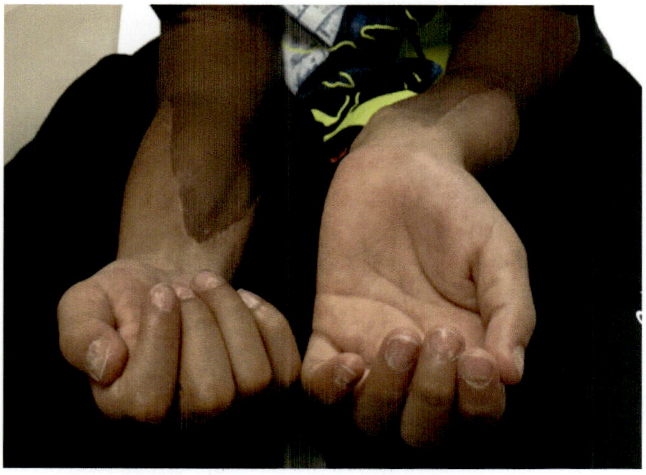

Fig. 18.3 Appearance of the bilateral hand transplants of Patient #3 four years post-operatively

At three years post-op, static two-point discrimination measured 8–9 mm for the left index finger, 10 mm for the left ring finger, and 12–14 mm for the thumb, small, and middle fingers. For the right hand, two-point discrimination measured 12–15 mm for all digits At five years post-transplantation, the patient is independent in most activities of daily living. He can successfully toilet, bathe, feed, and dress himself. He is able to don his prosthetic liners and legs without assistance. He can open a water bottle, tie his shoes, and cook a simple meal. He attends school, climbs rocks, and plays the cello. He is able to identify 70% of common items during stereognostic testing. Active range of motion at the wrist includes 30 degrees of extension and 20 degrees of flexion for the left and 30 degrees of extension and 90 degrees of flexion for the right. He has minimal radial and ulnar deviation at the wrist. Thumb opposition is better on the left, with the thumb reaching the small finger pulp, while thumb opposition on the right inconsistently reaches the index pulp only. He has achieved full digit extension with the wrist in neutral and fires extrinsic digit flexors for grasp and pinch.

18.3.7 Immunologic Outcomes

Our standard immunosuppression protocol was modified to address this patient's young age and prior renal transplant. Prior to limb transplantation, the patient was maintained on a regimen of tacrolimus and mycophenolate mofetil for his renal transplant. Induction was performed with six hours of solumedrol premedication, followed by intraoperative thymoglobulin. Post-operatively, the patient received four daily doses of thymoglobulin (1.5 mg/kg), as well as mycophenolate (600 mg/m^2/dose) every 12 h, tacrolimus (0.1 mg/kg/dose) every 12 h with a goal trough of 10–12 ng/mL, and solumedrol 2 mg/kg daily. A steroid taper to 0.2 mg/kg was performed over three months.

The patient has experienced multiple episodes of acute rejection, most frequently Banff Grades 1 and 2 with a single episode of Banff Grade 3 rejection, which were successfully mitigated through modulation of the immunosuppressive regimen, single doses or tapers of intravenous steroid, and application of topical tacrolimus and betamethasone. There has not been any evidence of chronic rejection. The patient's current immunosuppressive regimen includes tacrolimus, sirolimus, mycophenolate mofetil, and prednisone.

18.3.8 Other Outcomes and Challenges

Due to the young age at which our patient lost his hands, the brain accommodated and compensated with other organs such as the face and, more specifically, the mouth. We have followed our patient carefully with serial functional MRI scans to assess ongoing changes in his brain as they relate to the presence and increasing functionality of his transplanted hands.

While we have not encountered any significant technical, surgical, or immunologic challenges that differ from those in adults, pediatric transplantation adds an inherent level of complexity. For example, assessment of a patient's understanding of the surgical procedure and its consequences is limited and different communication techniques must be employed both for patient education and therapy.

18.3.9 Patient #3—8/22/2016

Our third recipient was a 28-year-old female who, at the age of 19, developed a streptococcal infection that resulted in sepsis and gangrene of both upper and lower extremities. She eventually underwent bilateral below-knee amputations and bilateral mid-forearm amputations.

The surgical procedure was performed per our standard protocol. The time from the start of procurement until reperfusion was 7 h and 17 min for the RUE and 7 h and 4 min for the LUE. While not performed standardly, the patient underwent division and re-insetting of the interface between her native skin and the VCA at 14 months and again at two years post-operatively.

In the immediate post-operative period, the patient returned to the operating room for evacuation of bilateral antecubital fossa hematomas nine days after transplantation. Arterial and venous anastomoses were examined and noted to be patent. At eleven days post-transplantation, the patient was taken once again to the operating room for evacuation of a recurrent hematoma at the right antecubital fossa. During exploration, an active bleeding was noted from a small artery and was controlled.

18.3.10 Functional Outcomes

The patient was discharged from the inpatient facility to a nearby private apartment 40 days after transplantation to continue intensive outpatient therapy. At seven months post-transplantation, she displayed 3 out of 5 strength on the Oxford scale bilaterally for wrist and digit flexion and extension, as well as forearm supination and pronation. No opposition or finger abduction was noted at that time. Sensation to light touch and temperature was present both volarly and dorsally. At fourteen months post-operatively, motor strength and sensation had improved and thumb abduction was present; however, the patient had no intrinsic function. At two years post-operatively, the patient recovered thumb opposition and function of her first dorsal interosseous muscle. At her most recent follow-up three years post-operatively, the patient had returned to work full-time and was living independently. She was able to shower and care for herself without assistance.

18.3.11 Immunologic Outcomes

The patient experienced an episode of rejection (Banff Grades 1 and 3) ten days after transplantation that responded to topical tacrolimus, plasmapheresis, and intravenous immunoglobulin, along with adjustment of immunosuppressive medication doses. Two months post-operatively, the patient had an episode of rejection that was treated successfully with an increased steroid dosage. She also experienced additional episodes of Banff Grade 1 rejection at 7, 14, and 24 months post-operatively; all episodes were treated successfully with topical agents. Currently, the patient's immunosuppressive regimen consists of azathioprine, sirolimus, and tacrolimus.

18.3.12 Other Outcomes and Challenges

This patient was the first international patient to undergo bilateral hand transplants at our facility. At 12 weeks post-transplantation, the patient returned to her home country. Rehabilitation and follow-up are monitored by a local team and the patient returns for a yearly visit at our outpatient clinic. Strong collaboration is required between teams in order for the Penn Hand Transplant Team to be aware of the patient's progress and stayed in the know of how patients are doing and management of the immunosuppressive regimen.

18.3.13 Patient #4—2/17/2019

Our most recent recipient was a 44-year-old female who had suffered septic shock after endometritis eight years prior, which resulted in hypoperfusion of her extremities. She underwent bilateral transtibial amputations, right mid-forearm amputation, and left transmetacarpal amputation. She subsequently received bilateral lower limb osseointegrated prostheses and was deemed an acceptable candidate for bilateral upper extremity VCA.

The patient underwent a right mid-forearm transplant and a left distal forearm transplant per our standardized protocol. The time from tourniquet placement on the recipient to re-establishment of inflow was 4 h and 14 min for the LUE and 4 h and 28 min for the right upper extremity. For the left upper extremity transplant, the ulnar artery was anastomosed first, to provide reperfusion. Other neurovas-

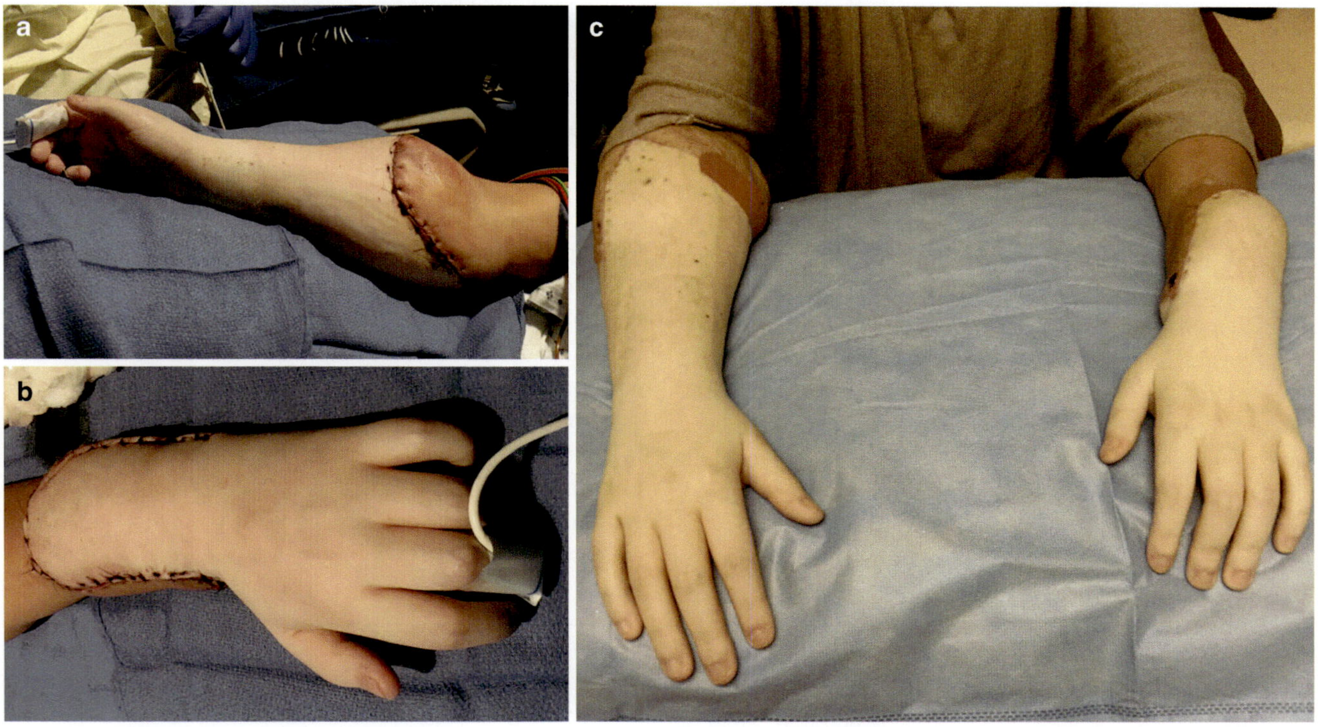

Fig. 18.4 Appearance of the bilateral hand transplants of Patient #4. (**a**) Right arm on post-operative day #3. (**b**) Left arm on post-operative day #3. (**c**) Bilateral hands five weeks post-operatively

cular and tendinous structures were repaired distally. There were no immediate surgical complications requiring a return to the operating room. Figure 18.4 shows the appearance of the patient's extremities on their third post-operative day.

18.3.14 Functional Outcomes

Nearly one month after transplantation, the patient reported paresthesias of the LUE and was able to perform active finger flexion and proximal interphalangeal joint extension with tenodesis. One year after transplantation, the patient is able to dress herself, but has difficulty with zippers and small hooks. She is able to drive and prepare meals, including opening boxes and cutting soft meats. Protective sensation is present on the right but diminished compared to the left. She is beginning to show improvements in lumbrical strength on the left and thumb opposition on the right but other intrinsic hand musculature has not yet shown significant function.

18.3.15 Immunologic Outcomes

Three weeks post-operatively, biopsies indicated Banff Grade 2 rejection which was successfully treated with topical tacrolimus. At discharge, her immunosuppressive regimen consisted of mycophenolate, tacrolimus, and prednisone. The patient's current regimen consists of her discharge regimen plus sirolimus.

18.3.16 Other Outcomes and Challenges

While the patient understands English, it is not her primary language and a translator is required for effective communication. In addition, the patient lives internationally and has recently returned to her home country. Contact was made with patient's primary physician for continuation of care and monitoring.

18.4 Lessons Learned

One of the strengths of the Penn Hand Transplant Program is that it is a team-based approach comprised of many different departments within our healthcare institution. Every team member's input is taken into consideration and suggestions are continually incorporated into the surgical planning. Over time, we have adapted the utilization of cutting guides for osteotomies and osteosynthesis and have become more comfortable managing Banff Grade 1 rejection. Ongoing cadaveric rehearsals and discussion of technical improvements have led to more efficient surgery and reliable functional outcomes throughout the program's development. Particularly, patients who have had proximal transplants at the level of the elbow have all recovered extrinsic and intrinsic motor function.

The evolution of this program has had its challenges. The logistics of international hand transplantations have been managed to increase the reach of our program. Two of our patients are internationally based, which requires us to work closely with colleagues abroad. Their follow-up has been seamless. This is made possible with technology such as FaceTime and Skype.

The field of VCA is still in its infancy, 24 years after the first-hand transplant. In addition to the challenges of reducing the toxicity of immunosuppression, the funding for this life altering care remains elusive. Current clinical research is directed toward validating the psychosocial benefits and functional advantages to the recipient, with hopes that demonstrated benefits will facilitate financial assistance.

Moving forward, cognizance of renal function prior to VCA, particularly in patients with multiorgan system failure, will influence our choice of immunosuppression. In the informed consent process, we now emphasize that post-transplant renal failure requiring renal allotransplantation may be a distinct possibility.

Over time, we hope to increase the opportunities for VCA in children and to utilize allogeneic vascularized bone and joint transplants for intractable problems of the upper extremity such as severe damage to the elbow joint in young patients.

Reference

1. Cendales LC, Kanitakis J, Schneeberger S, et al. The Banff 2007 working classification of skin-containing composite tissue allograft pathology. Am J Transplant. 2008;8(7):1396–400.

Upper Extremity Transplantation: The Massachusetts General Hospital Experience

19

Pierre Tawa, Marion Goutard, Elise Lupon, Philipp Tratnig-Frankl, Alexandre G. Lellouch, and Curtis L. Cetrulo Jr.

19.1 Introduction

The world's first documented attempt at hand transplantation was performed in Ecuador by Gilbert et al. in 1964 [1]. At the time, immunosuppressive therapy was still in its earliest stages of development, and the recipient's immunosuppression regimen consisted of only azathioprine, cortisone, and a single dose of local radiation. Due to the inadequate immunosuppression, the graft experienced irreversible acute rejection and required amputation within three weeks of transplantation. Despite the graft failure, they marked the beginning of vascularized composite allotransplantation (VCA) by demonstrating the technical feasibility of transplants involving multiple tissue types (composite grafts).

Developments in the field of immunosuppression paved the way for the first successful hand transplantation performed in France in 1998 [2]. The induction regimen included antithymocyte globulins (ATG), mycophenolic acid, tacrolimus (FK-506), and prednisone, while the maintenance therapy utilized this same regimen with the exception of ATG. This immunosuppression profile proved effective until non-compliance with the immunosuppression regimen resulted in graft rejection and removal 29 months post-transplantation. The first-hand transplant performed in the United States was carried out in Louisville, Kentucky, in 1999 and achieved long-term graft survival [3].

Since the beginning of the modern era of hand transplantation in 1998, the field of vascularized composite allotransplantation has expanded to include bilateral hand transplants, as well as transplants of the face, abdominal wall, larynx, penis, and uterus [4–10]. Hand and forearm transplants remain the most common type of VCA, with more than 60 (unilateral and bilateral) performed as of 2017 [11]. While hand transplantation has become a viable surgical option for amputees to restore form and function, acute rejection and the burden of current immunosuppressive regimens continue to pose major challenges to the surgical approach.

The program for vascularized composite allotransplantation at the Massachusetts General Hospital (MGH) was started in 2010, led by the plastic surgeon, Curtis L. Cetrulo Jr., MD and funded through an institutional grant. It took approximatively 2 years of intense practice and planning sessions to the team to prepare before the first unilateral upper extremity allotransplantation in Massachusetts was performed in October 2012. This first successful transplantation proved the feasibility of the program which is still active today and continues to screen potential candidates for hand transplantation.

Since the beginning, over 20 potential candidates have been screened in anticipation of becoming possible recipients for upper extremity transplantation. The screening protocol includes review of the medical charts, with the medical conditions of possible candidates. Inclusion criteria vary across different VCA transplant centers [12]. At MGH, the selection criteria include male or female patients aged between 18 and 65 years with a unilateral or bilateral upper limb loss, with a strong desire for functional improvement. Limb function is assessed with and without a prosthesis so that a functional risk/benefit ratio can be determined [13, 14].

For many years, prosthesis has been a reliable option for reconstruction of upper limb loss, with constant enhancement and innovations, including biomimetic robotic prosthesis that offer improved functional possibilities. However, upper extremity transplantation has become an alternative option for the treatment of upper limb loss, with highly encouraging functional outcomes and patient satisfaction [11, 15]. Both options have advantages and disadvantages that must be discussed with the patient. Once the benefits of hand transplantation over prosthesis have been established, potential contraindications that would prevent the patient

P. Tawa · M. Goutard · E. Lupon · P. Tratnig-Frankl
A. G. Lellouch · C. L. Cetrulo Jr. (✉)
Division of Plastic Surgery, Massachusetts General Hospital, Boston, MA, USA

Harvard Medical School, Boston, MA, USA
e-mail: elupon@mgh.harvard.edu; alellouch@mgh.harvard.edu; ccetrulo@mgh.harvard.edu

© Springer Nature Switzerland AG 2023

R. Gurunian et al. (eds.), *Reconstructive Transplantation*, https://doi.org/10.1007/978-3-031-21520-9_19

from being on a VCA waitlist are investigated. Usually, medical contraindications include current malignancy, chronic viral infection (HIV, hepatitis), chronic autoimmune diseases, peripheral neuropathies, blindness, and/or social or psychological issues. As in solid organ transplantation (SOT), the most important barrier to putting a patient on the waiting list for a hand transplant remains his/her ability to adhere to the recommended postoperative care in general and to lifelong immunosuppressive medication in particular [16].

This requirement is not obvious on a medical chart; hence, the surgeon and the rest of the team have to examine the patient thoroughly and dedicate as much time as necessary to discuss it with the candidate and his family. When consulting an upper limb amputee for a reconstruction solution, the patient and his entourage must be explained in the clearest way possible the extreme importance of care compliance for the rest of his life and be presented with major possible outcomes to make an informed decision. This discussion time is tremendously important in the screening process as non-compliance is the main postoperative default that leads to allograft rejection in VCAs [17, 18]. Thus, the patient–surgeon relationship must be truthful and transparent on the possible outcomes of the surgery, the complications, and the intense rehabilitation exercises it requires. The candidate must also be clear on the agenda of what to expect. For example, the misinformed patient might think that his new hand(s) will be functional as soon as the "visible" healing is complete and start using it inadequately, while the bone healing process takes several months [19]. Moreover, even though the rehabilitation process has been improved drastically with the help of specialized physical therapists, there is currently no solution to speed up the nerve regrowth time. Once all requirements are met, a few additional preoperative medical tests, including human leukocyte antigen (HLA) screening for better donor–recipient compatibility, are performed before the patient can be listed.

As of today, a total number of 2 patients were approved in the MGH upper limb transplantation program and currently 1 patient is on this list.

The COVID-19 pandemic has had a huge impact on public health and the global economy. The adaptation of health systems to this global challenge has required a redefinition of the role of plastic surgeons and surgical researchers in their communities. Current events call for a reassessment of clinical and research priorities in VCA, with a particular focus on patient safety. Little is known about COVID-19 in the transplant population, but recent evidence suggests an increased risk of serious disease associated with COVID-19 due to chronic immunosuppression and comorbidities [20]. However, we have highlighted the possibility of continuing VCA operations, despite COVID-19, by carrying out the major preparatory steps necessary for future operations through remote work that does not require a physical meeting of a group of people [21].

19.2 Patients

First, it is crucial to remind that almost no procedure in reconstructive surgery affords the opportunity for absolute preparation, especially in the VCA field. The donor operation needs to be rehearsed many times on cadavers before listing the patient, with particular attention to anatomic details relevant to each recipient listed for transplant—that is, technical details of the mid-forearm allograft recovery operation should be rehearsed specifically for a recipient with a mid-forearm amputation level. The donor procurement operation represents a culmination of months, or even years of planning to acquire the necessary approval processes from the Institutional Review Board (IRB), recipient hospital management, financial coordinators, public relations personnel, operating room staff, transplant surgery multidisciplinary staff, supporting surgical and anesthesiology physicians, nursing, and hand therapy to proceed with "listing" a potential hand transplant patient with the local Organ Procurement Organization (OPO). The regional OPO approval requires significant planning and commitment by the OPO to support a particular program. The "buy-in" by the regional OPO for a hand transplant program cannot be understated as the OPO will determine how and when a potential hand or arm allograft donor family should be approached. Despite concerns that a paucity of donors would limit the evolution of the field of hand transplantation, these fears have not been borne out as the expertise of the OPOs has led to relatively short waiting times for most hand transplant recipients. For example, the Massachusetts General Hospital patient was listed on September 11, 2012 and after receiving 3 calls for potential donors from the New England Organ Bank, the third call resulted in hand transplantation performed on October 6, 2012. In sum, a strong partnership with the OPO is paramount to success. Establishing a successful working partnership with the regional OPO and its network of regional coordinators results from understanding the "culture" of the world of transplantation, a tenet not always ingrained in the world of reconstructive surgery. For example, utilizing respectful terminology when referring to the donor procedure ("recovery" or "procurement" in lieu of "harvest") and integrating appropriate measures to show respect for the donor (e.g., a moment of respectful silence just before beginning the donor procedure to recognize the donor's gift) go a long way toward developing a successful and fruitful relationship with the OPO and the personnel who drive its mission. A critical component of this demonstration of respect for the donor is the postprocurement treatment of

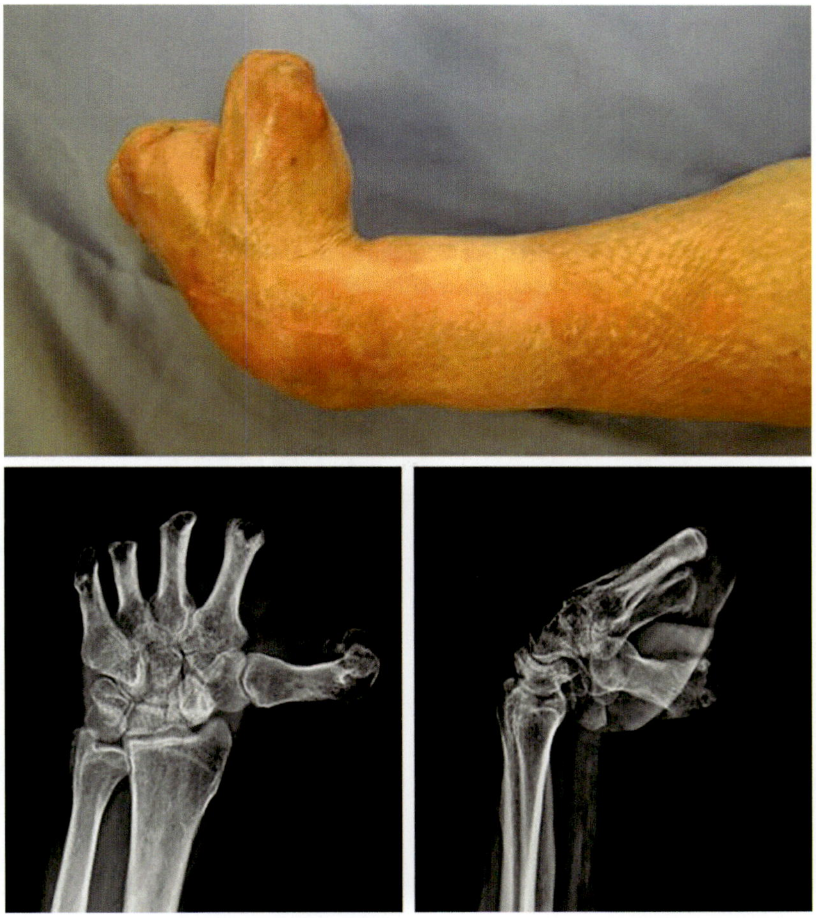

Fig. 19.1 Recipient arm with severe burn sequelae

the donor. Careful, watertight, and cosmetic closure of the amputation site is important for 2 reasons: embalming is more successful if the limbs are watertight, preventing the embalming solution from leaking when perfused. Second, an adequate soft-tissue taper facilitates prosthetic reconstruction of the limb(s) for the funeral service of the donor. Prosthetics can be obtained within a wide range of realism and cost and a number of options should be available to the surgical team. The prosthetic can be placed immediately after procurement, although some teams have suggested providing the funeral home with the prosthetic directly to avoid betadine—or worse, bloodstains—acquired in the OR during the procurement. It is important to realize that "postoperative care" of the donor family may also be required. Communication with the funeral home and regional OPO coordinator is necessary to assure that the donor family is happy with the color, size, and realism of the prosthetic that is brought to the funeral home.

The first upper extremity transplantation in Massachusetts occurred on October 6, 2012 at MGH. The recipient was a 44-year-old, left-hand-dominant man who had sustained 50 percent total body surface area burns after a tragic nightclub fire in 2003. This resulted in a metacarpal level amputation of his left hand with a truncated thumb, contracture of the first webspace, and a 45-degree flexion contracture of his wrist (Fig. 19.1).

In prior operations, the patient's forearm was debrided extensively to fascia or deeper and covered circumferentially with skin graft. Given the patient's preoperative deformity affecting both upper extremities, he was offered bilateral hand transplantation. Ultimately, he decided to pursue unilateral left-hand transplantation, as his right hand functioned as a helper limb, a function that he did not wish to jeopardize. The patency of the patient's cutaneous veins was a substantial preoperative concern given his extensive injury and surgical history, and ultrasound studies demonstrated an absence of cutaneous veins distal to the elbow suitable for anastomosis to donor veins during transplantation. To provide greater vessel caliber and more reliable venous outflow, a volar forearm extension was designed for the allograft to include the proximal basilic vein and larger vena comitans for outflow [22].

The donor was an 18-year-old brain-dead male, who was fatally injured after a traumatic accident that occurred in the northern Boston area. When arriving at the donor hospital, the team arranges the timing of hand allograft recovery relevant to the other organ procurement teams. The procurement was performed "in situ" on the donor, to allow reperfusion of the allograft before transport to the recipient hospital. The extremity of interest was prepped, a surgical time-out initiated, and a moment of silence was undertaken to acknowledge the donor's gift of life. At this time, a 5000 U IV heparin bolus was given systemically and after 3 min the tourniquet inflated to the extremity. The extremity allograft procurement was performed under tourniquet control, which included isolation of 5 cm of antecubital vein and brachial artery proximal to the elbow crease (Fig. 19.2).

The artery and vein were not yet cut, as reperfusion after the tourniquet run would be performed before the official beginning of ischemia time. All pertinent structures were dissected out and tagged with color-coded titanium tags with hole punches that were etched with the structures to be labeled (i.e., all nerves were gold tags, "median nerve"-etched tag was tagged to donor median nerve). Knots were tied down to each structure so long tails of suture that could become tangled were avoided. Once all structures were dis-

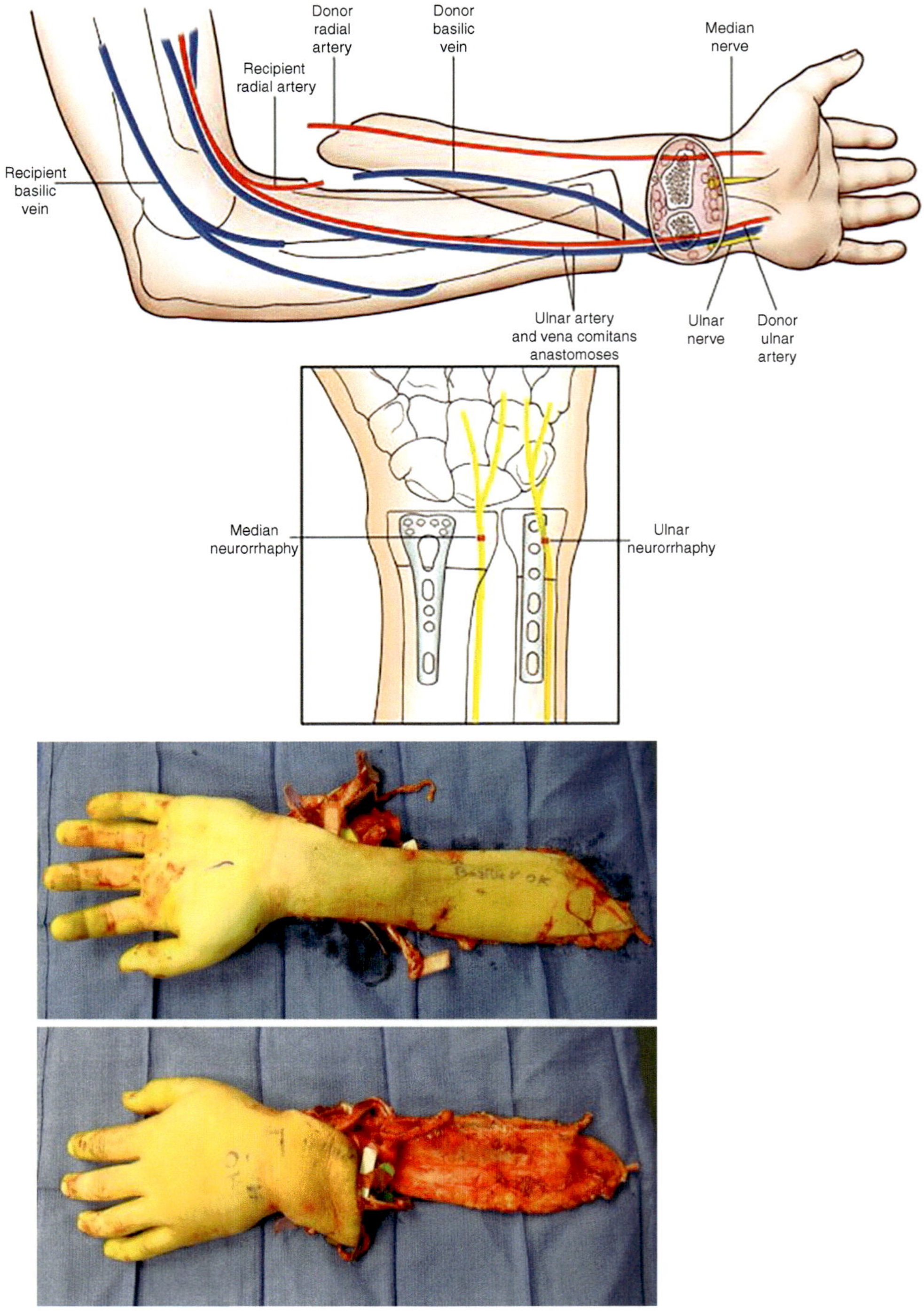

Fig. 19.2 Donor arm procurement

sected out and tagged, the tourniquet was let down and reperfusion appropriate to the length of time the extremity was under tourniquet occurs (e.g. 20 min for 2 h of dissection and tagging). This reperfusion period represented a good time to assess the progress of the recipient operation, which was proceeding concurrently at the recipient hospital with the recipient transplant team. Reperfusion was then followed by sharp disarticulation at the elbow joint. This time point marked the official beginning of ischemia time for the entire case. The extremity was then flushed on the back table, first through the brachial artery with heparin (100 U/mL) and then with a preservative solution. University of Wisconsin (UW) solution or HTK are commonly used for preservation—some teams prefer HTK because it is less viscous than UW, but has the disadvantage of being not readily available, expensive, and stocks need to be frequently replaced. OPOs do not commonly provide HTK, so the donor team would need to bring their own. In contrast, UW is commonly provided by the OPO. For this case, UW solution has been preferred. The allograft was then placed on ice in standard replant fashion inside a sealed bag that would prevent maceration or frostbite from the melting ice (i.e., wrapped in moist sterile gauze and placed in a sealed polyurethane bag) and transported in a sterile container with iced water at 4 to 6 °C. While the back table work occurred, other teammates closed the suture at the elbow disarticulation site in watertight fashion. The thoracic team could then give the standard 30,000 U of heparin and proceed with cross-clamp and organ recovery. The prosthesis to be attached to the elbow disarticulation site was provided at this time unless arrangements were to be made to deliver the prosthesis directly to the funeral home.

At the same time at MGH, the recipient left upper limb was prepared for transplantation. A cutaneous extension, incorporating the volar forearm fasciocutaneous paddle, was included with the allograft. The basilic vein was included with the fasciocutaneous extension, as it was confirmed to be patent, whereas the cephalic vein within the donor forearm was thrombosed. The forearm skin paddle was 8 cm in greatest width and designed immediately overlying the radial artery. Osteosynthesis was performed 3 cm proximal to the radiocarpal joint. The ulnar artery and vena comitans anastomoses were performed in the distal forearm proximal to the wrist crease. The radial artery, vena comitans, and basilic vein anastomoses were performed in the proximal forearm immediately distal to the antecubital fossa, providing inflow and reciprocal outflow through the volar forearm skin to and from the hand. The radial artery diameter in this region was approximately 2.5 mm and the basilic vein diameter was approximately 3.5 mm. Single-weave, "Brown" side-to-side tenorrhaphy was performed for all tendons [23]. Median and ulnar neurorrhaphies were performed distally at the wrist flexion crease. Total cold ischemia time was 5.5 h, and following vascular anastomosis, the hand was perfused without evidence of ischemia or venous congestion (Fig. 19.3).

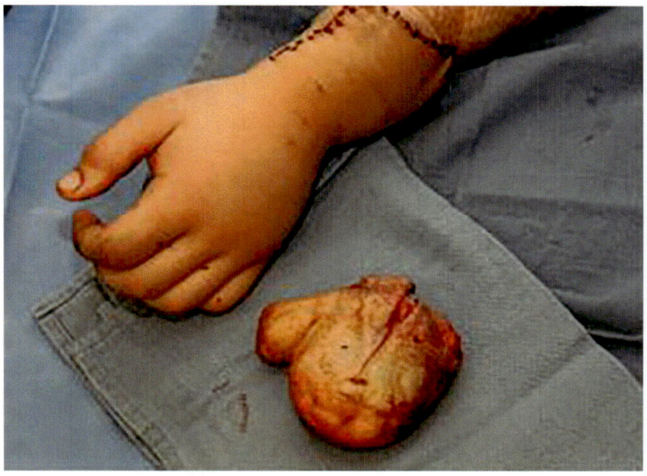

Fig. 19.3 Recipient hand after transplantation

The donor and recipient were of the same blood group and had 4/6 human leucocyte antigen (HLA) mismatches. The patient had no anti-HLA panel-reactive antibodies and retrospective cross-match was negative. The immunosuppression therapy was induced perioperatively with rabbit antithymocyte globulin, 75 mg administered intravenously; mycophenolate mofetil, 1000 mg administered orally; and methylprednisolone, 500 mg administered intravenously.

Immunosuppression was maintained postoperatively with tacrolimus (FK-506), steroids, and mycophenolate mofetil (MMF). After initial target levels of 10–15 ng of FK-506, levels were tapered down to 8–10 ng, in combination with 5 mg of steroids and MMF for maintenance therapy.

Postoperative monitoring included weekly routine skin biopsies for the first month, then once monthly for the first year. Blood work to observe infection values and kidney function was performed at the same time points. Patient was discharged at POD 14. Clinical consultations were performed routinely once a week for the first month after discharge, then monthly for the first year. With the second year the patient was seen every three months in our outpatient clinic.

For almost six years after surgery (Fig. 19.4), the patient did not experience any acute rejection (AR) episode, although AR usually occurs at least once for 85% of VCA recipients within first year [11]. At POY 6, the patient developed a bilateral polyneuropathy attributed to a side effect of tacrolimus (FK-506). The immunosuppression regimen was then modified, switching tacrolimus with cyclosporine-A (CsA). Six months later, the patient presented palmar vesicular rash on the graft combined with pain in the fingertips. The histological examination of the cutaneous biopsies revealed a grade III T-cell mediated rejection episode [24], confirming the diagnosis of atypical acute rejection episode [25]. Donor

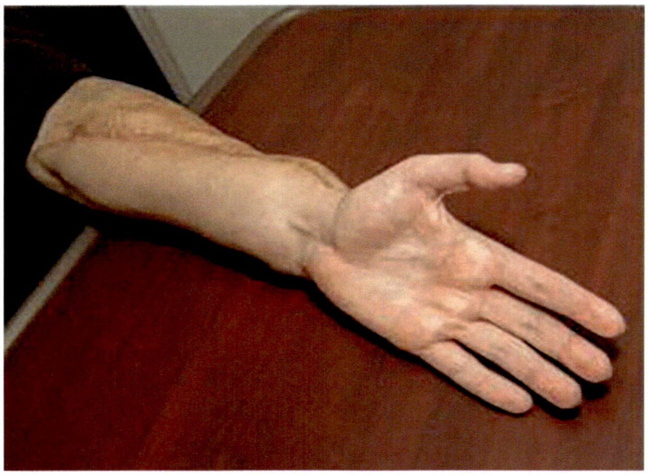

Fig. 19.4 Transplanted hand 6 years after surgery

specific antibodies (DSA) were not found in the C4d staining performed. This rejection was successfully treated with high doses of intravenous steroids, ATG, and belatacept. Another similar episode occurred six months later (Banff III atypical acute rejection) and was treated with high doses of steroids and ATG but no belatacept. Sirolimus was added to the maintenance therapy after this second acute rejection until a thrombotic episode made its discontinuation necessary. No other acute rejection episode occurred since then nor any other notable challenge.

19.3 Lessons Learned

It is crucial to have the resources and anatomic specimens to be able to practice with the team repeatedly before the operation. We learnt from other centers, and particularly Dr. Levin from University of Pennsylvania, the importance of having a step-by-step playbook that contains all the relevant organizational and operative information for both donor and recipient procedures. By following this playbook, and thanks to the resources available at MGH, we have been able to repeat the operation multiple times when the patient was still on the waiting list. These training sessions have been of great help, not only surgically but also in terms of team coordination between nurses, doctors, and residents. Collaboration with other VCA centers around the country and abroad has also been of major importance and allowed us to get some tips and tricks from different experts in this field. For instance, Dr. Kody Azari, from University of Pittsburg at the time, taught us how fixing the bones and tendons first allowed for proper tendon balance in a bloodless field prior to revascularization, thus optimizing this crucial operative step that directly impacts the patient's functional outcome.

The particularity of our case was that it was one of the first upper extremity transplantations made in a burned patient. As there were no remaining superficial veins in the recipient forearm, we had to go more proximally in order to get extra vein from uninjured tissue. We initially planned to make a cephalic sleeve, but the vein mapping made at the donor hospital showed that the cephalic vein was clotted from multiple previous IVs. We then opted for a volar forearm extension so the basilic vein could be used instead. This technique was first described by our team and really helped us deal with the additional defects of the recipient arm caused by the burns.

19.4 Perspective in VCA

Translational research in VCA from the laboratory will overcome the barriers currently present in VCAs, with the need for long-term immunosuppression at the forefront. Therefore, Dr. Cetrulo has a laboratory dedicated to VCA optimization. As a reconstructive plastic surgeon attending at the MGH, Dr. Cetrulo is also in an ideal situation to see this research translated directly from bench to bedside. Currently, lifelong immunosuppressive therapy is used to prevent acute and chronic rejection in hand transplant recipients, which can lead to a host of complications and profound side effects including predisposing patients to infections, cancer, and metabolic sequelae [26].

Kidney transplants performed at the MGH achieved mixed hematopoietic chimerism, so the recipient has no need of immunosuppressive drug regimens anymore, possibly overcoming the burden of lifelong medication [27]. Inspired by these achievements our laboratory is currently working on induction protocols in the field of VCA. Unlike in SOT, VCAs are skin containing transplants, which are considered the most immunogenic component due specifically to the important amount of antigen presenting cells present in the dermis, such as Langerhans cells and dermal dendritic cells, but also to the expression of MHC II molecules by keratinocytes upon stimulation, and the secretion of proinflammatory cytokines that attract lymphocytes to the epidermis [28–31]. To develop these kinds of protocols, our laboratory is working with a specially inbred swine herd with well-defined major histocompatibility complex (MHC), to be able to mimic clinical models [32]. We were able to induce mixed chimerism in haplo-mismatched donor–recipient scenario [33]. Later on, performing experiments, closer to the clinically more relevant full mismatch, our team was able to achieve tolerance in MHC class II mismatched swines, but failed within the MHC class I mismatch [34]. In the MHC class I group all components of the transplanted flaps were accepted by the donor, except the skin component. This phenomenon was called split-tolerances [34]. Recently we were able to demonstrate even in the MHC class I mismatch tolerance while overcoming the split-tolerance (data not published).

Current projects are focusing on enabling mixed chimerism in the full mismatched swines. Recently, another large animal study in non-human primates (NHP) was published using a delayed tolerance protocol [35]. Sixty days after the transplantation of a partial face graft, the recipients were irradiated (whole body and thymic) and then promptly received a bone marrow transplant (BMT). After the BMT, FK-506 was tapered and the recipients were checked for chimerism. Unfortunately, the protocol failed to induce chimerism and further modifications of the protocol are required. Once this barrier of immunogenicity is crossed clinical trials could be started.

Moreover, current protocols in clinical trials for mixed chimerism necessitate somewhere between 3 and 7 days to precondition the recipient, measured from initial donor graft recovery to recipient transplantation. Side stepping the need for preconditioning to induce mixed chimerism does not appear easy to achieve and failed in a clinical VCA transplant case when attempted by one team [36] Unfortunately, and contrary to kidney transplantation, in VCA there is no possibility of living donation, making advance recipient conditioning clinically unrealistic in most cases. Should donor organs be storable in the order of days, tolerance studies for VCA with current mixed chimerism protocols would be very feasible clinically. However, as with vital organs, ischemic time is an absolute technological constraint: permanent ischemic injury occurs within 6–8 h of cold ischemia in skeletal muscle, which is abundant in amputated limbs. In fact VCAs typically degrade even faster than vital organs [37]. In parallel, replantation of autografts, which is especially relevant in battlefield medicine, preserving/resuscitating the tissue after trauma to enable transportation to a surgical facility is absolutely critical but impossible with current technology. The current clinical standard in tissue preservation, static hypothermic preservation in ice-cold preservation solution (+4 °C), is insufficient to preserve tissue viability for more than a few hours, creating a technological bottleneck to realizing tolerance protocols in VCA transplantation.

Our laboratory recently developed a novel preservation protocol that enables viable preservation of rat livers for 3 days with 100% post-transplant survival, three times the maximum possible with current clinical standard [38]. This method relies on the use of supercooled temperatures below freezing point (−6 °C) to slow metabolism while avoiding freezing injury, preservative agents (PEG and 3OMG), and a rewarming step with 21 °C subnormothermic machine perfusion (SNMP), which ameliorates some of the cold ischemic injury. More recently, we developed a machine perfusion protocol for rodent hind limbs and were able to preserve rat limbs that were supercooled for 24 h in a viable state. These technologies provide our group unique readiness to extend "revolutionize ex vivo VCA tissue preservation strategies to extend the timeline between procurement and transplantation," as well as test its utility to enable tolerance induction in a clinically relevant large animal model.

To avoid the use of a damaging immunosuppressive therapy and the risk of rejection, the decellularization/recellularization strategy could also represent an interesting approach. Organ decellularization removes the native cells while preserving the extracellular matrix (ECM) molecules, in most cases by perfusing a detergent solution throughout the organ's native vasculature [39]. Recellularization consists of the repopulation of the decellularized tissue to render the organ "viable" and "transplantable" [40]. Thus, in 2018, Gerli et al. [41] performed the decellularization of a whole human limb. The main ECM components and the vasculature were preserved. The development of this human-scale acellular limb represented the first successful milestone toward the longer-term goal of constructing functional, vascularized, bioartificial reconstruction. The recellularization strategy of a native MEC could be the prerequisite to configure a very emerging and promising field, the 3D [42]. The fine structure of the tissue is not reproducible by bioprinting for the moment [43] and the decellularization/recellularization technology could be the key to solve this problem [44].

References

1. Gilbert Fernandez J, Febres-Cordero R, Simpson R. The untold story of the first hand transplant: dedicated to the memory of one of the great minds of the Ecuadorian medical community and the world. J Reconstr Microsurg. 2019;35(03):163–7.
2. Dubernard J-M, Owen E, Herzberg G, Lanzetta M, Martin X, Kapila H, et al. Human hand allograft: report on first 6 months. Lancet. 1999;353(9161):1315–20.
3. Jones JW, Gruber SA, Barker JH, Breidenbach WC. Successful hand transplantation—one-year follow-up. N Engl J Med. 2000;343(7):468–73.
4. Levi DM, Tzakis AG, Kato T, Madariaga J, Mittal NK, Nery J, et al. Transplantation of the abdominal wall. Lancet. 2003;361(9376):2173–6.
5. Strome M, Stein J, Esclamado R, Hicks D, Lorenz RR, Braun W, et al. Laryngeal transplantation and 40-month follow-up. N Engl J Med. 2001;344(22):1676–9.
6. Brännström M, Johannesson L, Bokström H, Kvarnström N, Mölne J, Dahm-Kähler P, et al. Livebirth after uterus transplantation. Lancet. 2015;385(9968):607–16.
7. van der Merwe A, Graewe F, Zühlke A, Barsdorf NW, Zarrabi AD, Viljoen JT, et al. Penile allotransplantation for penis amputation following ritual circumcision: a case report with 24 months of follow-up. Lancet. 2017;390(10099):1038–47.
8. Szafran AA, Redett R, Burnett AL. Penile transplantation: the US experience and institutional program set-up. Transl Androl Urol. 2018;7(4):639–45.
9. Cetrulo CL, Li K, Salinas HM, Treiser MD, Schol I, Barrisford GW, et al. Penis transplantation: first US experience. Ann Surg. 2018;267(5):983–8.
10. Devauchelle B, Badet L, Lengelé B, Morelon E, Testelin S, Michallet M, et al. First human face allograft: early report. Lancet. 2006;368(9531):203–9.

11. Petruzzo P, Sardu C, Lanzetta M, Dubernard JM. Report (2017) of the international registry on hand and composite tissue allotransplantation (IRHCTT). Curr Transplant Rep. 2017;4(4):294–303.
12. Mendenhall SD, Brown S, Ben-Amotz O, Neumeister MW, Levin LS. Building a hand and upper extremity transplantation program: lessons learned from the first 20 years of vascularized composite allotransplantation. Hand. 2020;15(2):224–33.
13. Salminger S, Roche AD, Sturma A, Mayer JA, Aszmann OC. Hand transplantation versus hand prosthetics: Pros and Cons. Curr Surg Rep. 2016;4(2):8. Available from: http://link.springer.com/10.1007/s40137-016-0128-3
14. Kubiak CA, Etra JW, Brandacher G, Kemp SWP, Kung TA, Lee WPA, et al. Prosthetic rehabilitation and vascularized composite allotransplantation following upper limb loss. Plast Reconstr Surg. 2019;143(6):1688–701.
15. Shores JT, Brandacher G, Lee WPA. Hand and upper extremity transplantation: an update of outcomes in the worldwide experience. Plast Reconstr Surg. 2015;135(2):351e–60e.
16. Dobbels F, Vanhaecke J, Dupont L, Nevens F, Verleden G, Pirenne J, et al. Pretransplant predictors of posttransplant adherence and clinical outcome: an evidence base for pretransplant psychosocial screening. Transplantation. 2009;87(10):1497–504.
17. Van Pilsum Rasmussen SE, Ferzola A, Cooney CM, Shores JT, Lee WA, Goldman E, et al. Psychosocial factors and medication adherence among recipients of vascularized composite allografts. SAGE Open Med. 2020;8:205031212094042.
18. Jowsey-Gregoire S, Kumnig M. Standardizing psychosocial assessment for vascularized composite allotransplantation. Curr Opin Organ Transplant. 2016;21(5):530–5.
19. Gabl M, Pechlaner S, Lutz M, Bodner G, Piza H, Margreiter R. Bilateral hand transplantation: bone healing under immunosuppression with tacrolimus, mycophenolate mofetil, and prednisolone. J Hand Surg. 2004;29(6):1020–7.
20. Akalin E, Azzi Y, Bartash R, Seethamraju H, Parides M, Hemmige V, et al. Covid-19 and kidney transplantation. N Engl J Med. 2020;382(25):2475–7.
21. Lupon E, Cetrulo CL, Lantieri LA, Lellouch AG. Comment on: composite allotransplantation in a post-COVID-19 pandemic vascularized world. Plast Reconstr Surg. 2021;148(2):315e–317e.
22. Eberlin KR, Leonard DA, Austen WG, Yaremchuk MJ, Mudgal CS, Winograd JM, et al. The volar forearm fasciocutaneous extension: a strategy to maximize vascular outflow in post-burn injury hand transplantation. Plast Reconstr Surg. 2014;134(4):731–5.
23. Brown SHM, Hentzen ER, Kwan A, Ward SR, Fridén J, Lieber RL. Mechanical strength of the side-to-side versus Pulvertaft weave tendon repair. J Hand Surg. 2010;35(4):540–5.
24. Cendales LC, Kanitakis J, Schneeberger S, Burns C, Ruiz P, Landin L, et al. The Banff 2007 working classification of skin-containing composite tissue allograft pathology: Banff CTA allograft pathology classification. Am J Transplant. 2008;8(7):1396–400.
25. Schneeberger S, Gorantla VS, van Riet RP, Lanzetta M, Vereecken P, van Holder C, et al. Atypical acute rejection after hand transplantation. Am J Transplant. 2008;8(3):688–96.
26. Schneeberger S, Khalifian S, Brandacher G. Immunosuppression and monitoring of rejection in hand transplantation. Tech Hand Up Extrem Surg. 2013;17(4):208–14.
27. Kawai T, Cosimi AB, Spitzer TR, Tolkoff-Rubin N, Suthanthiran M, Saidman SL, et al. HLA-mismatched renal transplantation without maintenance immunosuppression. N Engl J Med. 2008;358(4):353–61.
28. Lee WPA, Yaremchuk MJ, Pan Y-C, Randolph MA, Tan CM, Weiland AJ. Relative antigenicity of components of a vascularized limb allograft. Plast Reconstr Surg. 1991;87(3):401–11.
29. Sugita K, Kabashima K, Atarashi K, Shimauchi T, Kobayashi M, Tokura Y. Innate immunity mediated by epidermal keratinocytes promotes acquired immunity involving Langerhans cells and T cells in the skin. Clin Exp Immunol. 2007;147:176–83.
30. Uchi H, Terao H, Koga T, Furue M. Cytokines and chemokines in the epidermis. J Dermatol Sci. 2000;24:S29–38.
31. Gaspari AA, Katz SI. Induction and functional characterization of class II MHC (Ia) antigens on murine keratinocytes. J Immunol. 1988;140(9):2956–63.
32. Sachs DH, Leight G, Cone J, Schwarz S, Stuart L, Rosenberg S. Transplantation in miniature swine: I. fixation of the major histocompatibility complex. Transplantation. 1976;22(6):559–67.
33. Leonard DA, Kurtz JM, Mallard C, Albritton A, Duran-Struuck R, Farkash EA, et al. Vascularized composite allograft tolerance across MHC barriers in a large animal model: VCA tolerance in Miniature swine. Am J Transplant. 2014;14(2):343–55.
34. Shanmugarajah K, Powell H, Leonard DA, Mallard C, Albritton A, Harrington E, et al. The effect of MHC antigen matching between donors and recipients on skin tolerance of vascularized composite allografts. Am J Transplant. 2017;17(7):1729–41.
35. Lellouch AG, Ng ZY, Rosales IA, Schol IM, Leonard DA, Gama A-R, et al. Toward development of the delayed tolerance induction protocol for vascularized composite allografts in nonhuman primates. Plast Reconstr Surg. 2020;145(4):757e–68e.
36. Dubernard J-M, Lengelé B, Morelon E, Testelin S, Badet L, Moure C, et al. Outcomes 18 months after the first human partial face transplantation. N Engl J Med. 2007;357(24):2451–60.
37. Lin C-H, Aydyn N, Lin Y-T, Hsu C-T, Lin C-H, Yeh J-T. Hand and finger replantation after protracted ischemia (more than 24 hours). Ann Plast Surg. 2010;64(3):286–90.
38. Berendsen TA, Bruinsma BG, Puts CF, Saeidi N, Usta OB, Uygun BE, et al. Supercooling enables long-term transplantation survival following 4 days of liver preservation. Nat Med. 2014;20(7):790–3.
39. Orlando G, Remuzzi G, Williams DF, editors. Kidney transplantation, bioengineering, and regeneration: kidney transplantation in the regenerative medicine era. London: Elsevier, Academic Press, an imprint of Elsevier; 2017. p. 1225.
40. Badylak SF, Taylor D, Uygun K. Whole-organ tissue engineering: decellularization and recellularization of three-dimensional matrix scaffolds. Annu Rev Biomed Eng. 2011;13(1):27–53.
41. Gerli MFM, Guyette JP, Evangelista-Leite D, Ghoshhajra BB, Ott HC. Perfusion decellularization of a human limb: A novel platform for composite tissue engineering and reconstructive surgery. PLoS One. 2018;13(1):e0191497.
42. Duisit J, Maistriaux L, Taddeo A, Orlando G, Joris V, Coche E, et al. Bioengineering a human face graft: the matrix of identity. Ann Surg. 2017;266(5):754–64.
43. Varkey M, Visscher DO, van Zuijlen PPM, Atala A, Yoo JJ. Skin bioprinting: the future of burn wound reconstruction? Burns Trauma. 2019;7(1):4. Available from: https://academic.oup.com/burnstrauma/article/doi/10.1186/s41038-019-0142-7/5685906
44. Pati F, Cho D-W. Bioprinting of 3D Tissue Models Using Decellularized Extracellular Matrix Bioink. In: Koledova Z, editor. 3D cell culture. New York, NY: Springer New York; 2017. p. 381–90. (Methods in Molecular Biology; vol. 1612). Available from: http://link.springer.com/10.1007/978-1-4939-7021-6_27.

Upper Extremity Allotransplantation: Our Long-Term Experience in Lyon

20

Palmina Petruzzo, Jean Kanitakis, Aram Gazarian, Jean Michel Dubernard*, and Emmanuel Morelon

20.1 Introduction

Upper extremity transplantation (UET) was the first and remains the most commonly performed type of vascularized composite allotransplantation (VCA). The first successful hand transplantation was performed in Lyon in 1998 [1] and opened the VCA era, showing the feasibility of the surgical technique, efficacy of the immunosuppressive protocol, limited adverse events, and the importance of patient adherence to the immunosuppressive therapy and the rehabilitation program. The first right–hand transplantation was followed by the first bilateral hand transplantation performed in Lyon in 2000 [2] and then rapidly and successfully replicated in the United States, China, Italy, Austria, and Belgium [3].

In 2000 a prospective study including five cases of bilateral hand transplantation was approved in France by the "Comité de Protection des Personnes Participant à la Recherche Biomédicale" (CPPRB) and financed by a national grant (PHRC). It was then prolonged to 2003, including a total of seven patients. Because of ethical reasons, the French authorities allowed only bilateral hand transplantation.

At that time no set of indications for hand allotransplantation existed. Our team decided to transplant only young, otherwise healthy bilateral amputees who had used myoelectric prostheses with poor satisfaction. The goal of the study was to evaluate the efficacy and safety of the immunosuppressive protocol and the possibility of a satisfactory functional recovery.

Up till now one right-hand transplantation and seven bilateral UETs have been performed by our team. In the period of the inclusion of this cohort twenty amputees were screened. One candidate for bilateral proximal arm transplantation and one candidate for bilateral hand transplantation are on the waiting list. Both patients are included in two financed projects: DAMIE on bilateral arm transplantation (it will include 5 cases) and ARMEDIC on comparison between UET and prosthesis (it will include 15 cases).

20.2 Patients

20.2.1 Single Hand Transplantation

The recipient of the first single hand transplantation, a 48-year-old-man from New Zealand, whose right arm was accidentally amputated in 1984, received the hand of a 41-year-old brain-dead man on September 18, 1998. The donor and the recipient had the same blood group and 6 HLA (human leukocyte antigen) mismatches, negative T- and B-cell cross-match. The immunosuppressive protocol included an induction therapy based on antithymocyte globulins associated with prednisone, tacrolimus, and mycophenolate mofetil and a maintenance therapy based on prednisone 5 mg/day, tacrolimus with (blood levels between 5 and 10 ng/mL) and mycophenolate mofetil 2 g/day [1].

*Jean Michel Dubernard was deceased at the time of publication.

P. Petruzzo (✉)
Department of Transplantation, Hôpital Edouard Herriot, HCL, Lyon, France

Department of Surgery, University of Cagliari, Cagliari, Italy
e-mail: petruzzo@unica.it; palmina.petruzzo@chu-lyon.fr

J. Kanitakis
Department of Dermatology, Hôpital Edouard Herriot, HCL, Lyon, France
e-mail: jean.kanitakis@univ-lyon1.fr

A. Gazarian
Chirurgie de la Main et du Membre Supérieur, Hôpital Edouard Herriot, HCL, Lyon, France
e-mail: aram.gazarian@chu-lyon.fr

J. M. Dubernard
Department of Transplantation, Hôpital Edouard Herriot, HCL, Lyon, France
e-mail: jean-michel.dubernard@chu-lyon.fr

E. Morelon
Department of Transplantation, Hôpital Edouard Herriot, HCL, Lyon, France

Claude Bernard Lyon I University, Lyon, France
e-mail: emmanuel.morelon@chu-lyon.fr

© Springer Nature Switzerland AG 2023
R. Gurunian et al. (eds.), *Reconstructive Transplantation*, https://doi.org/10.1007/978-3-031-21520-9_20

In the first six months the patient adhered to his immunosuppressive treatment and physiotherapy protocol. He presented a well-vascularized hand graft with normal skin and nerve regeneration which resulted in protective and tactile sensation. He was able to perform the majority of daily activities (such as gripping a glass or writing) with his grafted hand. In the first post-transplant month he developed hyperglycemia and herpes virus infection as side effects of his immunosuppressive treatment. Eight weeks after transplantation, he suffered from an acute rejection episode, manifesting with erythematous maculopapular lesions disseminated on the transplanted hand, which regressed by increasing the oral dose of steroids and using topical immunosuppressants (tacrolimus and clobetasol creams).

Later, he did not always adhere to the treatment before discontinuing it completely. Fifteen months after transplantation signs of rejection appeared over the skin of the grafted hand and the lesions progressively worsened. They were remarkably similar to those seen in chronic lichenoid cutaneous graft-versus-host-disease. At the patient's request the allograft was amputated in London on March 2, 2001 (29 months after his transplantation). After amputation, various tissue specimens were studied [5] and showed that the most severe pathologic alterations (inflammatory infiltrate and necrosis) were present at the skin level. The other tissues showed milder, if any, alterations. A lymphocytic infiltrate of moderate density forming loose perivascular aggregates was shown in the vicinity of muscles and tendons [4].

20.2.2 Bilateral UET Cohort

Between 2000 and 2016 seven bilateral amputees received a bilateral UET at different levels. Table 20.1 outlines recipient and donor characteristics in bilateral upper extremity transplantation.

20.2.2.1 Pretransplant Investigations

All the recipients underwent routine pretransplant investigations and specific morphologic and functional tests of forearm stumps including angiography, functional magnetic resonance imaging (MRI), muscle and nerve charts, as well as brain functional magnetic resonance imaging (fMRI). Angiography was performed to study vascularization of both stumps; MRI to identify stump muscles, and electromyography to test nerve stimulation. To evaluate the impact of a double-hand transplantation on the hand cortical motor representation, fMRI was performed 1 month before transplantation and at 2, 4, 6, and 12 months thereafter.

20.2.2.2 Transplantation

The upper extremities were harvested from multiorgan brain-dead donors (family consent was always required and obtained), perfused with University of Wisconsin solution (in the first 2 cases) or with IGL-1 solution (in the remaining cases) and cold-stored. All patients were negative for anti-HLA antibodies before the transplantation and their T- and B-cell cross-match was negative.

The surgical procedure included bone fixation (plate and screws in all cases), vascular anastomoses (donor and recipient radial and ulnar arteries were anastomosed in all cases but in patients #6 and #7 where an end-to-side anastomosis was performed between recipient and donor humeral arteries; the number of sutured veins varied from 2 to 5), suture of 3 nerves in all patients (except for patient 1 who had only the ulnar and the median nerves sutured), and tendon suture.

The immunosuppressive protocol included induction therapy with antithymocyte globulins (ATG) and maintenance therapy with steroids (5 mg/day), tacrolimus (trough level between 5 and 10 ng/mL), and mycophenolate mofetil (2 g/day).

20.2.2.3 Rehabilitation Protocol

The rehabilitation protocol included physiotherapy, electrostimulation, and occupational therapy [2, 5]. It started 12–24 h after surgery twice daily for the first month, then it was performed daily for 4–5 h over a year. Different types of anti-claw splints were employed during the first year to protect hand allografts, avoid retractions, and facilitate the rehabilitation process. During the first 2 post-operative weeks,

Table 20.1 Recipient and donor characteristics in bilateral upper extremity transplantation

Patient	#1	#2	#3	#4	#5	#6	#7
Transplantation year	2000	2003	2007	2008	2009	2012	2016
Recipient age (years)	33	21	27	29	21	40	51
Donor age (years)	18	45	40	29	18	31	45
Level of amputation	R wrist L wrist	R mid forearm L distal forearm	R mid forearm L mid forearm	R palm L palm	R distal forearm L distal forearm	R mid forearm L mid forearm	R proximal forearm L mid forearm
Amputation cause	Explosion	Crush	Electrocution	Burn	Explosion	Crush	Sepsis
Amputation year	1996	2000	2004	2003	2004	2007	2010
HLA mismatches	5	4	4	3	5	6	6
Cold ischemia time	R 9 h 20 min L 8 h 40 min	R 8 h 10 min L 7 h 20 min	R 7 h 00 min L 7 h 00 min	R 7 h 30 min L 6 h 00 min	R 4 h 00 min L 4 h 00 min	R 2 h 55 min L 3 h 13 min	R 2 h 29 min L 2 h 34 min

R right, *L* left, *h* hours, *min* minutes

controlled-motion passive exercises were performed, then active exercises were added with respect of tenodesis effect between flexor and extensor muscles during the healing period. Electrostimulation of intrinsic muscles started after the first post-operative week to improve extrinsic muscle power and to avoid intrinsic muscle fibrosis. By the first month, exercises to improve forearm pronation, wrist and finger extension, and pinch strength were performed. By 2 months, occupational therapy was started to maintain extrinsic and intrinsic muscles, then, by six months, sensory re-education. After 9 months, the program worked on the balance of extrinsic and intrinsic muscles, fine-motor coordination, and a progressively complex program of somatosensory stimulation and retraining. At 12 months, the rehabilitation focused on all daily activities, aiming for autonomy, but also recovery of discriminative and tactile gnosis and further motor coordination.

20.2.2.4 Follow-Up

After transplantation, the medical conditions and functional results of the patients were evaluated at every annual follow-up. Macroscopic graft examination and 4-mm punch skin biopsies were performed at regular time points post-transplantation, including 1, 3, 6, and 12 months during the first year; thereafter, every 6 months over the following 2 years, then at every annual follow-up and whenever a rejection was clinically suspected. The specimens for histological examination were formalin-fixed and paraffin-embedded; 5 micron-thick sections were stained with hematoxylin-eosin and examined for the presence of pathological changes suggestive of rejection. AR severity was graded on the basis of the Banff 2007 rejection score [6]. Anti-HLA antibodies and blood lymphocyte subsets were monitored by LUMINEX and by fluorescence-activated cell sorting, respectively, at every annual follow-up and whenever an episode of AR was suspected. Metabolic, infectious, and neoplastic complications associated with the immunosuppressive treatment were carefully investigated. In addition, arterial and venous ultrasound Duplex assessment, radiological evaluation, and bone scintigraphy were performed at every annual follow-up, whereas an angiography was performed at 1 and 5 years post-transplantation and then each 5 years. From 2008 onwards, MRI of the grafted upper extremities and high-resolution peripheral quantitative computed tomographic scan were added in the study design and performed annually; in addition, from 2012 onward high-frequency ultrasonography was performed to investigate the intima-media thickness of radial and ulnar arteries. All recipients underwent an annual (intramuscular or surface) electromyogram, except for patient #3 who refused it after the first post-transplant year. Protective sensibility, touch sensation (Semmes–Weinstein test), and 2-point discrimination were investigated; active range of motion of wrist and metacarpophalangeal and interphalangeal joints was registered and grip and pinch strength was measured. Functional results were evaluated every year using the International Registry Score System (Hand Transplantation Score System, HTSS) [7], which includes graft appearance, nail and hair growth, sensibility and motion recovery, ability to perform daily activities and to work, as well as patient well-being, satisfaction, and quality of life. Moreover, the Disability of the Arm Shoulder and Hand (DASH) score [8] was calculated.

Patient #1

A 33-year-old man underwent bilateral UET in 2000. His treatment was based on the triple immunosuppressive protocol. One surgical re-intervention was performed (opposition tendon transfer at the level of the left thumb (Burkhalter's procedure). Three episodes of AR occurred (Table 20.2) and were easily reversed by increasing the dose of oral steroids. He never developed de novo donor specific antibodies (DSA).

Patient #2

A 21-year-old man underwent bilateral UET in 2003. His maintenance immunosuppressive treatment was based on the triple immunosuppressive protocol. On post-operative day 1, thrombosis of the right ulnar artery occurred and was treated by successful embolectomy. He underwent two skin revisions for cosmesis; FDP to index and long fingers were shortened to improve flexion, with benefit. During the first post-transplant year he developed two episodes of AR, which were easily reversed by increasing the oral steroid dose. In 2010 he developed de novo DSA (class II anti-HLA antibodies, 1900 MFI) which disappeared in 2013. In October 2013, signs of AR occurred and were successfully treated by increasing the dose of oral steroids; however, paraesthesia and hypoesthesia persisted in the right grafted hand. The immunosuppressive treatment was changed to avoid additional episodes of AR and the risk to develop CR; it included steroids (5 mg/day), tacrolimus (trough level between 4 and 7 ng/mL), sirolimus (trough level between 6 and 10 ng/mL), and mycophenolate mofetil (1 g/day). In 2014, DSA at very low levels reappeared (<500 MFI). In June 2014, necrosis of

Table 20.2 Acute rejection episodes

Patient	#1	#2	#3	#4	#5	#6	#7
#AR episodes	3	5	13	2	4	3	1
POD	53, 72	57, 86, 2759, 3830	16, 271,635, 951,1365, 1855,2250, 2340, 2695, 3270, 3585, 3879, 4070	65, 3034	10, 350, 930, 3950	20, 88, 154	35
Banff grade	2, 2	2, 2, 3, 3	2, 2, 3, 2, 3, 3, 3, 3, 2, 3, 3, 3, 2	2, 1	2, 2, 2, 3	2, 3, 3	2

AR acute rejection, *POD* post-operative day

the distal phalanx of the right third finger developed, followed by necrosis of other fingers. The grafts were completely removed on October 1, 2015. The histopathological study showed graft vasculopathy (GV) with luminal narrowing and arterial obstruction [9]. The day after the amputation DQ2 DSA reappeared (600 MFI). Three months later he was anti-HLA class I- and II-positive 91% and 49%, respectively.

Patient #3

A 27-year-old woman underwent bilateral UET in 2007. Her treatment was based on the usual triple immunosuppressive therapy during three years and was subsequently changed, because of several AR episodes, to steroids (5 mg/day), tacrolimus (trough level between 4 and 7 ng/mL), sirolimus (blood level between 6 and 10 ng/mL), and mycophenolate mofetil (1 g/day). Since 2016, Belatacept (375 mg/month) was introduced and sirolimus discontinued because the patient developed obesity, diabetes mellitus, and arterial hypertension. She developed 13 AR episodes (reversed by appropriate treatment such as increasing oral steroid dose, intravenous (IV) steroids, ATG, Campath-1H, and mesenchymal cells) but de novo DSA were never detected. She developed psychiatric disorders and many complications which prompted her to request graft removal; this was performed in 2018 [10].

Patient #4

A 29-year-old man underwent bilateral UET in 2008. The cause of amputation was burn injury, and therefore before transplantation he underwent bone biopsy to exclude infections and preparation of subcutaneous channels to place donor veins. His treatment was based on the usual triple immunosuppressive protocol. Two episodes of AR occurred and were successfully treated with IV steroids. He never developed de novo DSA.

Patient #5

A 21-year-old man underwent bilateral UET in 2009. His treatment was based on the usual immunosuppressive protocol. Several complications occurred during the first post-operative period including thrombosis of the right radial and the left ulnar arteries which was treated with heparin and then with a bypass between the left humeral and radial arteries. A burn occurred on the left metacarpal region from a hot pack, requiring cover with a pedicled groin flap, which was serially debulked. During the follow-up several re-interventions were performed: intrinsic release in the right hand which increased motion and function, but resulted in decreased grip; arthrodesis of the right carpometacarpal joint provided better position in the absence of intrinsic muscle recovery. On the left hand, a tendon release and tendon transfer improved thumb extension.

Four episodes of AR occurred and were reversed by IV steroids. The latest one (10.5 years after the transplantation) manifested initially with onychomadesis of both grafted hands. In January 2014 he developed de novo DSA (B56, MFI 900 and DQ2, MFI 500), in 2015 MFI were 330 and 300, respectively. The antibodies became undetectable afterwards.

Patient #6

A 40-year-old man underwent bilateral UET in 2012. His treatment was based on the usual triple immunosuppressive protocol. Three episodes of AR occurred in the early post-transplant period and were treated with IV steroids; the treatment was subsequently changed to steroids (5 mg/day), tacrolimus (trough level between 4 and 7 ng/mL), sirolimus (blood level between 6 and 10 ng/mL), and mycophenolate mofetil (1 g/day). He did not develop de novo DSA.

Patient #7

A 51-year-old man underwent bilateral UET in 2016. His treatment was based on the usual triple immunosuppressive protocol. An episode of AR occurred during the first post-transplant month and was successfully reversed by topical immunosuppressive treatment. The early post-transplant period was burdened by several infectious complications of skin and subcutaneous tissues with early plate removal in the early post-operative period. He did not develop de novo DSA.

20.2.2.5 Acute and Chronic Rejection

All patients experienced at least one episode of acute rejection (Table 20.2), which macroscopically manifested with erythematous macules over the graft skin. Microscopically, AR episodes were characterized mainly by the presence of a dermal perivascular lymphoid infiltrate made predominantly of CD3+/CD4+ T-cells occasionally reaching and penetrating the epidermis.

These episodes were reversed by increasing steroid oral dose or/and IV steroids; in patient #3 ATG and Campath-1 were used to treat some episodes of AR Banff grade 3 with capillary thrombosis and a lichenoid dermal inflammation [11]. In all patients topical immunosuppressants (clobetasol and tacrolimus ointments) were used.

Clinical signs of chronic rejection were only seen in patient #2 who developed GV leading to ischemic necroses of the graft necessitating transplant removal. However, in patient #3 pathological examination performed after the amputation revealed signs of GV, such as increased thickness of vessel wall resulting in some degree of luminal narrowing. Interestingly, in this patient the vascular changes were less severe and widespread compared with those reported in patients with clinical evidence of chronic rejection [10].

20.2.2.6 Functional Recovery

Functional recovery is the final goal in UET. It is a long and complex process, which not only involves preservation of the viability of neural, muscular, and sensory end-organ components but also requires appropriate and timely reinnervation of neural targets and several degrees of cortical reorganization. The functional outcome obtained in limb transplantation seems to be related to the level of amputation; indeed, our experience shows earlier results in the case of amputation at the wrist level. However, late functional outcome appears very encouraging also at the forearm level as demonstrated by the results achieved in the second and third recipient who presented a forearm amputation.

All the recipients showed a relevant sensorimotor recovery, which was evaluated using the HTSS and the DASH score (Figs. 20.1 and 20.2). All recipients showed recovery of protective and tactile sensibility; in addition, they regained partial discriminative sensibility as well as partial recovery of intrinsic muscles. Extrinsic and intrinsic muscle recovery enabled all patients, from 4 to 20 years of follow-up, to perform most daily activities, including eating, driving, grasping objects, stringing a needle, riding a bicycle, shaving, using the telephone and writing; they live a normal social life and patients #1 and #5 worked for three years and fifteen months after transplantation, respectively. Despite a remarkable functional recovery, all patients presented a limited

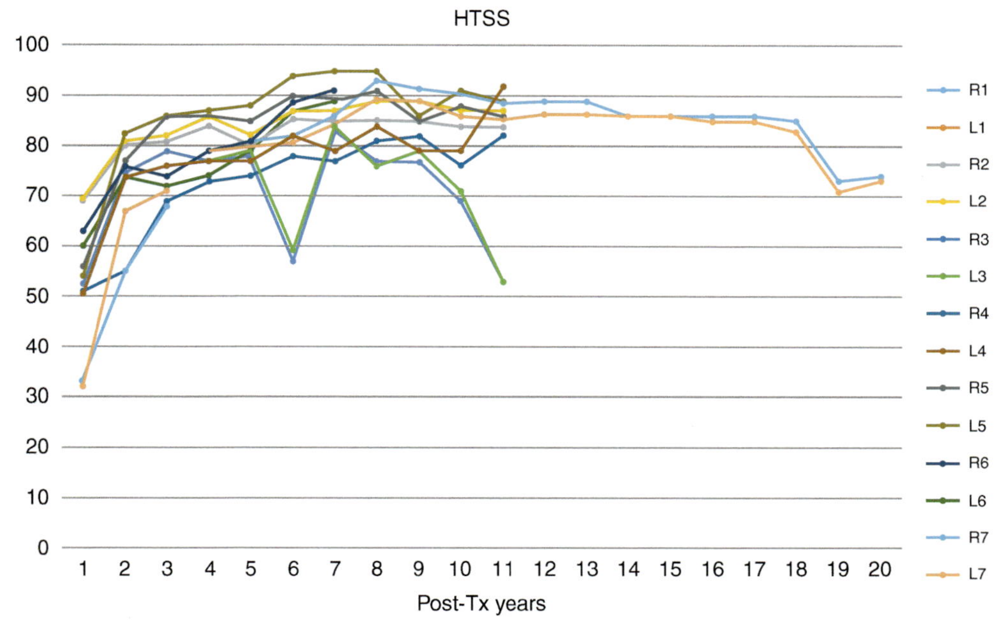

Fig. 20.1 The International Registry Hand Score System (HTSS) is represented by the curves of the right (R) and the left (L) transplanted upper extremity in the 7 recipients during the follow-up. Tx: Transplantation

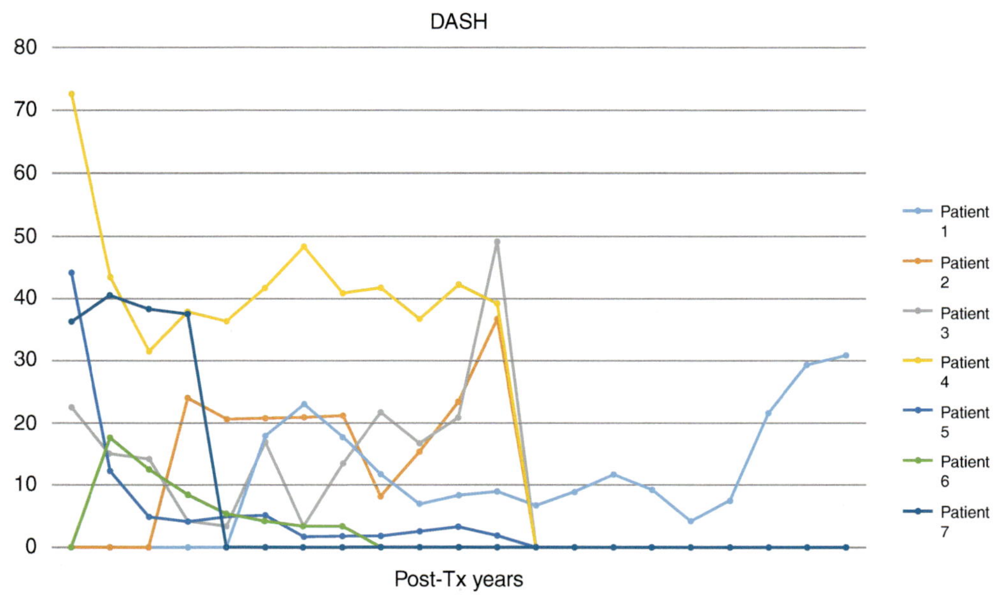

Fig. 20.2 The Disability of the Arm Shoulder and Hand (DASH) score is represented by a curve for each recipient during the follow-up

range of motion of their joints because of fibrosis and adherences, a variable degree of muscular hypotrophy and a diminished muscular power.

In all patients nerve conduction studies revealed motor reinnervation for median and ulnar nerves with an increase in motor action potentials during the first years. Cortical reorganization was shown by fMRI and transcranial magnetic resonance. Functional MRI was performed before and after transplantation at different time points of the follow-up in the bilateral hand-grafted patients showing that hand transplantation results in global remodeling of the limb cortical map, reversing the functional reorganization induced by the amputation [12]. Transcranial magnetic stimulation [12] showed a gradual reappearance of intrinsic hand-muscle representations in the motor cortex with distinct time courses for right and left muscles and also an asymmetry between the two upper extremities [13]. Although it is not yet possible to define how the level of amputation and the quality of peripheral reconnection interacted with central factors in determining the degree and extent of functional recovery, it is obvious that the process of motor cortical plasticity allows the recognition and integration of the transplanted muscles.

20.2.2.7 Complications

All the recipients presented some complications the majority of them being infectious and metabolic. Hyperglycemia occurred in the early post-transplant period in patients #1 and #5 (first 30 and 10 post-operative days, respectively; it required insulin therapy and then regressed), and in patient #6 who developed a post-transplant diabetes mellitus which still requires oral treatment with antidiabetic drugs. A transient increase in serum creatinine values occurred in patients #1 and #5. Hypercholesterolemia and various degrees of osteopenia/osteoporosis developed in the majority of patients. Arterial hypertension occurred in patients #5, #6, and #7. Osteitis of the left ulna occurred in patient #2 on day 152 and was successfully treated by antibiotics and removal of hardware. Herpes zoster infection occurred in patients #4 and #5. Patient #7 developed several infections (cutaneous and subcutaneous infection of the grafts in the first post-operative period, then pneumonia, scrotal abscess, and sepsis) also correlated to the previous splenectomy. Patient #1 developed serum sickness on day 7, tinea versicolor and scabies during the follow-up.

Patient #3 developed many metabolic and infectious complications (obesity, diabetes, hypertension, osteoporosis with bone fractures, bacterial and viral infections) correlated to the immunosuppressive treatment (particularly the therapy of the high number of AR episodes) and the psychiatric disorders which manifested after the transplantation.

20.2.2.8 Patient and Graft Survival

No death occurred. The unilateral hand transplantation recipient underwent graft removal due to active chronic rejection 29 months after transplantation; this was due to discontinuation of his immunosuppressive treatment. The transplants were removed in two bilateral UET recipients: in patient #2 it was due to progressive GV which occurred eleven years after transplantation and in patient #3 psychiatric disorders and many complications prompted her to request transplant removal nine years after transplantation.

20.3 Lessons Learned

In conclusion, although the results achieved in this first series showed the feasibility of UET, we also learned the paramount importance of patient motivation and adherence to the immunosuppressive treatment and physiotherapy.

UET not only provides sensory feedback, but is also more able to restore body image and a sense of wholeness by replacing "like with like." Nonetheless, the risks due to the life-long immunosuppressive treatment and the requirements of extensive hand therapy and long recovery and hospitalization periods are not to be underestimated. Our patients were satisfied with their transplanted UET, including patient #3 who considered the UET as a "benefit" even before the amputation, however pre-existing psychiatric conditions (i.e. depression, anxiety, post-traumatic stress disorder) and the impact of post-transplant complications on the patients' life might result in some patients in a decrease in QoL in the long-term follow-up. Their QoL is not only correlated to satisfaction, functional capacity, and functional demands but also to the patients' "well-being" which is in part correlated to the patients' capacity to overcome AR episodes, hospitalization, long-term constraints of the treatment.

In our experience patient selection influences UET outcomes with emphasis on medical, behavioral, psychological, and social factors. Moreover, the success of UET depends on the careful follow-up of the patients. This success relies also on the creation of a complex medical team, whose members can closely cooperate and contribute with their competence and enthusiasm to achieve these results.

On a final note, the paucity of donors is the main obstacle to a faster development of our program. Moreover, the COVID-19 pandemic is currently a further obstacle to the realization of VCA.

References

1. Dubernard JM, Owen E, Herzberg G, Lanzetta M, Martin X, Kapila H, Dawahra M, Hakim N. Human hand allograft: report on first 6 months. Lancet. 1999;353(9161):1315–20.
2. Dubernard JM, Petruzzo P, Lanzetta M, Parmentier H, Martin X, Dawahra M, Hakim NS, Owen E. Functional results of the first human double-hand transplantation. Ann Surg. 2003;238(1):128–36.
3. Petruzzo P, Sardu C, Lanzetta M, Dubernard JM. Report (2017) of the international registry on hand and composite. Curr Transpl Rep. 2017;4:294–303.

4. Kanitakis J, Jullien D, Petruzzo P, Hakim N, Claudy A, Revillard JP, Owen E, Dubernard JM. Clinicopathologic features of graft rejection of the first human hand allograft. Transplantation. 2003;76(4):688–93.
5. Petruzzo P, Gazarian A, Kanitakis J, Parmentier H, Guigal V, Guillot M, Vial C, Dubernard JM, Morelon E, Badet L. Outcomes after bilateral hand allotransplantation: a risk/benefit ratio analysis. Ann Surg. 2015;261(1):213–20.
6. Cendales L, Kanitakis J, Schneeberger S, Burns C, Ruiz P, Landin L, Remmelink M, Hewitt C, Landgren T, Lyons B, Drachenberger C, Solez K, Kirk A, Kleiner D, Racusen L. The Banff 2007 working classification of skin-containing composite tissue allograft pathology. Am J Transplant. 2008;8(7):1396–400.
7. Lanzetta M, Petruzzo P. A comprehensive functional score system in hand transplantation. In: Lanzetta M, Dubernard JM, editors. Hand transplantation. Milan, Italy: Springer-Verlag; 2007. p. 355–62.
8. Gummesson C, Atroshi I, Ekdahl C. The disabilities of the arm, shoulder and hand (DASH) outcome questionnaire: longitudinal construct validity and measuring self-rated health change after surgery. BMC Musculoskelet Disord. 2003;16(4):11.
9. Kanitakis J, Petruzzo P, Badet L, Gazarian A, Thaunat O, Testelin S, Devauchelle B, Dubernard JM, Morelon E. Chronic rejection in human vascularized composite allotransplantation (hand and face recipients): an update. Transplantation. 2016;100(10):2053–61.
10. Petruzzo P, Seulin C, Kanitakis J, Feugier P, Gazarian A, Badet L, Morelon E. Lessons learned from the amputation of a bilateral hand grafted patient due to psychiatric disorders. Plast Reconstr Surg Glob Open. 2020;8(10):e2905
11. Kanitakis J, Petruzzo P, Gazarian A, Karayannopoulou G, Buron F, Dubois V, Thaunat O, Badet L, Morelon E. Capillary thrombosis in the skin: a pathologic hallmark of severe/chronic rejection of human vascularized composite tissue allografts? Transplantation. 2016;100(4):954–7.
12. Giraux P, Sirigu A, Schneider F, Dubernard JM. Cortical reorganization in motor cortex after graft of both hands. Nat Neurosci. 2001;4(7):691–2.
13. Vargas CD, Aballéa A, Rodrigues EC, Reilly KT, Mercier C, Petruzzo P, Dubernard JM, Sirigu A. Re-emergence of hand-muscle representations in human motor cortex after hand allograft. Proc Natl Acad Sci U S A. 2009;106(17):7197–202.

Hand Transplantation: The Brigham and Women's Hospital Experience

21

Mario A. Aycart, Sarah E. Kinsley, Leonardo V. Riella, and Simon G. Talbot

Abbreviations

ADL	Activities of daily living
DASH	Disability of the arm, shoulder, and hand questionnaire
HTSS	Hand transplantation score system
IRHCTT	International registry on hand and composite tissue transplantation
VCA	Vascularized composite allotransplantation

21.1 Introduction

21.1.1 Program Inception

Brigham and Women's Hospital has a rich tradition in transplantation dating back to Dr. Joseph Murray's first successful human kidney transplantation in identical twins in 1954 [1]. Our VCA program began with our Institutional Review Board (IRB) approval of our face transplantation protocol in 2008 [2]. Our hand transplantation program followed closely thereafter in 2009 with our hand transplantation clinical trial (ClinicalTrials.gov #NCT01293214) under IRB-approved protocol #2009P01719. We have performed four bilateral upper extremity transplants since 2011. The program is still active, caring for post-transplantation patients and recruiting additional new patients.

M. A. Aycart · S. E. Kinsley
Division of Plastic Surgery, Brigham and Women's Hospital, Boston, MA, USA
e-mail: maycart@partners.org; skinsley@bwh.harvard.edu

L. V. Riella
Department of Medicine, Massachusetts General Hospital, Boston, MA, USA
e-mail: lriella@mgh.harvard.edu

S. G. Talbot (✉)
Upper Extremity Transplantation, Brigham and Women's Hosipital, Boston, MA, USA

Harvard Medical School, Boston, MA, USA
e-mail: sgtalbot@bwh.harvard.edu

21.1.2 Funding

Funding for the research aspects of the program was made possible through several Congressionally Directed Medical Research Program (CDMRP) grants from the U.S Department of Defense. Clinical care including surgery and immediate perioperative care for three months post-transplantation has been covered by Brigham and Women's Hospital. Ongoing immunosuppression is covered by patients' primary health insurance (and is pre-arranged prior to listing for transplantation). More recent Department of Defense grants cover clinical care for patients receiving novel immunosuppression protocols.

21.1.3 Patient Screening

Screening falls into several categories. Many potential candidates contact us by phone, email, or through our website to enquire about hand transplantation. This is then followed by a phone discussion. If the patient is a viable candidate and remains interested in transplantation, they are invited to meet a small subset of the team (surgeons, transplant physicians, and social worker). After this consultation, if they are felt to be a good candidate and wish to continue, they then proceed to meet the whole transplant team and undergo thorough screening. This includes a full medical evaluation, laboratory testing, imaging, electromyographic testing, and psychosocial screening. In 2015, we reported on our initial six-year experience with patient referrals and screening [3]. At that time, we had a total of 89 contacts, of which 25 underwent screening. Four of these patients were accepted and three

© Springer Nature Switzerland AG 2023
R. Gurunian et al. (eds.), *Reconstructive Transplantation*, https://doi.org/10.1007/978-3-031-21520-9_21

Table 21.1 Upper extremity transplant candidate criteria

Dominant or bilateral hand amputee
Age between 18 and 60 years
Strong motivation to proceed with transplant
Accepts dedicating >2 years to post-operative rehabilitation
Elapsed injury to transplant time >6 months, <15 years
History of current general health (e.g., no cardiopulmonary dysfunction, impaired renal and/or hepatic function; update age and family history-specific cancer screening, and no history of active cancer with or without metastases or within past 5 years)
Demonstrates record of medication compliance and social support system/family structure
Reports suboptimal outcome with myoelectric prosthesis for > 6 months, verified by occupational therapist
Must be able to receive adequate follow-up care and immunosuppression (without geographic or financial limitations)

Table 21.2 Upper extremity transplant Brigham and Women's Hospital patient screening transplant donor criteria

Similar phenotypic characteristics – e.g., skin color and tone; limb size and bone dimensions
Age (typically 18-60 years) and sex matching are considered
No history of unresolved sepsis, HIV/AIDS, active/untreated viral hepatitis or encephalitis, active CMV, active EBV, or active tuberculosis
No history of rheumatoid, or osteoarthritis of the transplanted limb(s)
No history of peripheral neuropathy, or other inflammatory or toxic neuropathy

Abbreviations: HIV human immunodeficiency virus, *AIDS* acquired immunodeficiency syndrome, *CMV* cytomegalovirus, *EBV* Epstein-Barr virus

Table 21.3 BWH cohort upper extremity transplant Brigham and Women's Hospital patient screening: upper extremity donor and recipient characteristics

Patient	1	2	3	4
Transplantation Date	May 2011	October 2011	October 2014	August 2016
Sex	F	M	M	M
Age at transplantation (years)	56	65	40	31
Years since amputation at time of transplantation	2	9	2	6
Cause of amputation	Animal attack	Sepsis	Sepsis	Improvised explosive device
Level of amputation	Left forearm, Right hand	Bilateral mid-forearm	Left above elbow, right below elbow	Left below elbow, right above elbow
Donor/recipient CMV status	+/+	–/–	–/–	–/–
Donor/recipient EBV status	+/+	+/+	+/+	+/+

Abbreviations: CMV cytomegalovirus, *EBV* Epstein-Barr virus, *M* male, *F* female

went on to transplantation, while the other was placed on the waiting list. Since then, we have had an additional 30 contacts, of which 11 were screened and one was accepted and ultimately went on to transplantation.

The purpose of evaluating potential recipients of upper extremity transplants is to identify risk factors that may pose a prohibitive risk to transplantation. Understandably, exclusion criteria of donors and recipients vary substantially among centers, and with advances in medical care, and experience gained in VCA, contraindications will continue to evolve and change with time. At present, our center like many others has absolute and relative contraindications (see Tables 21.1 and 21.2). We consider other potential barriers to transplantation on a case-by-case basis using a multidisciplinary approach. This includes a full psychiatric evaluation, which is performed to ensure that the patient is able to adapt to the psychological stressors associated with the complex intervention and recovery and to inquire into the patient's social support network.

Other important recipient screening practices include standard laboratory tests with the aim of excluding any malignancies, active infections, or other systemic illness that would preclude safe transplantation and long-term immunosuppressive therapy. Further, gender- or age-specific screening examinations such as colonoscopy, mammography, or prostate-specific antigen testing are performed according to standard national criteria during the screening process as is standard prior to solid organ transplantation. A pre-operative radiographic evaluation of the upper extremities is routinely performed, as this is a crucial component of the work-up to allow for pre-operative measurements of existing bony anatomy and allows for examination of the quality of the bone. A standard angiogram is also obtained to allow for exact visualization of the existing vasculature. Finally, we also obtain nerve conduction and electromyography studies to help determine the level and nature of muscle innervation.

Donor criteria in upper extremity transplantation are multifaceted and vary by institution. Whereas for most solid organ transplants, ABO blood group compatibility and absence of antibodies against donor human leukocyte antigen (HLA) are used as the main determinants of the immunologic compatibility, matching for upper extremity transplantation is more selective. In addition to above criteria, our center also uses other donor matching criteria, such as skin color, approximate age, size, and gender in addition to negative T- and B-cell cytotoxic cross matches. Other criteria are listed in Table 21.2. Donor and recipient characteristics are listed in Table 21.3.

21.1.3.1 Patient Approval and Current Waitlist

Five patients have been approved, four transplanted, one delisted, and none currently on the waiting list.

21.1.3.2 Obstacles to Program Expansion

Upper extremity transplantation continues through a transition from an experimental option to a mainstream treatment. Several obstacles exist (see Fig. 21.1):

1. Funding: Much of our clinical work continues to be funded internally by Brigham and Women's Hospital. Significant expansion seems unlikely without routine coverage by third-party payers.
2. Immunosuppression: The risk–benefit ratio between improved physical and psychosocial function versus lifelong immunosuppression (and its associated risks) continues to limit candidates to those most severely disabled and those willing to accept this tradeoff. Improved immunosuppression and decreased risks will allow further expansion.
3. Candidates: While there are significant numbers of upper extremity amputees, several factors limit the number who can undergo this complex surgery, including psychosocial issues, physical issues, and concurrent medical concerns. With improvements in technology and our healthcare system, the number of these patients who become appropriate candidates may increase.

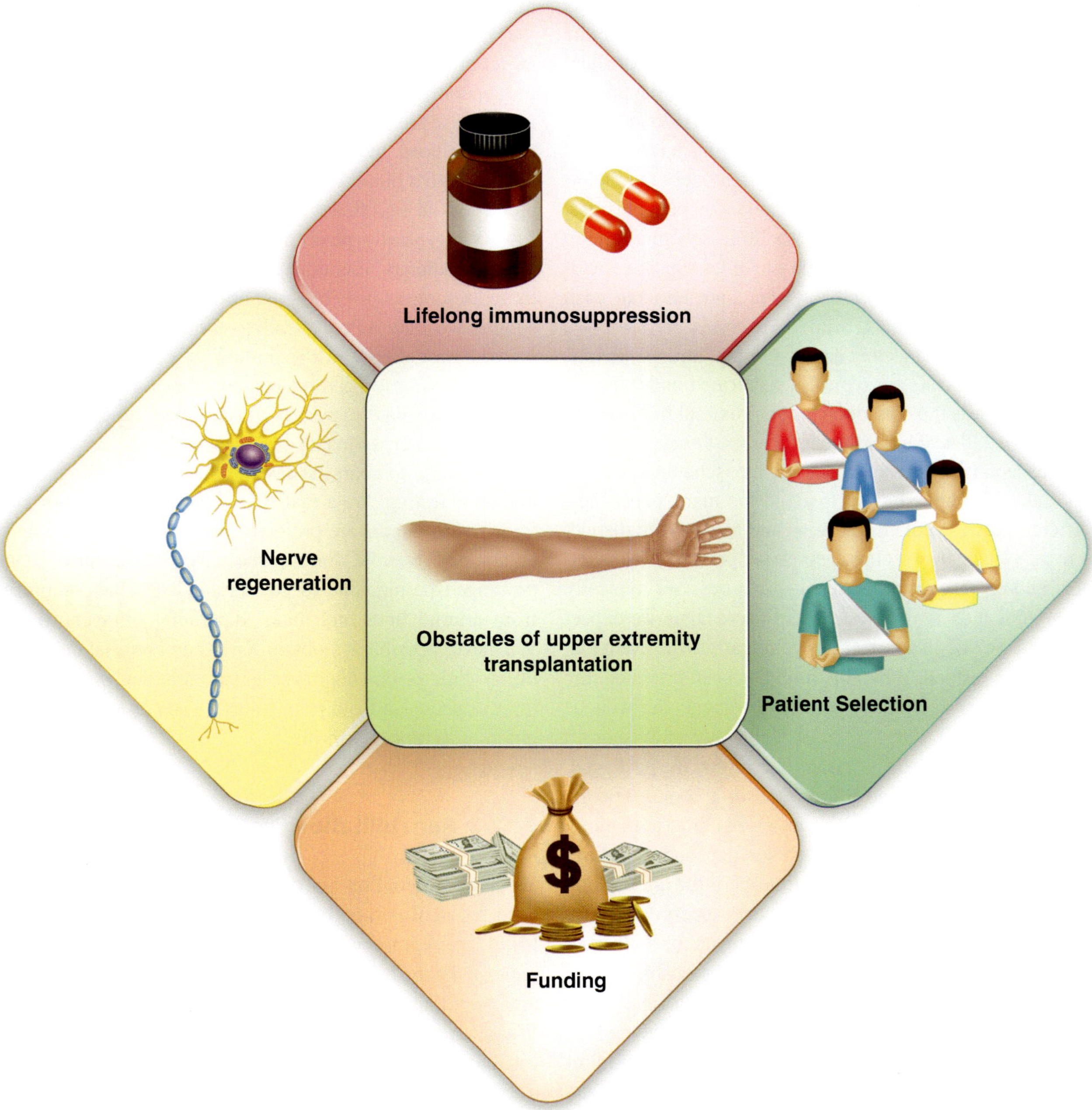

Fig. 21.1 Obstacles to upper extremity transplantation

4. Nerve regeneration: Recovery of nerves after transplantation remains the proverbial Achilles heel of upper limb transplantation, especially in those patients with high or trans-humeral amputations and those with associated brachial plexopathies. Improvements in nerve regeneration may broaden the list of potential candidates.

21.2 Patients

21.2.1 Surgical Technique

Similar to many centers, we utilize a two-team approach each with one lead surgeon dedicated to the limb procurement and the other to recipient preparation. Frequently the donor and recipient are in different hospitals and we use plaster molds, photographs, and radiographs of the recipient to help guide the location of incisions. Significant pre-planning has occurred including multiple cadaveric dissections to model each recipient and donor pair to ensure appropriate cutaneous incisions, bony length, and hardware fitting. We limit ischemia time to less than four hours including travel time of less than one-and-a-half hours. Whenever possible we prepare and tag each major structure of the donor, while the limb is perfused. We use waterproof paper tags that can be written intraoperatively. Our limb procurements are typically performed under tourniquet control unless the dissection is too proximal in the upper extremity. We deflate the tourniquet for at least twenty minutes before transecting the vessels to "reset" the ischemia duration. For the sake of simplicity, and to avoid too many paper tags, we differentially tag cutaneous veins and nerves with distinct clips (e.g., veins get two clips, nerves get one clip). To avoid tension and/or insufficient critical structures, we typically obtain significantly longer vessels and nerves than we expect to need, and we obtain a saphenous vein graft, in the event that vein grafts are needed. When the limb has been procured, the brachial artery is cannulated with a 16-gauge intravenous catheter and flushed with 500 cc of University of Wisconsin solution until the effluent is clear. The limbs are packaged, immersed in ice slurry, and transported in a cooler. For the transplantation, our order of repair follows similar to that of a replantation: osteosynthesis (plate choice dependent on level of amputation), microvascular anastomosis of the arteries and venae comitantes (and often at least one superficial vein), tenorrhaphies using a modified Kessler repair or Pulvertaft weave, muscle repairs using figure-of-eight absorbable sutures or joining GIA staple lines, neurorrhaphies, and finally soft tissue closure. We have found that interdigitating zig-zag skin flaps tailored to optimize a minimal tension closure and prevent a circumferential contracture with layered closure and use of closed-suction drains or a Penrose drain has worked well with very minimal complications.

As expected, preparation and organization are key. We practice dissections on cadaveric models simulating the level of transplantation planned. Planning for appropriate limb length, especially in patients with one above- and one below-elbow amputation is important, and we use normative limb length data from the forensic literature in determining the anticipated limb lengths and appropriate donor size. We prepare a bag of disposable equipment to travel with us to each donor hospital to avoid not having necessary equipment. We bring additional surgical headlights to facilitate multiple concurrent surgeons. Ahead of each case we discuss with our solid organ procurement colleagues to ensure that we will not impact their surgery, and typically we procure the limbs ahead of the visceral procurement. We have a strict time schedule to ensure that we minimize ischemia time and have the procured limbs available at the time that the recipient limbs are ready. We have considerable pre-operative discussions with our anesthesiologists including development of a protocol so that intraoperative immunosuppression, antibiotics, and blood product use are clear ahead of time. To limit exposure to additional antigens and to minimize hypercoagulability, we use intraoperative blood collection instruments ("Cell Saver") if blood loss is significant and have a high threshold to transfuse. We typically place central venous lines and brachial plexus catheters immediately pre-operatively and remove these as soon as possible post-operatively. Months ahead of surgery we place a Port-a-Cath to allow easy blood draws and medication delivery in the immediate post-operative period without having to perform venipuncture on the transplanted limbs. Immediately pre-operatively, we repeat laboratory testing and a cross-match if not recently on file. We have a low threshold to abort the case if concerning findings on pre-operative testing. We are also very careful with donor selection. Young donors are preferred, without identifiable tattoos or marks. We avoid donors who have been in an ICU for a prolonged period, due to edema and vascular compromise from arterial lines and many superficial intravenous lines. Whenever possible we obtain X-rays and arterial and venous ultrasounds of our donors to ensure absence of occult fractures or sequelae from prior injuries such as a scaphoid non-union or advanced arthritis.

21.2.2 Rehabilitation Protocol

We have reported on our detailed rehabilitation protocol and each protocol is modified according to each patient's needs [4]. As is common with other centers, our protocol uses principles from the replantation literature, using multimodal therapy including splinting, edema and scar management, range of motion and activities of daily living (ADL) exercises, electrical stimulation, cognitive training, and strengthening [5]. The protocol is divided into four phases of care. This includes pre-operative, and three post-operative phases: initial (days 0–14), intermediate (3–8 weeks), and late (week 9 onward). We administer formal testing including quantitative measures and video assessments pre-operatively and at specific time

Table 21.4 BWH upper extremity transplants: patient-reported outcome measures

Patient	2	3	4
Follow-up (years)	8	5	3.5
Level of amputation	Bilateral mid-forearm	Left above elbow, right below elbow	Left below elbow, right above elbow
DASH	50	41.7	39
HTSS	R 63 L 67	R 69 L 69	R 75 L 75
Carroll test	R 55 L 57	R 55 L 55	R 63 L 62

DASH Disability of the arm, shoulder, and hand questionnaire, *HTSS* Hand transplantation score system
DASH scale score ranges from 0 (no disability) to 100 (most severe disability)
HTSS: 81–100 points is graded as an excellent outcome, 61–80 as good, 31–60 as fair and 0–30 as poor

Table 21.5 Range of motion, total active motion, grip strength, and Semmes-Weinstein sensation of BWH upper extremity transplant recipients

Patient	2	3	4
Follow-up (years)	8	5	3.5
Level of amputation	Bilateral mid-forearm	Left above elbow, right below elbow	Left below elbow, right above elbow
Forearm Pronation/ supination, range/degrees	R 75°/55° L 80°/30°	R 40°/–20° L 65°/35°	R 90°/0° L 90°/0°
Wrist extension/ flexion, range/ degrees	R 60°/0° L 0°/55°	R 15°/65° L 75°/55°	R 80°/45° L 65°/65°
Thumb TAM, degrees	R 50 L 40	Not measured	R 80 L 40
Other digits TAM, degrees	R 122 L 46	Not measured	R 230 L 152
Grip strength, lbs	R 1 lbs L 2 lbs	Not measured	R 3 lbs L 4 lbs
Sensation	R dorsum & volar: Loss of protective sensation L dorsum & volar: Diminished protective sensation	R dorsum & volar: Diminished light touch L dorsum & volar: Diminished light touch	R dorsum: Diminished light touch R volar: Diminished protective sensation L dorsum: Intact L volar: Diminished protective sensation

Abbreviations: TAM total active motion, *lbs* pounds

points at 6, 12, and 24 weeks post-transplant and every six months thereafter. We use several standardized global upper extremity scoring systems such as the Disability of the Arm Shoulder and Hand (DASH) questionnaire [6, 7], Hand Transplantation Score System (HTSS) [8], and the Carroll Test [9]. We undertake routine, standard occupational therapy measurements including range of motion testing, Semmes-Weinstein monofilament evaluation, and grip/pinch strength. As part of our evaluation of functional outcomes, we also videotape assessments in the clinic and have patients send videos of their ADLs and when accomplishing important milestones. We have found that video evaluations have been a useful addition to standardized testing and allow for a more complete evaluation of improvements and changes in function [10]. Patient-reported outcome measures and objective measures are listed in Tables 21.4 and 21.5, respectively.

21.2.3 Immunosuppression Protocol

Currently, there is no standard immunosuppressive regimen for upper extremity transplantation recipients. Our immunosuppression protocols, as with many other VCA centers, are based on years of work and success in solid organ transplantation. At our institution, induction therapy consists of thymoglobulin and high-dose steroids followed by maintenance immunosuppression consisting of tacrolimus, mycophenolate mofetil, and a tapered prednisone regimen. Episodes of acute rejection, pending clinical condition of the patient, severity, and type of rejection are typically managed with pulse-dose steroids (solumedrol 500 mg/day for 3 days) and maintenance immunosuppression is temporarily increased if trough levels are deemed insufficient. In addition, topical steroids or tacrolimus are used in some patients as adjuvant therapy. In cases of no response to the aforementioned treatment, anti-thymocyte globulin or alemtuzumab (patient #4) is administered as rescue therapy. For antibody-mediated rejection, plasmapheresis and intravenous immunoglobulin are considered. Appropriate *Pneumocystis* prophylaxis with trimethoprim-sulfamethoxazole and cytomegalovirus prophylaxis with valganciclovir are given for 6 months post-transplantation, or longer with treatment for acute rejection(s).

While we have previously reported on our successful steroid withdrawal [11], this is not uniform for all of our VCA patients and each has a specific regimen tailored to their immunologic profile. Those with donor-specific antibodies remain on low dose prednisone. After transplantation, the patient's general medical condition and functional results are monitored closely. We perform 4 mm punch biopsies at 3, 6, and 12 months and then annually as well as during suspected rejection episodes (such as presentations with rashes, suspicious exanthemas, or new cutaneous lesions). Specimens are formalin-fixed and paraffin-embedded for further analysis by our Dermatopathology Section at Brigham and Women's Hospital. All samples are assessed according to the most recent Banff 2007 Working Classification of Skin-Containing Composite Tissue Allograft Pathology [12]. We have not seen evidence of chronic rejection in our

Table 21.6 Acute rejection episodes of upper extremity transplant recipients

Patient	2	3	4
Number of AR episodes	3	2	3
Timepoint (months)	10, 36, 38	7 days, 3	1, 2, 3
Banff grade	I, III, II	II with DSA, II	II/III, II/III, III
Treatment	All three episodes: increased IS, topical steroid/tacrolimus	1. plasmapheresis + IVIG 2. IV steroids, increased IS	1. Increased IS, IV steroids 2. IV steroids, ATG 3. Alemtuzumab, steroid taper, topical steroid/tacrolimus

Abbreviations: AR acute rejection, *IS* immunosuppression, *ATG* anti-thymocyte globulin, *IV* intravenous, *IVIG* intravenous immunoglobulin, *DSA* donor specific antibody

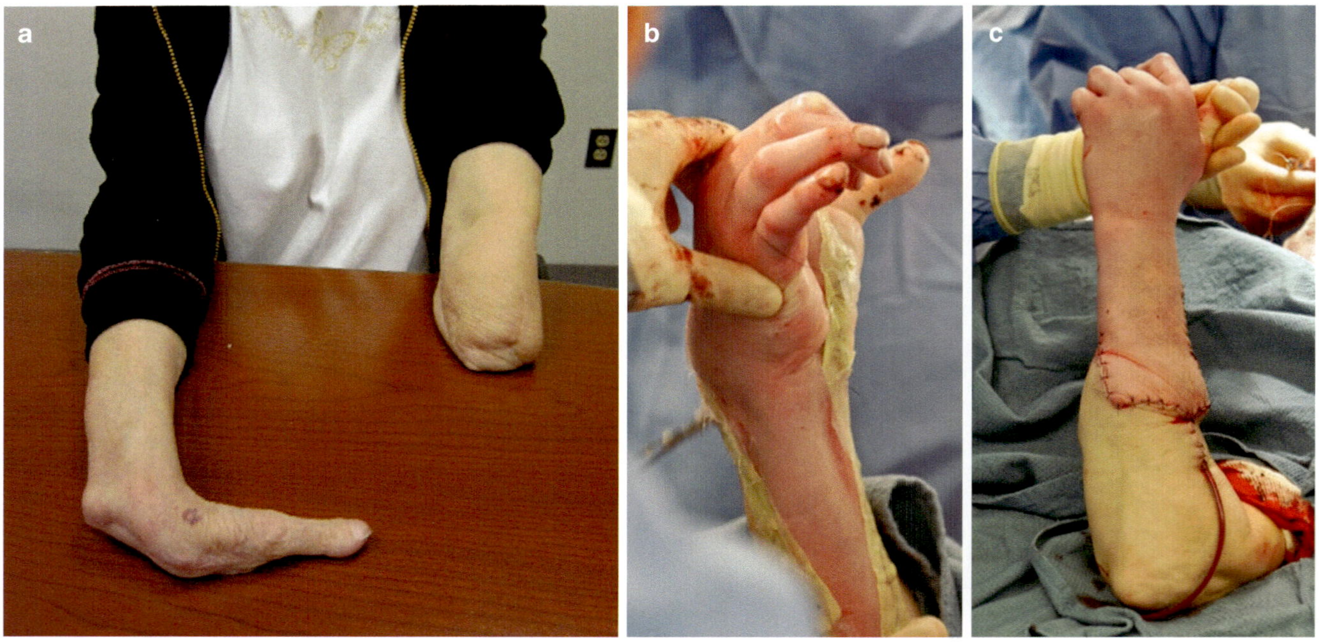

Fig. 21.2 Recipient #1 pre-operative (**a**) and post-operative photos (**b**, **c**)

upper extremity transplant cohort. Experience and recognition of longitudinal changes in pathologic evaluation are critical; we are fortunate to have an experienced group of dermatopathologists who are interested and have seen many samples from both our face and hand transplant cohorts. A summary of all rejection episodes and respective treatments is listed in Table 21.6.

21.2.4 Patients

21.2.4.1 Recipient #1

At the time of transplantation, our patient was a 56-year old female who was attacked by a chimpanzee in February of 2009 sustaining severe injuries to face and bilateral upper extremities. She was stabilized and treated at an outside facility and was referred to us for consideration of combined upper extremity and face transplantation in May 2010. In May of 2011, she underwent left mid-forearm and right partial hand transplantation in addition to a full-face transplant. The donor was a brain-dead female of similar age. Though the multi-VCA transplant was a surgical success, both upper extremity VCAs were lost in the post-operative period secondary to pulmonary sepsis [13]. See Fig. 21.2 for pre-operative and post-operative photos.

21.2.4.2 Recipient #2

At the time of transplantation, our patient was a 65-year-old formerly left-hand dominant man, who lost all four limbs in 2002 secondary to sepsis and disseminated intravascular coagulation related to pyelonephritis. The donor was a brain-dead male in his 40s. In October 2011, he underwent bilateral hand transplantation at the mid-forearm level. At his 8-year post-operative follow-up, he remained mostly independent with his ADLs, save for opening tight jars and

Table 21.7 Complications after upper extremity transplantation

Patient 1	Patient 2	Patient 3	Patient 4
• VCA loss secondary to pulmonary sepsis immediately post-operatively	• Acute appendicitis (5 years postop) • Pneumonia (5 years postop) • Olecranon fracture requiring ORIF complicated by Mycobacterial SSI, ROH	• Influenza • Avascular necrosis of the right humeral head • Multiple cutaneous SCC, HPV lesions, molluscum contagiosum	• Longstanding rash minimally responsive to changes in IS

Abbreviations: ORIF open reduction internal fixation, *SSI* surgical site infection, *ROH* removal of hardware, *SCC* squamous cell carcinoma, *HPV* human papilloma virus, *IS* immunosuppression

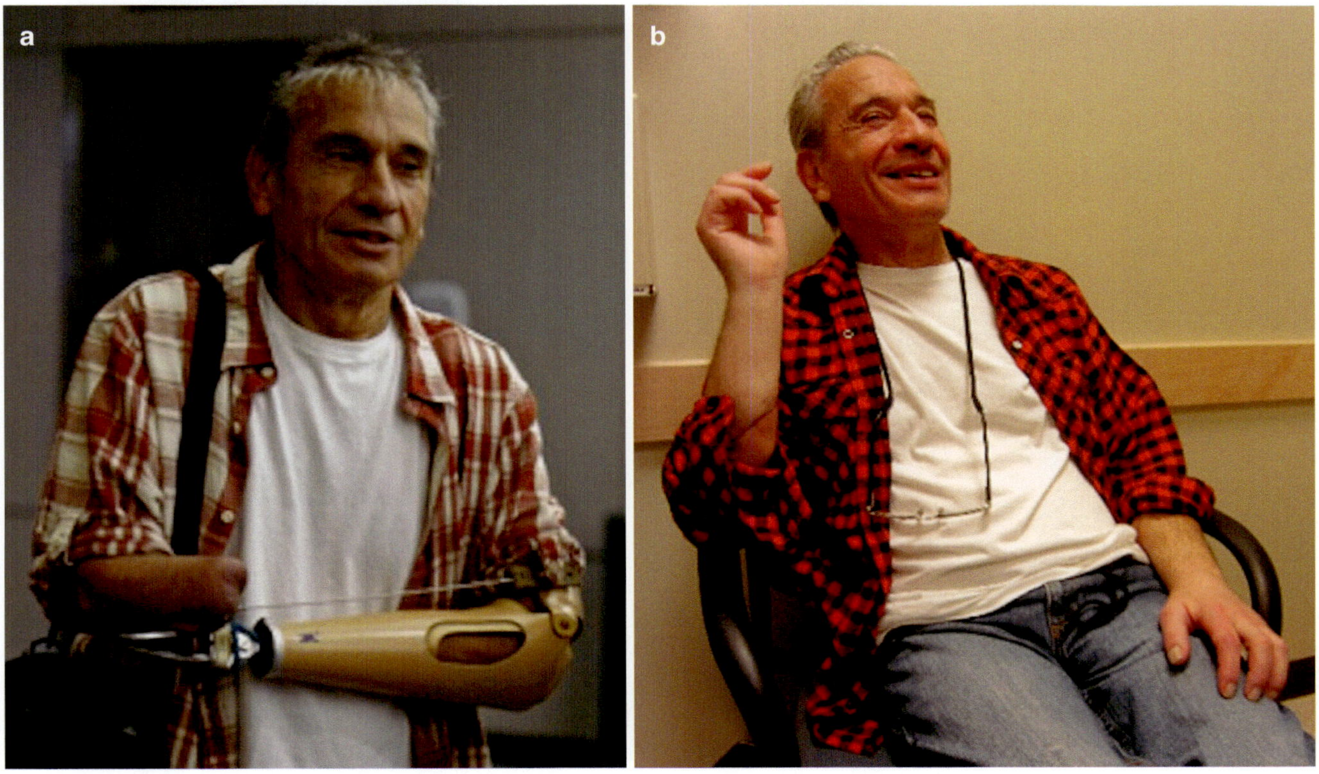

Fig. 21.3 Recipient #2 pre-operative (**a**) and post-operative photos (**b**)

using a knife to cut his food. He enjoys playing the piano and guitar in addition to painting. We have previously reported on the use of video clips demonstrating the functional outcomes in this patient [10]. Secondary surgeries for this patient have included bilateral forearm extensor tenolysis at 7 months and left-sided Royle-Thompson opponensplasty (left ring finger FDS tendon to the thumb abductor tendon transfer) and step lengthening of left small finger FDP tendon at 20 months. With regard to sensory recovery, 8 years post-transplant, he has mostly Semmes-Weinstein grade 4 out of 6 (diminished protective sensation) in all fingertips. He is overall pleased with his results in comparison to his previous results with his prosthetics and likes to see skin of his hands when wearing long-sleeved shirts. He has had a very stable post-operative course in terms of general health, psychosocial factors, and immunosuppression. He has had several complications (see Table 21.7) which are now resolved. See Fig. 21.3 for pre-operative and post-operative photos.

21.2.4.3 Recipient #3

At the time of transplantation, our patient was a 40-year-old, formerly left-hand dominant male, who lost all four limbs in 2012 due to sepsis secondary to a group A streptococcal infection. The donor was a brain-dead male in his 20s. In October 2014, he underwent left above-elbow and right below-elbow upper extremity transplantation. Thirteen months post-transplant, he underwent a right forearm corrective osteotomy (to allow for improved pronation) and bilateral debulking of soft tissues four years post-transplant. At his 5-year follow-up, he continued to make steady progress in becoming independent in his ADLs (feeding, hygiene, and dressing) and continues to compensate for limitations in his range of motion. With regard to sensation, he has achieved

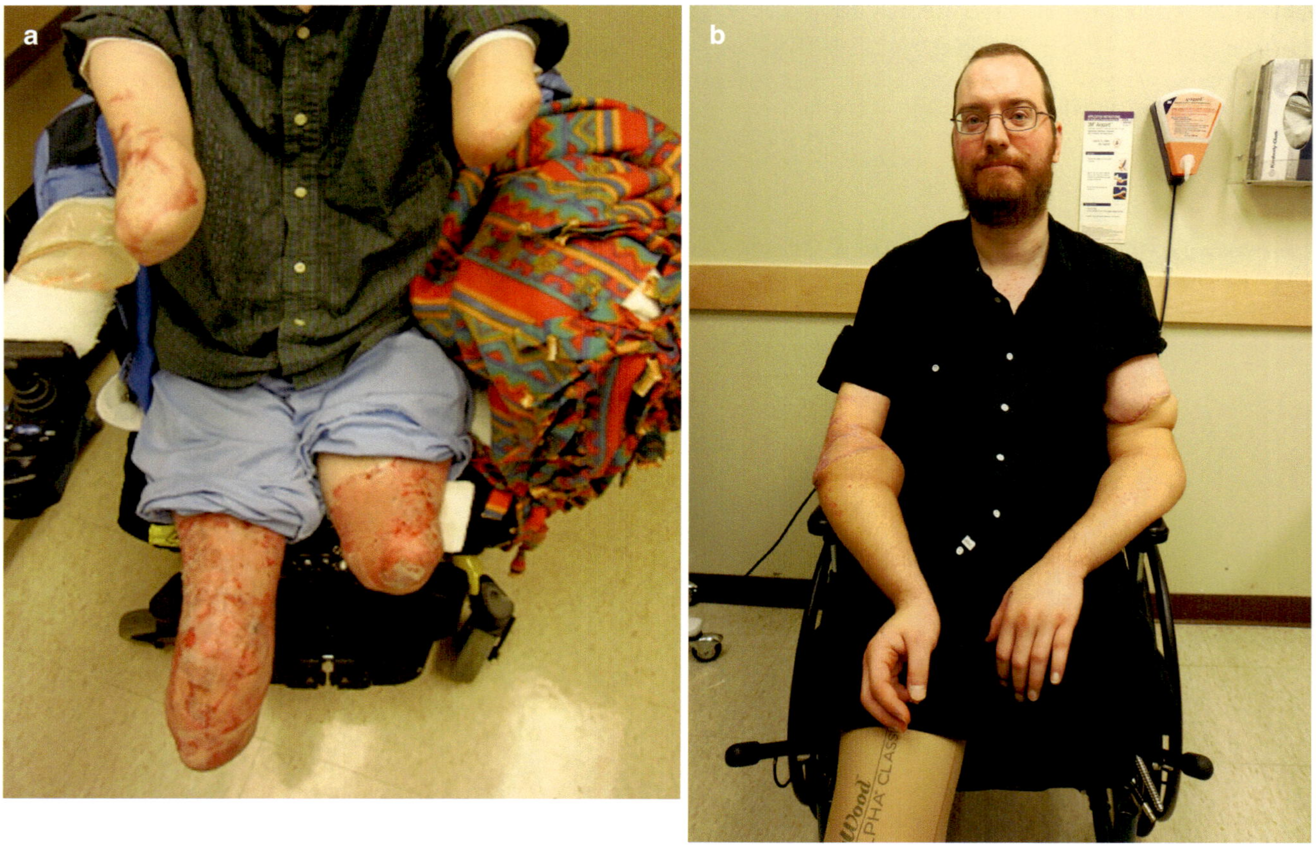

Fig. 21.4 Recipient #3 pre-operative (**a**) and post-operative photos (**b**)

Semmes-Weinstein grade 5 out of 6 (diminished light touch) sensation, with his left digits and right dorsal thumb testing inconsistently in the 6 out of 6 (normal) range. Overall, he is pleased with his ongoing improvements in ADLs and this remains a strong motivating factor in his recovery. He has had a very stable post-operative course regarding general health, psychosocial factors, and immunosuppression. See Fig. 21.4 for pre-operative and post-operative photos.

21.2.4.4 Recipient #4

At the time of transplantation, our patient was a 31-year-old, formerly right-hand dominant male, who became a quadruple amputee in 2010 after an improvised explosive device detonation in Afghanistan while on military service. In August of 2016, he underwent left below-elbow and right above-elbow transplantation. He underwent debulking of his right upper extremity at 19 months post-transplant. The

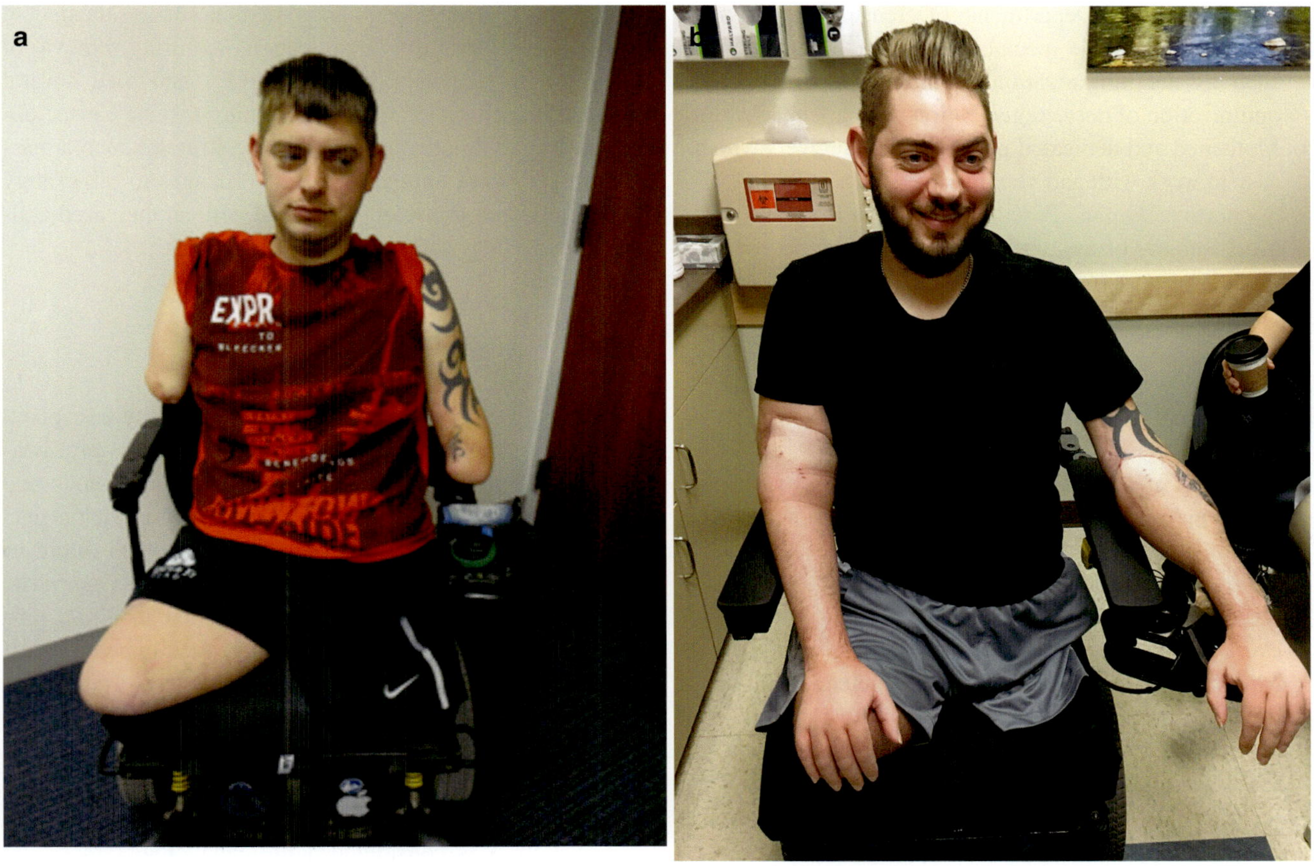

Fig. 21.5 Recipient #4 pre-operative (**a**) and post-operative photos (**b**)

donor was a brain-dead male of similar age. At his 3.5-year follow-up he was independent in his ADLs (feeding, hygiene) and had made improvements in patient-reported outcome measures and functional measures including the Carroll test. With regard to sensory recovery, he has patchy recovery ranging from diminished light touch to diminished protective sensation. Overall, he is pleased with his recovery and looks forward to ongoing improvements and is proud of his ability to now perform push-ups. His immunosuppression has been challenging, with difficulty in stabilizing his tacrolimus dosing, ultimately requiring a conversion to extended-release tacrolimus (Envarsus XR, Veloxis Pharmaceuticals). He has had a chronically low white cell count, which we believe to be related to his immunosuppression, responsive to regular G-CSF and prompting a later conversion from tacrolimus to basiliximab. A chronic rash was thought to be an ongoing low-grade rejection but has improved significantly with his normalizing white blood cell count and empirical antibiotic treatment, suggesting that this rash was not related to rejection. His latest biopsies have been normal. See Fig. 21.5 for pre-operative and post-operative photos.

21.3 Lessons Learned

21.3.1 Program Strengths

1. Teamwork: VCA is the epitome of interdisciplinary research and patient care. There are several team members working together for a common goal. A corollary here was our response to the Boston Marathon bombings, where our experience working together in VCA helped us to fast-track management of these complex cases [14].
2. Experience and breadth of expertise: We established our VCA program in 2008 and to date have performed 9 face and 4 bilateral upper extremity transplants. We have a full complement of surgical, medical, anesthesia, pathology, occupational therapy, dermatology, nursing, and ICU colleagues with vast experience in VCA since the program's inception.
3. Support: Support and funding are critical to the advancement of the field. As previously mentioned, much of our clinical work is made possible through institutional support and several research studies are funded through sev-

eral grants by the Department of Defense. There are many aspects that deserve special attention in the field of VCA such as the minimization of immunosuppression and optimization of nerve regeneration and patient selection.
4. Motivated and dedicated patients and caregivers who are easy to work with and very involved in their care.
5. Supportive Organ Procurement Organization: spearheaded many of the discussions and protocols for VCA procurement across the USA in order to establish a national network for VCA donation.

21.3.2 Modifications

1. Thorough and strict selection of donors and recipients: Seemingly minor issues are magnified with such a life-changing event as transplantation that can lead to failure in this patient population.
2. Development of patient-specific checklists to ensure every plan is implemented correctly.
3. Minimization of ischemia time: This includes limiting the geographical area for donors and extensive pre-operative planning of every step prior to vascular anastomosis.
4. Increased involvement of multiple specialists throughout the entire spectrum of care (e.g., social work, occupational therapy).
5. Pre-operative placement of a Port-a-Cath to avoid venipuncture of newly transplanted limbs.
6. Adoption of waterproof labels to identify structures instead of metal tags to mitigate issues with counts, finding the right tag, and obviate tangled tags.
7. Emphasis and use of video clips to document recovery over traditional objective occupational therapy measurements [10].
8. Pre-operative training of family and caregivers in rehabilitation protocols to allow them to perform some of the therapy at home and lessen the burden of the already multiple hospital and clinic visits that are required in the early post-operative period.
9. Decreased threshold for revision operations: We have found that these provide substantial functional improvement (e.g., opponensplasty or debulking) and have proven to be safe in the context of maintenance immunosuppression.

With the successful reproducibility of upper extremity transplantation, there remains considerable debate on the feasibility of multi-VCA transplantation. There have been two cases of concomitant facial and bilateral upper extremity transplantation, with one case resulting in loss of life and the other in the loss of bilateral upper extremity transplants [13]. The other multi-VCA transplant (bilateral upper extremity and single lower extremity) occurred in Turkey in 2012 and though this was heralded as an immediate success the patient went on to suffer from complications requiring removal of one limb immediately post-operatively and died several months thereafter [15, 16]. At this time, it is unclear the etiologies of the failure, and whether the stress of such a massive surgery (and trauma), profound changes to physiology with multi-limb transplants, coupled with an increased antigenic load can be safely tolerated by patients.

21.3.3 Future of VCA

Over twenty years since the first upper extremity transplant, the field of VCA continues to evolve. As the long-term benefits remain unknown, the reporting of all outcomes and complications that extend beyond basic demographic data and opinion remains a critical component to the future of VCA. The International Registry on Hand and Composite Tissue Transplantation (IRHCTT), founded in 2002, provides an opportunity for centers to share their experiences. It is our responsibility to share and report honest and consistent outcomes. Collaboration is vital and only through these registries can we potentially move upper extremity VCA from experimental to a procedure accepted and covered by third-party payers [17].

Since VCA is considered a life-enhancing, rather than life-saving procedure, the inherent risks of immunosuppression remain one of the several obstacles to the widespread adoption of upper extremity transplantation. Immune tolerance remains the holy grail in the field of transplantation. There are several ongoing trials in the induction of tolerance (ClinicalTrials.gov #NCT01459107) and minimization of immunosuppression to mitigate their deleterious effects while maintaining immunocompetence (ClinicalTrials.gov #NCT03241719). Upper extremity transplants have several unique physical and immunologic characteristics, none more obvious and important than the presence of skin. Visual inspection of the skin represents a powerful clinical tool to detect acute rejection at earlier stages than is possible with solid organ transplants. However, the accurate and timely diagnosis of acute rejection can at times be confounded by external conditions and non-rejection skin exanthemas. Therefore, the development and discovery of novel non-invasive biomarkers to detect rejection before physical manifestations remain an active area of research with promising pilot findings from our research group [18].

Functional outcomes in upper extremity transplantation remain in large part driven by the extent of nerve regeneration. This remains a challenge to more proximal transplantations and current intrinsic hand muscle reinnervation. Improvements in nerve regeneration and preservation of motor endplates remain vital to the future of VCA. There are several promising modalities under investigation such as the local delivery of growth factors [19] and FK-506 [20], systemic growth hormone therapy [21], and electrical stimulation [22]. One can imagine some or all of these techniques being applicable in the setting of upper extremity transplantation.

Another integral aspect to a successful outcome is the psychosocial well-being and strong social support of our transplant recipients. We have recently conducted qualitative studies to understand psychosocial factors associated with perceived success in upper extremity transplantation [23]. We have found that patients setting realistic expectations, maintaining a positive perspective on the experience and strong community and caregiver support were integral themes in the perceived success of the transplant. These findings have also been confirmed using data from the IRHCTT [24].

We have seen some remarkable results in upper extremity transplantation and some incredible work by countless clinicians and researchers. We are optimistic that upper extremity transplantation will remain a viable treatment option for select patients with otherwise devastating disabilities. As our technology and science evolve, we look forward to the broadening of indications and a tipping of the risk–benefit ratio toward safer and more commonplace surgery. Furthermore, we envisage the integration of bioengineering to allow more advanced prosthetics and assist devices to complement transplantation and perhaps a combining of these fields to create bioengineered limbs for transplantation. This future is very exciting.

References

1. Guild W, Harrison J, Merrill J, Murray J. Successful homotransplantation of the kidney in an identical twin. Trans Am Clin Climatol Assoc. 1955;67:167–73.
2. Pomahac B, Aflaki P, Chandraker A, Pribaz JJ. Facial transplantation and immunosuppressed patients: a new frontier in reconstructive surgery. Transplantation. 2008;85(12):1693–7.
3. Kiwanuka H, Aycart MA, Bueno EM, Pomahac B, Talbot SG. Experience with patient referrals for upper extremity transplantation at a U.S. Academic Medical Center. J Hand Surg Am. 2017;42(9):751.e1–e6.
4. Bueno E, Benjamin MJ, Sisk G, Sampson CE, Carty M, Pribaz JJ, et al. Rehabilitation following hand transplantation. Hand. 2014;9(1):9–15.
5. Heineman J, Bueno EM, Kiwanuka H, Carty MJ, Sampson CE, Pribaz JJ, et al. All hands on deck: hand replantation versus transplantation. SAGE Open Med. 2020;8:2050312120926351.
6. Gummesson C, Atroshi I, Ekdahl C. The disabilities of the arm, shoulder and hand (DASH) outcome questionnaire: longitudinal construct validity and measuring self-rated health change after surgery. BMC Musculoskelet Disord. 2003;4:11.
7. Beaton DE, Katz JN, Fossel AH, Wright JG, Tarasuk V, Bombardier C. Measuring the whole or the parts? Validity, reliability, and responsiveness of the disabilities of the arm, shoulder and hand outcome measure in different regions of the upper extremity. J Hand Ther. 2001;14(2):128–46.
8. Lanzetta M, Petruzzo P, Dubernard JM, Margreiter R, Schuind F, Breidenbach W, et al. Second report (1998-2006) of the international registry of hand and composite tissue transplantation. Transpl Immunol. 2007;18(1):1–6.
9. Carroll D. A quantitative test of upper extremity function. J Chronic Dis. 1965;18:479–91.
10. Singh M, Benjamin MJ, Turenne M, Lang G, Li H, Bueno E, et al. Use of video clips to assess the outcomes of bilateral hand transplantation. Plast Reconstr Surg Glob Open. 2015;3(11):e553.
11. Diaz-Siso JR, Fischer S, Sisk GC, Bueno E, Kueckelhaus M, Talbot S, et al. Initial experience of dual maintenance immunosuppression with steroid withdrawal in vascular composite tissue allotransplantation. Am J Transplant. 2015;15(5):1421–31.
12. Cendales LC, Kanitakis J, Schneeberger S, Burns C, Ruiz P, Landin L, et al. The Banff 2007 working classification of skin-containing composite tissue allograft pathology. Am J Transplant. 2008;8(7):1396–400.
13. Carty MJ, Hivelin M, Dumontier C, Talbot SG, Benjoar MD, Pribaz JJ, et al. Lessons learned from simultaneous face and bilateral hand allotransplantation. Plast Reconstr Surg. 2013;132(2):423–32.
14. Carty MJ, Caterson EJ, Caterson SA, Chun YS, Erdmann-Sager J, Hadad I, et al. Why we are here: early reflections on the role of reconstructive plastic surgery in the 2013 Boston marathon bombings. Plast Reconstr Surg. 2013;132(6):1623–7.
15. Shores JT, Brandacher G, Lee WP. Hand and upper extremity transplantation: an update of outcomes in the worldwide experience. Plast Reconstr Surg. 2015;135(2):351e–60e.
16. Fraser S Turkish hospital performs triple limb transplant 2012 [Available from: https://medicalxpress.com/news/2012-01-turkish-hospital-limb-transplants.html.
17. Breidenbach WC, Meister EA, Turker T, Becker GW, Gorantla VS, Levin LS. A methodology for determining standard of care status for a new surgical procedure: hand transplantation. Plast Reconstr Surg. 2016;137(1):367–73.
18. Kollar B, Uffing A, Borges TJ, Shubin AV, Aoyama BT, Dagot C, et al. MMP3 is a non-invasive biomarker of rejection in skin-bearing vascularized composite allotransplantation: a multicenter validation study. Front Immunol. 2019;10:2771.
19. Raimondo TM, Li H, Kwee BJ, Kinsley S, Budina E, Anderson EM, et al. Combined delivery of VEGF and IGF-1 promotes functional innervation in mice and improves muscle transplantation in rabbits. Biomaterials. 2019;216:119246.
20. Tajdaran K, Chan K, Shoichet MS, Gordon T, Borschel GH. Local delivery of FK506 to injured peripheral nerve enhances axon regeneration after surgical nerve repair in rats. Acta Biomater. 2019;96:211–21.
21. Lopez J, Quan A, Budihardjo J, Xiang S, Wang H, Koshy K, et al. Growth hormone improves nerve regeneration, muscle re-innervation, and functional outcomes after chronic denervation injury. Sci Rep. 2019;9(1):3117.
22. Gordon T. Electrical stimulation to enhance axon regeneration after peripheral nerve injuries in animal models and humans. Neurotherapeutics. 2016;13(2):295–310.
23. Kinsley SE, Lenhard NK, Lape EC, Shah SB, Edwards RR, Katz JN, et al. Perceived success in upper extremity vascularized composite allotransplantation: a qualitative study. J Hand Surg Am. 2021;46(8):711.e1–711.e35.
24. Kinsley SE, Song S, Petruzzo P, Sardu C, Losina E, Talbot SG. Defining psychosocial predictors of upper extremity transplantation outcomes: a review of the international registry 1998-2016. Plast Reconstr Surg Glob Open. 2020;8(9):e3133.

Double Hand Transplant Monza

22

Massimo Del Bene, Gaetano Musumarra,
and Antonio Peri di Caprio

22.1 Introduction

Our program started in 2008 at Ospedale S. Gerardo Monza. The program is still active and we have included four patients. Two patients were screened for transplantation, one patient was excluded for oncological reasons and another patient is waiting for the transplant at this time.

At present, we do not have patients on the waiting list for transplantation. We excluded many patients because we do not perform unilateral transplants and transplants in children. The principal obstacle for the expansion of our program is the immunosuppression therapy because of the long term side effects in young patients.

22.2 Patient 1

22.2.1 Donor

A 58-year-old female suffering from cerebral accident, who did not present comorbidities.

22.2.2 Recipients

A 52-year-old female undergoing double hand amputation for septic shock for hydronephrosis (July 2007) (Fig. 22.1). The patient was hospitalized in our hospital so we performed the amputation with great care and with the plan to perform a hand transplant in the future. It was a very important step because frequently we evaluate patients that are amputated in other hospitals. The patient after the transplantation began to move her fingers and her wrists initially with very small movements during day 1 after the transplantation and after, with recovery of sensibility and functionality of fingers and wrist (Fig. 22.2).

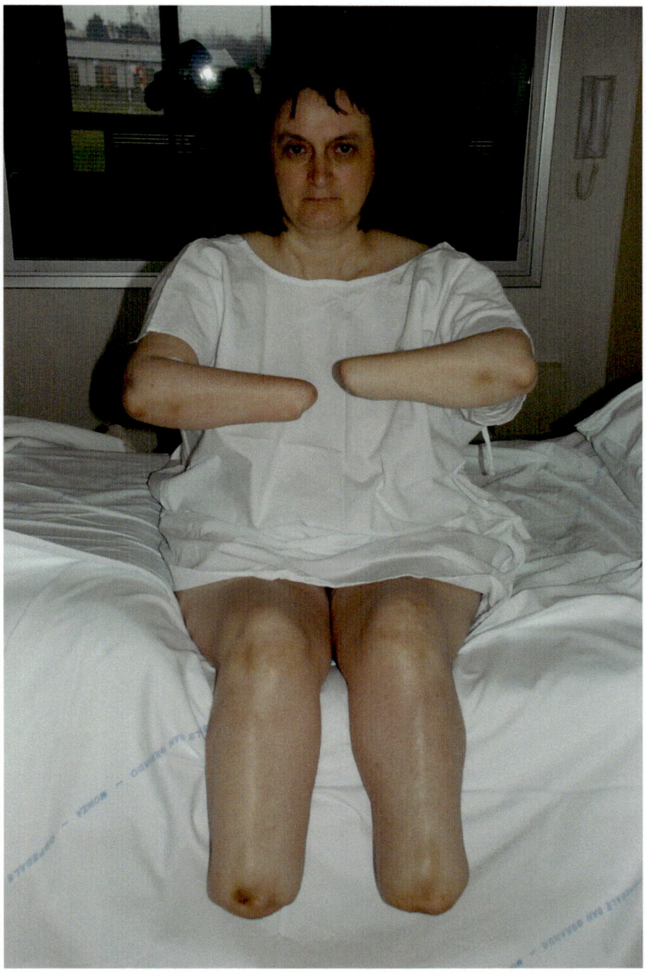

Fig. 22.1 Patient before transplantation

We evaluated this recovery with clinical tests and with functional MRI before the transplant with small activation areas that became larger during the rehabilitation (Figs. 22.3a, b and 22.4a, b).

M. Del Bene
Plastic Surgery, Monza, Italy
e-mail: m.delbene@asst-monza.it

G. Musumarra · A. P. di Caprio (✉)
Ospedale San Gerardo—Monza, Monza, Italy

© Springer Nature Switzerland AG 2023
R. Gurunian et al. (eds.), *Reconstructive Transplantation*, https://doi.org/10.1007/978-3-031-21520-9_22

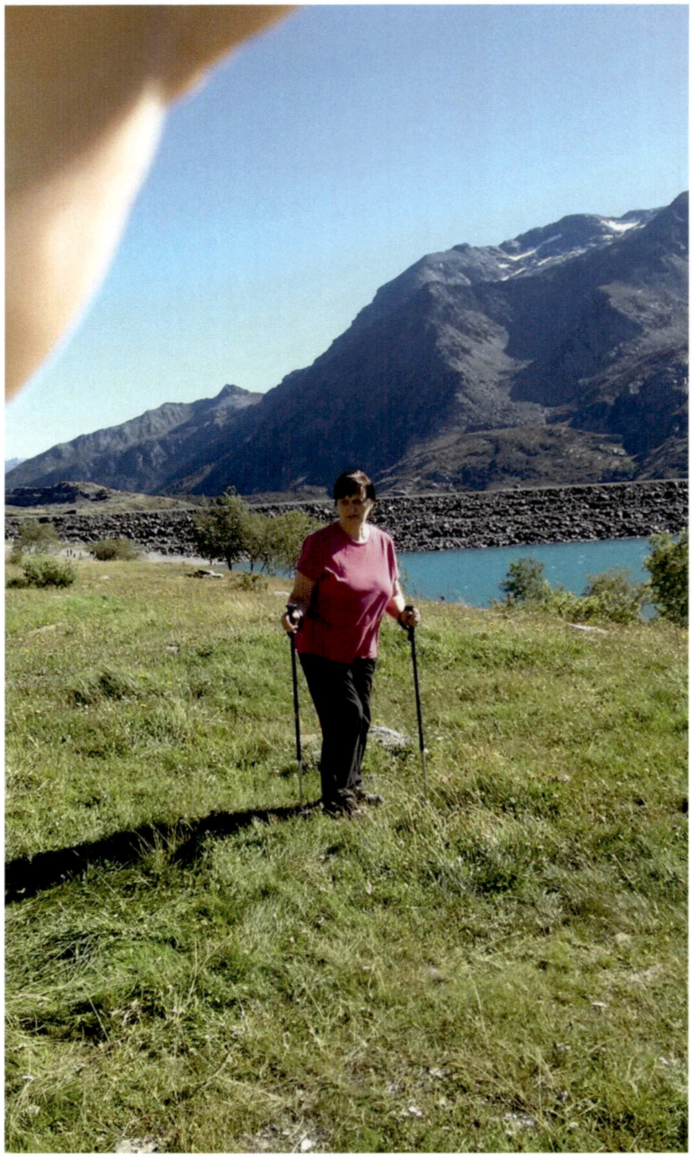

Fig. 22.2 Patient after transplantation

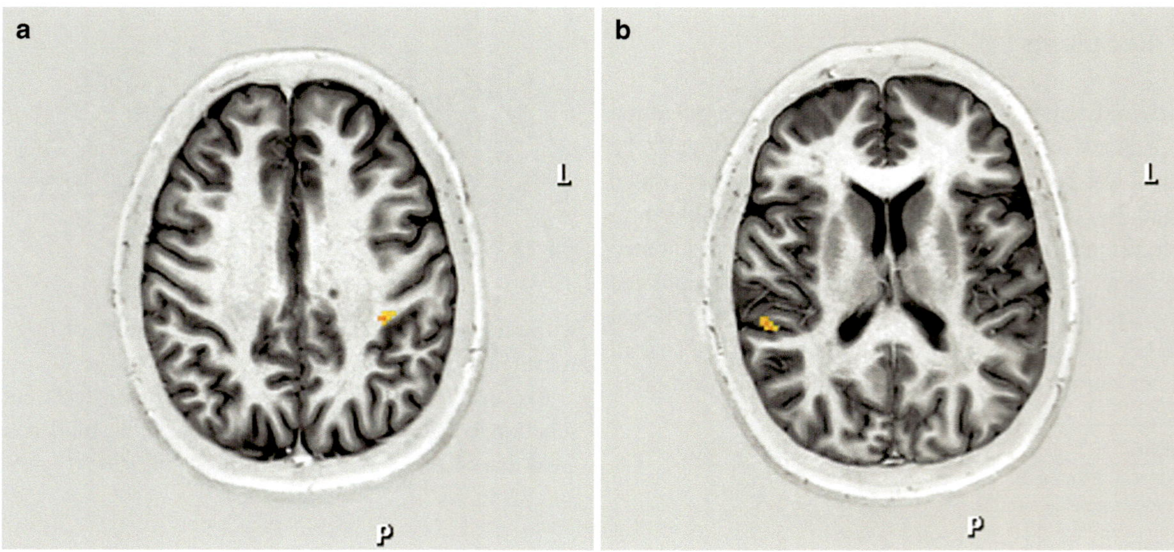

Fig. 22.3 (**a**, **b**) Brain MRI before transplantation (right and left)

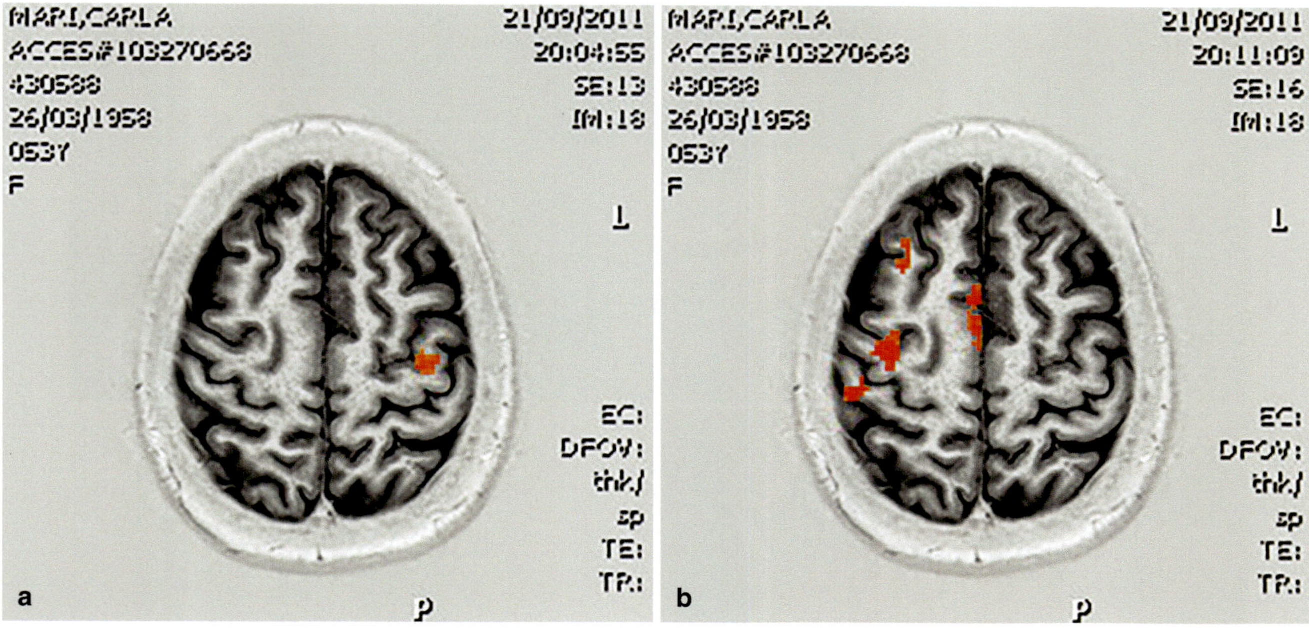

Fig. 22.4 (**a**, **b**) Brain MRI one year post-transplantation (right and left)

Now the patient can use the phone, a pen and she is completely independent. Now we are at 10 years of follow-up and the patient has not had any episodes of rejection.

22.3 Surgical Technique

In October 2010, a donor was found. The transplant team went to another hospital to harvest both hands. For the bone we performed an amputation at the distal third of the radius and ulna. For vascular anastomosis we performed a dissection from distal to cranial until the brachial artery was dissected, because our idea was to perform an anastomosis at a proximal level to prevent to perform the anastomosis at the level where the vessels could have been damaged during insertion of arterial lines in the radial artery in the ICU. After the hands were harvested, we used the University of Wisconsin solution to wash the vessels (Fig. 22.5a–c).

Once the hands were transported to our hospital, first a team of two plastic surgeons prepared the left wrist recipient site. The osteosynthesis was performed at the distal radius and ulna with two six-hole plates using a total of twelve 12 mm screws, the brachial artery was anastomosed first followed by the collateral veins and cephalic vein (Fig. 22.6a–d). We coapted the ulnar and median nerves, sutured the extensor and flexor tendons (only deep flexors), and finally we closed the skin directly. Skin graft was used for the residual defect (Fig. 22.7a, b).

At the level of the right hand we performed the preparation of the stump, osteosynthesis of radius and ulna with two five hole plates with a total of ten 12 mm screws. Vascular anastomoses were performed at the level of the brachial artery first and then the collateral veins and cephalic vein were anastomosed. We sutured the ulnar and median nerves, extensor and flexor tendons (only deep flexors), and finally we closed the skin directly and we used a skin graft for the residual defect.

In this technique we prefer to perform the anastomosis of veins before the anastomosis of the artery, this is very important because when we start the perfusion of the hand we do not have to stop the revascularization to perform the vein anastomosis.

At the end of the procedure X-rays showed good fixation of the bone (Fig. 22.8a, b).

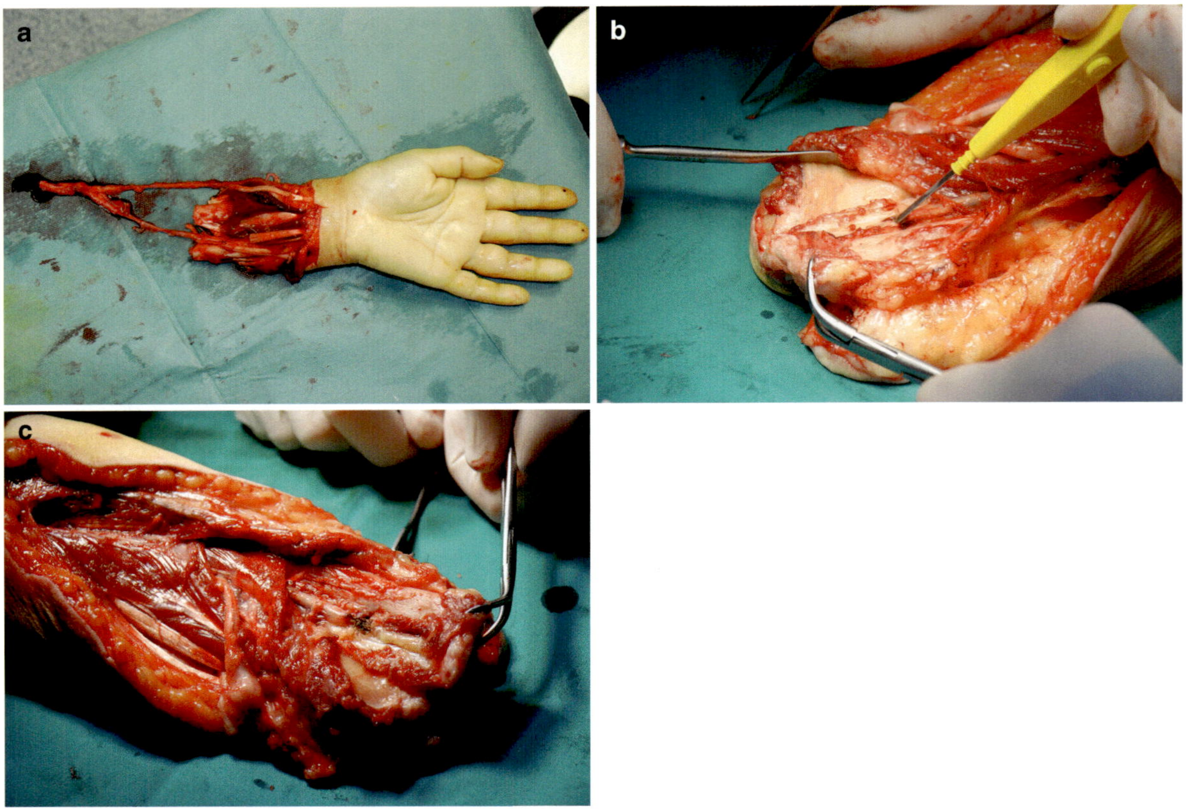

Fig. 22.5 (**a**) Hand harvest with vessel preparation (**b** and **c**). Preparation of the amputation stump

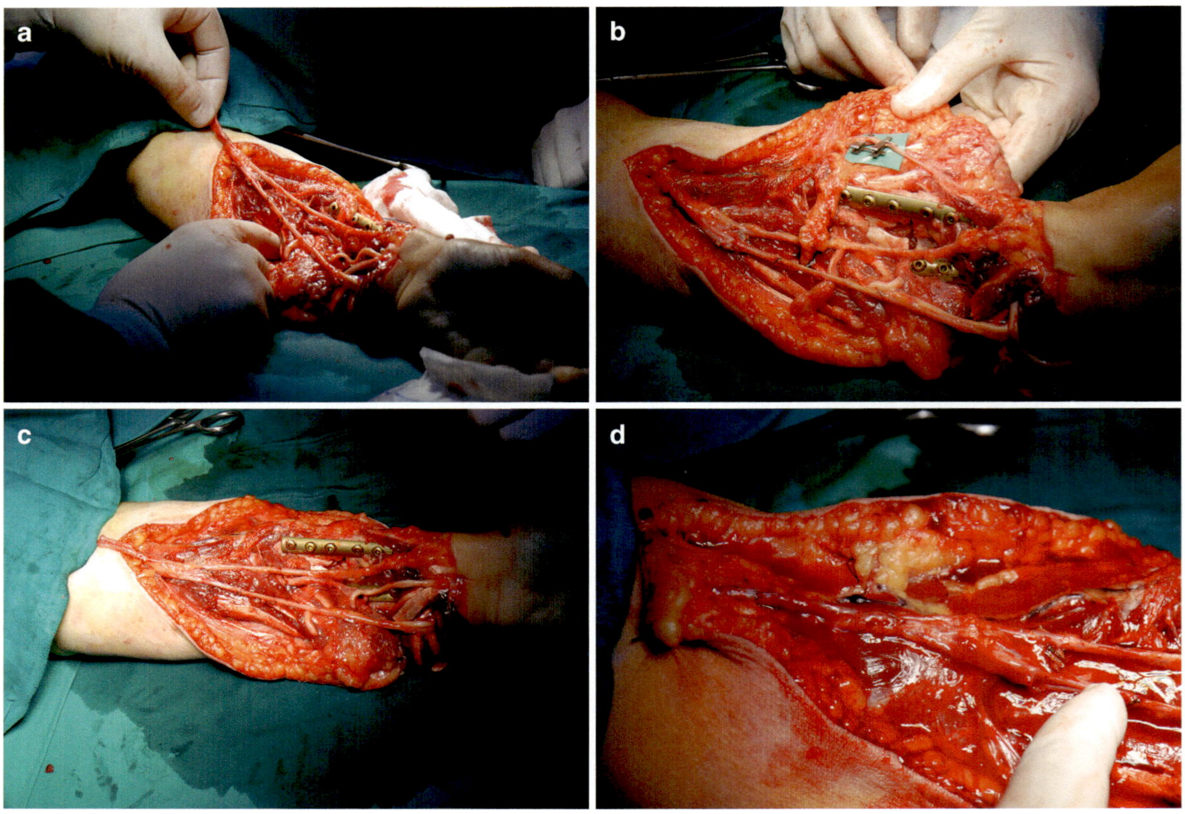

Fig. 22.6 (**a**, **b**, **c**, **d**) Vascular stage in which we used the brachial artery, collateral veins, and cephalic vein for anastomoses

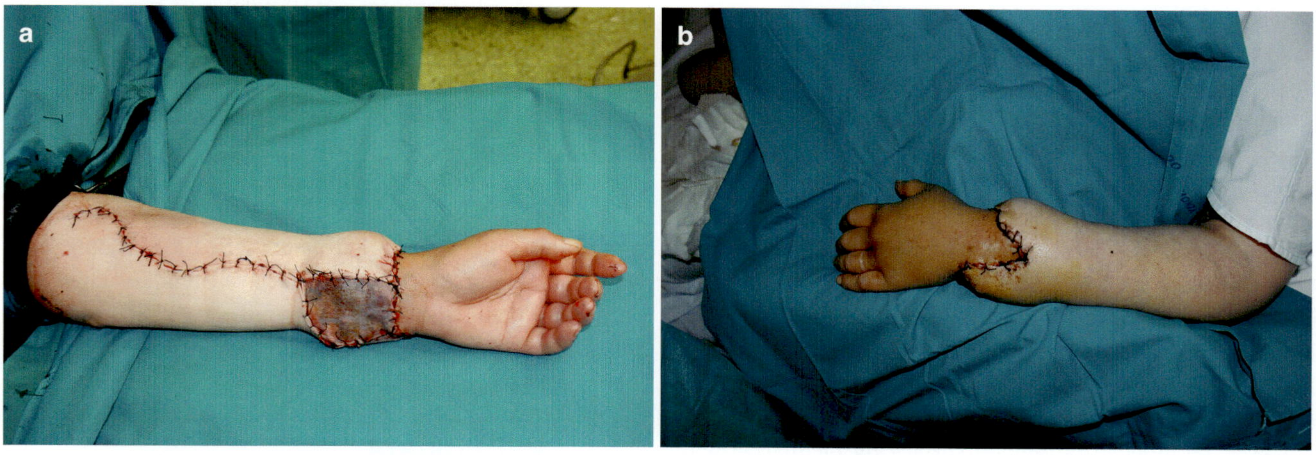

Fig. 22.7 (**a**, **b**) Left hand at the end of transplant volar and dorsal views

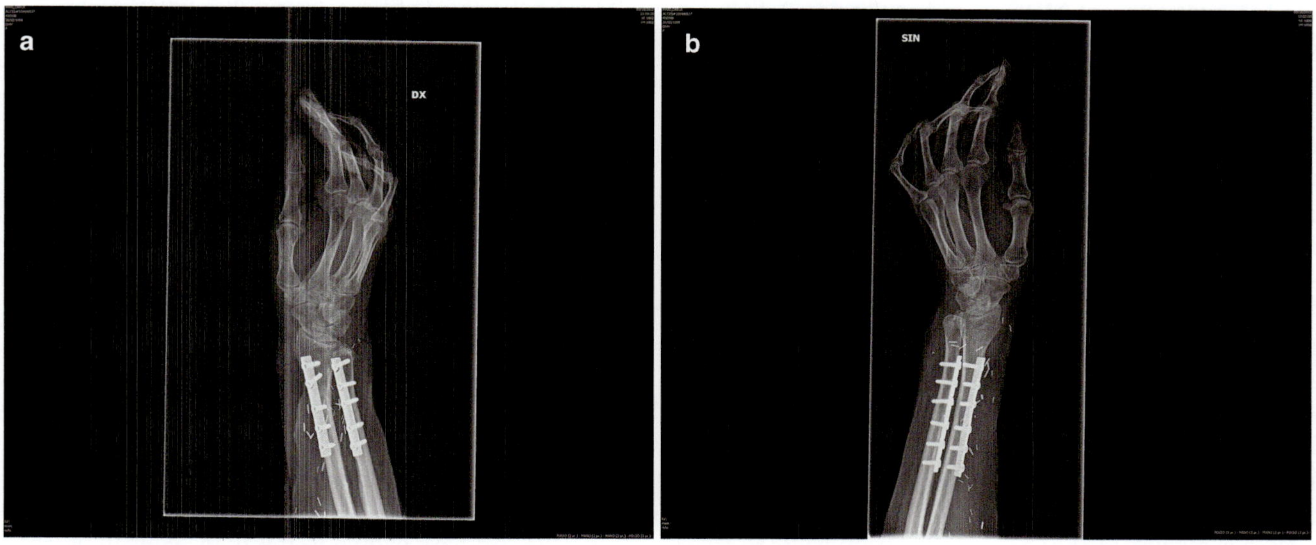

Fig. 22.8 (**a**, **b**) X-rays showing osteosynthesis

22.4 Multipotent Mesenchymal Stromal Cells

22.4.1 The Active Principle of Multipotent Mesenchymal Stromal Cells (MSCs)

Human MSCs are adherent cells with elongated spindle shape fibroblast-like morphology [1]. Human MSCs are somatic cells of mesodermal origin, which are known to constitute the bone marrow (BM) stroma and help hematopoietic stem cells engraftment [2, 3]. Furthermore, they show immunosuppressive activity in vitro and in vivo. In particular, they are able to inhibit the proliferation of human T-cells in vitro in response to antigenic or mitogenic stimuli. The mechanism for immunosuppression is not completely understood but may depend on their capacity to release immunosuppressive cytokines and/or interact with specific immune cells. MSCs expanded in culture conditions show the expected morphology and phenotype and are able to suppress human T-cell proliferation.

The internationally accepted criteria to define human MSCs must be:

- Plastic adherence when maintained in culture.
- Fibroblastic morphology (spindle shape).
- Expression of cd105, cd73, and cd90.
- Lack of expression of CD45, CD34,CD14 or CD11b,CD79, or CD19 or HLA-DR.

The MSCs generally reside in the BM and indeed, they have a multipotent differentiation potential and differentiate in appropriate condition in vitro osteoblasts, adipocytes, chondroblasts. Certainly most of the present popularity of MSCs must be attributed to the more recent discovery of their immune-modulatory properties. While, initially, most studies investigated the effects of MSCs on T-lymphocytes, with accumulating data on their T-cell suppressing properties, it has become later evident that MSCs may display their effect on all the cells involved in an immune response, including B-lymphocytes, dendritic cells, and NK cells. MSCs express low level of human HLA class I molecules and normally do not express class II molecules. These can, however, be induced in the cell surface by incubation with interferon-gamma. In addition, MSCs do not express CD40, CD80, or CD 86 co-stimulatory molecules and are unable to induce proliferation of allogenic lymphocytes. Because of the low expression of MHC class I molecules, MSCs can escape detection by T-cells. Several independent groups have shown that cultured MSCs can suppress T-cell proliferation induced by allogenic peripheral blood mononuclear cells and by mitogens, such as phytohemagglutinin, concanavalin A, and anti-CD3/anti-CD28 antibodies, in a dose-dependent manner [4–8]. Inhibition of lymphocyte proliferation by MSCs has not been associated with the induction of apoptosis but is thought to be due to inhibition of cells division. This prevents T-lymphocyte capacity to respond to antigenic triggers while maintaining these cells in a quiescent state [9]. MSCs also strongly inhibit in vitro activation of alloantigen-specific cytotoxic lymphocytes at the higher ratio of MSCs than effector cells. At a low ratio, they may either decrease or increase alloantigen-specific cell-mediated cytotoxic activity [5, 10]. Inhibition of T-cell proliferation and cytotoxicity does not require MHC compatibility between MSCs and responder lymphocytes. This supports the hypothesis that MSCs can be considered as universal suppressors. Most human MSCs-mediated immune suppression on activated T-Lymphocytes has been attributed to the secretion of anti-proliferative soluble factors, such as hepatocyte growth factor, prostaglandin E2, transforming growth factor-beta1 (TGF-beta1), indoleamine2, 3-dioxygenase (IDO), which causes depletion of tryptophan, an essential factor for lymphocyte proliferation, nitric oxide, and interleukin IL-10 [11]. However, published data do not exclude that a part of the immunosuppressive effect exerted by human MSCs on alloantigen-induced T-cell activation could be dependent on cell-to-cell contact mechanisms. Interestingly, the calcineurin inhibitors, cyclosporine-A, and tacrolimus, currently employed to prevent or treat GvHD, enhance the immune suppressive effect of human MSCs. As already mentioned, the effect played by MScs on the immune system is pleiotropic. In fact, it has been recently reported that MSCs co-cultured with purified CD19+ B cells in the presence of a cocktail of stimuli significantly inhibit B-cell proliferation and that this effect is mainly due to soluble factors [12]. Human MSCs display an inhibitory effect on alloantigen-induced dendritic cell differentiation and on antigen presenting cell maturation [13]. This could be related to their capacity to produce anti-inflammatory cytokines, such as TGF-beta, known to inhibit in vitro activation and maturation of dendritic cells [14]. To summarize MSCs have been shown to favor hematopoiesis, to have immunosuppressive properties against a variety of immune cells, and to play a role in tissue repair.

22.5 MSC Protocol

MSC from allogenic donors is expanded in platelet lysate (PL) in cell factories under good manufacturing practice (GMP) laboratory conditions. In case the clinical center is an external site the MSC lots will be shipped as a frozen material according to GMP procedure, then thawed at 37 °C, and immediately slowly infused. If the clinical center is inside the San Gerardo Hospital the MSCs will be transported at the clinical department by personnel of Laboratorio Verri. In any case, MSCs are infused within 15 min after thawing.

The final medical product is composed of recipient human MSCs resuspended in clinical grade human albumin (Kedroin) and 10% clinical grade DMSO (WAK-Chemie) and 10% anticoagulant ACD. Numbers of MSCs/vial are approximately 25×10^6. MSCs have already been the subject of several clinical trials. At the beginning of the clinical experience, final products were infused directly into the patients without freezing. Subsequently, it has been demonstrated that frozen MSCs are equally active as freshly prepared cells. We have chosen to freeze the cells in order to allow quarantine to be performed and to allow execution of all the quality control tests before release. Ten percent of DMSO is a standard additive amount for freezing human cells, including hematopoietic stem cells for clinical use and has been demonstrated to allow cryopreservation of cells for long periods in liquid nitrogen. The number of cells/vial is calculated on the basis of an average weight of an adult or pediatric patient of 50 kg and 30 kg and of the planned administration of doses of $1 \pm 0.5 \times 10^6$/kg. This dosage has been used so far in most of the clinical GvHD studies ([15, 16]).

The immunosuppressive protocol involved administration of 20 mg basiliximab prior to reperfusion and 4 days post-transplant; The tacrolimus was administrated at dosages such as to maintain the target blood levels (from 12 to 15 ng/ml during first two weeks to 4–6 ng/ml one year post-transplantation); at reperfusion methylprednisolone 100 mg was administered and, for 7 days at 25 mg/day; after 7 days we used prednisone PO in decreasing dosage until complete suspension at 7 months after transplant. Mycophenolate was administrated 1 g twice a day until 7 months post-transplant. The dosage was halved and completely suspended at 31 months after transplant. This immunosuppressive protocol was associated with MSCs administration at 12 h post-transplant administrated at the dosage of 2 × 10^6/kg, MSCs were previously prepared and stored at Cell Factory "Stefano Verri." We did not have validated plasma markers, so the response to MSCs administration was evaluated, at +24 h, +48 h, +7 days, by measuring Elafin, a marker validated for cutaneous graft versus host disease (GVHD) > 2 degree. We detected high level Elafin of this molecules after transplant, and his drastic reduction at all time points analyzed, this reduction suggests a reduction of skin inflammatory state. Further studies will be needed to confirm the role of Elafin as a response marker. Second and third administration at dosage of 2 × 10^6/kg of MSCs was administered at 722 and 729 days post-transplant for histological aspect of low-grade rejection (Grade1 Banff classification). This low-grade rejection was clinically unresponsive to increase in dosage of tacrolimus and to administration of prednisone at dosage of 2 mg/kg. After administration of MSC we had a good clinical response with resolution of edema and reduction of periungual hyperemia. At 10 years post-transplant we use a single drug immunosuppressive regimen with tacrolimus, in range between 4 and 6 ng/ml. This approach is unheard of for composite transplant, which is usually treated with triple immunosuppressive therapy. Actually functional and esthetic results are good for both hands. It is not completely clear to what extent this result is attributable to the MSCs, rather than a good matching donor/recipient. If this protocol proves to be really effective in the future, composite transplant could be performed with the possibility of extending transplantation to very young patients.

22.6 Immunosuppression Protocol

We use a protocol developed with our hematologist colleagues. We use simulect (basiliximab) 20 mg at reperfusion and 20 mg four days post-operation; prograf (tacrolimus) 0.6–0.8 mg/kg/day in Tao somministrati in 24 h to maintain: 1–3 week 12–15 ng/ml; 4–8 week 10–12 ng/ml; 3–6 month 8–10 ng/ml; after sixth months 6–8 ng/ml. 100 mg methylprednisolone at reperfusion; day 1–6: 25 mg methylprednisolone; day 7–20: 25 mg prednisone; day 21–34: 20 mg/day prednisone; day 35–third month: 15 mg/day prednisone per os; month 4th–6th: 10 mg/day prednisone and after 10 mg alternate day until suspension attempt.

22.7 Treatment of Rejection

Methylprednisone 500 mg for three days until maximum dosage of 1500 mg.

22.8 Antibiotic Prophylaxis

Before transplant: Ceftriazone 2 g and after 1 g/day for 7 days.

First three months after transplant: Fluconazol 50 mg/day.

Twelve months after transplant: Aspirin: 100 mg/day.

Twelve months after transplant TMP/SMX: 1 tablet every other day.

Ganciclovir 10 mg/kg/day twice/day for 1 week and afterward ganciclovir 1000 mg × 3 times/day for 9 months after transplantation.

22.9 Monitoring Protocol (Table 22.1)

1. Before transplant:

   Two months before, start the program for stem cell collection.

   Blood tests: CBC, coagulation, blood gas, C-reactive protein (CRP), hemoglobin A1c, fructosamine.

   Complete urine examination with urine culture.

   Serology: EBV-DNA, antibodies anti-EBV, CMV-PCR, antibodies anti-CMV, antibodies anti-herpes, toxo, varicella, HAV, HBV, HCV.

   Instrumental examination:

Table 22.1 Monitoring protocol panel. PT: post-transplant, MSC: mesenchymal stromal cell

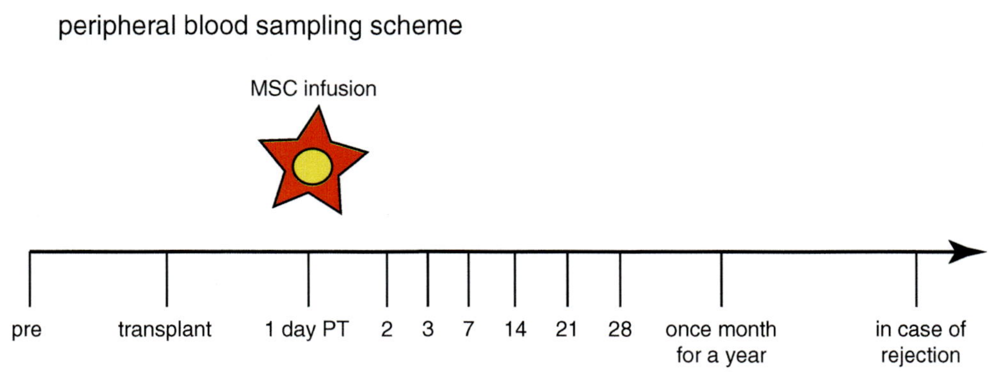

Abdominal ultrasound, chest X-ray, echocardiogram with ECG.

Anesthesia evaluation.

Neurologic evaluation + possible cerebral MRI.

Blood group and blood sampling for Nord Italian Transplant (NIT).

2. After three months:

   Blood tests: CBC, coagulation, blood gas, C-reactive protein (CRP), hemoglobin A1c, fructosamine.

   Complete urine examination with urine culture.

   Serology: EBV-DNA, antibodies anti-EBV, CMV-PCR, antibodies anti-CMV, antibodies anti-herpes, toxo, varicella, HAV, HBV, HCV.

   Instrumental examination:

   Abdominal ultrasound, chest X-ray, echocardiogram with ECG.

   Anesthesia evaluation.

   Neurologic evaluation + possible cerebral MRI.

   Blood group + blood sampling for NIT.

3. After 6 months (Fig. 22.9a, b):

   Blood tests: CBC, coagulation, blood gas, C-reactive protein (CRP), hemoglobin A1c, fructosamine.

   Complete urine examination with urine culture.

   Serology: EBV-DNA, antibodies anti-EBV, CMV-PCR, antibodies anti-CMV, antibodies anti-herpes, toxo, varicella, HAV, HBV, HCV.

   Instrumental examination:

   Abdominal ultrasound, chest X-ray, echocardiogram with ECG.

   Anesthesia evaluation.

   Neurologic evaluation + possible cerebral MRI.

   Blood group + blood sampling for NIT.

4. Every year post-transplantation (Fig. 22.10a, b, follow-up at 1 year).

   Blood tests: CBC, coagulation, blood gas, C-reactive protein (CRP), hemoglobin A1c, fructosamine.

   Complete urine examination with urine culture.

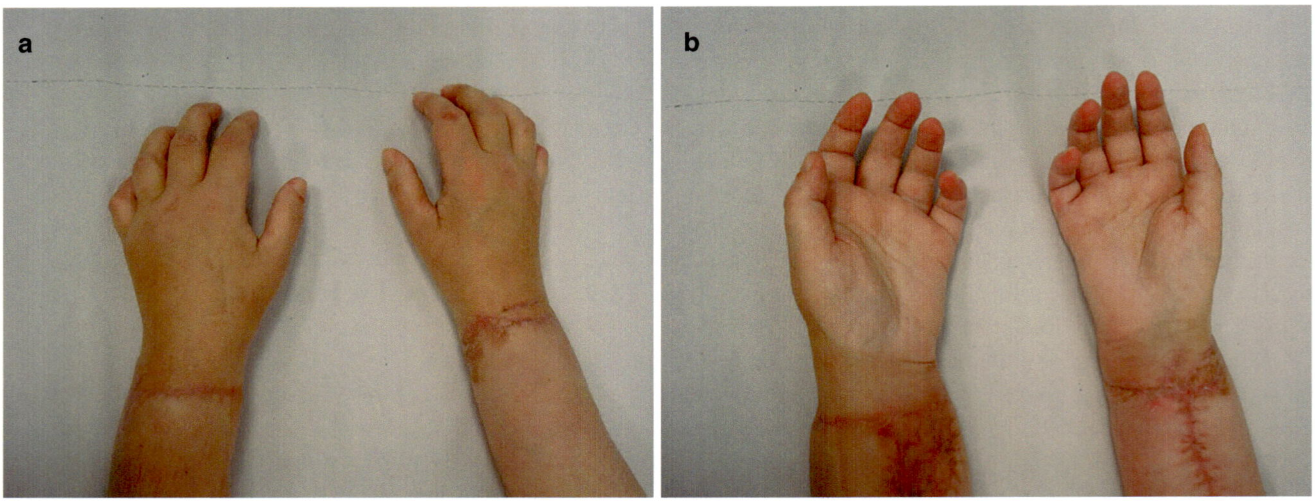

Fig. 22.9 (**a**, **b**) Follow-up at 6 months

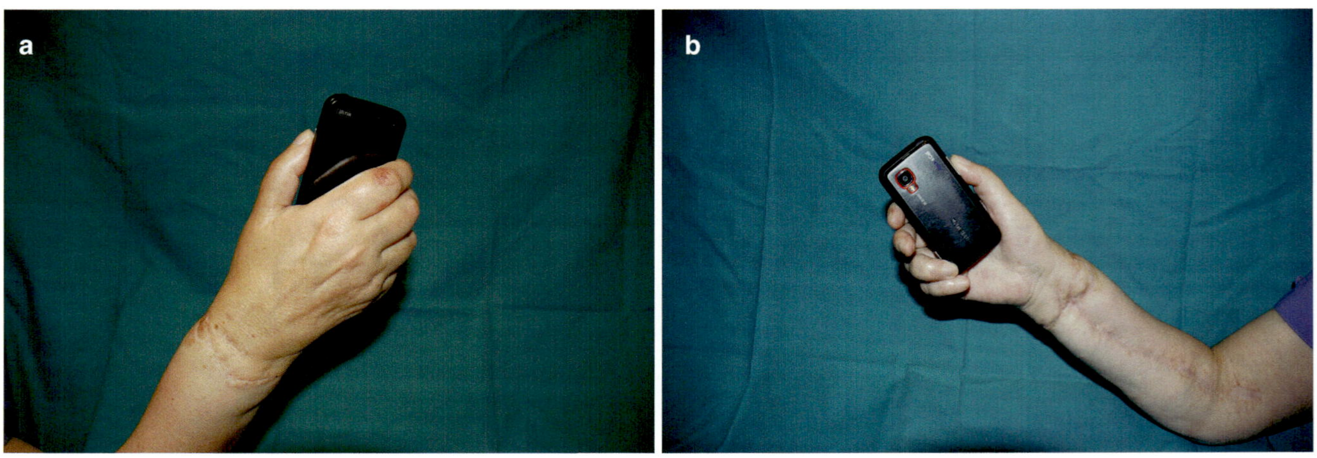

Fig. 22.10 (**a**, **b**) Follow-up at one year

Serology: EBV-DNA, antibodies anti-EBV, CMV-PCR, antibodies anti-CMV, antibodies anti-herpes, toxo, varicella, HAV, HBV, HCV.

Instrumental examination:

Abdominal ultrasound, chest X-ray, echocardiogram with ECG.

Anesthesia evaluation.

Neurologic evaluation + possible cerebral MRI.

Blood group + blood sampling for NIT.

22.10 Rehabilitation Protocol

The rehabilitation starts on day 1 after transplant with mobilization of finger and wrist with rehabilitation every day for one year with splinting and active and passive mobilization. After one year three times/week for 6 months and afterward 2 times/week.

22.11 Problems Encountered

We did not encounter any particular problem. We only had very little dermal reaction on the fingers and palm at 5 years but it regressed very rapidly with topical therapy. We had a transplant loss in the second recipient because of the mismatch between donor and recipient vessels with severe venous stasis.

22.12 Lessons Learned

The strength of our program is the use of stem cells with reduction of immunosuppressive therapy. In our experience this approach allows to reduce or remove the transplant therapy with evident advantages. In the future we will be more careful in the selection of donor. The future of VCA is the use of stem cells instead of immunosuppression therapy with the possibility to increase the indications and improve long term results without chronic rejection overtime.

References

1. Müller I, Kordowich S, Holzwarth C, Spano C, Isensee G, Staiber A, Viebahn S, Gieseke F, Langer H, Gawaz MP, Horwitz EM, Conte P, Handgretinger R, Dominici M. Animal serum-free culture conditions for isolation and expansion of multipotent mesenchymal stromal cells from human BM. Cytotherapy. 2006;8(5):437–44. https://doi.org/10.1080/14653240600920782.
2. Friedenstein AJ, Petrakova KV, Kurolesova AI, Frolova GP. Heterotopic of bone marrow. Analysis of precursor cells for osteogenic and hematopoietic tissues. Transplantation. 1968;6(2):230–47.
3. Friedenstein AJ, Deriglasova UF, Kulagina NN, Panasuk AF, Rudakowa SF, Luriá EA, Ruadkow IA. Precursors for fibroblasts in different populations of hematopoietic cells as detected by the in vitro colony assay method. Exp Hematol. 1974;2(2):83–92.
4. Krampera M, Glennie S, Dyson J, Scott D, Laylor R, Simpson E, Dazzi F. Bone marrow mesenchymal stem cells inhibit the response of naive and memory antigen-specific T cells to their cognate peptide. Blood. 2003;101(9):3722–9. https://doi.org/10.1182/blood-2002-07-2104. Epub 2002 Dec 27
5. Maccario R, Podestà M, Moretta A, Cometa A, Comoli P, Montagna D, Daudt L, Ibatici A, Piaggio G, Pozzi S, Frassoni F, Locatelli F. Interaction of human mesenchymal stem cells with cells involved in alloantigen-specific immune response favors the differentiation of CD4+ T-cell subsets expressing a regulatory/suppressive phenotype. Haematologica. 2005;90(4):516–25.
6. Di Nicola M, Carlo-Stella C, Magni M, Milanesi M, Longoni PD, Matteucci P, Grisanti S, Gianni AM. Human bone marrow stromal cells suppress T-lymphocyte proliferation induced by cellular or nonspecific mitogenic stimuli. Blood. 2002;99(10):3838–43. https://doi.org/10.1182/blood.v99.10.3838.
7. Rasmusson I, Le Blanc K, Sundberg B, Ringdén O. Mesenchymal stem cells stimulate antibody secretion in human B cells. Scand J Immunol. 2007;65(4):336–43. https://doi.org/10.1111/j.1365-3083.2007.01905.x.
8. Aggarwal S, Pittenger MF. Human mesenchymal stem cells modulate allogeneic immune cell responses. Blood. 2005;105(4):1815–22. https://doi.org/10.1182/blood-2004-04-1559. Epub 2004 Oct 19
9. Uccelli A, Pistoia V, Moretta L. Mesenchymal stem cells: a new strategy for immunosuppression? Trends Immunol. 2007;28(5):219–26. https://doi.org/10.1016/j.it.2007.03.001. Epub 2007 Apr 2
10. Rasmusson I, Ringdén O, Sundberg B, Le Blanc K. Mesenchymal stem cells inhibit the formation of cytotoxic T lymphocytes, but not activated cytotoxic T lymphocytes or natural killer cells. Transplantation. 2003;76(8):1208–13. https://doi.org/10.1097/01.TP.0000082540.43730.80.
11. Le Blanc K, Tammik C, Rosendahl K, Zetterberg E, Ringdén O. HLA expression and immunologic properties of differentiated and undifferentiated mesenchymal stem cells. Exp Hematol. 2003;31(10):890–6. https://doi.org/10.1016/s0301-472x(03)00110-3.
12. Corcione A, Benvenuto F, Ferretti E, Giunti D, Cappiello V, Cazzanti F, Risso M, Gualandi F, Mancardi GL, Pistoia V, Uccelli A. Human mesenchymal stem cells modulate B-cell functions. Blood. 2006;107(1):367–72. https://doi.org/10.1182/blood-2005-07-2657. Epub 2005 Sep 1
13. Beyth S, Borovsky Z, Mevorach D, Liebergall M, Gazit Z, Aslan H, Galun E, Rachmilewitz J. Human mesenchymal stem cells alter antigen-presenting cell maturation and induce T-cell unresponsiveness. Blood. 2005;105(5):2214–9. https://doi.org/10.1182/blood-2004-07-2921. Epub 2004 Oct 28
14. Strobl H, Knapp W. TGF-beta1 regulation of dendritic cells. Microbes Infect. 1999;1(15):1283–90. https://doi.org/10.1016/s1286-4579(99)00256-7.
15. Lucchini G, Introna M, Dander E, Rovelli A, Balduzzi A, Bonanomi S, Salvadè A, Capelli C, Belotti D, Gaipa G, Perseghin P, Vinci P, Lanino E, Chiusolo P, Orofino MG, Marktel S, Golay J, Rambaldi A, Biondi A, D'Amico G, Biagi E. Platelet-lysate-expanded mesenchymal stromal cells as a salvage therapy for severe resistant graft-versus-host disease in a pediatric population. Biol Blood Marrow Transplant. 2010;16(9):1293–301. https://doi.org/10.1016/j.bbmt.2010.03.017. Epub 2010 Mar 27
16. Introna M, Lucchini G, Dander E, Galimberti S, Rovelli A, Balduzzi A, Longoni D, Pavan F, Masciocchi F, Algarotti A, Micò C, Grassi A, Deola S, Cavattoni I, Gaipa G, Belotti D, Perseghin P, Parma M, Pogliani E, Golay J, Pedrini O, Capelli C, Cortelazzo S, D'Amico G, Biondi A, Rambaldi A, Biagi E. Treatment of graft versus host disease with mesenchymal stromal cells: a phase I study on 40 adult and pediatric patients. Biol Blood Marrow Transplant. 2014;20(3):375–81. https://doi.org/10.1016/j.bbmt.2013.11.033. Epub 2013 Dec 7

United States Military Hand Allotransplantation

23

Jennifer Cooley and Dmitry Tuder

23.1 Introduction

The San Antonio project was unique in its development. A team of military and civilian surgeons and specialists was formed to perform not only the first female VCA in the United States but also the first VCA at a military facility on a military service member [1]. The unilateral hand transplant was performed on February 17, 2010, at Wilford Hall Medical Center on Lackland Air Force Base in San Antonio, Texas. The transplant team was formed approximately a year and a half prior to the transplant and included physicians from across San Antonio, Texas.

The patient was a United States Air Force (USAF) Master Sergeant. She was a victim of a package bomb explosion at Lackland Air Force Base in July 2001 and suffered a traumatic left wrist disarticulation, lost three fingers on her right hand, and lost her right eye [2]. She was 50 years old at the time of injury, in good physical health prior to the event, and was left-hand dominant. For the following nine years, despite undergoing multiple surgical revisions of her left wrist disarticulation and trialing multiple prosthetics, she continued to have suboptimal results. She underwent numerous procedures on her right hand as well, resulting in amputation of her distal third through fifth fingers.

The patient approached her medical team after reading about hand allotransplantation to see if she was a candidate for the procedure. The hook prosthesis negatively impacted her psychological health. She felt it interfered with her job as a teacher because it frightened her students. At that time, the Hand and Upper Extremity Services at Wilford Hall Medical Center obtained permission from the United States military to pursue a unilateral hand allotransplantation for the patient. After obtaining approval from the department of defense, a team of military and civilian surgeons and specialists was formed. The transplant, postoperative medical care, and immunosuppressive therapy were funded by the department of defense. The patient underwent extensive medical and psychological screening prior to the transplant [3]. An appropriate donor was found after 8 months [2]. The transplant was performed nine years after the initial injury, in February 2010.

After transplantation, the patient faced multiple challenges, including 13 episodes of acute rejection, multiple episodes of acute renal failure, cytomegalovirus (CMV) reactivation, and she underwent one reoperation on the transplanted hand. Despite these challenges, she had improved Disabilities of the Arm, Shoulder, and Hand (DASH) scores post-operatively. She was able to return to activities she enjoyed prior to the incident including horseback riding. Ten years post-operatively, at age 70, she elected for amputation of the transplanted hand. She chose to have the hand amputated because she no longer wanted to be on immunosuppressive therapy. Overall, the operation was successful in affording the patient a functional left hand for ten years. It allowed her to enjoy multiple activities before voluntarily electing for removal due to the adverse effects of immunosuppressive therapy.

The project is no longer active at this time. It was an individualized endeavor setup specifically for the patient. There are currently no plans for future VCA procedures at United States military installations. Current clinical VCA research is funded outside of the military system. This was the only patient screened and no current waiting list exists. The United States military clinical medical missions have been refocused toward providing immediate combat care, as well as maintenance of the fighting force with preventative treatments and procedures. Higher level treatments such as VCA are referred to specialized civilian centers at this time.

The United States military continues to collaborate and conduct research for amputees and VCA patients. Restorative Endeavor for Servicemembers Through Optimization of Reconstruction (RESTOR) is a preclinical translational research program for tissue preservation and immunomodu-

J. Cooley
USAISR - The United States Army Institute of Surgical Research, San Antonio, TX, USA

D. Tuder (✉)
Alamo Orthopedics, San Antonio, TX, USA

© Springer Nature Switzerland AG 2023
R. Gurunian et al. (eds.), *Reconstructive Transplantation*, https://doi.org/10.1007/978-3-031-21520-9_23

lation. They are also a part of the Transplantation Outcomes Research Collaborative for the Hand (TORCH) project. This was developed to create a new measurement system for major extremity trauma and amputations. TORCH conducts qualitative research concerning quality of life issues for hand transplant patients at major hand transplant centers across the United States. Comprehensive Advanced Restorative Effort (CARE) is a partnership network the Naval Medical Center in San Diego, California, has with civilian academic centers. It helps wounded soldiers obtain evaluations, logistical support, and aftercare.

23.2 Donor

Donor screening included the following criteria: female gender, caucasian ethnicity, age 18–60 years old, weight 120–250 lbs., CDC low risk, no history of surgery or recent trauma to the left upper extremity, no history of diabetes or peripheral vascular disease, no tobacco use, and ABO compatibility. It took 8 months to find an appropriately matched donor. The donor was a 24-year-old caucasian female. She was CMV positive. The donor hand skin color was matched to the recipient. She was declared brain dead secondary to multiple intracranial hemorrhages following a single car collision 2 months prior. The donor harvest was performed at University of Texas Health Science Center at San Antonio. It was conducted by a 2 surgeon team including Dr. Mark Bagg and Dr. Dmitry Tuder. The procedure consisted of a left elbow disarticulation. The donor arm was infused with 1 L of Lactated Ringer's Solution with 18 mg of mannitol and 2000 units of heparin for preservation. Reconstruction of the donor arm with an available prosthetic was performed to allow for an open casket if desired.

23.3 Recipient

The recipient was a 59-year-old female, USAF Master Sergeant. She suffered a traumatic left wrist disarticulation secondary to a package bomb explosion 9 years prior to the hand transplant. The patient tolerated the operation well. She had multiple complications detailed below including CMV reactivation, acute renal failure, acute rejection, and need for a second operation on the left hand.

23.4 Surgical Technique

The patient underwent a left-hand allotransplantation on February 17–18, 2010. The procedure took a total of nine and a half hours. The donor operation consisted of a left elbow disarticulation with prosthetic reconstruction. The details of the donor operation are further described above in the "Donor" section. The recipient site preparation and the transplantation operations were performed at Lackland's Wilford Hall Medical Center in San Antonio. Preparation of the recipient site was performed by a four surgeon team. The transplantation was then performed by a team of six surgeons. Internal fixation of the radius and ulna was performed with plate and screw constructs. Tendon fixation and transfer was performed using the Pulvertaft weave technique and included the following: extensor carpi radialis longus (ECRL) to flexor digitorum profundus (FDP), extensor carpi radialis brevis (ECRB) to ECRB, brachioradialis (BR) to extensor pollicis longus (EPL), extensor digitorum communis (EDC) to EDC, flexor carpi radialis (FCR) to flexor pollicis longus (FPL), and flexor carpi ulnaris (FCU) to FCU. Median and ulnar nerves were coaptated. End-to-side donor radial to recipient brachial artery coaptation was performed. Total tissue ischemia time was 3 ½ h. Total surgical time was 9 ½ h.

23.5 Immunosuppression Protocol

Induction immunotherapy consisted of the following:

1. 100 mg (1.5 mg/kg) of thymoglobulin on days 0, 1, 2, 4, and 6.
2. 250 mg of solumedrol on days 0 and 1.
3. 4 mg of tacrolimus twice daily was started on day 0.
4. 500 mg of mycophenolate mofetil twice daily was started on day 1. This was increased to 1000 mg twice a day throughout the patient's postoperative period.

Maintenance immunotherapy consisted of the following:

1. 2 mg of tacrolimus twice daily.
2. 5 mg of prednisolone daily.
3. Initially 500 mg of mycophenolate mofetil twice daily. This was increased to 750 mg twice daily 3 ½ years postoperatively due to an episode of acute rejection. It was increased a final time to 1000 mg twice daily at 5 years and 10 months post-transplant due to another acute rejection episode.
4. Septra DS three times a week.
5. Protopic ointment three times a day.
6. Clobetasol ointment three times a day.

23.6 Episodes of Acute Rejection

The patient experienced 13 episodes of acute rejection. The timing of these episodes and the treatments performed are detailed in Table 23.1.

Table 23.1 Episodes of acute rejection

Postoperative date	Treatment
Day 19	• Topical tacrolimus and triamcinolone • 250 mg IV solumedrol for 3 days
Day 29	• Topical tacrolimus and triamcinolone • 500 mg IV solumedrol for 3 days
Day 103	• Topical tacrolimus and triamcinolone • 500 mg IV solumedrol for 3 days
Day 194	• Topical tacrolimus and triamcinolone • 500 mg IV solumedrol for 3 days
2 years 4 months	• Topical tacrolimus and triamcinolone • 500 mg IV solumedrol for 3 days
3 years 6 months	• Topical tacrolimus and triamcinolone • 500 mg IV solumedrol for 2 days • Mycophenolate mofetil increased to 750 mg twice daily
4 years 9 months	• Prednisone PO 50 mg for 10 days
5 years 5 months	• Prednisone PO 50 mg for 10 days
5 years 10 months	• 500 mg IV solumedrol for 2 days • Mycophenolate mofetil increased to 1000 mg twice daily
6 years 3 months	• Prednisone PO 100 mg for 4 days
6 years 7 months	• Prednisone PO 50 mg for 5 days
6 years 11 months	• 500 mg IV solumedrol for 2 days
8 years 6 months	• Prednisone PO 50 mg for 5 days

23.7 Monitoring

Monthly tacrolimus levels were obtained.

23.8 Rehabilitation Protocol

The following protocol was developed for post-operative rehabilitation.

23.8.1 Starting 3 Days Post-Op

- Fabricate a volar forearm based resting hand splint in safe position:
  - Wrist extension = 30 degrees.
  - MCP flexion = 45–60 degrees.
  - IPs = 0 degrees.
  - Thumb in mid-radial and palmar abduction.
- Perform passive range of motion exercises every two hours off tension (passive tenodesis with digits and thumb) with forearm in neutral supination and pronation.
  - MP extension with IP extension and wrist in gentle flexion.
  - MP flexion with IP flexion with wrist in gentle extension.
  - Thumb passive flexion and extension as available while positioned in mid-radial palmar abduction.
  - Intrinsic stretching: MPs extended and IPs flexed, MPs flexed and IPs extended.
- Edema management.
  - Elevation day and night.

    Night elevation with two pillows and two bath towels.
  - Retrograde massage.
- Maintain range of motion at the shoulder and elbow.
  - Complete shoulder and elbow active range of motion with resting splint donned.
- Educate on sensory loss, susceptibility to injury, and compensatory strategies to prevent injury to transplanted hand.
- Daily clinic treatment.
  - Heat under supervision with hand postured in safe position.
  - Passive range of motion as described above.
  - Place and hold exercises with tenodesis 15 repetitions, 5 s hold.

    Instruct to complete gentle place and hold every 2 waking hours, 15 repetitions each, 5 s hold.
  - Gentle active supination and pronation to forearm.
  - Sensory re-education.
  - Transcutaneous electrical nerve stimulation (TENS) for neurogenic pain ("conventional" TENS or "acupuncture-like" TENS).

23.8.2 At 3 Weeks Post-Op

- Full digit and thumb active range of motion with wrist and forearm in neutral position.
  - Increase effort level of all exercises as appropriate to the level of healing.
- Active range of motion for differential tendon gliding and blocking exercises to digits and thumb.
- Incorporate use of electrical stimulation for neuromuscular re-education.
- Fabricate splints as needed to promote differential tendon gliding and/or blocking exercises; splints to be worn only for exercise.
- Fabricate anti-claw splint with C-bar for thumb and wrist in neutral position to be used with light non-resistive functional activities to promote functional grip patterns.
- Continue with protective resting splint and edema management when not exercising.
- Perform scar massage.
- Advance home exercise program with increased effort level of all active range of motion exercises.
- Continue with TENS, sensory re-education, and edema management.

23.8.3 At 6 Weeks Post-Op

- Discontinue protective resting splint.
- Fabricate hand based anti-claw splint with C-bar to be worn with activity.
- Fabricate flexor tenodesis and/or extensor tenodesis splint as needed and include C-Bar in splints.
- Extension splinting for nightwear if extensor lag is present.
- Initiate grip and pinching program with hand based anti-claw splint, advancing strengthening program with increased effort level as appropriate.
- Increase functional level light strengthening through work and leisure simulation activities with hand based anti-claw splint.
  - May use BTE for eccentric and concentric exercises of wrist and digit flexors and extensors as well as forearm rotators.
  - Incorporate light functional strengthening activities.

23.8.4 At 9–12 Weeks Post-Op

- Initiate functional wrist strengthening while wearing hand based anti-claw splint.
  - May fabricate dynamic wrist extension and/or flexion splints that incorporate the anti-claw splint to increase strength of the agonist and antagonist muscle groups in the wrist.

23.8.5 Other Considerations

Depending on condition of donor arm (i.e. arthritic) consider a resting splint at night and a day splint for functional gripping (MPs blocked, IPs free, and thumb positioned in functional opposition).

23.9 Follow-Up

The recipient was followed for 10 years post-transplantation. Her DASH score improved from 37.5 preoperatively to 8.3 at 9 years 6 months post-operatively. This self-reported questionnaire evaluates the patient's ability to perform physical activities involving the arm, shoulder, and hand, the severity of their symptoms including pain, paresthesias, and weakness, and the effect it has on their social functioning, work life, and psychological status [4]. A score of zero represents no disability, while a score of 100 represents severe disability [4]. She showed marked improvement postoperatively compared to her preoperative score.

23.10 Sensory Function

At 9 years 6 months the patient had 2 point discrimination as follows: thumb 6 mm, index finger 6 mm, middle finder 6 mm, ring finger 8 mm, and small finger 12 mm. Two-point discrimination of 6 mm for the fingertip is considered in the normal range [5]. Her Semmes-Weinstein at this time was 3.61gm. This denotes a grade 4/5, representing diminished light touch. Grade 5 is normal sensation, while grade 1 represents deep pressure sensation only [6]. She had hot and cold sensation in her fingers and palm.

23.11 Motor Function

The patient had no intrinsic motor function of the left hand. She had proximal interphalangeal joint fixed flexion contractures. Her index finger was fixed at 45 degrees, middle finger at 45 degrees, ring finger at 90 degrees, and small finger at 90 degrees. In all metacarpophalangeal joints she had active range of motion from 0 to 90 degrees. She had active dorsiflexion of the wrist from 0 to 80 degrees. She had no active palmar flexion of the wrist, but had passive palmar flexion between 0 and 45 degrees.

23.12 Complications

23.12.1 CMV Reactivation

The donor was tested and found to be CMV positive. The patient experienced CMV reactivation on post-operative days 67, 114, and 920. Each episode was treated with ganciclovir. After 2 ½ years she had no further episodes of CMV reactivation.

23.12.2 Acute Renal Failure

The patient experienced two episodes of acute renal failure on days 138 and 233 post-transplantation. Each episode was treated with IV hydration. Her baseline creatinine in 2019 was stable at 1.2.

23.12.3 Return to Operating Room

The patient was taken back to the operating room 20 months postoperatively for wrist and finger extensor tenolysis, Zancolli lasso of the index finger, middle finger, ring finger, and small finger, and thumb static tenodesis to the radius. Prior to the take back, the patient had 0 degrees of wrist flexion. Post-operatively, the patient had initial marked improvement in metacarpophalangeal joint hyperextension and proximal interphalangeal joint active range of motion. The patient subsequently developed progressive proximal interphalangeal joint fixed flexion contractures.

23.12.4 Unrelated Injuries

The patient also had two traumatic injuries not involving the hand allotransplantation, which are included for completion. At 22 months post-transplant, the patient fell from her horse and was found to have multiple rib fractures as well as multiple thoracic and lumbar spine transverse process and vertebral process fractures. At 8 years post-transplant, the patient fell from her horse a second time and sustained a rotator cuff tear. At 2 years and 6 months post-transplant and 3 years 1 month post-transplant the patient underwent bilateral total hip arthroplasties. At the time of surgery there was no evidence of osteonecrosis.

23.13 Unique Challenges

At age 70, the patient elected to have her hand amputated. The amputation was performed in January 2021. She enjoyed 10 years of life with a hand that had both motor and sensory functions. She was able to continue her passion of horseback riding during this time. She was also able to continue teaching. Overtime she developed progressive proximal interphalangeal joint fixed flexion contractures and had no active palmar flexion at the wrist. She made the decision to voluntarily undergo amputation due to the adverse effects of the immunosuppressive therapy. She desired to no longer require lifelong medication. The amputation was uncomplicated.

23.14 Lessons Learned

This was an individualized project that was undertaken at the request of the patient. It was the first female VCA in the United States. It was also the first VCA performed on a military servicemember at a military facility. This case is unique in the fact that it was not done at a specialized VCA center. The patient had a successful hand transplant and had 10 years with improved functionality. This demonstrates that this procedure can successfully be performed outside of specialized centers.

This case as well as the eight other documented cases worldwide of servicemembers undergoing vascularized composite allotransplantation have demonstrated similar outcomes for servicemembers compared to the civilian population [3]. The initial concerns with VCA in the military population have not been demonstrated in these cases. Some of these concerns include immunologic sensitization and latent infections [3]. Though there are no longer VCA cases being performed at military facilities, there are programs to assist servicemembers in finding VCA programs at civilian academic centers. The military continues to fund and perform research for the improvement of VCA.

The patient's immunosuppression regimen was adjusted over time based on her episodes of acute rejection. With current immunosuppressive therapy, close monitoring and frequent medication adjustments are necessary for success. The patient eventually decided to have her hand amputated due to the adverse effects of immunosuppressive therapy and the desire to no longer require lifelong medication. This highlights an important area of VCA research. Lifelong immunosuppression is one of the largest drawbacks to VCA. This has been a highly researched topic, but as demonstrated in this case, it continues to be an area in need of improvement.

References

1. Fries CA, Tuder D, Gorantla VS, Chan RK, Davis MR. Military VCA in the world. Curr Transpl Rep. 2020;7:246–50. https://doi.org/10.1007/s40472-020-00294-y.
2. WellSpan surgeon participated in rare hand transplant. WellSpan Health 2010, Mar 14. https://www.wellspan.org/news/story/wellspan-surgeon-participated-in-rare-hand-transplant/N4117
3. Fries CA, Tuder D, Iyer S, Gorantla VS, Davis MR, Rickard RF. Upper limb reconstruction transplantation in military recipients: summary of world experience. J Roy Nav Med Serv. 2018;104(1):6–1. http://jrnms.com/JournalArticle.ashx?ID=12535
4. Williams NDASH. Occup Med. 2013;64(1):67–8. https://doi.org/10.1093/occmed/kqt130.
5. McGee S. Examination of the sensory system. Evidence-Based Physical Diagnosis. 2018;4:569–582.e3. https://doi.org/10.1016/B978-0-323-39276-1.00062-7.
6. Suda M, Kawakami M, Okuyama K, Ishii R, Oshima O, Hijikata N, et al. Validity and reliability of the Semmes-Weinstein monofilament test and the thumb localizing test in patients with stroke. Front Neurol. 2021; https://doi.org/10.3389/fneur.2020.625917.

Part V

Lower Extremity Transplantation

Lower Extremity Transplantation by Ozkan Team (Turkey)

24

Özlenen Özkan, Mustafa Gökhan Ertosun, and Ömer Özkan

24.1 Introduction

Our program started in January 2012, with the first lower extremity transplant in Turkey with special permission from the government. As in hand, face, and uterus transplantation, lower extremity transplantation was performed by our center for the first time in our country [1–7]. Lower extremity transplantation program is still active.

The preoperative, operative, and postoperative costs associated with vascularized composite allotransplants are very high. Reconstruction costs for Turkish citizens with social security in our country are covered by the state. Similarly, expenses related to lower extremity transplant are covered by the state, like any other reconstruction and transplantation operation.

Six patients have applied to our center for consideration of lower extremity transplantation. After screening, 4 candidates met the lower extremity transplantation criteria. Since one of our candidates had a lower extremity transplant, we currently have 3 candidates on our waiting list.

In lower extremity transplantation ensuring gender compatibility between the recipient and the donor, which is also applied in other composite tissue transplantations in our country, has been one of the challenges hindering the expansion of the program. Another significant factor in our country limiting the expansion has been the fact that lower extremity transplantation had to be performed simultaneously with upper extremity transplantation. Therefore, patients who needed both upper and lower extremity transplantation could be selected as candidate. Thus, individuals who only need lower extremity transplantation are excluded from this program.

Another criterion is related to the level of amputation. The indication for lower extremity transplantation in our country is below the amputation. However, the prostheses used for amputations at this level have been proven successful in maintaining near to normal activity. Patients can carry on their daily lives successfully by the use of prosthesis, and also they can avoid serious side effects of immunosuppressive drugs Lifelong need for immunosuppressive therapy after transplantation is associated with secondary viral and fungal infections as well as malignancy. For the aforementioned reasons, lower extremity transplantation alone is not performed in our country but is applied to individuals with arm transplantation.

24.2 Patients

The Donor: This was a 39-year-old male patient with brain death who sustained an accident.

The Recipient: The patient, born in 1978, had an electric burn injury in 1989. As a result of this accident, both arms were amputated from the proximal level and the right leg was amputated below the knee. The patient underwent arm and lower extremity transplantation in the same surgery. The transplanted lower extremity was removed 18 h after the operation due to venous insufficiency.

24.3 Surgical Technique

The accepted indication in our country is the recipient sill also have an upper extremity transplantation. Lower extremity transplantation alone is contraindicated. A prosthetic copy of the extremity to be harvested as a donor is taken and donor integrity planning is made with a suitable prosthesis after amputation. After the removal of the upper extremities, the lower extremities are harvested and prepared for transfer. In order not to risk the removal of other solid organs, the extremity can be harvested quickly after all solid organs have been harvested. However, since the muscle load in the lower extremities is high, attention should be paid to the ischemia

Ö. Özkan (✉) · M. G. Ertosun · Ö. Özkan
Department of Plastic, Reconstructive, and Aesthetic Surgery, Akdeniz University School of Medicine, Antalya, Turkey

© Springer Nature Switzerland AG 2023
R. Gurunian et al. (eds.), *Reconstructive Transplantation*, https://doi.org/10.1007/978-3-031-21520-9_24

time. The tourniquet may or may not need to be used depending on the general condition of the donor and whether other solid organs have been removed yet. If other solid organs have been removed and the heartbeat has stopped, amputation can be achieved very quickly with a guillotine-like method. In any case, while the donor extremity is being prepared, an extremity longer than the specified need should be harvested in order to aid skin, muscle, and bone tissue adaptation for possible edema that may occur after transplantation. The repair of vessels and nerves should be performed without tension. After the skin incision level is determined in the donor, the main muscle groups are marked with appropriate long sutures and transected and separated. The vascular and nerve pedicles are dissected proximally (up to the superficial femoral artery and femoral vein above the knee, as well as the great saphenous vein, sciatic nerve and, if the level is appropriate, up to the femoral nerve) by marking. Again, osteotomies are (femur above the knee) performed to obtain slightly longer than the required length (to be adapted during osteosynthesis). After the extremity is removed, the prosthesis team places the appropriately prepared prosthesis on the amputated leg for donor integrity. The prepared lower extremity is quickly placed on a large operating table and perfused with the perfusion fluid (Wisconsin, UW solution) using arterial catheterization. Perfusion is continued until transparent liquid comes out of the venous pedicle. By providing cold ischemia conditions suitable for the extremity, the recipient is taken to the operating room as quickly as possible. If upper extremity transplantation is planned simultaneously (which is the accepted indication), a second team must be ready for lower extremity transplantation, and even the donor extremity should be prepared simultaneously when the extremity is taken from the donor. In the amputation stump, it is planned to preserve the vascularity of the skin tissue in the most appropriate way. Anterior and posterior skin flaps are created and dissected to expose the muscles and mark their appropriate anatomical alignment at the amputated tip. The muscular ends are prepared to be compatible with the transferred muscles. Neurovascular structures, the femoral artery and vein anteriorly and, if appropriate, the great saphenous vein and nerve pedicle are prepared by dissecting them to the most appropriate level to allow reliable anastomosis and coaptation point. Posteriorly, the sciatic nerve is prepared and marked in the same way. The bone (femur above the knee) is dissected from the place where it appears most healthy and prepared for osteosynthesis with a proper osteotomy. When the lower extremity allotransplant is brought to the recipient extremity, the excess part of the femur is properly removed by osteotomy, considering the bilateral femur length with preoperative plain X-ray. Rigid osteosynthesis is provided with an appropriate plating with the recipient femur. Very quickly, the previously marked donor and recipient muscles are approximated with simple sutures and muscle continuity is ensured.

At this stage, it is very important for the anesthesia team to decrease cardiac output with close monitoring. Depending on the major extremity replantation experience of the surgical team, after the femoral artery and vein anastomoses, the vascular clamp in the femoral artery is opened, and some venous blood flow of the great saphenous vein is permitted by close hemodynamic monitoring. Vascular clamp in the femoral vein is opened without disturbing hemodynamics and great saphenous vein anastomosis is provided. After bleeding control, femoral nerve (if proximal muscle transplantation is also performed) (may not be necessary in distal amputations) and sciatic nerve coaptations are provided with appropriate tension (considering that tension may occur with postoperative edema) without leaving too long donor nerves. The skin flaps are excised and sutured at appropriate tension and levels where reliable circulation is ensured. Skin grafts are prepared from excess skin and stored for use if necessary. Below-knee fasciotomies can be performed depending on the duration of the operation and the follow-up possibilities. When extremity perfusion is ensured, the operation is terminated.

In our case, although revision of vascular anastomoses was performed in the same session due to circulatory problems, the transplanted tissue was removed on the same day because of the change in skin color, the appearance of petechiae, and worsening of kidney functions. The general condition of the patient recovered after the amputation and the follow-up of the transplanted upper extremity was continued in the floor after the completion of his treatment in the intensive care unit.

24.4 Immunosuppression Protocol (Induction, Maintenance, and Variations; Treatment of Rejection)

The patient underwent bilateral forearm transplantation and lower extremity transplantation. If the transplanted lower extremities were not removed, the initial induction and maintenance immunosuppression protocol we used in arm transplantation was going to be continued in the same way [1].

Initial Induction Treatment: Anti-thymocyte globulin and prednisolone were administered. Anti-thymocyte globulin was initiated intraoperatively at a dose of 2.5 mg/kg per day. Prednisolone was started on the day of surgery, at 1000 mg and tapered down to 20 mg, 1-week post-op. On post-op day four, tacrolimus (0.2 mg/kg Prograf per day with blood levels 15–20 ng/mL) was started. Anti-thymocyte globulin was stopped on day 7–10, depending on blood CD3 level and the achievement of the desired tacrolimus blood levels.

Maintenance Treatment: Prednisolone (20 mg/day) tapering to 10 mg/day six months postoperatively, tacrolimus (blood levels between 15 and 20 ng/ml for the first three months, tapered to 7–10 ng/ml 6 months postoperatively) and mycophenolate mofetil (MMF) (2 g/day).

In Rejection Attacks: We increase the dose of tacrolimus, and we use topical tacrolimus treatment in addition to systemic tacrolimus. In addition to tacrolimus, we also use pulse steroid therapy in rejection attacks.

Although it was planned to be this way, the dose of immunosuppression might need to be increased due to the high amount of tissues with high antigenic load in the transplanted tissues.

24.5 Monitoring Protocol

Mucosal biopsies would be scheduled on the transplanted oral mucosa biweekly for three months and then monthly for six months. Skin biopsies near the incision marks were planned to be performed monthly for the first six months and then quarterly in the most inconspicuous area. Biopsy samples were planned to be analyzed according to the Banff 2007 scale.

24.6 Unique Problems or Challenges

In our patient, major problems were experienced in the recipient vascular structures during the operation, since the cause of the limb loss was an electrical burn. Due to the venous insufficiency that developed during this period, the transplanted lower extremities of the patient were surgically removed 18 hours after the operation.

The patient had a disseminated cerebral and renal aspergillosis due to immunosuppressive therapy. Despite the proper treatments against this infection, the patient died.

24.7 Lessons Learned

24.7.1 What Are the Strengths of Your Program?

Below the knee amputation is an indication for lower extremity transplantation in Turkey. As mentioned before, prosthetic fit of individuals with below the knee amputation is quite good in terms of functionality. Also, below the knee amputation alone is not an indication for lower extremity transplantation. Lower extremity transplantation is applied to patients with an indication for upper extremity transplantation. Transplantation gives better results than prostheses in the upper extremity due to the high number of minor movements in social life, unlike the lower extremity. For this reason, side effects that may occur during and after transplantation can be considered. When these conditions are evaluated, lower extremity transplantations are applied to patients simultaneously with upper extremity transplantations.

Since patients will use lifelong immunosuppressive agents with potential risk of malignancy and infection, it is very important that the patient has a strong desire to pursue with the transplantation understanding its consequence. Even if the patient has the slightest hesitation, it is imperative to avoid the transplantation.

24.7.2 What Will you Not Repeat in the Future?

The extremity loss was due to electrical burn injury in the patient who underwent the transplantation. It is necessary to be more careful in planning transplantation in individuals who have had amputations as a result of electrical burn injury. Electrical injuries affect the vessels with significant fibrosis. For this reason, angiography should be applied to prospective recipients in the pre-op period and the possibility of fibrosis in the vessels should not be overlooked.

Due to the large bulk of muscles contained in the transplanted extremities the time to withstand ischemia is quite limited. In addition, in our country, as mentioned before, lower extremity transplantation is performed together with upper extremity transplantation. Therefore, the ischemia time is much more critical when multiple extremities are involved in the transplantation. When planning the lower extremity transplantation, it is very important that the recipient and the donor are in the same hospital, and operations are conducted in the operating rooms that are next to each other to minimize the ischemia time. For this reason, in the next lower extremity transplant operation, it is planned that the recipient and the donor will be in the same hospital, procedures will be performed in the operating rooms that are close proximity to each other, if possible.

It should not be forgotten that the priority is to remove the lower extremity when ischemia is suspected in lower extremity transplantation surgeries performed together with upper extremity transplantation.

References

1. Ozkan O, Demirkan F, Ozkan O, Dinckan A, Hadimioglu N, Tuzuner S, et al. The first (double) hand transplantation in Turkey. Transplant Proc. 2011;43(9):3557–60.
2. Ozkan O, Ozkan O, Ubur M, Hadimioglu N, Cengiz M, Afsar I. Face allotransplantation for various types of facial disfigurements: a series of five cases. Microsurgery. 2018;38(8):834–43.
3. Ozkan O, Akar ME, Erdogan O, Ozkan O, Hadimioglu N. Uterus transplantation from a deceased donor. Fertil Steril. 2013;100(6):e41.

4. Erman Akar M, Ozkan O, Aydinuraz B, Dirican K, Cincik M, Mendilcioglu I, et al. Clinical pregnancy after uterus transplantation. Fertil Steril. 2013;100(5):1358–63.
5. Ozkan O, Akar ME, Ozkan O, Erdogan O, Hadimioglu N, Yilmaz M, et al. Preliminary results of the first human uterus transplantation from a multiorgan donor. Fertil Steril. 2013;99(2):470–6.
6. Ozkan O, Ozkan O, Dogan NU, Bahceci M, Mendilcioglu I, Boynukalin K, et al. Birth of a healthy baby 9 years after a surgically successful deceased donor uterus transplant. Ann Surg. 2022;275(5):825–32.
7. Ertosun MG, Ozkan O, Celen E, Ozkan O, Yoldas B. Correlation of miRNAs with prognosis in composite tissue allotransplantation. Exp Clin Transplant. 2021;19(11):1212–23.

Quadruple Extremity Transplantation

25

Serdar Nazif Nasir and Arda Küçükgüven

25.1 Introduction

The lower extremity transplantation has not been popular compared to the other vascularized composite allotransplantations. However, the major lower limb losses are seen 15 times higher compared to the major upper limb losses [1]. Bilateral above-knee amputations cause severe functional impairment. The hesitancy to perform lower extremity transplantations can be attributed to its uncertain outcomes and immunosuppressive risks. The concept of lower extremity transplantation lies in the fact that lower extremity prosthetics lack proprioceptive and protective sensation needed for balance. Moreover, improved postoperative functional capacity and restored body image are other invaluable benefits of vascularized lower extremity allotransplantations.

Increasing evidence gathered from upper extremity allotransplantations indicates that excellent anatomical replacement and satisfactory restoration of motor and sensory functions are possible and achievable with current techniques and immunosuppression strategies. Far fewer immunosuppression-related problems have been encountered than initially expected among recipients which may be attributed to the need for less aggressive regimens compared to the treatment protocols initially used [2]. Outcomes of upper extremity composite allotransplantations have been promising and laid the ground for the potentially favorable outcomes in lower extremity allotransplantation.

In 2006, the first case of composite lower limb allotransplantation was performed by Zuker et al. in ischiopagus conjoined twins without the need for immunosuppression [3]. A functioning lower limb of one twin with a lethal cardiac anomaly was transplanted to the other. Six years after the transplant, the patient regained good sensory and motor recovery. The patient was able to ambulate well and attend sports activities at school [4].

In 2011, Cadavas et al. performed the second case of bilateral above-knee transplantation of lower limbs in a 21-year-old male patient. They presented good functional outcomes at 1-year follow-up. The patient was able to walk between parallel bars using rigid ankle-foot orthoses [5]. The patient was diagnosed with primary central nervous system posttransplant lymphoproliferative disease. Therefore, the immunosuppressive therapy was discontinued and the legs were removed [6].

Despite recent developments in immunosuppressive therapy, lifelong immunosuppression continues to be a significant risk factor for these patients. In light of limited experience with lower limb allotransplantation cases performed to date, it can be postulated that vascularized composite allotransplantation may be a reasonable alternative with the potential to restore sensory and motor function as well as esthetics in lower extremity amputees in the future. However, there are currently several concerns and questions related to the ideal immunosuppression protocol and lower extremity allotransplantation indications which have yet to be answered and clarified.

In our institution, we commenced the composite allotransplantations after obtaining the Composite Tissue Transplant Center License from Turkish Ministry of Health in 2011. First, we performed a total face transplantation. The patient gained full face mimic muscle activity as well as sensorial innervations after six months postoperatively [7]. Then, we performed a quadruple extremity transplantation on a 27-year-old male who had lost his upper and lower extremities after a high-voltage electrical accident 14 years ago. The patient died on the fourth day after transplantation in a clinical condition of severe systemic inflammatory response [8]. We had two patients on the lower extremity transplantation waiting list during that period. These patients were approved by the Institutional Composite Tissue Allotransplantation Council regarding the transplantation

S. N. Nasir (✉)
Department of Plastic, Reconstructive and Aesthetic Surgery, Hacettepe University Faculty of Medicine, Ankara, Turkey

A. Küçükgüven
Plastic, Reconstructive and Aesthetic Surgery Clinic, University of Health Sciences, Ankara Training and Research Hospital, Ankara, Turkey

© Springer Nature Switzerland AG 2023
R. Gurunian et al. (eds.), *Reconstructive Transplantation*, https://doi.org/10.1007/978-3-031-21520-9_25

indications. After finding a male brain-dead donor, his extremities were procured and transferred to our institution. The whole process was covered by the government health insurance program since the indications were approved by the Institutional Composite Tissue Allotransplantation Committee, and we had the Composite Tissue Transplant Center License. Other than the face and quadruple extremity transplantations we have not performed any other allotransplantations. Our institutional composite tissue allotransplantation program is not active at present because we do not have the license currently.

25.2 Case Presentation

The recipient patient was a 27-year-old male. He had all four extremities amputated following a high-voltage electrical injury 14 years ago (Fig. 25.1). The amputations were at the level of shoulder on the right arm, at the level of mid-humerus on the left arm, and above-knee level on the legs. National Organization for Organ Transplantation and institutional review board approvals were granted for the operation. Institutional Composite Tissue Allotransplantation Council also evaluated the patient and indications in detail and approved the surgery. A thorough preoperative blood testing was performed. The patient was evaluated by the nephrology, cardiology, pulmonology, gastroenterology, endocrinology, and psychiatry departments of our institution preoperatively. This multidisciplinary team did not find any medical problems or contraindications that would prohibit surgery. The simultaneous procurement of 4 extremities from a 47-year-old male brain-dead heart-beating donor was performed by our team in another institution. The recipient and donor had a 0/6 HLA match and were blood group compatible (A and O).

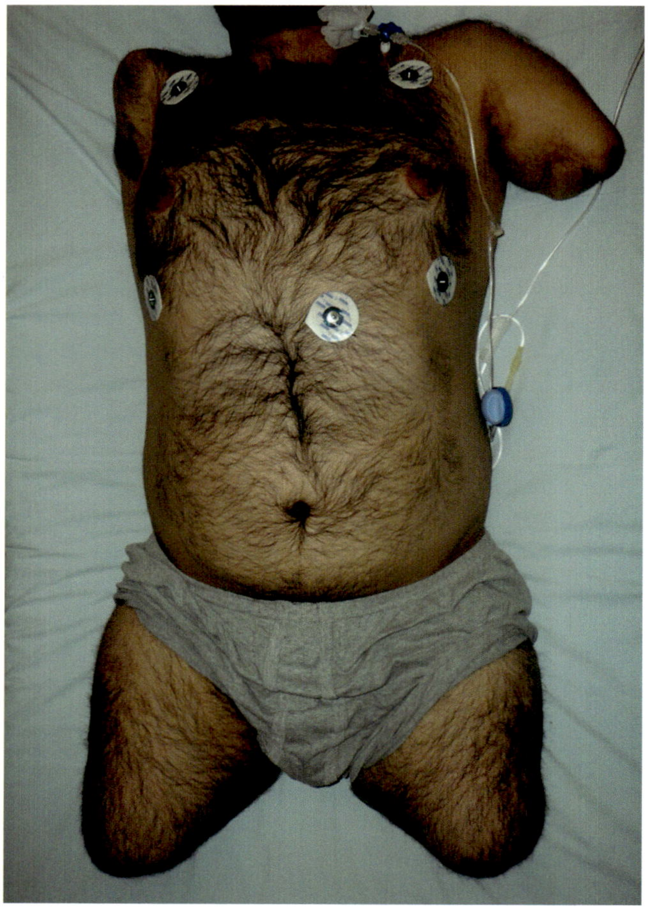

Fig. 25.1 A quadruple extremity transplantation was performed on a 27-year-old male who had lost his upper and lower extremities after a high-voltage electrical accident 14 years ago

25.2.1 Transplant Procurement

Solid organs and all 4 extremities of the donor were procured simultaneously by multiple surgical teams. The extremities were perfused by using the University of Wisconsin solution [9].

25.2.2 Irradiation of the Procured Extremities

Irradiation of the extremities was performed preoperatively based on the promising outcomes of the study conducted by our radiation oncology team. They showed that the antigenic load of an allotransplant could be reduced by preoperative irradiation [10].

25.2.3 Immunosuppression

In our immunosuppressive protocol, ATG (antithymocyte globulin) and a standard triple therapy including mycophenolate mofetil, tacrolimus, and corticosteroids were given to the patient 1 h before the surgery for induction.

25.2.4 Operative Details

We aimed to shorten the duration of cold ischemia time by increasing the number of microsurgery teams and using temporary shunts. The upper extremity transplantations were performed simultaneously by different surgical teams. During that period, temporary shunts were placed between the stumps of femoral vessels to reestablish the circulation of lower extremities (Fig. 25.2). Surgicel was applied to raw surfaces of the lower extremities to prevent excessive bleeding during upper extremity transplantations. The total cold ischemia time of each extremity was

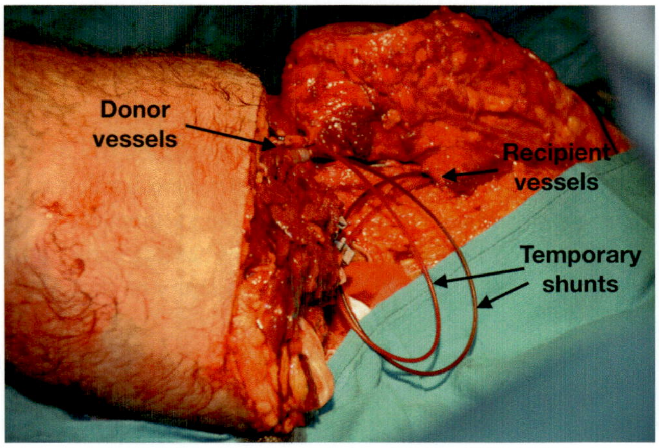

Fig. 25.2 Temporary shunts were placed between the stumps of femoral vessels to reestablish the circulation of lower extremities and reduce ischemia during the upper extremity transplantations

around 8 h. The whole transplantation surgery was completed in approximately 12 h.

Arterial and venous microsurgical anastomoses were performed with satisfactory patency of each anastomosis. Unconventional strategies were performed to achieve sufficient vascular access for fluid resuscitation, monitoring, and anastomosis of one vascular stump of right upper extremity. Since we used the femoral and subclavian vessels for vascular anastomoses, they were not available for monitoring and fluid resuscitation. For fluid resuscitation, the left internal jugular vein was used during the surgery. The right inferior epigastric artery was dissected and used for a period of 3 h for invasive blood pressure monitoring. However, it was occluded after that period. Based on this observation, it can be proposed that any artery or vein proximal to the femoral vessels should not be used in lower extremity transplantations. This might interfere with the success of the operation. Then, we placed an internal iliac artery cannula for invasive blood pressure monitoring.

Intraoperatively, we realized that the injured segment of the right subclavian vein was quite long due to the nature of the previous injury. Because of the fact that its stump was found just below the costoclavicular segment at the thoracic inlet, we opted to use the right external jugular vein after dissecting and transposing it under the clavicle for anastomosis with the allotransplant's right subclavian vein. Before beginning the microsurgical work for each extremity, arthrodesis of the right shoulder, internal fixation of the left upper extremity at the mid-humerus level, and internal fixation of the lower extremities at the level of proximal 1/3 of the femoral bones were performed by orthopedic surgeons. Then, we performed the vascular anastomoses and nerve coaptations with 8.0 nylon sutures. At the end of the surgery, revascularization of all extremities was established successfully after 12 h (Fig. 25.3).

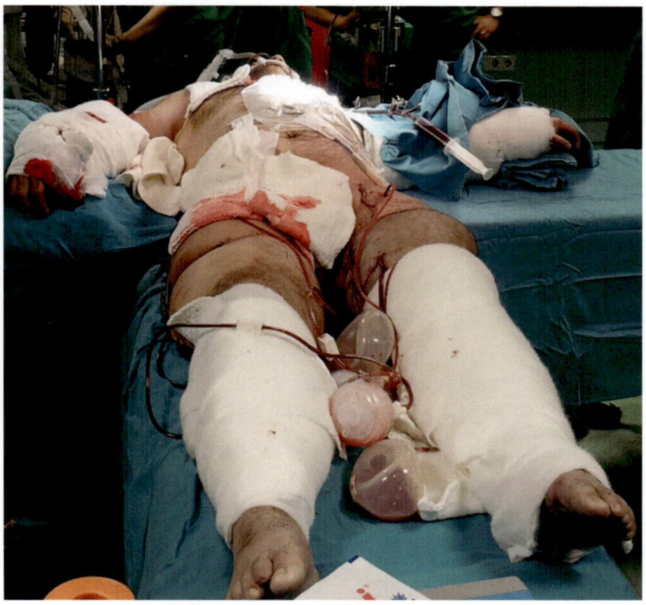

Fig. 25.3 Revascularization of all extremities was established successfully at the end of the surgery. The whole surgery was completed in 12 h

Metabolic and hemodynamic parameters of the patient were closely monitored during the surgery. Mild hyperkalemia and slight metabolic acidosis were present during the first half of the operation. This metabolic condition was managed, and the patient was stable during the initial phases of the surgery. Despite all fluid replacement and supportive treatments, the metabolic acidosis worsened close to the end of the surgery. Progressive bradycardia and subsequent cardiac arrest occurred one hour after the transplantation of the last extremity. After a short period of cardiopulmonary resuscitation which required sternotomy, the patient was stabilized after reestablishing spontaneous circulation. At that point, blood tests revealed that the patient had metabolic acidosis, hyperphosphatemia, and hyperkalemia. Therefore, intermittent plasmapheresis and continuous hemodialysis were performed to improve the patient's worsening metabolic condition. Despite all supportive efforts, metabolic acidosis could not be reversed resulting in increased transfusion requirements. A total of 200 units of erythrocyte suspension and other blood products were transfused for a period of 4 days. Following the sequential amputation of the extremities, the patient died on the fourth day despite all supportive therapies.

25.3 Discussion and Lessons Learned

Although the lower extremity prostheses have satisfactory outcomes and there are increased risks of lifelong immunosuppression in transplantation patients, these patients report an increased interest for composite lower extremity allotransplantations [11]. Despite the increasing number of sophisticated high-tech lower extremity prostheses, it is clear that these assist devices lack tactile and proprioceptive responses which are essential for normal lower extremity function [12]. Studies have shown that there are no differences between the high-tech and low-tech prostheses in terms of activity level regardless of the level of amputation [13, 14]. These findings suggest that indications for composite tissue allotransplantations should continue to be explored and will be the subject of clinical studies in the future.

The justification for replantation in cases of lower extremity amputations remains controversial. The significance of peripheral nerve regeneration and hence restoration of function remains to have a pivotal role in lower extremity replantation, which is highly affected by the level of amputation and degree of injury [15, 16]. Therefore, replantation, allotransplantation, and prosthesis associated risks must be weighed carefully against their sensory, motor, and esthetic outcomes in deciding which treatment option to follow in lower limb amputees.

We believe that the composite lower extremity allotransplantations should be reserved for patients who had lost their both lower limbs. Since patients having a single lower extremity can carry out most daily activities, such as walking, with the help of prosthetics or an orthopedic walker, composite tissue transplantations should be considered as overtreatment for these patients. In our case, we aimed to enable the patient to walk with the aid of a walker and external knee stabilizers.

There is significant controversy regarding the indications of quadruple composite tissue transplantation currently. The concept of simultaneous vascularized composite tissue allotransplantation is still in its infancy. However, it is a reality that patients who had lost all four extremities need quadruple extremity transplantations to improve the quality of life and regain their daily activities.

Our transplantation team conducted several experimental studies about composite tissue allotransplantations. The senior author demonstrated several experimental composite allotransplantation models and the induction of permanent immunotolerance using various therapeutic strategies. In those studies, the main objective was to improve the standards of composite tissue allotransplantations by achieving permanent immunosuppression, obviating the lifelong use of immunosuppressive drugs [17–24]. We also performed the sixth full-face composite allotransplantation in the world. This patient had the activity of all mimic muscles at the postoperative 6 months [7].

As the experimental and clinical studies have showed promise in the composite tissue allotransplantation, the idea of multiple transplantations gained popularity. Although the concomitant transplantations are hypothetically possible and intriguing, controversy on indications is still present and clinical experience is insufficient. One of the most complicated technical difficulties we faced during the surgery was the need for adequate length of vascular stumps. The high-voltage electrical injury was responsible for the vascular damage extending beyond the level of amputation which was uncommon in acute traumatic cases that we are familiar with in common practice. We had dissected long segments of vascular stumps in all four donor extremities bearing in mind the possible adverse effects of the electrical injury on the recipient vessels.

Ischemia and reperfusion injury are of major importance in the success of composite tissue allotransplantations. This challenge begins with the procurement of composite tissue and continues intraoperatively and postoperatively. Especially, metabolic load created by the reperfusion of the allotransplants might pose a life-threatening risk to patients. Simultaneous multi-organ harvesting from a donor sounds logical but it is very challenging for multiple teams to work together in a confined space during that period [25]. Therefore, these teams should be aware of this intraoperative difficulty and be prepared preoperatively. If multiple composite tissues are planning to be transplanted, it is vital to have multiple surgical teams to reduce ischemia (Fig. 25.4). Another useful tip is the use of temporary shunts to decrease the extent of reperfusion injury and shorten the ischemic period. Despite all medical and technical precautions, the metabolic load caused by the transplantation of four extremities exceeded the amount that could be reversed and was more than we expected. Hemodialysis was efficient for the management of hyperkalemia and metabolic acidosis in the early stages of the operation. However, it was not possible to reverse the worsened metabolic acidosis by continuous hemodialysis and intermittent plasmapheresis after a certain point in the operation. This might have been caused by the metabolic overload that increased suddenly after the transplantation of all extremities.

The clinical scenario that we encountered was similar to the clinical conditions characterized by severe systemic inflammatory process and increased vascular permeability. Several measures should be taken to prevent or decrease these harmful effects. Performing the composite tissue allotransplantations with almost zero ischemia should be the ultimate goal. To achieve this, either harvesting or transplantation of the composite tissues should be performed in a single center or an extracorporeal perfusion machine should be utilized during the transport of extremities which was developed by Vogel et al. for solid organ transplantations [26]. Constantinescu et al. conducted an experimental study regarding the effectiveness of this extracorporeal perfusion concept which showed promising results [27]. Further clinical studies are needed to improve the standards of interinstitutional transport and decrease ischemia to prevent metabolic overloading related problems. Selecting a heart-beating

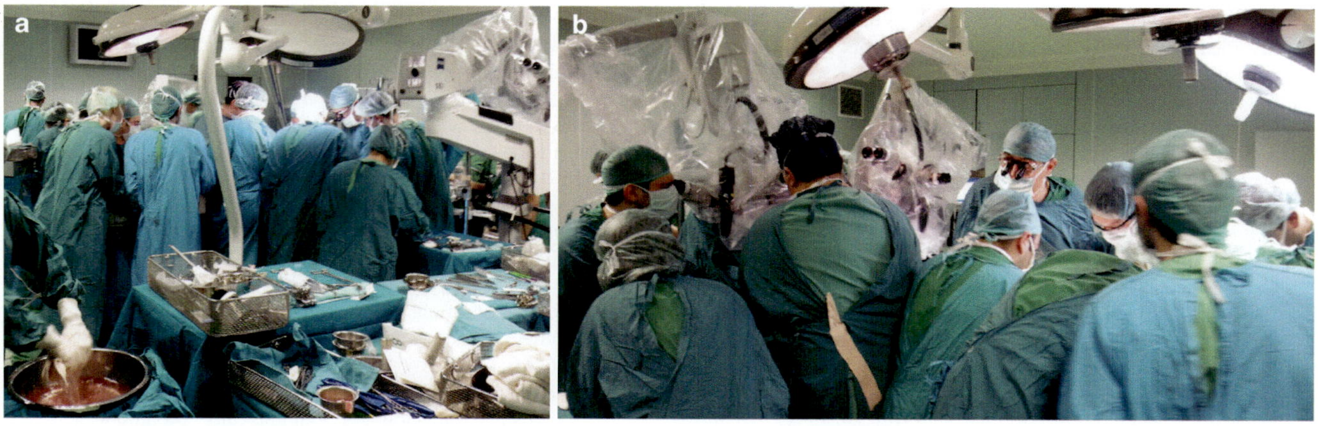

Fig. 25.4 (**a**, **b**) If multiple composite tissues are planned to be transplanted, it is vital to have multiple surgical teams to reduce ischemia

donor is another factor decreasing ischemia but this is not always possible.

We believe that continuous hemodialysis should be performed prophylactically and continued during intraoperative and early postoperative period until the patient's metabolism is stabilized. This helps us be prepared for sudden increase in metabolic load after multiple simultaneous transplantations.

In two experimental studies, we showed that the volume and number of composite tissue allotransplants might increase the antigenic load and have an effect on induction and maintenance of chimerism [20, 23]. However, there is little evidence to support the idea that increased antigenic burden might put the patient at high risk in concomitant composite tissue allotransplantations.

Graft-versus-host disease can be seen in recipient patients if the composite tissue includes bone marrow [28]. Bone marrow irradiation can be used to prevent this in lower extremity transplantations which have high antigenic load. Adjustment of the irradiation dosage is an important subject to get optimum results in extremity transplantations. Our coworkers presented the safe dosage of irradiation that does not cause endothelial injury in an experimental study [10]. After extrapolating their results into human, we applied 6 Gy of radiation for 15 min to all extremities to reduce the antigenic load. We believe that this dosage can safely be used to induce immunosuppression in composite tissue allotransplantations.

Despite continuous hemodialysis, serum K levels reached 7 mg/dL. Subsequently, the patient had a cardiac arrest which indicates metabolic overloading. Echocardiography was not performed intraoperatively but the need for extracorporeal pump support indicates that a state of cardiac failure was present intraoperatively. Unfortunately, autopsy examination was not performed to investigate the causes of death.

Considering the high amount of blood product infusion requirement and similarity of the patient's intraoperative hemodynamic profile to distributive shock, it can be proposed that the main problem causing mortality was an immunologically triggered acute severe systemic inflammatory response. This argument can also be supported by the fact that the amount of blood loss during surgery alone is insufficient to explain the magnitude of blood transfusion. Disseminated intravascular coagulation might be another underlying mechanism of metabolic overloading caused by intravascular hemolysis as a component of acute severe systemic inflammatory response. Based on our experience, we believe that the quadruple extremity allotransplantation is going to be performed successfully in the future with improved composite tissue allotransplantation standards such as reduced ischemic period and better immunosuppressive strategies.

References

1. Ziegler-Graham K, MacKenzie EJ, Ephraim PL, Travison TG, Brookmeyer R. Estimating the prevalence of limb loss in the United States: 2005 to 2050. Arch Phys Med Rehabil. 2008;89(3):422–9.
2. Petruzzo P, Dubernard JM. The international registry on hand and composite tissue allotransplantation. Clin Transpl. 2011:247–53.
3. Zuker RM, Redett R, Alman B, Coles JG, Timoney N, Ein SH. First successful lower-extremity transplantation: technique and functional result. J Reconstr Microsurg. 2006;22(4):239–44.
4. Fattah A, Cypel T, Donner EJ, Wang F, Alman BA, Zuker RM. The first successful lower extremity transplantation: 6-year follow-up and implications for cortical plasticity. Am J Transplant. 2011;11(12):2762–7.
5. Cavadas PC, Thione A, Carballeira A, Blanes M. Bilateral transfemoral lower extremity transplantation: result at 1 year. Am J Transplant. 2013;13(5):1343–9.
6. Cavadas PC, Thione A, Blanes M, Mayordomo-Aranda E. Primary central nervous system posttransplant lymphoproliferative disease in a bilateral transfemoral lower extremity transplantation recipient. Am J Transplant. 2015;15(10):2758–61.
7. Nasir S Total mimic muscle movements of full face transplant at postoperative 1.5 year. 2020. Available at: https://www.youtube.com/watch?v=lnvr1m2SNdM. Accessed August 30 2021.
8. Nasir S, Kilic YA, Karaaltin MV, Erdem Y. Lessons learned from the first quadruple extremity transplantation in the world. Ann Plast Surg. 2014;73(3):336–40.

9. Southard JH, van Gulik TM, Ametani MS, Vreugdenhil PK, Lindell SL, Pienaar BL, et al. Important components of the UW solution. Transplantation. 1990;49(2):251–7.
10. Yavas G, Yildiz F, Guler S, Sargon MF, Yildiz D, Yolcu T, et al. Concomitant trastuzumab with thoracic radiotherapy: a morphological and functional study. Ann Oncol. 2011;22(5):1120–6.
11. Carty MJ, Duclos A, Talbot SG, Tullius SG, Pribaz JJ, Pomahac B. Attitudes regarding lower extremity allotransplantation among lower extremity amputees. Plast Reconstr Surg. 2014;134(6):1334–42.
12. Carty MJ, Zuker R, Cavadas P, Pribaz JJ, Talbot SG, Pomahac B. The case for lower extremity allotransplantation. Plast Reconstr Surg. 2013;131(6):1272–7.
13. MacKenzie EJ, Bosse MJ, Castillo RC, Smith DG, Webb LX, Kellam JF, et al. Functional outcomes following trauma-related lower-extremity amputation. J Bone Joint Surg Am. 2004;86(8):1636–45.
14. Klute GK, Berge JS, Orendurff MS, Williams RM, Czerniecki JM. Prosthetic intervention effects on activity of lower-extremity amputees. Arch Phys Med Rehabil. 2006;87(5):717–22.
15. Tukiainen E, Suominen E, Asko-Seljavaara S. Replantation, revascularization, and reconstruction of both legs after amputations. A case report. J Bone Joint Surg Am. 1994;76(11):1712–6.
16. Schmidhammer R, Huber W, Pelinka LE, Haller H, Kroepfl A. Simultaneous bilateral lower leg replantation: evaluation by different scoring systems--a critical analysis. J Trauma. 2004;57(3):648–52.
17. Hivelin M, Klimczak A, Cwykiel J, Sonmez E, Nasir S, Gatherwright J, et al. Immunomodulatory effects of different cellular therapies of bone marrow origin on chimerism induction and maintenance across MHC barriers in a face allotransplantation model. Arch Immunol Ther Exp. 2016;64(4):299–310.
18. Siemionow M, Rampazzo A, Gharb BB, Cwykiel J, Klimczak A, Madajka M, et al. The reversed paradigm of chimerism induction: donor conditioning with recipient-derived bone marrow cells as a novel approach for tolerance induction in vascularized composite allotransplantation. Microsurgery. 2016;36(8):676–83.
19. Bozkurt M, Klimczak A, Nasir S, Zor F, Krokowicz L, Siemionow M. Composite osseomusculocutaneous sternum, ribs, thymus, pectoralis muscles, and skin allotransplantation model of bone marrow transplantation. Microsurgery. 2013;33(1):43–50.
20. Nasir S, Klimczak A, Sonmez E, Bozkurt M, Gibson S, Siemionow M. New composite tissue allograft model of vascularized bone marrow transplant: the iliac osteomyocutaneous flap. Transpl Int. 2010;23(1):90–100.
21. Nasir S, Bozkurt M, Krokowicz L, Klimczak A, Siemionow M. Correlation of chimerism with graft size and revascularization in vascularized and nonvascularized skin allografts. Ann Plas Surg. 2009;62(4):430–8.
22. Siemionow M, Nasir S. Impact of donor bone marrow on survival of composite tissue allografts. Ann Plas Surg. 2008;60(4):455–62.
23. Nasir S, Bozkurt M, Klimczak A, Siemionow M. Large antigenic skin load in Total Abdominal Wall transplants permits chimerism induction. Ann Plas Surg. 2008;61(5):572–9.
24. Siemionow M, Nasir S. Chimerism and bone marrow based therapies in transplantation. Microsurgery. 2007;27(5):510–21.
25. Carty MJ, Hivelin M, Dumontier C, Talbot SG, Benjoar MD, Pribaz JJ, et al. Lessons learned from simultaneous face and bilateral hand allotransplantation. Plast Reconstr Surg. 2013;132(2):423–32.
26. Vogel T, Brockmann JG, Coussios C, Friend PJ. The role of normothermic extracorporeal perfusion in minimizing ischemia reperfusion injury. Transplant Rev-Orlan. 2012;26(2):156–62.
27. Constantinescu MA, Knall E, Xu XF, Kiermeir DM, Jenni H, Gygax E, et al. Preservation of amputated extremities by extracorporeal blood perfusion; a feasibility study in a porcine model. J Surg Res. 2011;171(1):291–9.
28. Jagasia M, Arora M, Flowers MED, Chao NJ, McCarthy PL, Cutler CS, et al. Risk factors for acute GVHD and survival after hematopoietic cell transplantation. Blood. 2012;119(1):296–307.

Vascularized Knee Joint Allotransplantation

26

Michael Diefenbeck, Martin H. Kirschner, Frithjof Wagner, and Gunther O. Hofmann

26.1 Introduction

Extensive destruction of the knee joint after high-velocity trauma is a real challenge in reconstructive trauma and orthopedic surgery. Worst-case scenario is the combination of bone and cartilage loss, destruction of the extensor mechanism, and skin/soft tissue defects. The extensor mechanism consists of the quadriceps tendon, patella, and patella ligament. If it is completely destructed, active extension of the knee is not possible anymore. Treatment options include arthrodesis, above knee amputation, or an attempt to reconstruction of the joint.

Knee joint fusion results in a stable extremity, but motion is lost, and segmental bone loss can lead to a shortening of the leg [1]. To avoid shortening, the bone loss might be addressed by large alloplastic diaphysis implants or tumor endoprosthesis devices. Above knee amputation with rehabilitation is effective, but is associated with an increased risk of limp, dependence on walking aids, anxiety, and possibly a loss of independence in the long term [2]. Reconstruction of a mangled knee joint requires a combination of total knee arthroplasty [3], reconstruction of the extensor mechanism (e.g., by a tendon-muscle flap [4], allograft [5], or synthetic material [6]), and a local [7] or free flap [8] for skin and soft tissue management. Each of these approaches is technically achievable, but each has inherent risks and limitations. The outcome of a combination of all three techniques has a high risk of failure. As an alternative treatment option, we developed the concept of vascularized knee allotransplantation as a synergism of transplant and orthopedic surgery. Results in animal models [9, 10] and also the results of our first vascularized transplantations of human femoral diaphyses [11–13] had been very encouraging. Thus, after growing experience in vascularized composite allotransplantation (VCA) and intense ethical discussions at the Louisville Symposium on Composite Tissue Allotransplantation (VCT) [14] we started our clinical allotransplantation program of vascularized knee joints in 1996 [15, 16]. Since then, six transplantations have been performed by our group, the last in 2002.

26.2 Patients and Methods

A vascularized knee joint allotransplant was performed in five male and one female patients. All patients had extensive loss of bone and cartilage combined with destruction of the extensor mechanism of the knee joint. In one case, an additional soft tissue defect was present.

All patients underwent routine pre-transplantation examinations with radiographs, angiographs, HLA typing, exclusion of preformed antibodies, and microbiological testing. The sterile osseous defect of the knee joint was temporarily stabilized with a hinge arthroplasty fixed in the femur and tibia by intramedullary nails or a long intramedullary nail in the case of a long diaphyseal defect of the femur (Fig. 26.1a, b). Isometric exercises and/or assisted passive motion were possible. These exercises were necessary to avoid contractions and muscular atrophy. Informed consent was obtained, and the patients were placed on a waiting list for the procedure.

M. Diefenbeck (✉)
Scientific Consulting in Orthopedic Surgery, Hamburg, Germany
e-mail: diefenbeck@wibe-ortho.com

M. H. Kirschner
Ludwig-Maximilians-University of Munich Klinikum Großhadern, Munich, Germany
e-mail: martin@kirschner-hamburg.com

F. Wagner
Berufsgenossenschaftliche Unfallklinik Murnau, Murnau am Staffelsee, Germany
e-mail: info@fdawagner.de

G. O. Hofmann
Klinik für Unfall-, Hand- und Wiederherstellungschirurgie, Universitätsklinikum Jena, Jena, Germany

Klinik für Unfall- und Wiederherstellungschirurgie, Berufsgenossenschaftliches Klinikum Bergmannstrost, Halle (Saale), Germany
e-mail: gunther.hofmann@med.uni-jena.de; gunther.hofmann@bergmannstrost.de

© Springer Nature Switzerland AG 2023

R. Gurunian et al. (eds.), *Reconstructive Transplantation*, https://doi.org/10.1007/978-3-031-21520-9_26

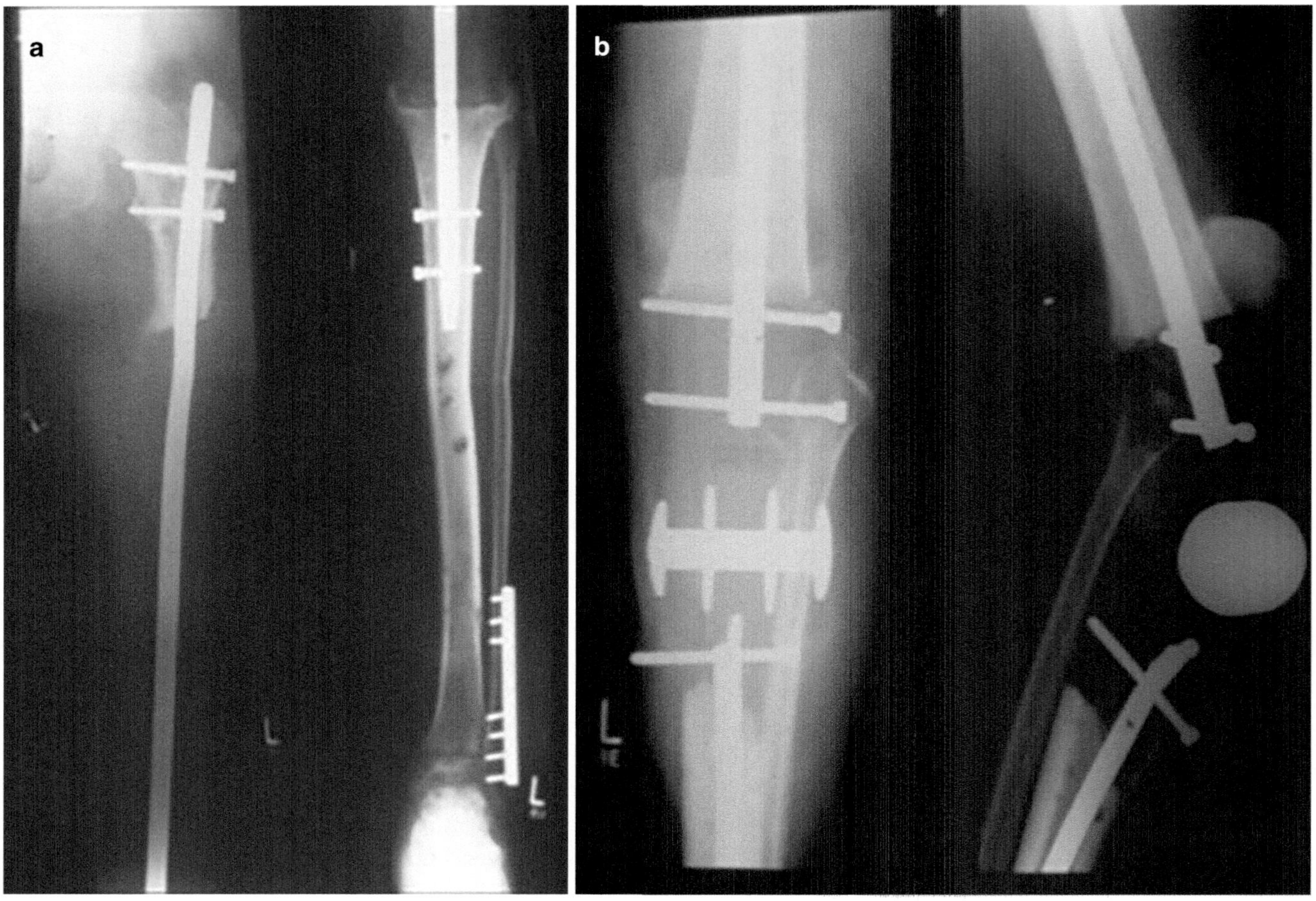

Fig. 26.1 (**a**, left) Radiograph in anteroposterior view of left femur and tibia with hip, knee, and ankle joint: Osseous defect including femur, knee joint, and prox. Tibia (length 44 cm), temporally stabilized with an intramedullary arthrodesis nail. (**b**, right) Radiograph in anteroposterior and lateral view of left knee joint: Osseous defect stabilized with a hinge arthroplasty

26.3 Bone Allograft Procurement

The knee joints were harvested in compliance with standard organ procurement guidelines used in multiorgan donation (MOD). Authorization for knee donation was obtained from the donor's family. MODs older than 45 years or those who had an accident involving the graft were excluded. For additional safety reasons, MODs who had received blood substitutes or fresh frozen plasma were excluded as well.

Harvesting of the knee joint began with the perfusion of the external iliac artery with 4 l University of Wisconsin (UW) solution at 4 °C, followed by dissection of the femoral artery and vein according to our own anatomical studies [17–19] in order to preserve the superior and the inferior genicular artery with a long vascular pedicle of the femoral artery. The muscles were divided, and an osteotomy of the femur and the tibia was performed. The graft was stored in sterile conditions in three layers of plastic bags at 4 °C. Cold ischemic time ranged from 18 to 25 h.

26.4 Back-Table Allograft Preparation

The allograft was dissected from surrounding soft tissue while ligating the muscular vessels and preserving the superior and inferior genicular arteries, which are the two main vessels for the tibial and femoral blood supply [17–19]. The quadriceps tendon and the articular capsule remained intact. All vessels perfusing the muscles were ligated. The vessels to the bone and surrounding tissues were prepared according to our anatomical studies to ensure the optimal vascular supply of the knee joint allograft. Finally, the allograft's arterial pedicle was injected with methylene blue in order to confirm the adequate perfusion of the graft (Fig. 26.2).

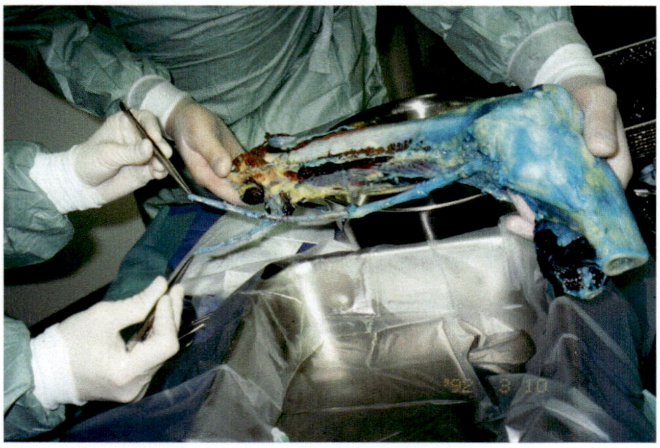

Fig. 26.2 Intraoperative view of the allograft consisting of the knee joint with intact capsule, femur, tibia, quadriceps tendon, vascular pedicle, and sentinel skin graft

26.5 Transplantation Procedure

The surgical procedure started with the removal of the spacer and the intramedullary nails. The allograft was then inserted and fixed by an anterograde femoral and a retrograde tibial interlocking compression nail. The technique of retrograde tibial nailing had been developed previously by members of our group [20]. The allograft vessels were anastomosed to the recipient's superficial femoral artery and vein using an end-to-side technique. Reperfusion started immediately, while the quadriceps tendon was reconstructed.

26.6 Histocompatibility and Immunosuppression

AB0-compatibility and negative crossmatch were confirmed in all transplantations. HLA profiles were determined but not matched due to logistical restrictions in donor acquisition.

Immunosuppressive therapy was started immediately after reperfusion of the allograft. It consisted in the first five cases of ATG (anti-thymocyte globulin), 4 mg/kg BW (body weight) IV as an induction therapy and Cyclosporin A (CsA), 1, 5 mg/kg BW IV/azathioprine, 1.5 mg/kg BW IV/methylprednisolone, 250 mg IV for the first 3 days.

During the first two weeks, methylprednisolone was tapered down in a stepwise manner. Immunosuppression was continued with an oral double-drug maintenance therapy using CsA (6 mg/kg BW; blood level 100–150 ng/ml) and azathioprine (1.0 mg/kg BW).

In patient 6, tacrolimus (Prograft, 10 mg p.o.) and mycophenolate mofetil (MMF; 2 g p.o.) were used instead of CsA and azathioprine, following the immunosuppressive regimen used in hand transplantation [21, 22]. Oral double-drug maintenance therapy was continued with MMF (2 g p.o.; serum level 2–6 lg/ml) and tacrolimus with a serum level between 8 and 10 lg/ml from the beginning of the third week. A heparin infusion was administered for the first 3 days. Subsequently, it was continued as subcutaneous to maintain partial thromboplastin times (PTT) within the range of 60–80 s.

26.7 Postoperative Follow-up

Postoperative monitoring included clinical examinations, routine laboratory tests, Duplex sonography, radiographical assessment of the bones, digital subtraction angiography (DSA) for the arterial blood supply, and single photon emission computerized tomography (SPECT). Local inflammation of the knee and fever were the only clinical indicators of infection or rejection in the first five cases. Whereas the sentinel skin graft was used to monitor rejection in patient 6.

Laboratory studies included differential white blood cell count, erythrocyte sedimentation rates, C-reactive protein as well as CsA and tacrolimus serum levels and PTT.

Later CsA and Tacrolimus levels were monitored twice a week.

Radiographs were used to demonstrate bone healing. DSA was employed to monitor the macrocirculation of the allograft vascular pedicle during the first postoperative day and thereafter as needed to investigate clinical symptoms and possible complications. Duplex sonography was performed daily during the first week.

99 m-Tc-MDP scintigrams demonstrated perfusion, metabolism, and viability of the allograft. Also, SPECT was used to exclude tracer uptake from the overlying soft tissue [23, 24]. If clinical signs of rejection were observed, an arthroscopy was performed along with biopsies for histological examination.

After discharge from hospital, patients were seen weekly by a designated general practitioner (GP) and every two months at our outpatient department.

26.8 Results

Six allotransplantations of vascularized knee joints have been performed to date. Preliminary outcomes and follow-ups have been published in detail elsewhere [15, 16, 25–30]. In the following, each patient is described separately. After the first five cases, the treatment protocol was changed, as mentioned above.

26.9 Patient 1

The first knee joint allotransplantation was performed on April 26, 1996 in a 17-year-old male. There was no intraoperative or early postoperative complication. Adequate perfusion of the allograft was demonstrated by duplex sonography and angiography. Microcirculation and intact cellular metabolism were demonstrated by scintigraphy and via SPECT. Incisions healed with no complications. The patient was discharged from hospital at 2 weeks postoperatively, ambulating with two crutches and partially weight-bearing. Radiographs demonstrated complete osseous integration of the transplanted knee at 6 months postoperatively. Full range of motion was achieved on clinical examination at 12 months. 15 months post-grafting, the patient complained of pain and reduced range of motion of the transplanted joint. The knee showed clinical signs of inflammation. Rejection of the graft was suspected. SPECT showed an increased accumulation of tracer in the subcartilaginous zone of the graft. Biopsy of the synovial membrane revealed viable and perfused tissue; however, there were signs of perivascular infiltration of lymphocytes. Duplex sonography showed occlusion of the allograft vascular pedicle with transplant failure. Immunosuppression was discontinued. The patient underwent a total knee arthroplasty (TKA) using the graft as bone stock that resulted in good stability as well as mobility.

The patient was lost to follow up against our advice. We understand from written correspondence that a periprosthetic joint infection occurred in 2002. Despite surgical and antibiotic treatment, a chronic infection of the TKA developed. With severe sepsis and imminent multiorgan failure (MOF), an above knee amputation was performed in 2004.

26.10 Patient 2

The second knee joint allotransplantation was performed in November 1996 in a 35-year-old male without postoperative complications. At 12 months, the patient had a stable joint. He was able to ambulate, engage in sports activities, and had returned to work. During an acute psychiatric crisis in 1999, the patient discontinued his immunosuppressive medication. Acute rejection occurred and most parts of the graft were lost. A TKA was performed, using the remaining graft as bone stock. Later a periprosthetic joint infection was diagnosed. On request of the patient, above knee amputation was performed in 2001.

26.11 Patient 3

A surgical site infection of the allograft was detected in a female patient one week after grafting procedure in December 1996. Despite antibiotic therapy, reduction of the immunosuppressive regimen, and aggressive surgical debridement, infection persisted. Immunosuppression was discontinued and the allograft was removed 5 weeks post-transplantation. With infection controlled, a temporary, articulating spacer was implanted, and the patient rescheduled for transplantation. Due to difficulties in the size match (small size of the recipient's knee), a donor could not be found within a year. A number of options were discussed with the patient and her family. Arthrodesis of the knee, bridging the bone defect with a callus distraction in Ilizarov's technique was performed in 1997.

26.12 Patient 4

The fourth knee joint allotransplantation was performed in July 1997 in a 47-year-old male. Two years following transplantation the patient developed a stress fracture of the tibial plateau of the grafted knee joint. SPECT revealed no tracer uptake of the whole graft. A TKA using parts of the remaining allogeneic bone as bone stock was performed. Postoperatively the patient had a stable joint, good mobility, was able to walk, and returned to work. In March 2000, 3 years post-transplantation, a periprosthetic joint infection occurred. The patient rejected further surgical treatment for control of the infection and an above knee amputation was performed.

26.13 Patient 5

The first year after vascularized knee joint allotransplantation in February 1998 was uneventful in a 22-year-old male. At 14 months a stress fracture of the lateral tibia plateau was detected. A TKA was performed, using the remaining graft as bone stock. At discharge the patient had a full range of motion at the knee joint and no signs of infection. Eighteen months later a periprosthetic fracture following a fall onto the knee was diagnosed. The femoral component of the TKA was removed and a custom designed femoral component implanted. At 5 years the patient reinjured his grafted knee sustaining a patella fracture. Open reduction and internal fixation with screws failed. The patella ligament was reconstructed using autologous fascia lata. Late rejection resulted in necrotic bone stock and infection. The transplant was removed and an intramedullary arthrodesis performed, resulting in an 8 cm shortening of the leg.

26.14 Patient 6

The latest allotransplantation was performed in April 2002 in a 41-year-old male. An island of donor skin and subcutaneous tissue was harvested with the allograft. It was inserted into the skin of the recipient on the lateral thigh to

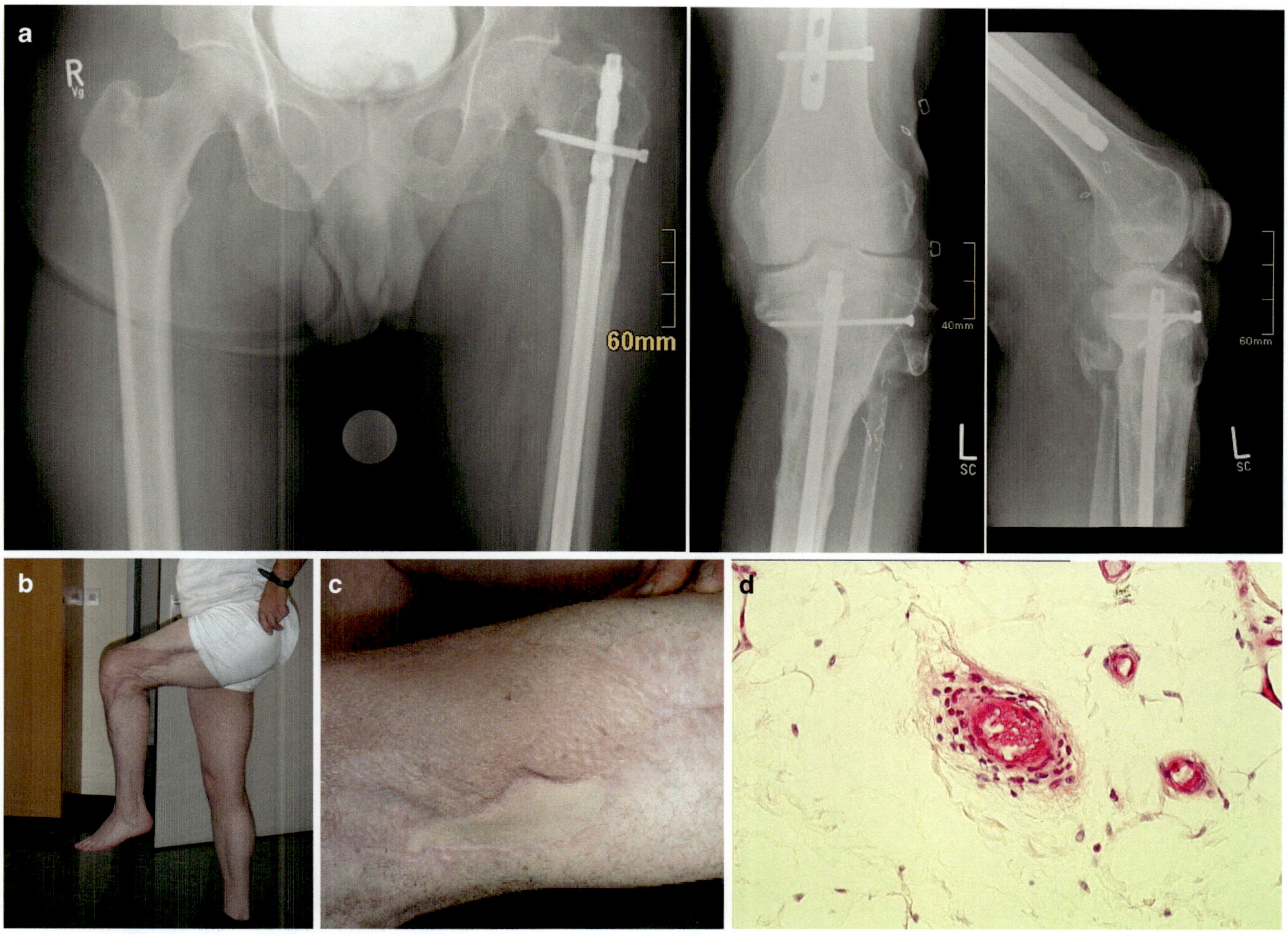

Fig. 26.3 (**a**): Radiograph of left femur with hip and knee joint: control after 1.5 years following transplantation. The graft is completely osseous integrated. (**b**, **c**): Clinical examination after 1.5 years showing good range of motion and (**c**) completely integrated allogeneic sentinel skin graft. (**d**): Synovial biopsy 18 months after transplantation: mild proliferation of the intima, H&E stain

monitor graft rejection or insufficient perfusion (sentinel skin graft (SSG)).

Eighteen months post-transplantation the patient was ambulating, fully weight-bearing, and had returned to his previous job. Radiographs showed complete osseous integration of the graft (Fig. 26.3a). Range of motion (ROM) of the left knee joint was 0-0-90 (Fig. 26.3b). The SSG was fully integrated within the recipient skin (Fig. 26.3b). At that time, the tibial nail was removed, and biopsies of the cartilage, bone, and synovia were taken, which showed vital tissue without necrosis. In the synovial vessels, a mild proliferation of the intima with infiltration of mononuclear cells was found (Fig. 26.3d). This was read as a mild rejection with no need for treatment. Arthroscopy showed vital cartilage without degeneration, intact menisci, and ligaments.

At 28 months, erythematous papules on the SSG were noticed by the patient (Fig. 26.4). Suspecting acute rejection, skin biopsies of the SSG were taken. Histology showed acute cellular rejection (Fig. 26.5a). Synovial biopsies, taken via an arthroscopy, confirmed these findings (Fig. 26.5b) [31]. Treatment with methylprednisolone (250 mg i.v. for 3 days) was initiated and resulted in restitution of normal skin histology. This remained the sole episode of a visible AR on the SSG.

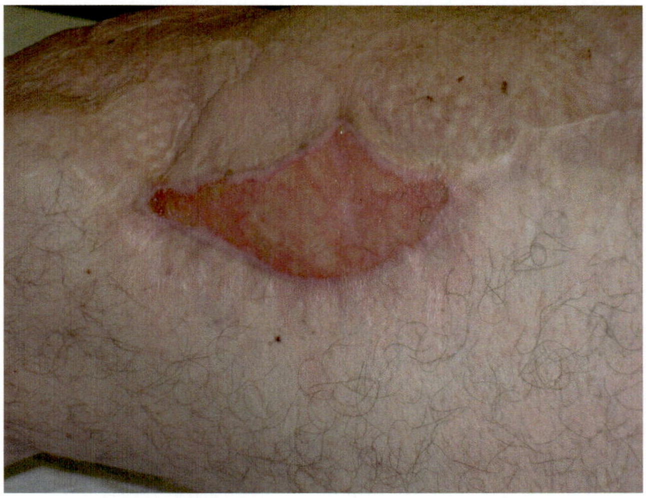

Fig. 26.4 Clinical examination at 18 months: erythematous papules on the sentinel skin graft at the lateral tight

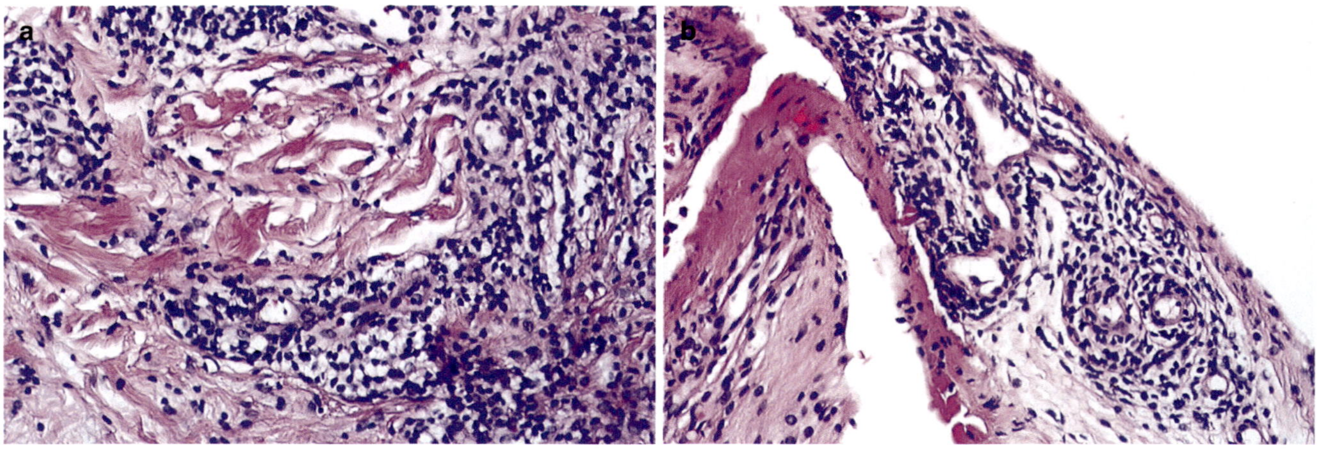

Fig. 26.5 (**a**) Histology of sentinel skin graft: extensive peri- and intravascular infiltration of the dermal stoma by activated mononuclear lymphatic cells (H&E stain). (**b**) Histology of synovia: infiltration by activated mononuclear lymphatic cells consistent with acute rejection (H&E stain)

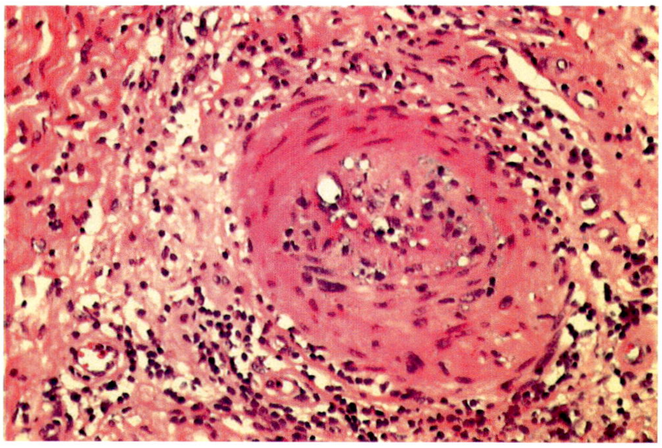

Fig. 26.6 Biopsy of sentinel skin graft (SSG) 36 months after transplantation: Concentric narrowing of small arterial vessels by fibrotic proliferation of the intima, H&E stain

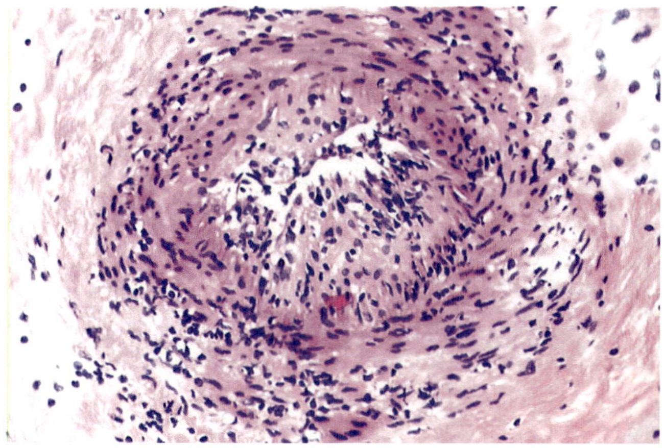

Fig. 26.7 Synovial biopsy 50 months after transplantation: Concentric fibroses of the intima with subtotal occlusion of the lumen, H&E stain

At 36 months after transplantation, a proportion of the SSG became necrotic. Biopsies of the SSG showed superficial skin necrosis. In the deeper layers, concentric intima proliferation in small arteries with luminal occlusion was found (Fig. 26.6). Subsequently, biopsies of the allograft were taken. Synovial and soft tissue samples revealed perivascular mononuclear cell infiltrates, intimal proliferation with mononuclear cell infiltration, and concentric subtotal obliteration of small vessels [32]. In some sections, complete occlusion and fibrosis of the surrounding tissue were observed.

At 50 months, knee function (ROM) decreased from 0-0-90 to 0-10-40 and an anterior instability developed. In allograft biopsies, articular cartilage and bone necrosis were found. Vessels showed severe concentric hyperplasia of the intima with variable degrees of lumen obliteration (Figs. 26.7 and 26.8). A deep surgical site infection, descending from the necrotic SSG to the allograft developed. This infection caused by Pseudomonas aeruginosa persisted despite therapy with antibiotics, surgical debridement, and vacuum assisted closure therapy (VAC; Kinetic Concepts Inc., San Antonio, TX, USA). After a detailed discussion of the situa-

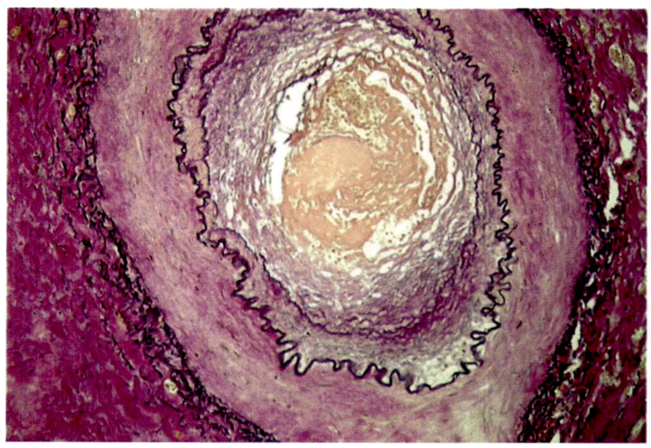

Fig. 26.8 Soft tissue biopsy 50 months after grafting: Hypertrophic intima with an intact internal elastica lamina, Elastica-van Gieson stain

tion with the patient and the lack of treatment alternatives, he decided for an above knee amputation, which was performed at 56 months after transplantation.

The patient died due to an acute heart failure at the age of 64. An autopsy confirmed the heart disease. The femoral allograft, which was left after the above knee amputation in situ to gain a longer bony stump, was found to be partial necrotic. Patient was normally ambulating with his exoprosthesis.

26.15 Discussion

26.15.1 Surgical Technique

We developed and introduced the surgical technique of a vascularized knee joint allotransplantation, which is based on the ex-vivo anatomical studies published by our group [17–19]. There were no complications related to the surgical technique. Cold ischemia time (CIT) ranged from 18 to 25 h. This is longer than CIT in other VCAs, e.g., human hand transplantation (from 310 min [22] to 12.5 h [33]). In our cases, the same team harvested, prepared, transported, and transplanted the allograft. We attribute the longer CIT to having a single team compared to transplantations performed by two teams. In all cases bone healing and osseous integration of the allograft were completed after 6 months under immunosuppression. There was no delayed bone healing or non-union. This relates with the results of bone healing in hand transplants [33], where no adverse effect of immunosuppression on bone healing was found.

Although there was no microbiological evidence of infection in biopsies taken from all recipients prior to grafting, one case (patient 3) developed a surgical site infection in the immediate postoperative period. In this case the indication for grafting was an extensive bone and joint destruction after a post-traumatic osteomyelitis. Likely postoperative immunosuppression caused reactivation of the osteomyelitis. To curtail this risk, previous bone and joint infections should be considered as an exclusion criterion for transplantation.

26.15.2 Psychological Assessment

One patient (patient 2) discontinued the immunosuppressive medication 3 years post-transplantation during an acute psychosis leading to rejection of the well-functioning transplant. Kanitakis and co-workers reported a similar case of a non-compliant patient [34]. This emphasizes that a comprehensive set of psychological tests is necessary to assess the recipients and to evaluate their ability to understand the potential risks and complications of the procedure [14, 35].

26.15.3 Lifelong Immunosuppression and its Consequences

Preceding studies showed that strong immunological reactions in the recipient of vascularized allogenic bone have to be expected [36–38]. Both cases mentioned above indicate that lifelong immunosuppression is necessary in VCA of extremities.

VCA is considered to improve the quality of life, but is not a lifesaving procedure as with standard organ transplantations. Therefore, the question arises, if the risks posed by the immunosuppressive drugs, i.e., opportunistic infections, end-organ toxicity, and malignancy [39], justify the benefits of VCA procedures. It is difficult to assess the "relative risk" of VCA. Brouha et al. published a study outlining the relative risk that individuals were willing to accept in order to receive the benefits of VCA procedures [40]. They used the Louisville Instrument for Transplantation (LIFT) Questionnaire [41]. The authors concluded that VCA procedures convey benefits to recipients, which outweigh the risk of immunosuppression. Other authors see the subject more critically, with the incidence of neoplasms among the organ transplant recipient population increasing, estimated to be between 4 and 18% [42]. Therefore, the ultimate goal in VCA is to minimize the risk of immunosuppression. This could be achieved by induction of tolerance without long-term immunosuppression. So far, tolerance in VCA has only been reported in animal models [43].

26.15.4 Late Rejection and Sentinel Skin Graft (SSG)

In four patients (patients 1, 4, 5, 6) late rejection of the graft was found after 15, 16, and 24 months, respectively. Unlike the transplantation of parenchymal organs, where graft failure is noticed immediately by reduced organ function and laboratory testing, it seems impossible to detect graft rejection in knee joints early enough to initiate appropriate increased immunosuppression. Our patients presented late with reduced function of the transplanted joint. Radiographs showed stress fractures of the allotransplants. In surgical exploration of the grafts, necrosis of bone and soft tissue was seen. Histologic study showed ischemic necrosis.

To monitor rejection, we harvested a vascularized island of skin and subcutaneous tissue with a vascular pedicle together with the graft and integrated the allogeneic skin in the recipient skin in patient 6 [31]. A similar technique had previously been used by Lanzetta et al. in their hand transplantation project, where an additional full-thickness skin was transplanted onto the left hip area [44]. The skin served as a source of biopsies and as an additional area to monitor rejection, hence called "distant sentinel skin graft" [33]. In patient 6, the first sign of rejection was redness of the SSG 3 years post-transplantation. Biopsies of the SSG and synovia, taken 2 days later by arthroscopy, showed the same signs of acute cellular rejection. This indicates that the grafted skin can be used as a monitor of rejection. In this patient, this rejection episode was overcome by treatment with steroids [31].

In 12 of 18 patients with hand transplants, acute rejection episodes were seen [45] and all of them were reversible. After the experience of late rejection in three cases and one surgical site infection, we changed our immunosuppressive regime to tacrolimus (10 mg p.o.) and mycophenolate mofetil (MMF; 2 g p.o.) with omission of steroids after 2 weeks. We speculate that this immunosuppressive regimen is a major factor along with the SSG for the longest graft survival so far in case 6. In the hand transplants a similar effect was seen with this immunosuppressive regime [33]. However, there is no clear evidence—neither experimentally nor clinically as to whether which regimen of immunosuppressive drugs is the optimal combination in VCA transplantation.

26.15.5 Allograft Vasculopathy

We described for the first time in a case of allograft vasculopathy in VCA, appearing as a myointimal proliferation, probably as the consequence of repetitive acute rejection [32].

The hand and face transplantations performed in the last decade showed that skin of a VCT is not immediately or irreversibly rejected but might serve as a useful monitor tool for such a graft [46]. Acute rejection episodes of the skin occurred in 85% of patients with hand transplants within the first year [47] and were treated successfully with topical treatment or steroids, basiliximab, ATG, and alemtuzumab [48]. In the first five cases of knee allografts, no episodes of AR had been detected. However, without an SSG, these grafts could not be adequately monitored. Taking skin biopsies of the SSG in patient 6, AR was detected and adequately treated [31, 49].

Signs of a progressive vasculopathy became apparent at 36 months after transplantation as described above. Unadkat et al. published findings from an orthotopic hind limb allotransplantation model in rats, where multiple AR episodes resulted in the development of myointimal proliferation and morphologic signs for chronic rejection [50]. In this model, repeated AR episodes were treated with CsA and dexamethasone. At postoperative day 90 animals had gone through 19 episodes of AR, and myointimal proliferation associated with concentric luminal occlusion and perivascular fibroses was observed.

We clearly see parallels between this animal study and the case of patient 6 presented here with similar histologic alterations in vessels and bones. However, since we have only recognized one single AR in our follow-up compared with up to five in the first year after hand allotransplantation, multiple AR might have been missed because of the lack of adequate monitoring tools.

Histopathologic features of composite tissue vasculopathy are morphologically comparable with cardiac allograft vasculopathy after cardiac transplantation [51–53].

Two years after our report on allograft vasculopathy in vascularized knee allotransplantation, Kaufman et al. published their experience of graft vasculopathy in clinical hand transplantation [54]. They found that the vessels, both arteries and veins may also be a primary target of rejection in the hand. Two of their recipients developed severe intimal hyperplasia and vasculopathy early post-transplant [54].

The exact mechanisms of chronic rejection are not fully understood [55]. The Banff 2007 and 2011 classifications did not include any characteristics of chronic rejection [56, 57]. Clinicopathologic features suggestive of chronic rejection could include myointimal proliferation of arterioles, loss of adnexa, nail changes, skin and muscular atrophy, and fibrosis of deep tissues [56]. Clearly, there is an urgent need for appropriate animal models to study the underlying immune and non-immune mechanisms involved in chronic rejection pathogenesis [55].

As treatment options in case of a vasculopathy are very limited, we suggest careful monitoring and immediate treatment of AR episodes. Our clinical knee allotransplantation program is on hold until better tools to monitor rejection are available and more knowledge about the risks of allograft vasculopathy has been gained.

26.15.6 Osteochondral Allograft (OCA) Transplantation to Reconstruct Focal Osteochondral Defects

In the six above mentioned cases, the whole knee joint including the extensor mechanism was completely destroyed; the only other promising treatment options remaining were above knee amputation or knee joint fusion.

If the damage to the knee joint is less severe, i.e., resulting only in focal osteochondral defects, different surgical techniques for the reconstruction of these osteochondral lesions are available to the orthopedic surgeon. These include chondroplasty, microfracture, autologous matrix induced chondrogenesis (AMIC), osteochondral autograft transplants (OATS), mosaicplasty, and autologous chondrocyte implantation (ACI) [58].

In some cases, defects are so large that concerns of donor-site morbidity can prevent reconstruction via OATS or mosaicplasty procedures. For such cases, the use of osteochondral allograft (OCA) transplants has been suggested [58]. Fresh,

fresh frozen, or cryopreserved cadaveric samples are used to fill the focal osteochondral defects. The grafts are harvested, procured, and distributed by tissue banks. Unfortunately, the processing and storage techniques of fresh frozen and cryopreserved treatments risk loss of up to 95% of chondrocytes in the sample [59].

The main difference to the vascularized knee joint allotransplantation technique described by us above is that the osteochondral allograft transplants are much smaller in size and not vascularized. They are not connected to the recipient's circulation via arterial and venous anastomosis. The perfusion of the graft depends on vascular ingrowth from the recipient's transplant bed to keep the OCA vital. The upside is that no immunosuppression is needed; the downside is the risk that vascular ingrowth is insufficient, and the OCA becomes necrotic. A case report by Krettek et al. describes in detail, how an OCA transplant was used to reconstruct a large osteochondral defect of the lateral tibial plateau [60].

In general, OCA has demonstrated favorable outcomes with radiographic union in 86% and excellent or good results in 86–89% at 2 years [61]. However, long-term results show a significant deterioration with survival rates falling from 95% at 5 years to 80–85% at 10 years and 65–74% at 15 years [62–64], while reoperation rates requiring revision or arthroplasty procedures of 32–47% in the first 10 years have been reported [62]. More research is required to better understand the long-term results of OCA transplantation.

26.16 Conclusion

Critical evaluation of our experience presents some limitations, which need to be addressed. First, the indication for transplantation needs to be a combination of extensive loss of cartilage and bone, deficient extensor mechanism, and soft tissue and skin defects. In this indication, the joint can be replaced, and the soft tissue defect covered with a vascularized composite allograft in a one-stage procedure. Transplantation should only be performed as a last option before above knee amputation. Patients with postinfectious joint defects should be excluded to minimize the risk of a postoperative surgical site infection.

Psychologic assessment of candidates for knee transplantation and psychological support after transplantation are mandatory, as recommended by the Louisville group for VCT [14, 35]. Monitoring of immunosuppression and the use of the sentinel skin graft needs to be refined, e.g., regular skin biopsies should be carried out. Finally, the risks of allograft vasculopathy need to be better understood.

Unless these criteria are met, a vascularized knee allotransplantation cannot be recommended for the reconstruction of an extensively damaged knee joint.

References

1. Klinger HM, Spahn G, Schultz W, Baums MH. Arthrodesis of the knee after failed infected total knee arthroplasty. Knee Surg Sports Traumatol Athrosc. 2006;14:447.
2. Pardasaney PK, Sullivan PE, Portney LG, Mankin HJ. Advantage of limb salvage over amputation for proximal lower extremity tumors. Clin Orthop Relat Res. 2006;444:201.
3. Anract P, Missenard G, Jeanrot C, Dubois V, Tomeno B. Knee reconstruction with prosthesis and muscle flap after total arthrectomy. Clin Orthop Relat Res. 2001;384:208.
4. Kubota Y, Tsubo K, Toh S, Ogawa T. Vastus medialis muscle flap and hemi v-y skin flap for knee extensor and soft tissue reconstruction. Ann Plast Surg. 2006;56:196.
5. Burnett RS, Berger RA, Paprosky WG, Della Valle CJ, Jacobs JJ, Rosenberg AG. Extensor mechanism allograft reconstruction after total knee arthroplasty. A comparison of two techniques. J Bone Joint Surg Am. 2004;86(12):2694–9.
6. Sherief TI, Naguib AM, Sefton GK. Use of Leeds-Keio connective tissue prosthesis (L-K CTP) for reconstruction of deficient extensor mechanism with total knee replacement. Knee. 2005;12:319.
7. Ries MD, Bozic KJ. Medial gastrocnemius flap coverage for treatment of skin necrosis after total knee arthroplasty. Clin Orthop Relat Res. 2006;446:186.
8. Markovich GD, Dorr LD, Klein NE, McPherson EJ, Vince KG. Muscle flaps in total knee arthroplasty. Clin Orthop Relat Res. 1995;321:122.
9. Lee WP, Pan YC, Kesmarky S, et al. Experimental orthotopic transplantation of vascularized skeletal allografts: functional assessment and long-term survival. Plast Reconstr Surg. 1995;95:336.
10. Fricker R, Schafer D, Rosso R, et al. Surgical technique in vascularized auto- and allotransplantation of the knee joint a dog model. Helv Chir AVCT. 1994;60:1015.
11. Hofmann GO, Kirschner MH, Bühren V, et al. Allogeneic vascularized transplantation of a human femoral diaphysis under cyclosporine a immunosuppression. Transpl Med. 1995;8:418–9.
12. Kirschner MH, Hofmann GO. Vorläufige Ergebnisse der Transplantation allogener gefäßgestieleter Femurdiaphysen unter Immunosuppression. Transplantation. 1996;8:48–53.
13. Kirschner MH, Wagner FD, Nerlich A, Land W, Bühren V, Hofmann GO. Allogenic grafting of vascularized bone segments under immunosuppression. Clinical results in the transplantation of femoral diaphyses. Transpl Int. 1998;11(3):195–203.
14. Tobin GR, Breidenbach WC, Klapheke MM, Bentley FR, Pidwell DJ, Simmons PD. Ethical considerations in the early composite tissue allograft experience: a review of the Louisville ethics program. Transplant Proc. 2005;37:1392.
15. Hofmann GO, Kirschner MH, Wagner FD, et al. First vascularized knee joint transplantation in man. Tx Med. 1996;8:46.
16. Hofmann GO, Kirschner MH, Wagner FD, et al. Allogeneic vascularized grafting of a human knee joint with postoperative immunosuppression. Arch Orthop Trauma Surg. 1997;116:125–8.
17. Kirschner MH, Menck J, Hofmann GO. Anatomical bases of a vascularized allogenic knee joint transplantation: arterial blood supply of the human knee joint. Surg Radiol Anat. 1996;18(4):263–9.
18. Kirschner MH, Menck J, Nerlich A, Walser R, Bühren V, Hofmann GO. The arterial blood supply of the human patella. Its clinical importance for the operating technique in vascularized knee joint transplantations. Surg Radiol Anat. 1997;19(6):345–51.
19. Kirschner MH, Menck J, Hennerbichler A, Gaber O, Hofmann GO. Importance of arterial blood supply to the femur and tibia for transplantation of vascularized femoral diaphyses and knee joints. World J Surg. 1998;22(8):845–51; discussion 852.

20. Hofmann GO, Gonschorek O, Bühren V, Retrograde tibial nailing. Anatomical considerations and first clinical experiences. Osteosynthesis Int. 1999;7:162–9.
21. Dubernard JM, Owen E, Lefrancois N, et al. First human hand transplantation. Case report. Transpl Int. 2000;13(Suppl. 1):S521.
22. Jones JW, Gruber SA, Barker JH, Breidenbach WC. Successful hand transplantation. N Engl J Med. 2000;343:468.
23. Kirschner MH, Manthey N, Tatsch K, Nerlich A, Hahn K, Hofmann GO. Use of three-phase bone scans and SPECT in the follow up of patients with allogeneic vascularized femur transplants. Nuc Med Commun. 1999;20:517–24.
24. Manthey N, Kirschner MH, Nerlich A, Hofmann GO, Tatsch K, Hahn K. 3-phase bone imaging and SPECT in the follow up of patients with allogenic vascularized knee joint transplants. Nuklearmedizin. 2001;40(6):187–92.
25. Hofmann GO, Kirschner MH, Wagner FD, et al. Allogeneic vascularized transplantation of human femoral diaphysis and total knee joints – first clinical experiences. Transplant Proc. 1998;30:2754–61.
26. Hofmann GO, Kirschner MH, Brauns L, Wagner FD, Land W, Bühren V. Vascularized knee joint transplantation in men: a report on the first cases. Transpant Int. 1998;11:487.
27. Hofmann GO, Kirschner MH, Wagner FD, Brauns L, Gonschorek O, Bühren V. Allogeneic vascularized grafting of human knee joints under postoperative immunosuppression of the recipients. World J Surg. 1998;22:818–23.
28. Kirschner MH, Brauns L, Gonschorek O, Bühren V, Hofmann GO. Vascularized knee joint transplantation in man: the first two-year experience. Eur J Surg. 2000;166:320–7.
29. Hofmann GO, Kirschner MH. Clinical experience in allogeneic vascularized bone and joint allografting. Microsurgery. 2000;20:375–83.
30. Diefenbeck M, Wagner F, Kirschner MH, Nerlich A, Mückley T, Hofmann GO. Outcome of allogeneic vascularized knee transplants. Transpl Int. 2007;20(5):410–8.
31. Diefenbeck M, Wagner F, Kirschner MH, Nerlich A, Mückley T, Hofmann GO. Management of acute rejection 2 years after allogeneic vascularized knee joint transplantation. Transpl Int. 2006;19:604–6.
32. Diefenbeck M, Nerlich A, Schneeberger S, Wagner F, Hofmann GO. Allograft vasculopathy after allogeneic vascularized knee transplantation. Transpl Int. 2011;24(1):e1–5.
33. Lanzetta M, Petruzzo P, Vitale G, et al. Human hand transplantation: what have we learned? Transplant Proc. 2004;36:664.
34. Kanitakis J, Jullien D, Petruzzo P, et al. Clinicopathologic features of graft rejection of the first human hand allograft. Transplantation. 2003;76:688.
35. Klapheke MM, Marcell C, Taliaferro G, Creamer B. Psychiatric assessment of candidates for hand transplantation. Microsurgery. 2000;20:453.
36. Hofmann GO, Falk C, Wangemann T. Immunological transformations in the recipient of grafted allogeneic human bone. Arch Orthop Trauma Surg. 1997;116(3):143–50.
37. Hofmann GO. Immunologischer und hygienischer Stellenwert der allogenen Kniegelenkstransplantation für die Wiederherstellungschirurgie. Akt Chir. 1991;26:126–33.
38. Hofmann GO, Kirschner MH, Wangemann T, Falk C, Mempel W, Hammer C. Infections and immunological hazards of allogeneic bone transplantation. Arch Orthop Trauma Surg. 1995;114(3):159–66.
39. De Mattos AM, Olyaei AV, Benett WM. Nephrotoxicity of immunosuppressive drugs: long term consequences and challenges for the future. Am J Kidney Dis. 2000;35:333.
40. Brouha P, Naidu D, Cunningham M, et al. Risk acceptance in composite-tissue allotransplantation reconstructive procedures. Microsurgery. 2006;26:144.
41. Cunningham M, Majzoub R, Brouha PCR, et al. Risk acceptance in composite tissue allotransplantation reconstructive procedures – instrument design and validation. Eur J Trauma. 2004;30:12.
42. Veroux M, Puliatti C, Flamingo P, et al. Early de novo malignancies after kidney transplantation. Transplant Proc. 2004;36:718.
43. Hettiaratchy S, Melendy E, Randolph MA, et al. Tolerance to composite tissue allografts across a major histocompatibility barrier in miniature swine. Transplantation. 2004;77:514.
44. Lanzetta M, Petruzzo P, Margreiter R, et al. The international registry on hand and composite tissue transplantation. Transplantation. 2005;79:1210.
45. Gabl M, Pechlaner S, Lutz M, Bodner G, Piza H, Margreiter R. Bilateral hand transplantation: bone healing under immunosuppression with tacrolimus, mycophenolate mofetil and prednisolone. J Hand Surg [Am]. 2004;29:1020.
46. Schneeberger S, Gorantla VS, Hautz T, Pulikkottil B, Margreiter R, Lee WPA. Immunosuppression and rejection in human hand transplantation. Transplant Proc. 2009;41:472.
47. Petruzzo P, Lanzetta M, Dubernard JM, et al. The international registry on hand and composite tissue transplantation. Transplantation. 2008;86:487.
48. Lanzetta M, Petruzzo P, Dubernard JM, et al. Second report (1998–2006) of the international registry of hand and composite tissue transplantation. Transpl Immunol. 2007;18:1.
49. Brauns L, Hofmann GO, Kirschner MH, Wagner FD, Nehrlich A, Bühren V. Abstossungsmonitoring und immunosuppressive Therapie nach gefäßgestielter allogener Kniegelenkstransplantation. Transpl Med. 1997;9:148–52.
50. Unadkat JV, Schneeberger S, Horibe EH, et al. Composite tissue vasculopathy and degeneration following multiple episodes of acute rejection in reconstructive transplantation. Am J Transplant. 2010;10:251.
51. Johnson DE, Gao SZ, Schroeder JS, DeCampli WM, Billingham ME. The spectrum of coronary artery pathologic findings in human cardiac allografts. J Heart Transplant. 1989;8:349.
52. Pucci AM, Forbes RD, Billingham ME. Pathologic features in long-term cardiac allografts. J Heart Transplant. 1990;9:339.
53. Billingham ME. Histopathology of graft coronary disease. J Heart Lung Transplant. 1992;11(3 Pt 2):S38.
54. Kaufman CL, Ouseph R, Blair B, Kutz JE, Tsai TM, Scheker LR, Tien HY, Moreno R, Ozyurekoglu T, Banegas R, Murphy E, Burns CB, Zaring R, Cook DF, Marvin MR. Graft vasculopathy in clinical hand transplantation. Am J Transplant. 2012;12(4):1004–16.
55. Sarhane KA, Tuffaha SH, Broyles JM, Ibrahim AE, Khalifian S, Baltodano P, Santiago GF, Alrakan M, Ibrahim Z. A critical analysis of rejection in vascularized composite allotransplantation: clinical, cellular and molecular aspects, current challenges, and novel concepts. Front Immunol. 2013 Nov;25(4):406.
56. Cendales LC, Kanitakis J, Schneeberger S, Burns C, Ruiz P, Landin L, Remmelink M, Hewitt CW, Landgren T, Lyons B, Drachenberg CB, Solez K, Kirk AD, Kleiner DE, Racusen L. The Banff 2007 working classification of skin-containing composite tissue allograft pathology. Am J Transplant. 2008;8(7):1396–400.
57. Mengel M, Sis B, Haas M, Colvin RB, Halloran PF, Racusen LC, Solez K, Cendales L, Demetris AJ, Drachenberg CB, Farver CF, Rodriguez ER, Wallace WD. Glotz D; Banff meeting report writing committee. Banff 2011 meeting report: new concepts in antibody-mediated rejection. Am J Transplant. 2012;12(3):563–70.
58. Howell M, Liao Q, Gee CW. Surgical Management of Osteochondral Defects of the knee: an educational review. Curr Rev Musculoskelet Med. 2021;14(1):60–6.
59. Pisanu G, Cottino U, Rosso F, Blonna D, Marmotti AG, Bertolo C, et al. Large osteochondral allografts of the knee: surgical technique and indications. Joints. 2018;6(1):42–53.
60. Krettek C, Clausen J, Omar M, Noack S, Neunaber C. Two-stage late reconstruction with a fresh large osteochondral shell allograft

transplantation (FLOCSAT) for a large osteochondral defect in a non-union after a lateral tibia plateau fracture 2-year follow up. Injury. 2017;48(7):1309–18.
61. Chahal J, Gross AE, Gross C, Mall N, Dwyer T, Chahal A, et al. Outcomes of osteochondral allograft transplantation in the knee. Arthroscopy. 2013;29(3):575–88.
62. Gross AE, Shasha N, Aubin P. Long-term follow-up of the use of fresh osteochondral allografts for posttraumatic knee defects. Clin Orthop Relat Res. 2008;466(8):1863–70.
63. Aubin PP, Cheah HK, Davis AM, Gross AE. Long-term follow-up of fresh femoral osteochondral allografts for posttraumatic knee defects. Clin Orthop Relat Res. 2001;391:S318–27.
64. Levy YD, Gortz S, Pulido PA, McCauley JC, Bugbee WD. Do fresh osteochondral allografts successfully treat femoral condyle lesions? Clin Orthop Relat Res. 2013;471:231–7.

Part VI

Abdominal Wall Transplantation

Abdominal Wall Transplantation

27

Andrew Atia, Andrew Hollins, Jorge Andres Hernandez, and Detlev Erdmann

27.1 Introduction and History

Abdominal wall vascularized composite allotransplantation (AW-VCA) has emerged as a technically feasible option for abdominal wall reconstruction in patients whose abdomen cannot be closed using traditional methods [1–3]. Innovations and advances in the fields of vascular surgery and solid organ transplantation were instrumental in making vascularized composite allotransplantation possible. In the late nineteenth century, the first successful vascular anastomoses were being performed by directly apposing or invaginating vessels end-to-end and suturing with fine silk. Then in 1902, Alexis Carrel reported the triangulation method of end-to-end anastomosis that is still routinely used today. He was awarded the Nobel prize for his work in 1912. In 1916, heparin was discovered by a medical student named Jay McLean, and this was critical in the development of microsurgery. Finally, the introduction of the operating microscope in the 1920s helped to usher in modern microvascular surgery. From there, microsurgical instruments and suture were refined. In the 1950s, the field of solid organ transplantation was rapidly gaining traction. The first successful kidney transplant took place in 1954. A decade later, in 1964, a team of surgeons attempted the first documented account of vascularized composite allotransplantation (VCA)—a hand transplant. Unfortunately, this surgery failed with rejection of the transplant due to lack of adequate immunosuppression. Over the next 30 years, the field of solid organ transplantation made significant advances, and this coincided with the development of enhanced immunosuppressive drugs including calcineurin inhibitors and the antimetabolite, mycophenolate mofetil. These advancements in technique and immunosuppression renewed interest in VCA. Abdominal wall transplantation (AWT) was introduced in 1999 in the context of reconstruction of complex abdominal wall defects in conjunction with intestinal/multi-visceral organ transplantation in patients who could not be reconstructed with biomaterials or autologous tissue [1]. In such cases, factors including prior trauma, repeat laparotomies, enterocutaneous fistulae, multiple ostomy revisions, and exhaustion of local reconstructive options often lead to loss of domain, extensive scarring, and overall poor local tissue quality [4, 5]. Since that time, approximately 40 abdominal wall transplants have been performed. All cases of abdominal wall transplantation to date have been performed in conjunction with intestinal or visceral organ transplantation. In the following text, a comprehensive overview of AW-VCA will be presented including surgical considerations in abdominal wall transplantation, a case report from the authors' experience, and postoperative follow-up with discussion of complications.

27.2 Surgical Considerations

27.2.1 Abdominal Wall Anatomy

The anterior abdominal wall is composed of skin, subcutaneous tissue, fascia, and muscle. As a functional unit, it serves to protect the visceral organs and aids in posture and respiration. The arterial vascular perfusion of the abdominal wall can be divided into three zones as described by Huger in 1979 [6]. Recently, Light et al. performed anatomical cadaveric perfusion studies and proposed a classification system for harvesting abdominal wall allografts based on recipient defect [2]. They determined that the entire abdominal wall could be reperfused based on the iliofemoral system which captures the deep inferior epigastric vessels, superficial inferior epigastric vessels, deep circumflex iliac vessels, and superficial circumflex iliac vessels. They noted that perfusion of the extended abdominal wall allograft which extends laterally to include the obliques and transversus abdominis is significantly improved by inclusion of the deep circumflex iliac vessels. Per their classification system, Type 1 defects

A. Atia (✉) · A. Hollins · J. A. Hernandez · D. Erdmann
Division of Plastic, Maxillofacial, and Oral Surgery, Department of Surgery, Duke University Medical Center, Durham, NC, USA
e-mail: andrew.atia@duke.edu; andrew.hollins@duke.edu; j.andres.hernandez@duke.edu; detlev.erdmann@duke.edu

© Springer Nature Switzerland AG 2023
R. Gurunian et al. (eds.), *Reconstructive Transplantation*, https://doi.org/10.1007/978-3-031-21520-9_27

defined as minor defects can be reconstructed using traditional methods including component separation, tissue expansion, and regional flaps. Type 2 defects are central abdominal defects which can be reconstructed with abdominal wall allografts containing the bilateral rectus abdominis muscles. Adequate perfusion for this graft can be achieved by utilizing an allograft pedicle of the bilateral deep inferior epigastric vessels or femoral vessels. Types 3 and 4 defects involve the hemiabdomen or total abdomen, respectively. These defects benefit from inclusion of the obliques and are revascularized with an allograft pedicle consisting of the iliofemoral system to ensure adequate perfusion of the lateral tissues. Detailed understanding of this anatomy is critical for successful procurement and revascularization of abdominal wall grafts.

27.2.2 Surgical Allograft Harvest

At present, the technique for abdominal wall allograft harvest used by groups performing abdominal wall vascularized composite allotransplantation is as described by Levi et al. in their original manuscript [1]. The harvest begins with a median sternotomy and bi-subcostal incision. Longitudinal incisions are then made following the lateral edges of the rectus sheath and extended into the groins bilaterally. The common femoral vessels are identified through subcutaneous dissection in the inguinal region. Finally, a transverse suprapubic incision is made, connecting the existing two longitudinal incisions to create and en-bloc abdominal wall harvest. Techniques have been described for extended flap harvest for reconstruction of larger defects; however, use of these techniques has not been reported to date [7].

27.2.3 Revascularization of Abdominal Wall Allografts

Successful initial abdominal wall revascularization in the setting of visceral organ transplantation can pose a major challenge. Surgeons must balance the importance of graft ischemia time of both the visceral organs and abdominal wall while operating in a limited surgical field and adjusting to variable recipient and donor anatomy. Several techniques have been reported to accomplish abdominal wall revascularization. Previously published techniques include the following [8]:

Macrovascular anastomosis of donor deep inferior epigastric vessels in continuity with the iliac and femoral vessels to recipient common iliac vessels

In their landmark paper published in 2003, Levi et al. demonstrated that abdominal wall transplantation (AWT) is a feasible approach for complex abdominal wall reconstruction in patients with inadequate soft tissue to achieve abdominal closure after visceral transplantation using conventional methods [1]. The technique consisted of procuring the deep inferior epigastric system in continuity with the iliac and femoral vessels and a short segment of distal aorta and inferior vena cava from the donor at the time of procurement. The AW-VCA vasculature was then anastomosed in an end-to-side fashion to the common iliac vessels of the recipient as is routinely performed in renal transplantation (Fig. 27.1) [9]. This method of revascularization is advantageous in that it is a common technique for surgeons who perform visceral transplants and avoids the need for microsurgery. However, this approach may not be feasible when other procurement teams require retrieval of the iliac and femoral vessels for vascular grafts. This described method also prevents the ability for simultaneous revascularization of both the visceral organ transplant and the AWT. The visceral organ transplant team must complete their portion of the procedure and inset prior to allowing the start of the abdominal wall transplantation. This increases cold ischemia time of the AW-VCA and total operative time. In addition, in the case of MVT with concurrent kidney transplantation, the

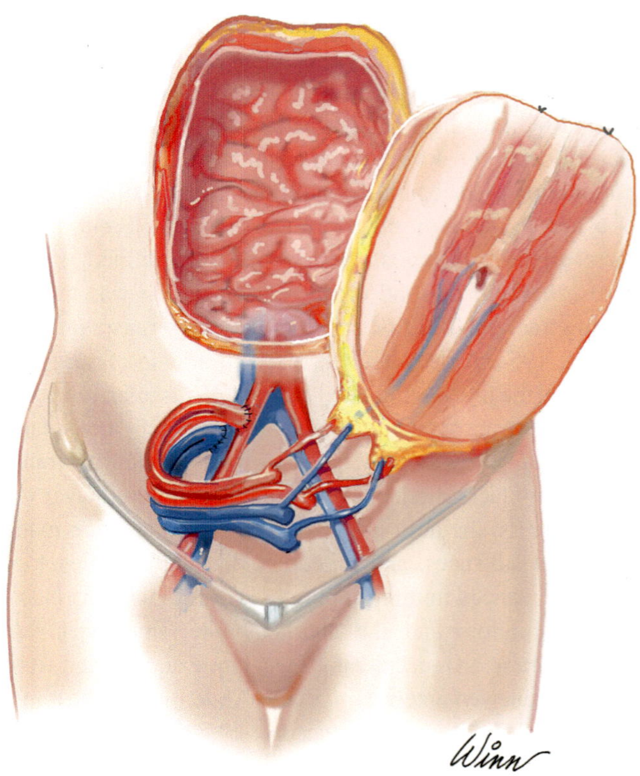

Fig. 27.1 Technique performed by Levi et al. with macrovascular anastomosis of donor deep inferior epigastric vessels in continuity with the iliac and femoral vessels to recipient common iliac vessels. (Figure originally published in the Journal of Reconstructive Microsurgery)

technical difficulty and reliability of an anastomosis to the recipient iliac vessels may be problematic due to pre-existing anastomosis of the renal vessels at the same site.

Microvascular anastomosis of donor inferior epigastric vessels to recipient inferior epigastric vessels or deep circumflex iliac vessels

In 2007, Cipriani et al. published an alternate technique for revascularization of AW-VCA utilizing a microsurgical approach [10]. In this method, the donor inferior epigastric vessels were dissected to their origin at the external iliac vessels and anastomosed end-to-end with the recipient inferior epigastric vessels (Fig. 27.2). The authors reported an overall similar time to revascularization and time to completion of surgery as compared to the original technique described by Levi et al. once visceral organ transplantation was complete. Both groups reported an average time to revascularization of 1 h and required one additional hour of operative time to perform definitive closure, extending the case overall by 2 h after completion of visceral transplantation. The authors note that they did not experience technical failures and were able to spare the donor iliac and femoral vessels which could then be utilized as vascular grafts. While this technique is certainly valuable, it also presents significant limitations. Dissection of the recipient deep inferior epigastric vessels may be difficult or impossible as patients receiving AW-VCAs commonly have extensive scarring and significant past surgical history which compromises and distorts abdominal wall vascular anatomy. The authors noted that one of the three patients reported in their series required microvascular anastomosis to the deep circumflex iliac vessels due to prior resection of the inferior epigastric vasculature. Compared to the technique described by Levi et al., this technique did not shorten total operative time or prevent prolonged cold ischemia.

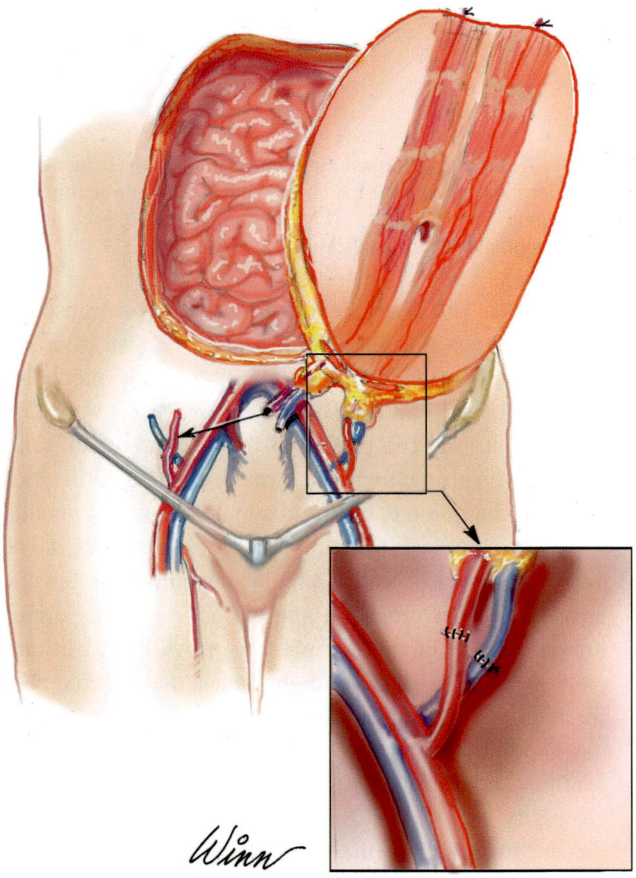

Fig. 27.2 Technique performed by Cipriani et al. with microvascular anastomosis of donor inferior epigastric vessels to recipient inferior epigastric vessels or deep circumflex iliac vessels. (Figure originally published in the Journal of Reconstructive Microsurgery)

Remote revascularization using forearm banking

In 2014, Giele et al. published the first revascularization technique which could address factors including prolonged cold ischemia time and recipient instability during transplantation. The authors utilized temporary "banking" of the abdominal wall allograft at the forearm prior to transfer and inset of the flap in situ [11]. To perform the remote revascularization, the allograft inferior epigastric vessels are anastomosed to the recipient forearm vessels (Fig. 27.3). Ideally, upon completion of the visceral transplant and assessing the recipient's ability to tolerate additional operative time, the AW-VCA is detached from the forearm vessels and anastomosed to the donor inferior epigastric vessels. Finally, an additional anastomosis is performed at the forearm to restore arterial continuity of the forearm vasculature. This method is advantageous in that it prevents prolonged cold ischemia time by allowing immediate revascularization of the AW-VCA upon arrival of the allograft to the operative institution. In addition, in the event that the recipient becomes unstable during the operation, the flap may remain perfused by the forearm vessels and secured in situ. While these are unique advantages of the technique, disadvantages include additional donor site morbidity at the forearm, the need to perform multiple anastomoses leading to increased total operative time, possible prolonged immobilization of the forearm to the abdominal wall if unable to transfer the vascular pedicle at the time of index operation, and the potential need for additional operative interventions. In their series, Giele et al. were able to transfer the pedicle at the time of index operation in 4 of 6 cases. If the patient could not tolerate additional operative time and the pedicle could not be transferred, perfusion of the abdominal wall allograft was maintained using the forearm vasculature. The forearm was immobilized by securing it to the abdominal wall for 4–6 weeks and subsequently reassessed at that time for sufficient neovascularization by using a tourniquet to occlude the brachial artery. If ade-

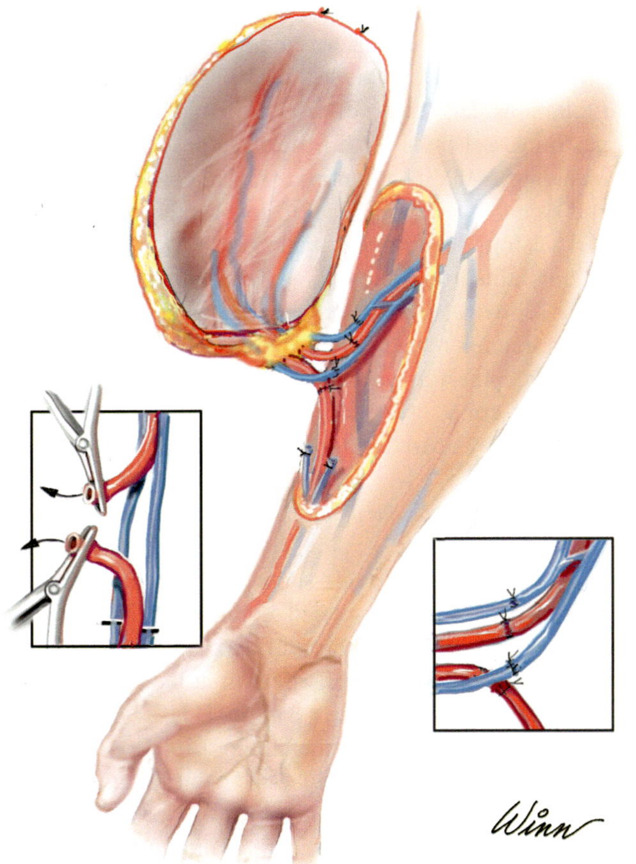

Fig. 27.3 Technique performed by Giele et al. with remote revascularization using forearm banking prior to in situ transfer and re-anastomosis to recipient inferior epigastric vessels. (Figure originally published in the Journal of Reconstructive Microsurgery)

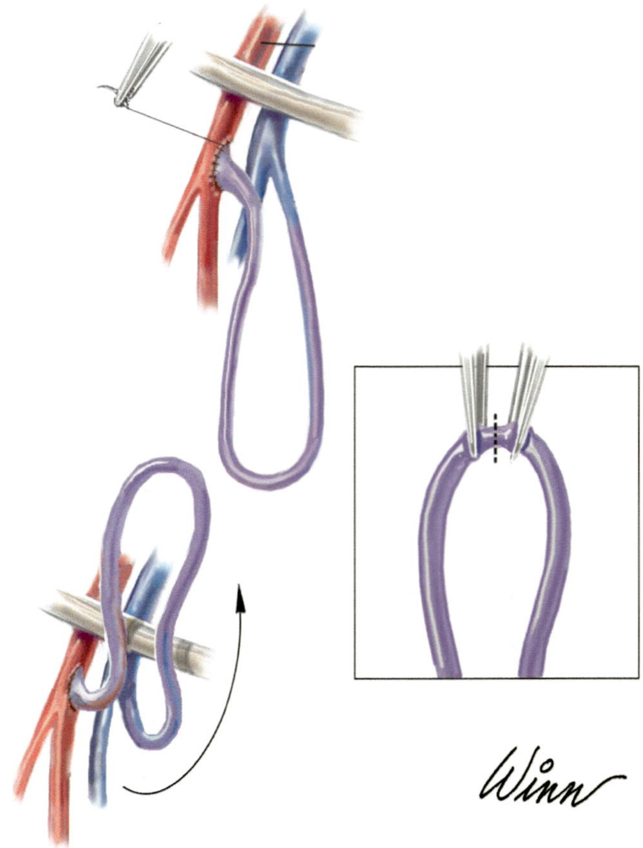

Fig. 27.4 Technique performed by Erdmann et al. with creation of an arteriovenous loop using saphenous vein with end-to-side anastomosis with common femoral artery. (Figure originally published in the American Journal of Transplantation)

quate perfusion was noted, the forearm was separated from the abdominal wall; however, if the AW-VCA was not clinically well perfused, an additional microsurgical anastomosis was performed in situ. While this method allows for synchronous revascularization of the visceral and abdominal wall grafts, the additional steps required using this technique likely increase the total length of surgery, though this outcome is not reported in their work.

Creation of arteriovenous loop using saphenous vein to common femoral artery and anastomosis of donor inferior epigastric vessels to transected AV loop

In 2019, Erdmann et al. reported a novel technique for synchronous in situ revascularization of visceral and abdominal wall allografts utilizing the creation of an arteriovenous loop, a well-established technique in plastic surgery [12]. During cold ischemia time, an incision was made from the inferior aspect of the abdominal incision to the level of the mid-thigh. The saphenous vein was then transected distally and rotated proximally to allow an end-to-side anastomosis with the common femoral artery (Fig. 27.4). The arteriovenous loop was then transected and anastomosed to the donor inferior epigastric vessels under loupe magnification (Fig. 27.5). This procedure was performed bilaterally. The AW-VCA was then secured until the completion of the visceral organ transplant at which time final inset was performed. Utilization of this technique has several distinct advantages, including minimizing cold ischemia time of the AW-VCA and decreasing total operative time as synchronous revascularization is performed in situ. In addition, this option improves ease of anastomosis by providing additional recipient pedicle length and eliminates the possible need for additional operative interventions to divide or transfer the vascular pedicle associated with forearm banking. Limitations of this technique include additional donor site morbidity due to thigh incision and possible risk of seroma formation at the level of the groin or thigh. In addition, this procedure must be modified if the saphenous vein has been previously compromised or used for other procedures.

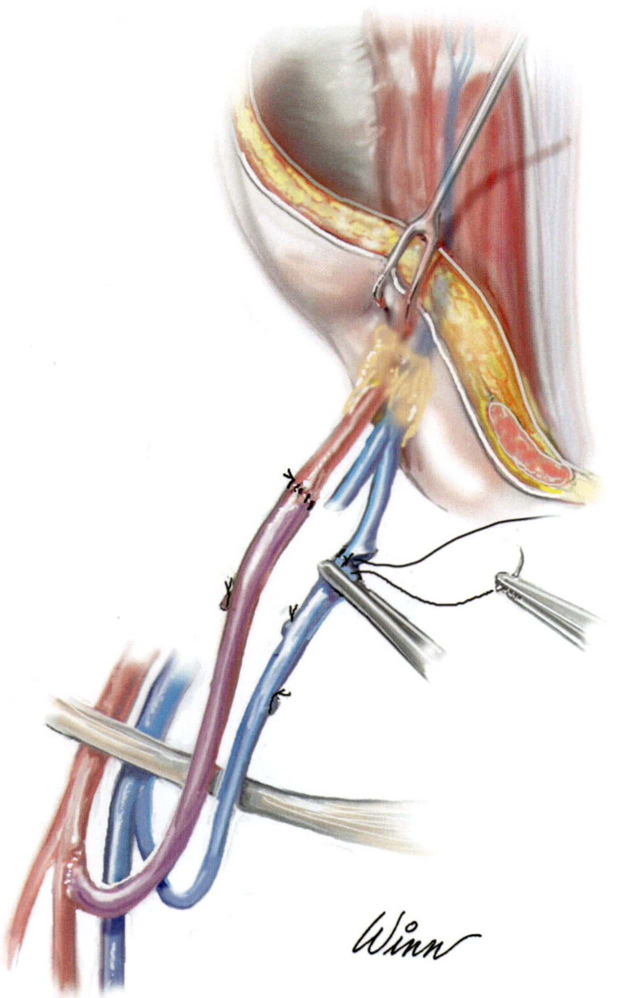

Fig. 27.5 The matured arteriovenous loop is then transected and anastomosed end-to-end to the donor inferior epigastric vessels. (Figure originally published in the American Journal of Transplantation)

27.2.4 Technical Considerations

The allocation of donor organs and operative factors may influence which AW-VCA revascularization technique is preferred. In the case of MVT combined with AW-VCA in the same recipient, the iliac vessels are available to the abdominal wall transplant team and revascularization may be performed as described by Levi et al., if no operative factors necessitate prompt synchronous revascularization. If the donor liver, pancreas, and small bowel are utilized in different recipients, the iliac vessels will not be available to the AW-VCA team. In such cases, or if prompt synchronous revascularization is required, a different technique is necessary. In general, when possible, delaying donor cross-clamp until recipient surgery is underway to minimize cold ischemia time of the AW-VCA is recommended. The demands of multiple procurement teams or geographical constraints may prohibit delayed cross-clamp; however, in the case of MVT combined with AW-VCA, this consideration should be taken into account. In addition, recipient factors including intraoperative stability and available vascular anatomy should inform the transplant team as to which technique is optimal in any given case. For example, many patients who are planned to undergo IT have been on parenteral nutrition for extended periods and may have occluded femoral, saphenous, and iliac veins. In those patients, peripheral venous drainage of the abdominal wall transplant through the distal inferior epigastric veins may be possible. Alternatively, venous drainage into the mesenteric system or by interposition grafts onto the superior mesenteric vein may be used. As such, the reconstructive team must carefully consider both donor and recipient variables to perform the ideal operation.

27.3 Case Report

We present the following case report from recent experience of the senior author of this text. The patient, a 37-year-old army veteran with a history of perforated appendicitis during early childhood, underwent several laparotomies for lysis of adhesions and intestinal obstruction over two decades. In 2014, he developed a small bowel obstruction and presented to an outside hospital. An emergently initiated lysis of adhesions resulted in multiple inadvertent enterotomies and led to the catastrophic scenario of discontinuation of his gastrointestinal tract by proximal stapling and an open abdomen. He was transferred to our institution at that time for further management. The patient became dependent on total parenteral nutrition (TPN) and developed multiple high-output small bowel enterocutaneous fistulas. He underwent several failed attempts of fistula takedown and ventral hernia repair by component separation and use of biologic mesh. The patient was diagnosed with short bowel syndrome and a recurrent high-output small bowel enterocutaneous fistula. During a prior laparotomy, 100 cm or more of native small bowel remained; however, it was considered non-functional given the dense adhesions and partial high-grade obstructions observed throughout the remnant native intestine. He required recurrent hospital admissions for treatment of life-threatening bloodstream infections. In May of 2018, the patient was hospitalized for dehydration due to high-output enterocutaneous fistula and was considered for a small bowel transplantation. Because of extensive scarring and the estimation that 25–30% of the native abdominal wall would be compromised with an additional laparotomy, there was major concern that his native abdominal wall would not be sufficient to support an anticipated small bowel transplant (Fig. 27.6). The patient was enrolled under an Institutional Review Board (IRB)-approved protocol for AWT in conjunction with small bowel transplantation. The procedure was performed in October 2018 after a suitable donor became

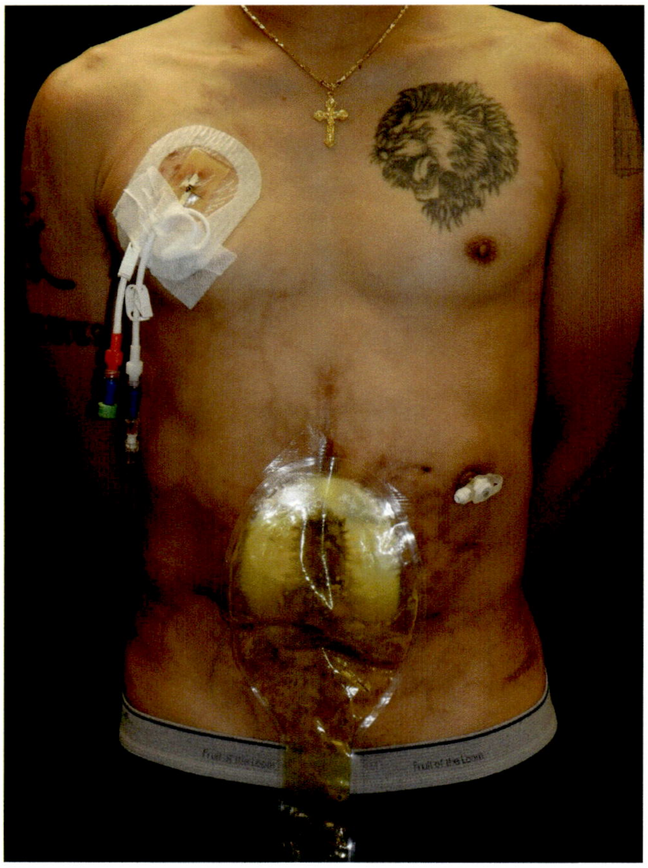

Fig. 27.6 Abdominal wall of patient following multiple laparotomies with extensive scarring and multiple recurrent enterocutaneous fistulas. It was determined that the use of conventional methods for soft tissue closure after intestinal transplant would not be sufficient to provide adequate coverage. (Figure originally published in the American Journal of Transplantation)

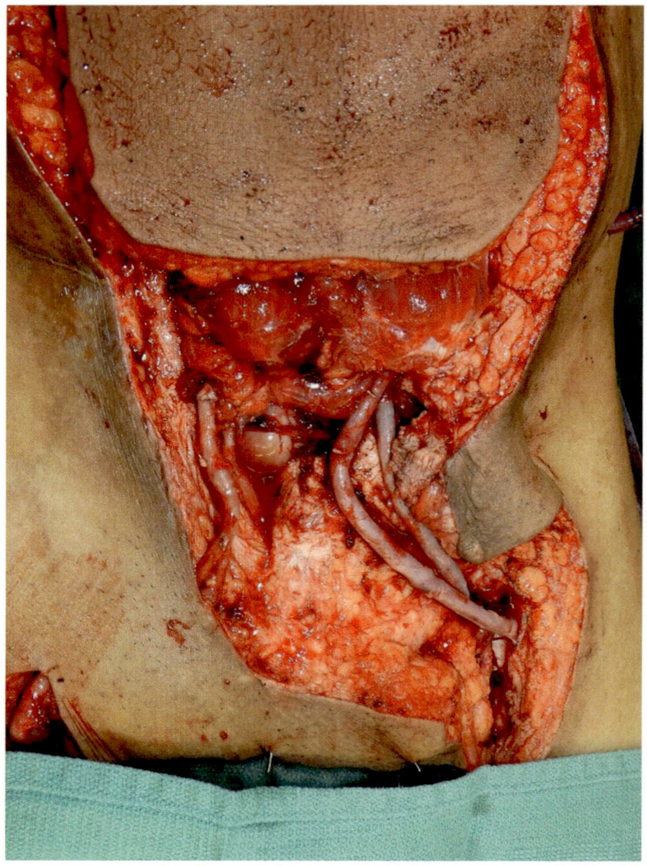

Fig. 27.7 Abdominal wall-vascularized composite allograft after dual revascularization at the groin level. (Figure originally published in the American Journal of Transplantation)

available. The donor family agreed to donate the abdominal wall at the time of the visceral organ recovery. A standard approach to abdominal wall allograft harvest was used and synchronous revascularization was performed as detailed above. After completion of the intestinal transplant including revascularization and bowel anastomoses, the AW-VCA was transferred in situ and a right-sided revascularization was performed in the same technique to augment perfusion resulting in dual perfusion to the abdominal wall allograft (shown in Fig. 27.7). The anastomosis time of the AW allograft was 45 min. Following dual revascularization, intraoperative angiography demonstrated an entirely vascularized AW-VCA. Finally, the compromised native AW was excised and the AW-VCA was secured in multiple layers. The overall cold ischemia time of the small bowel graft was 4 h 56 min and the cold ischemia time of the AW allograft was 5 h. The patient tolerated the 14-h operation well. The immediate on-table result after reperfusion is shown in Fig. 27.8. The patient received Thymoglobulin® induction (1.5 mg/kg × 4 doses) and maintenance immunosuppression consisting of Tacrolimus (Prograf®), Mycophenolate mofetil, MMF (CellCept®), and prednisone, which is the standard immunosuppression regimen given to patients who undergo intestinal transplantation at the operative institution. The patient was extubated on postoperative day 1 and tolerated a regular diet by postoperative day 14. A clinical photograph 8 weeks after synchronous small intestine and abdominal wall-vascularized composite allograft transplantation is shown in Fig. 27.9.

27.3.1 Postoperative Course

In the immediate postoperative setting, the AW-VCA was monitored for rejection and vascular compromise using frequent clinical exam, implantable Doppler probes, and tissue

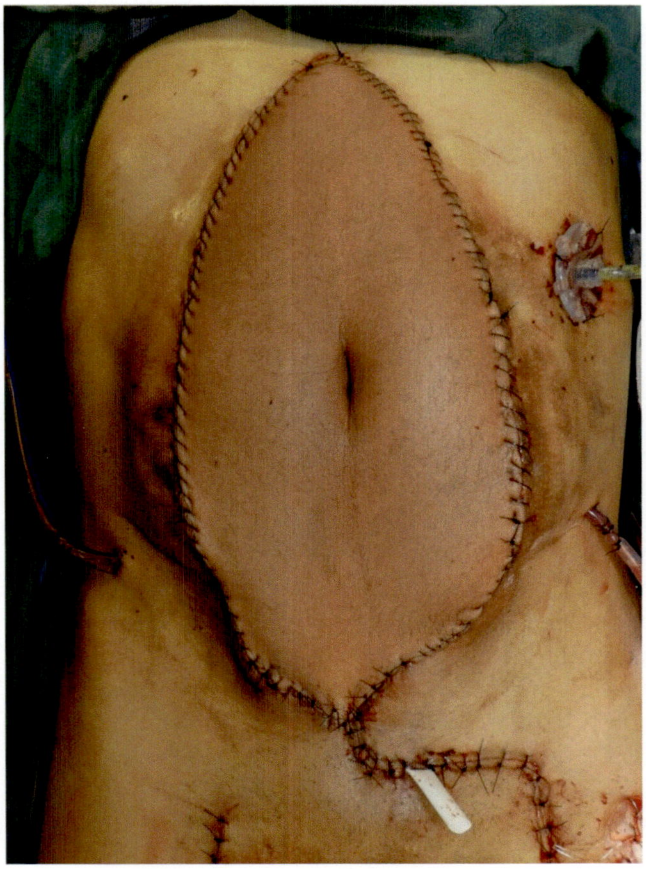

Fig. 27.8 Abdominal wall-vascularized composite allograft in situ after completion revascularization and inset. (Figure originally published in the American Journal of Transplantation)

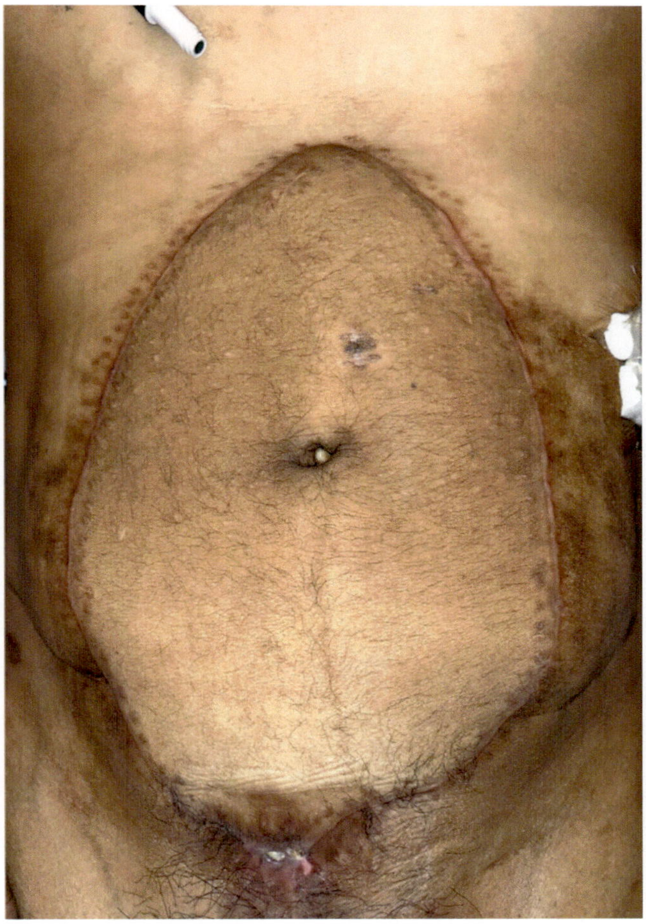

Fig. 27.9 Clinical exam at 8 weeks after synchronous small intestine and abdominal wall-vascularized composite allograft transplantation. (Figure originally published in the American Journal of Transplantation)

oximetry. After recovery, the patient was scheduled for examinations including skin biopsies per standard institutional protocol and in the event he reported any rash or other skin changes of the AW. Standard immunosuppression continued with tacrolimus (Prograf®), goal trough level: 15–18 ng/mL × 3 months, mycophenolic mofetil, MMF (CellCept®) 1000 mg Q12 h, and steroid taper per protocol (prednisone 20 mg daily). A standard prophylactic antibiotic and antifungal regimen given to all intestinal transplant patients at the home institution was initiated which included piperacillin/tazobactam (Zosyn®) and fluconazole for 2 weeks, followed by clotrimazole for 3 months and sulfamethoxazole/trimethoprim (Bactrim®) for 1 year. At the same time, IT biopsies were performed to screen for rejection. In addition, the patient underwent scheduled skin biopsies per IRB-approved protocol for AW transplantation that led to an unnecessary amount of clinic visits and insult to the AW skin (scars). Interestingly, there was only one questionable episode of mild intestinal rejection but multiple episodes of AW-VCA rejection on biopsy according to the Banff Classification [13]. The clinical and histologic appearance of an acute Banff III rejection of the AW-VCA skin is shown in Figs. 27.10 and 27.11. Although IT rejection could not be detected in specimens, the AW-VCA rejection was treated with high doses of steroids in addition with Thymoglobulin® and clobetasol propionate gel (one event).

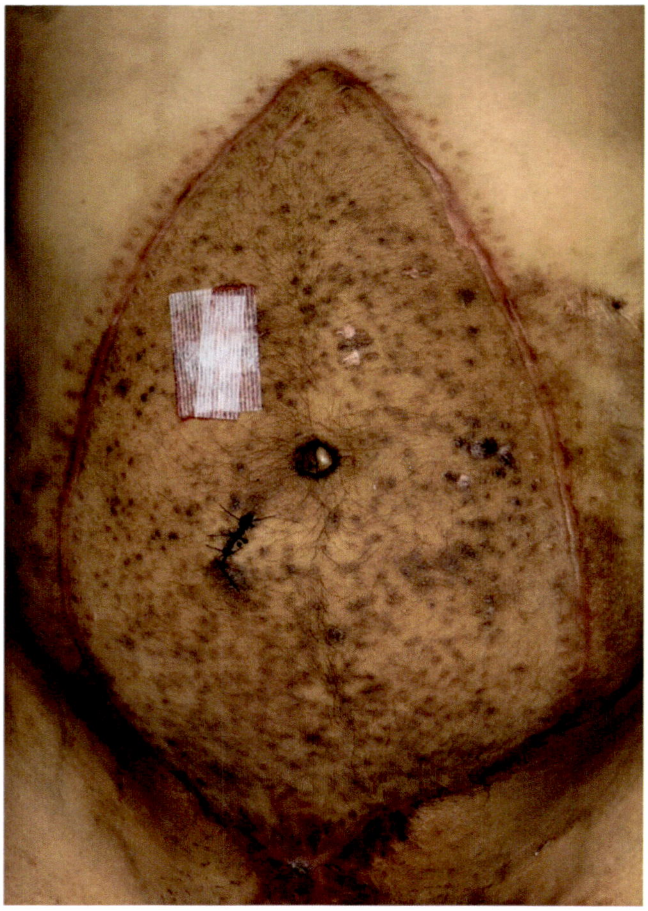

Fig. 27.10 Representative findings of abdominal wall allograft during BANFF III rejection episode. The abdominal wall demonstrates multiple scars from frequent skin biopsies. (Figure originally published in Plastic and Reconstructive Surgery Global Open)

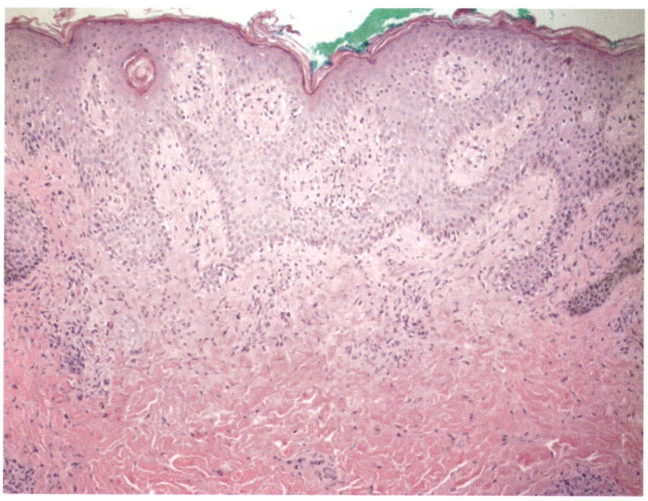

Fig. 27.11 Biopsy of abdominal wall demonstrating severe inflammation and epidermal involvement with epithelial apoptosis, dyskeratosis, and keratinolysis consistent with BANF III rejection. (Figure originally published in Plastic and Reconstructive Surgery Global Open)

27.4 Future Directions

27.4.1 Defining Indications

One of the first challenges that needs to be addressed with any surgical procedure is to define indications for the procedure. In the case of AW-VCA, the reconstructive team must determine when an abdominal wall allograft is needed. Currently, abdominal wall VCA is performed for reconstruction of complex abdominal wall defects in patients who cannot be reconstructed with biomaterials or autologous tissue. However, there are no defined indications or objective preoperative assessments in the literature to establish which patients should be considered for abdominal wall transplantation at the time of multi-visceral or intestinal transplant. Prior studies have evaluated pre- and postoperative CT scans of patients who had received intestinal or multi-visceral organ transplants to determine if there is a predictable change in abdominal volume after transplantation which can be used to predict the need for a concurrent abdominal wall transplant [14]. While several preoperative risk factors were identified that are linked to abdominal wall complications in patients receiving IT or MVT, no predictable change in abdominal wall volume could be determined. At present, the reconstructive team must rely on clinical judgment to determine who will benefit from abdominal wall transplantation, and this remains an important question for future research.

27.4.2 Neurotization

There remains debate regarding the importance and possibility of improved functional outcomes with neurotization of abdominal wall allografts. While neurotization has not been performed in AW-VCA to date, Broyles et al. recently published a cadaveric anatomical study to assess the feasibility of innervating abdominal wall allografts [15]. The authors successfully isolated thoracolumbar nerves with full-thickness abdominal wall allografts from three cadavers. They identified an average of five thoracolumbar nerves on each side of the allograft and found that the nerves were of adequate length and caliber to perform tension-free coaptation. While several clinical barriers to neurotization remain including prolonged operative time and extensive scarring of the native recipient abdominal wall leading to difficult dissection, further evidence is needed to determine if neurotization will lead to improved outcomes in AW-VCA.

27.4.3 Immunosuppression

As surgical techniques have improved, without doubt, the most pressing challenge remaining in AW-VCA today is optimizing immunosuppression. Specifically in abdominal wall transplantation, all reported immunosuppression protocols have followed institutional norms for immunosuppression of intestinal or liver transplantation. The Oxford working group reported outcomes regarding immunosuppression in the largest cohort of AW-VCA [16]. This protocol includes alemtuzunab (Campath®) as induction therapy with tacrolimus as maintenance therapy. The outcome of the study demonstrated a 36% rate of rejection. Their rejection monitoring protocol included endoscopy multiple times a week for 6 months, followed by bi-monthly monitoring. There were no scheduled skin biopsies; however, biopsies were taken if a change in clinical exam was noted. This regimen may be an alternative immunosuppression protocol that could be considered. An additional consideration to minimizing immunogenicity is removal of the skin, if possible. As the AW-VCA heals and IT edema resolves during the postoperative course, AW skin redundancy is noted. Therefore, excision of redundant skin along the periphery of the AW-VCA may be considered. Given that skin is the most antigenic component of VCA [17], excision of excess skin may theoretically decrease the antigenic load associated with AW-VCA while improving the AW appearance [18]. The central skin component should remain, which continues to allow for noninvasive monitoring (clinical examination).

27.5 Conclusion

The field of vascularized composite allotransplantation continues to grow with the advancements in immunotherapy and solid organ transplantation. Refinement of the presented methods will continue to evolve with greater available evidence and outcomes. We must continue to critically review surgical techniques, postoperative management, and outcomes to improve long-term patient results.

References

1. Levi DM, Tzakis AG, Kato T, et al. Transplantation of the abdominal wall. Lancet. 2003;361(9376):2173–6. https://doi.org/10.1016/S0140-6736(03)13769-5.
2. Light D, Kundu N, Djohan R, et al. Total abdominal wall transplantation: an anatomical study and classification system. Plast Reconstr Surg. 2017;139(6):1466–73. https://doi.org/10.1097/PRS.0000000000003327.
3. Giele H, Vaidya A, Reddy S, Vrakas G, Friend P. Current state of abdominal wall transplantation. Curr Opin Organ Transplant. 2016;21(2):159–64. https://doi.org/10.1097/MOT.0000000000000276.
4. Carlsen BT, Farmer DG, Busuttil RW, Miller TA, Rudkin GH. Incidence and management of abdominal wall defects after intestinal and multivisceral transplantation. Plast Reconstr Surg. 2007;119(4):1247–55. https://doi.org/10.1097/01.prs.0000254401.33682.e9; discussion 1256-8.
5. Alexandrides IJ, Liu P, Marshall DM, Nery JR, Tzakis AG, Thaller SR. Abdominal wall closure after intestinal transplantation. Plast Reconstr Surg. 2000;106(4):805–12.
6. Huger WE Jr. The anatomic rationale for abdominal lipectomy. Am Surg. 1979;45(9):612–7.
7. Hollenbeck ST, Senghaas A, Turley R, et al. The extended abdominal wall flap for transplantation. Transplant Proc. 2011;43(5):1701–5. https://doi.org/10.1016/j.transproceed.2011.01.176.
8. Atia A, Hollins A, Shammas R, et al. Surgical techniques for revascularization in abdominal wall transplantation. J Reconstr Microsurg. 2020;36(7):522–7. https://doi.org/10.1055/s-0040-1709481.
9. Selvaggi G, Levi DM, Kato T, et al. Expanded use of transplantation techniques: abdominal wall transplantation and intestinal autotransplantation. Transplant Proc. 2004;36(5):1561–3. https://doi.org/10.1016/j.transproceed.2004.05.037.
10. Cipriani R, Contedini F, Santoli M, et al. Abdominal wall transplantation with microsurgical technique. Am J Transplant. 2007;7(5):1304–7. https://doi.org/10.1111/j.1600-6143.2007.01798.x.
11. Giele H, Bendon C, Reddy S, et al. Remote revascularization of abdominal wall transplants using the forearm. Am J Transplant. 2014;14(6):1410–6. https://doi.org/10.1111/ajt.12724.
12. Erdmann D, Atia A, Phillips BT, et al. Small bowel and abdominal wall transplantation: a novel technique for synchronous revascularization. Am J Transplant. 2019;19(7):2122–6. https://doi.org/10.1111/ajt.15370.
13. Cendales LC, Kanitakis J, Schneeberger S, et al. The Banff 2007 working classification of skin-containing composite tissue allograft pathology. Am J Transplant. 2008;8(7):1396–400. https://doi.org/10.1111/j.1600-6143.2008.02243.x.
14. Hollins AW, Napier K, Wildman-Tobriner B, et al. Using radiographic domain for evaluating indications in abdominal wall transplantation. Ann Plast Surg. 2021;87(3):348–54. https://doi.org/10.1097/SAP.0000000000002708.
15. Broyles JM, Berli J, Tuffaha SH, et al. Functional abdominal wall reconstruction using an innervated abdominal wall vascularized composite tissue allograft: a cadaveric study and review of the literature. J Reconstr Microsurg. 2015;31(1):39–44. https://doi.org/10.1055/s-0034-1381958.
16. Gerlach UA, Vrakas G, Sawitzki B, et al. Abdominal wall transplantation: skin as a sentinel marker for rejection. Am J Transplant. 2016;16(6):1892–900. https://doi.org/10.1111/ajt.13693.
17. Jones ND, Turvey SE, Van Maurik A, et al. Differential susceptibility of heart, skin, and islet allografts to T cell-mediated rejection. J Immunol. 2001;166(4):2824–30. https://doi.org/10.4049/jimmunol.166.4.2824.
18. Atia A, Hollins A, Erdmann RF, et al. Synchronous abdominal wall and small-bowel transplantation: a 1-year follow-up. Plast Reconstr Surg Glob Open. 2020;8(7):e2995. https://doi.org/10.1097/GOX.0000000000002995.

Abdominal Wall Transplantation with Microsurgical Technique

28

Riccardo Cipriani, Valentina Pinto, Federico Contedini, Chiara Gelati, Maria Elisa Lozano Miralles, Chiara Zanfi, Antonio Daniele Pinna, and Matteo Cescon

Abbreviations

ACR	Acute cellular rejection
ALT	Anterolateral thigh
AW	Abdominal wall
AWTX	Abdominal wall transplantation
CA	Cerebral aspergillosis
CMV	Cytomegalovirus
CRF	Chronic renal failure
DIEA	Deep inferior epigastric artery
DIEV	Deep inferior epigastric vein
GVHD	Graft versus host disease
ITX	Intestinal transplantation
MA	Mycotic aneurysm
MVTX	Multivisceral transplantation
NPT	Negative pressure therapy
PTLD	Lymphoproliferative disease
SG	Skin graft
UNOS	United network for organ sharing
VCA	Vascularized composite graft

R. Cipriani · V. Pinto (✉) · F. Contedini · C. Gelati
Plastic Surgery, IRCCS Azienda Ospedaliero-Universitaria di Bologna, Bologna, Italy
e-mail: riccardo.cipriani@aosp.bo.it; valentina.pinto@aosp.bo.it; federico.contedini@aosp.bo.it; chiara.gelati@aosp.bo.it

M. E. L. Miralles
Plastic Surgery, IRCCS Azienda Ospedaliero-Universitaria di Bologna, Bologna, Italy

Plastic Surgery, Policlinico di Modena, University of Modena and Reggio Emilia, Modena, Italy

C. Zanfi · M. Cescon
General Surgery and Transplantation Unit, IRCCS Azienda Ospedaliero-Universitaria di Bologna, Bologna, Italy
e-mail: chiara.zanfi@aosp.bo.it; matteo.cescon@unibo.it

A. D. Pinna
Abdominal Transplant Center, Weston, FL, USA
e-mail: antoniodaniele.pinna@unibo.it

28.1 Introduction

Abdominal wall closure is of paramount importance to avoid the loss of the recipient's abdominal domain in intestinal (ITx) and multivisceral transplantation (MVTx); a safe and reliable soft tissue coverage for transplanted organs is critical to reduce postoperative complications and mortality rate. But, to date, it is still the most important challenge. The main causes requiring stable soft tissue reconstruction are past history of complete bowel removal with loss of the abdominal domain or severely damaged abdominal wall due to repeated laparotomies or enterocutaneous fistulae. These conditions result in an abdominal cavity that is too contracted to receive transplanted organs. Also, because organs are often more edematous at the end of the visceral transplantation, a tight closure could increase morbidity and mortality risk, leading to intestinal failure. The patients who are candidates for intestinal or multivisceral transplantation could have several problems that may lead to difficult abdominal wall closure [1–3]. The main indications are listed in Table 28.1.

Conventional techniques for traditional abdominal wall closure, such as simple tension-free closure, component separation, use of synthetic or biological meshes (better absorbable), staged tissue expanders, local or free flaps, are not always possible. A prosthetic mesh for definitive primary closure or combined with a pedicled flap can be considered in partial abdominal wall defect. The prosthetic material allows a quick recovery, but, unfortunately, it may be com-

Table 28.1 Common indications to abdominal wall transplantation (AWTx)

Indications for abdominal wall transplantation (AWTx)
Multiple scars and fibrosis due to previous abdominal surgery
Multiple enterocutaneous fistulas
Ostomies
Donor/recipient size mismatch (donor to recipient unfavorable weight ratio)
Loss of bowel length for previous bowel resection
Postoperative oedema of the intestinal loops

© Springer Nature Switzerland AG 2023
R. Gurunian et al. (eds.), *Reconstructive Transplantation*, https://doi.org/10.1007/978-3-031-21520-9_28

plicated by infection of the mesh and formation of enterocutaneous fistulae [4].

Abdominal reconstruction using pedicled flap allows one stage closure avoiding the placement of alloplastic materials, but it requires longer operative time and an additional donor site morbidity. Any attempt to close under tension might result in a wide range of abdominal complications, such as wound dehiscence, infections, necrosis of bowel loops, vascular thrombosis of the graft, abdominal compartment syndrome, and respiratory complications. Different strategies have been proposed to overcome these problems, such as the reduction of the graft size, use of prosthetic meshes, abdominal wall expansion, NPT (negative pressure therapy), pedicled flaps, free flaps [5–8], and, in selected cases, abdominal wall transplantation [9]. The pedicled anterolateral thigh (ALT) flap is the gold standard for medium and large sized defects, as proposed by Kimata et al. in 1999 [10]; it does not require microsurgical anastomosis, but it can be used only for lower abdominal defects. Fascia lata can be incorporated to prevent hernia formation [11]. ALT flap is a fasciocutaneous or cutaneous flap from the thigh, supplied by perforators of the descending branch of the lateral circumflex femoral artery that can be used also as a free flap for defects involving upper abdomen.

Abdominal closure under tension might result in a wide range of complications, such as wound dehiscence, infections, necrosis, exposure of bowel loops, vascular thrombosis of the microsurgical flap, abdominal compartment syndrome, and respiratory complications [9]. In patients with complete loss of the abdominal domain, undergoing visceral organ transplantation, two main strategies have been proposed to overcome these potential risks. One option to reduce donor graft size, choosing smaller donor, but this procedure can extend the waiting time, increasing the risk of mortality in the waiting list. Then, the preferred approach is abdominal domain enlargement, as described for the first time by Levi et al. in 2003 [12], with the introduction of abdominal wall transplantation simultaneously to intestinal or multivisceral transplantation. Abdominal wall transplantation is a feasible and safe procedure: it allows primary closure of the abdomen, avoids the potential morbidity of exposed viscera, and allows early mobilization and recovery of these patients [13]. Abdominal wall transplantation (AWTx) is a full-thickness vascularized composite allograft included as a VCA (vascularized composite allotransplantation) in the UNOS (United Network for Organ Sharing) Registry [14] Table 28.2.

The main advantage to use abdominal composite tissue allograft in such patients is the fact that there is need for further immunosuppression. The ideal candidates to AWTx present with heavily scarred abdominal wall due to previous multiple intestinal resections, or, more often, have a "virtual" abdominal cavity [1, 15] precluding a primary abdominal closure for donor/recipient size mismatch. Fishbein et al. [16] reported that the most acceptable donor/recipient weight ratio is between 1.1 and 0.76. Multiple previous laparotomies and of partial/total enterectomy were predictive of difficult closure of the abdomen, even if the reported ratio is respected. In these selected cases, AWTx is the gold standard.

Over-resuscitation with fluids should be avoided, and colloid solutions should be used if possible. Moreover all dysfunctional remaining bowels should be removed, and all adhesions should be lysed to enlarge intraperitoneal space. Other options to control donor/recipient size discrepancy

Table 28.2 Abdominal wall transplantation (AWTx): type of transplant, tissue composition, main features

Type of transplant	VCA (Vascularized composite allotransplantation)	Included in the UNOS registry (United Network for Organ Sharing)
Tissue composition	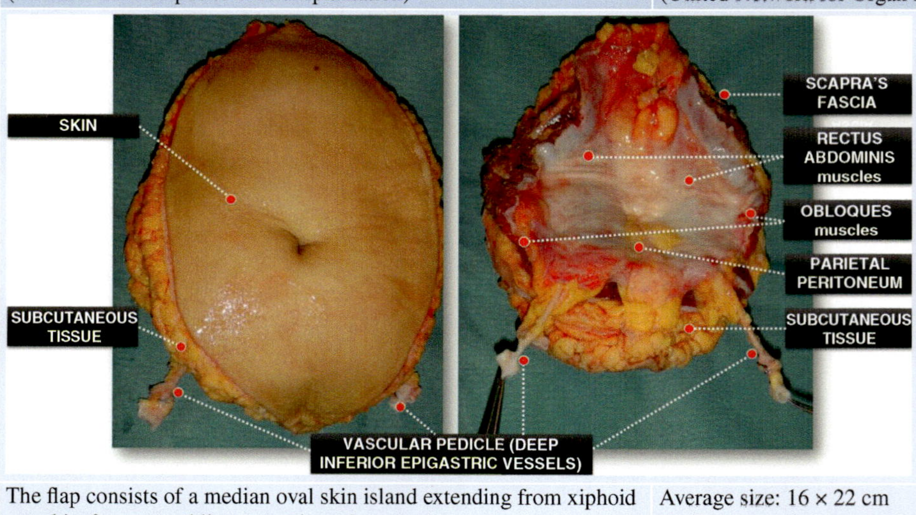	
Main features	The flap consists of a median oval skin island extending from xiphoid to pubis, from one oblique muscle to the other	Average size: 16 × 22 cm

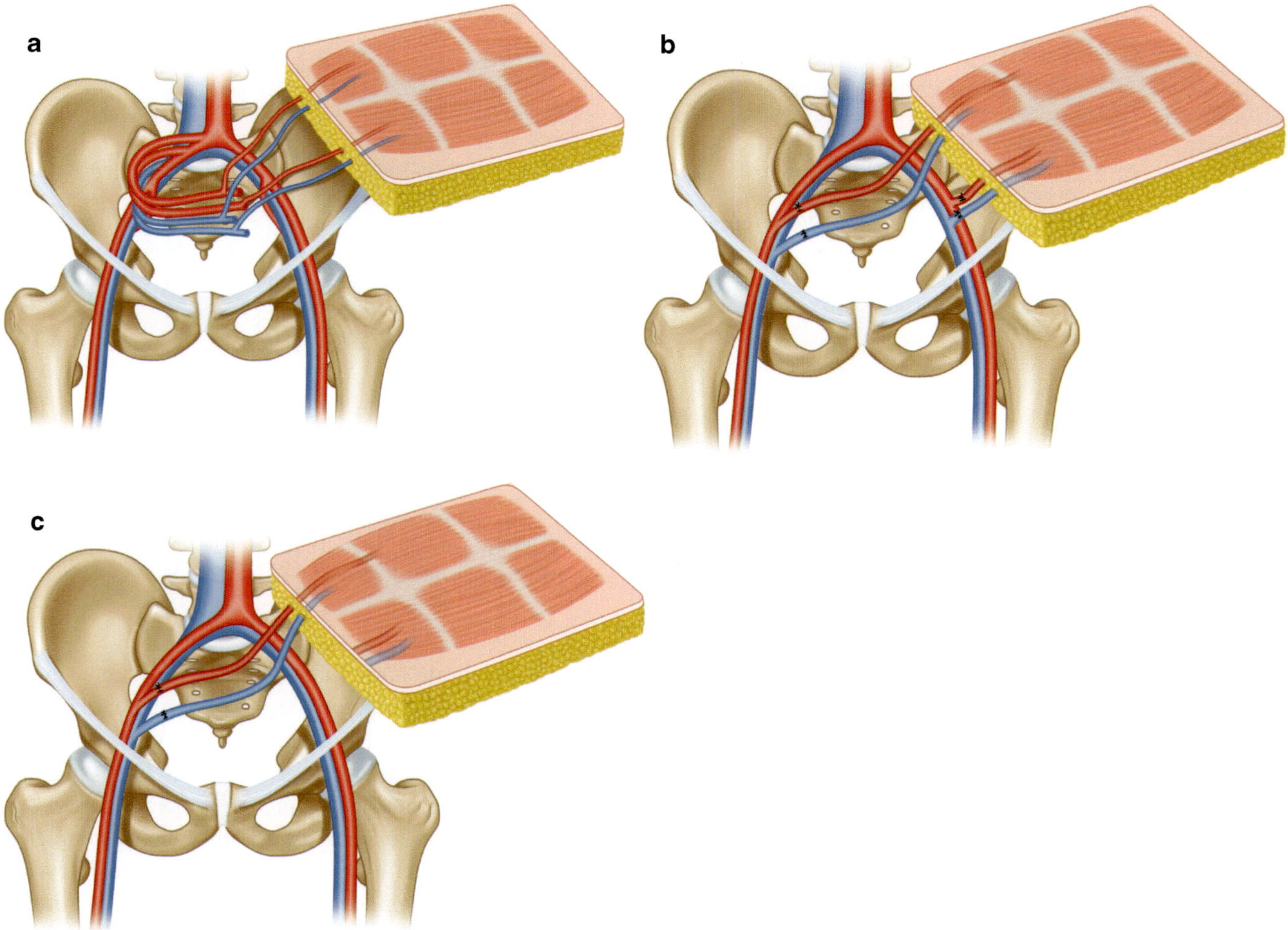

Fig. 28.1 Comparison between traditional macrosurgical procedure (**a**) (Levi) (12) and microsurgical technique (Cipriani) (17) using bilateral (**b**) or monolateral (**c**) deep inferior epigastric pedicles for microvascular anastomoses

include splenectomy (but this procedure increases the risk for sepsis) and partial transplanted bowel resection (but it can cause inadequate absorption and function).

Recruitment of the abdominal wall graft does not interfere with the procurement of other organs and tissues. Transplantation of the abdominal wall composite graft can take place during the intestinal transplant procedure or, in selected cases, several days later, with a graft from a different donor. Delayed abdominal wall transplant allows reduction of perioperative edema and stabilization of patient's condition, before abdominal closure. This strategy may be preferable in wide abdominal recipient defect; a temporary negative pressure therapy (NPT) is applied to reduce the infection risk in these cases. To date, both traditional macrosurgical procedure [9] and microsurgical approach [17] are well described and used worldwide (Fig. 28.1, Table 28.3).

When did the program start?

Since 2006, Cipriani et al. applied microsurgical technique to AWTx, modifying traditional macroanastomoses on the iliac vessels proposed by Levi [9], with microanastomoses on deep inferior epigastric system [17, 18].

28.1.1 Procurement of AWTx Graft

The AW graft was retrieved at heart-beating donor during the multiorgan procurement from selected donor after certification of brain death [17, 18].

The abdominal flap consists of a median oval cutaneous paddle (average size: 16 × 22 cm), extended from xiphoid to pubis, including the full length of both rectus abdominis muscles. The AWTx is composed of cutaneous and subcutaneous tissues, both rectus abdominis muscles and a small part of the oblique ones, the deep muscular fascia, and parietal peritoneum, raised on the inferior epigastric arteries and associated venae comitantes isolated bilaterally, if possible.

The flap is planned and harvested by a microsurgeon. The procedure starts with a cranial subcostal incision of the skin

Table 28.3 Abdominal wall transplantation (AWTx): differences between traditional and microsurgical technique

Abdominal wall transplantation (AWTX)		
The harvesting of the abdominal wall graft is performed at heart-beating donor		
	Traditional technique	Microsurgical technique
First description	*Levi DM,* et al. "Transplantation of the abdominal wall" Lancet. *2003*;361:2173	*Cipriani R,* et al. "Abdominal wall transplantation with microsurgical technique" Am J Transplant. *2007*;7(5):1304–7
Type of transplant	*VCA vascularized composite allotransplantation*	*VCA vascularized composite allotransplantation*
Vascular pedicle	Bilateral deep inferior epigastric vessels, *connected with the iliac vessels* (+/– short segment of distal aorta and inferior vena cava)	Bilateral deep inferior epigastric vessels *isolated from iliac origin* (Deep circumflex iliac vessels are a second choice)
Type of anastomosis	End-to-Side *MACRO*-ANASTOMOSIS	End-to-End *MICRO*-ANASTOMOSIS
Immunosuppression	*NO* further immunosuppression	*NO* further immunosuppression
Advantages	• NO microsurgical skills • NO microscope	• Anastomoses on extra peritoneal vessels mean no compression on transplanted organs • The anastomosed vessels are more superficial than iliac ones and are rarely involved in scar tissue • Donor iliac vessels are available for other surgeons (vascular graft for vascular surgeons)

and subcutaneous tissues, including the deep fascia under rectus muscles; then the dissection proceeds laterally, including rectus muscles and preserving a small part of oblique muscles. The dissection is stopped at the inferior edge of the flap, where a transverse suprapubic incision is performed connecting longitudinal ones. The abdominal flap is turned downward to allow the recruitment of the abdominal viscera. During this time, abdominal graft is packed with cold water and ice, while the other organs are flushed with preservation solution during their harvesting.

After this step, the epigastric pedicles of the abdominal wall flap are sectioned at the origin from iliac vessels. A further cold perfusion is performed through incannulation of the two epigastric arteries; the abdominal graft is then stored in a container with ice and Celsior solution for the transport. Primary closure can be performed in the donor site by wide undermining of the residual lateral abdomen and flanks flaps.

28.1.2 Microsurgical Technique for AWTx

The AWTx revascularization is performed after abdominal organ transplantation. Microsurgical approach consists of bilateral end-to-end anastomoses between donor and recipient deep inferior epigastric vessels [17, 18]. Deep circumflex iliac arteries and veins are a second choice for recipient vessels. According to the current anatomical knowledge, monolateral anastomosis of DIEA and DIEV are sufficient to guarantee perfusion for a conventional abdominal graft. Monolateral anastomosis allows to perform AWTx when previous surgeries, vessel injuries, or trauma on the donor's abdomen could alter donor graft vessels.

Abdominal graft harvesting and microanastomoses on deep inferior epigastric system require approximatively the same operative time, without impairment to other organs or pedicles, without vascular complications or increasing the risk of vascular thrombosis, saving the donor's iliac vessels to use as vascular grafts. The surgical procedure is completed with ileostomy and multilayer suture tension-free. Dressing leaves an inspection window to monitor flap vitality. Sutures are removed after 15–20 days, Figs. 28.2 and 28.3. Sequential steps in abdominal wall flap dissection, microanastomosis, and postoperative management of the microsurgical AWTx procedure are summarized in Table 28.4. Ischemia time is reported in Table 28.5.

28.1.3 Immunosuppressive Protocol

The baseline immunosuppressive agent is tacrolimus [17–20].

Immunosuppressive protocol consisted of:

- Induction: A first phase with alemtuzumab 0.03 mg/kg (Campath®) before transplant, at the time of the reperfusion and at third and seventh postoperative days;
- Maintenance: Tacrolimus monotherapy with a target level of 8–12 ng/mL (Prograf®: 0.075 mg/kg).

The majority of the VCA patients received either polyclonal (antithymocyte globulins, ATG) or monoclonal (alemtuzumab, basiliximab) plus antibody preparation as an induction agent followed by a high dose of tacrolimus and steroids for maintenance therapy. No antimetabolites

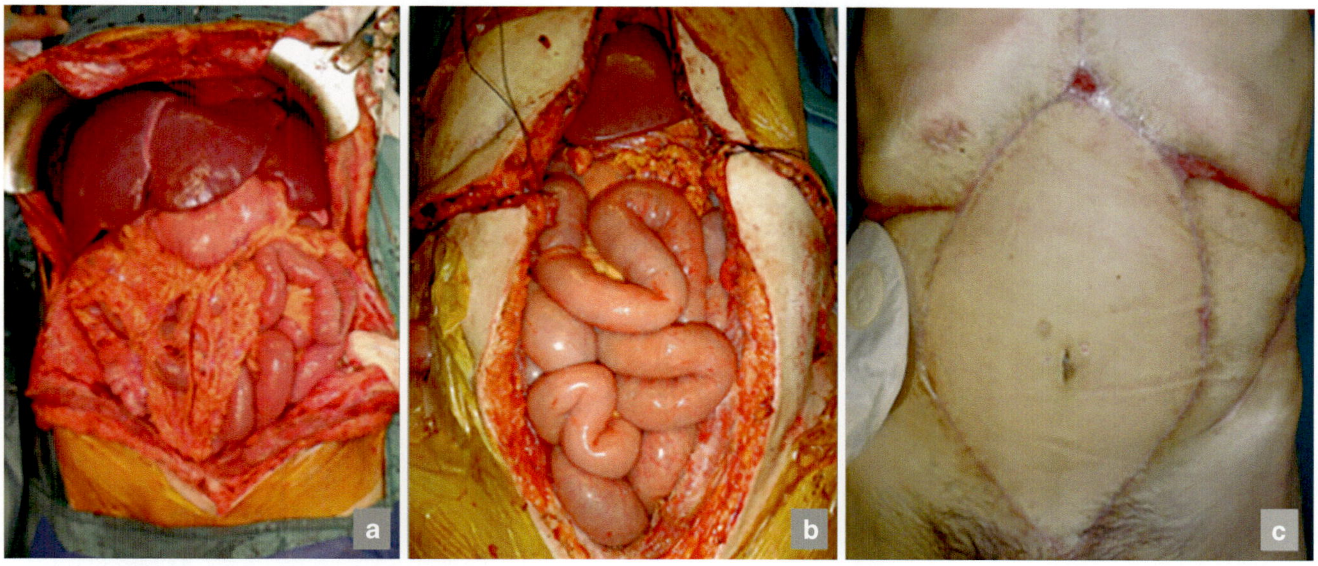

Fig. 28.2 A 33-year-old man underwent MVTx (1**a**, 1**b**) and simultaneous AWTx (1**c**) for multiple enterocutaneous fistulas due to Crohn's disease. Microanastomoses of abdominal graft were performed on bilateral deep inferior epigastric artery and vein. Three months after transplantation, patient died from mycotic aortic aneurysm

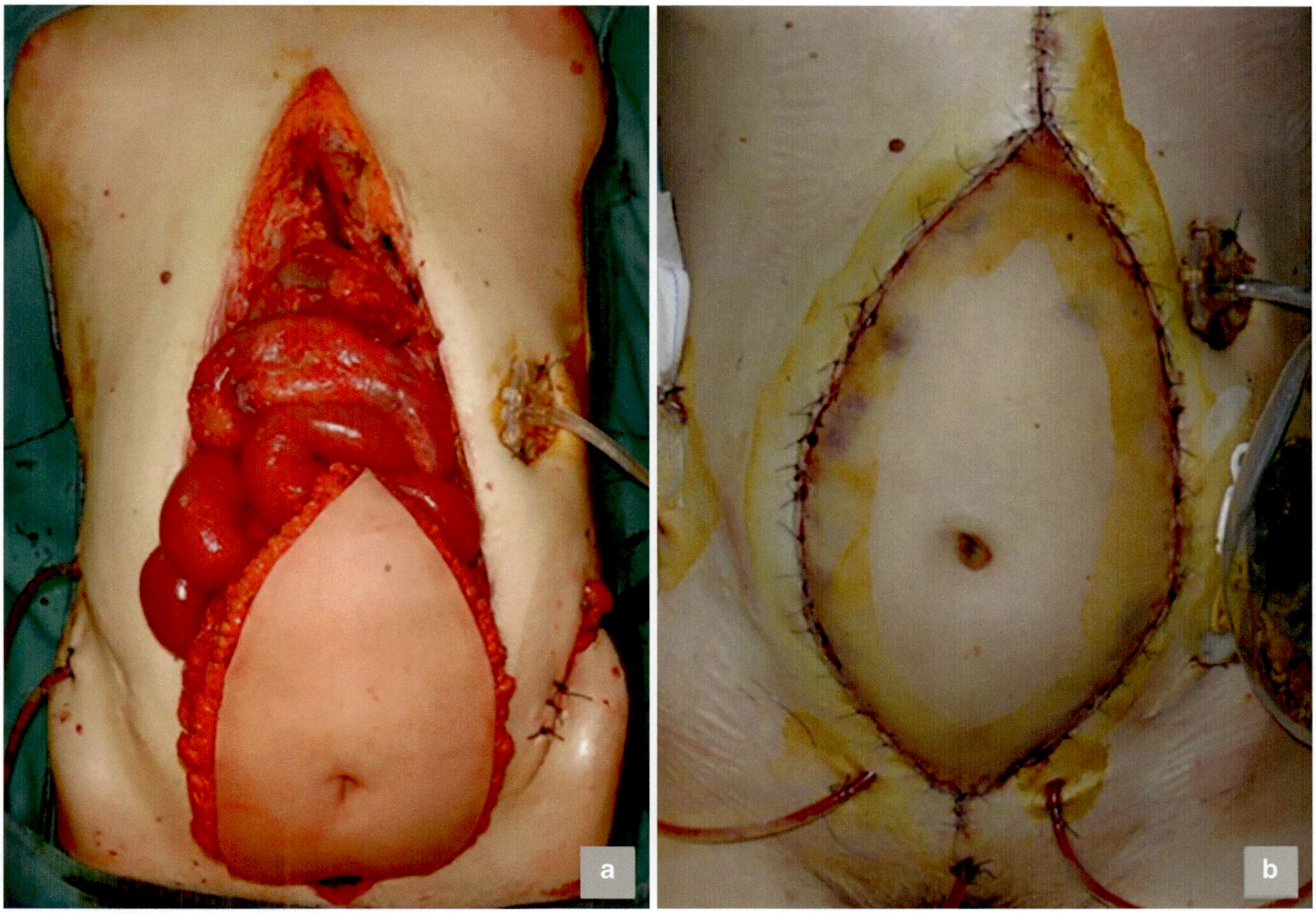

Fig. 28.3 A 16-year-old girl affected by complete bowel atony has been treated with total ITx (2**a**) combined to AWTx. (2**b**), by using microsurgical procedure. Recurrent episodes of GVHD were successfully treated by corticosteroids. At 25 months after transplantation, death occurred due to cerebral aspergillosis

Table 28.4 Microsurgical technique for AWTx, performed in Bologna University Hospital since 2007

Bologna microsurgical technique: how we do it		
Preoperative planning		
Step 1	The graft consists of a median oval cutaneous composite flap, extended from xiphoid to pubis, from one oblique muscle to the other (average size: 16 × 22 cm)	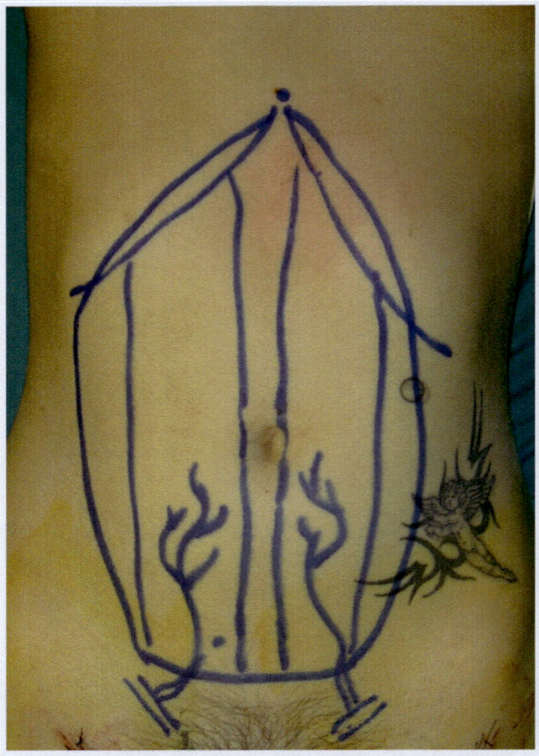
Sequential steps in abdominal wall flap dissection		
Step 2	Bi-subcostal incisions continuing the lateral edges of the rectus muscles till groins bilaterally	
Step 3	Identification of external iliac vessels and of the DIEav	
Step 4	Transverse suprapubic incision	
Step 5	Abdominal flap turning downward to harvest abdominal organs	
Step 6	Dissection of the inferior epigastric pedicles of the abdominal wall flap at the origin from iliac vessels and their section	
Abdominal wall flap storage and donor site closure		
Step 7	Cold perfusion cannulation of the DIEav	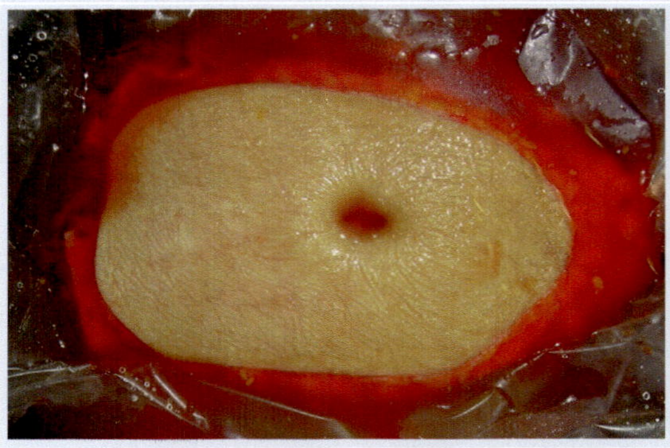
Step 8	Storage with ice and celsior solution	
Step 9	Primary closure of the donor	
Abdominal wall flap microanastomosis and defect closure		
Step 10	The AWT is performed after abdominal organs transplantation	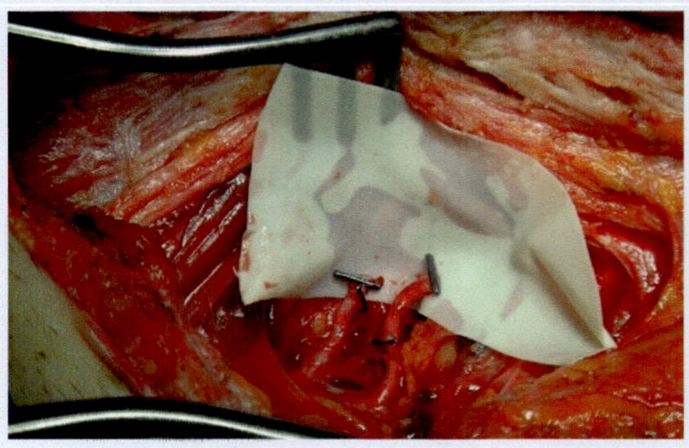
Step 11	End-to-End anastomoses between donor epigastric pedicles and recipient deep inferior epigastric vessels (Nylon monofilament 9.0—Interrupted sutures)	
Step 12	Ileostomy	
Step 13	NO tension multilayers recipient suture	

Table 28.4 (continued)

Bologna microsurgical technique: how we do it		
Postoperative management		
Step 14	*AWTx monitoring:*	
	• Clinical observation of the skin perfusion (color and the temperature of the skin paddle, capillary refill, SatO2)	
	AWTx/intestinal viability and rejections	
	• Punch biopsies (1/biopsy every week for the first month)	
	Immunosuppressive postoperative therapy	
	• Tacrolimus baseline agent	

How we do it: pre-operative planning, sequential steps in abdominal wall dissection, graft storage and donor site closure, microanastomosis and recipient closure, postoperative management

Table 28.5 Ischemia time

	Time (min)
Surgical procedure (*average*)	720
Cold ischemia graft (*average*)	376
Warm ischemia graft (*average*)	24
Total ischemia graft (*average*)	400

were currently used for combination therapy in our standard immunosuppressive protocol. Compared with other centers, we did not observe a higher acute or chronic rejection rate, so this regimen was maintained as standard immunosuppression.

28.1.3.1 Monitoring Protocol

Apart from achieving a primary abdominal closure after intestinal and multivisceral transplantation, abdominal wall graft was used as a sentinel to detect immunologic rejections, allowing an early and easier evaluation of the overall transplant survival and avoiding misdiagnosis (rejection vs. infection). Abdominal skin is extremely valuable to study rejection in the AWTx before it manifests in the intestinal graft; once clinically relevant, intestinal rejection is clearly more difficult to control than skin rejection in terms of controlling severe graft injury, septic peritonitis, clinical deterioration, and dehydration. Standard monitoring was performed by using clinical examination of the skin paddle (color, temperature, capillary refill) to identify adequate perfusion. The flow through the inferior epigastric vessels of the graft was monitored with a handheld Doppler ultrasound. Histology of mucosal specimen remains the gold standard for detecting rejection. Punch biopsies of the skin of the graft were undertaken randomly (1 biopsy every week for the first month) and further when rejection was suspected on clinical grounds (clinical symptoms like diarrhea, abdominal distension, and hyperpyrexia were often seen and treated preemptively as surrogate markers of rejection) [17, 18].

Is the program still active?

To date, our experience has reached 6 consecutive abdominal wall transplantation applying microsurgical technique [8]. In all cases the microsurgical technique for vessel anastomosis was used (Table 28.6).

Abdominal graft harvesting and microanastomoses on deep inferior epigastric system require approximatively the same operative time, without impairment to other organs or pedicles, without vascular complications or increasing the risk of vascular thrombosis, saving the donor's iliac vessels to use as vascular grafts [17, 18]. The main features and additional advantages of these surgical techniques are reported in Table 28.7.

How were the transplants funded?

Intestinal (ITx) and multivisceral transplantation (MVTx), combined with abdominal wall transplantation (AWTx) are fully provided by the National (Italian) Government Insurance.

How many patients were approved and how many are on the waiting list?

All the patients approved for ITx/MVTx and AWTx were treated. Nowadays only two patients are still in the waiting list to receive combined ITx/MVTx and AWTx.

Is there any obstacle to the expansion of the program? Describe.

To date, abdominal wall transplantation has always been used as a coverage flap in intestinal transplantation (ITx) or multivisceral transplantation (MVTx). In these cases, graft survival rates are still the lowest in comparison to other solid organ transplants. One of the main reasons is the frequent occurrence of acute cellular rejection (ACR) and its complications.

Table 28.6 Data collection of Bologna's experience on six consecutive AWTx

	1	2	3	4	5	6
Aetiology	Churg strauss vasculitis	Chronic intestinal pseudo-obstruction	Gardner SDR	Bowel atony	Crohn disease	Short gut SDR
Recipient gender	M	M	F	F	M	F
Recipient age	41	33	38	16	33	39
Donor gender	F	F	F	M	M	M
Donor age	23	37	38	11	15	10
Tx	ITx	ITx	ITx	ITx	MVTx	MVTx
Waiting list time (days)	243	1191	357	85	208	72
Complications						
Immediate	Recurrent sepsis					
Intermediate					Wounds dehiscence	
Long-term						Abdominal muscular atrophy
Treatment					TPN + SG	
Immunological outcomes	Mild ACR	Moderate ACR		Recurrent episodes of GVHD		
Treatment	Steroids	Steroids		Steroids + extracorporeal photopheresis		
Follow up	Deceased	Deceased	Deceased	Deceased	Deceased	Alive
Days	331	4775	844	742	103	**1433**
Cause of death	PTLD ✗	CRF + SEPSIS ✗	Bladder squamous cell carcinoma lung neoplasia ✗	CA ✗	MA ✗	Alive ✓

Table 28.7 The main features and additional advantages of abdominal wall transplantation (AWTx)

General advantages of the AWTx	Additional specific advantages of AWTx microsurgical technique
Safe coverage of the multivisceral graft	→ Safe coverage of the multivisceral graft
NO further immunosuppression	→ NO further immunosuppression
Reduction of morbidity and mortality	→ Reduction of morbidity and mortality
	Anastomoses on extra peritoneal vessels mean no compression on transplanted organs
	More superficial vessels than iliac ones are rarely involved in scar tissue
	Donor iliac vessels are available as vascular graft for other surgeons

28.2 Future Perspectives

At the moment abdominal wall transplantation has always been used as a coverage flap allowing good esthetic results. In literature there is not any report of successful reinnervation of the abdominal graft muscles that is definitely advisable in the future, in order to improve in the long term the organs contention and patient's everyday activities [21]. Lessons learned has been summarized in Table 28.8.

Table 28.8 Lesson learned

Lesson learned	
What are the strengths of your program?	The main advantage to use a composite abdominal allograft is no need for further immunosuppression Microsurgical procedure performing anastomosis on deep inferior epigastric vessels requires the same operative time of the traditional procedure proposed by Levi The recruitment of the abdominal flap does not compromise viscera or other vascular pedicles, does not involve complications, saving the donor's iliac vessels to use as vascular grafts
What did you change over time?	The knowledge of the blood supply is important when planning the transplantation of the anterior abdominal wall and help surgeons to choose which vessels to anastomose to adequately perfuse the whole abdominal graft. According the current anatomical knowledge, the anastomosis of a single DIEA and DIEV are sufficient to guarantee perfusion for a conventional abdominal graft. Monolateral anastomosis allows to perform AWTx when previous surgeries, vessel injuries or trauma on the donor's abdomen could alter donor graft vessels
What will you not repeat in the future?	I would avoid abdominal graft from male donors for female recipients and vice versa
How do you see the future of VCA?	About AWTx, new protocols in immunomodulation and progress in neurotized transplant, could expand surgical indications far beyond the ITx/MVTx, as in wide abdominal defects or large hernias, including abdominal wall transplantation for an elective non-lifesaving procedure

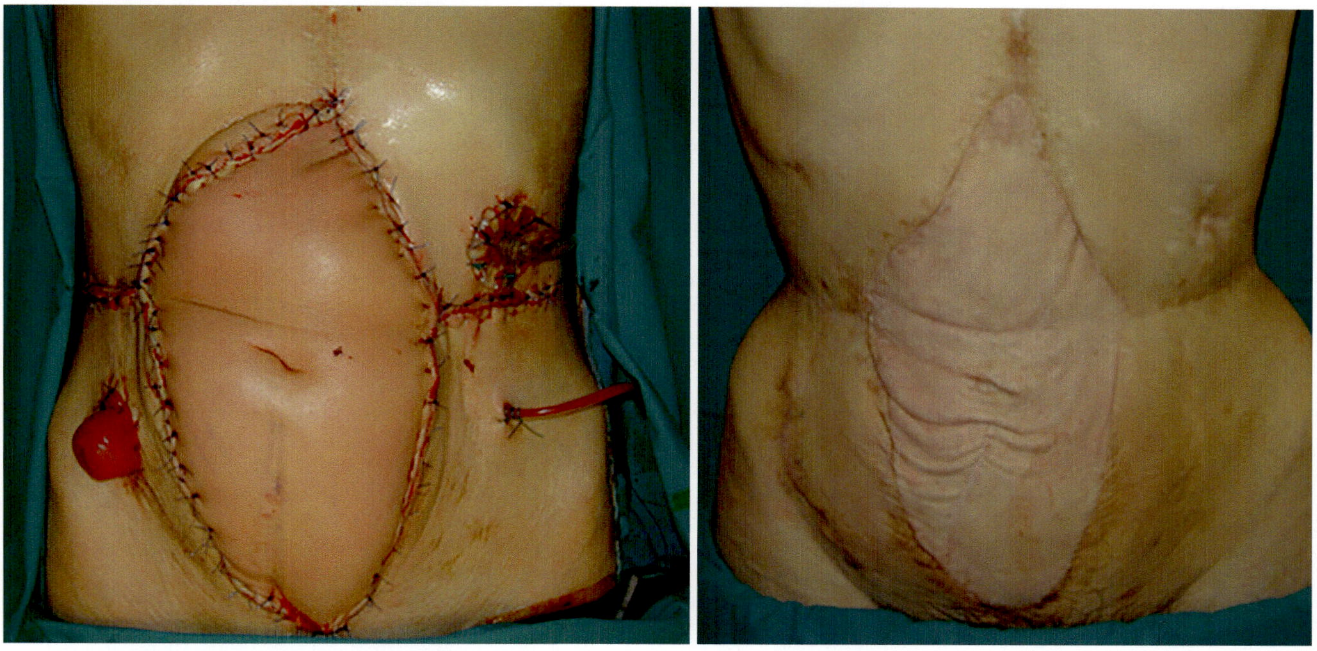

Fig. 28.4 Appearance of the hypotrophic abdominal wall without reinnervation of the graft

The role of the innervation of the abdominal wall graft in achieving a functional result is to date unclear. Every AW-VCA performed to date has been nonfunctional, non-neurotized composite allograft with consequent loss of strength and ability to maintain muscle mass, to resist atrophy, to provide dynamic support and movements, to optimize respiratory mechanism (Fig. 28.4) [2].

Current research on cadavers and animals is exploring the potential for reinnervation to maintain muscle viability and function, but to date, no functional and neurotized composite abdominal allograft was performed in vivo [22]. About AWTx, new protocols in immunomodulation and progress in neurotized transplant could expand surgical indications far beyond the ITx/MVTx, as in wide abdominal defects or large hernias, where traditional abdominal reconstruction is not possible, including abdominal wall transplantation for an elective non-lifesaving procedure.

28.3 Conclusions

Abdominal wall transplantation (AWT) is nowadays the gold standard for the complete loss of the domain or multiple scars in patients undergoing visceral organ transplantation, where no alternatives for traditional wall repair are possible. Both traditional macrosurgical procedure and microsurgical approach are well described and used worldwide. AWTx, based on microanastomosis on deep inferior epigastric vessels is a safe and reliable procedure.

Despite the potential advantages and acceptable outcomes (AWTx risk of rejection and graft versus host disease, GVHD, appear to be similar to ITx without AWTx), AWTx remains an uncommonly performed procedure, and it is not a solution for wide abdominal wall defects in patients not receiving visceral transplant.

References

1. Zanfi C, Cescon M, Lauro A, Dazzi A, Ercolani G, Grazi GL, Del Gaudio M, Ravaioli M, Cucchetti A, La Barba G, Zanello M, Cipriani R, Pinna AD. Incidence and management of abdominal closure-related complications in adult intestinal transplantation. Transplantation. 2008;85(11):1607–9.
2. Berli JU, Broyles JM, Lough D, Shridharani SM, Rochlin D, Cooney DS, Lee WP, Brandacher G, Sacks JM. Current concepts and systematic review of vascularized composite allotransplantation of the abdominal wall. Clin Transpl. 2013;27(6):781–9.
3. Alexandrides IJ, Liu P, Marshall DM, Nery JR, Tzakis AG, Thaller SR. Abdominal wall closure after intestinal transplantation. Plast Reconstr Surg. 2000;106(4):805–12.
4. Di Benedetto F, Lauro A, Masetti M, Cautero N, De Ruvo N, Quintini C, Diago Uso' T, Romano A, Dazzi A, Ramacciato G, Cipriani R, Ercolani G, Grazi GL, Gerunda GE, Pinna AD. Use of prosthetic mesh in difficult abdominal wall closure after small bowel transplantation in adults. Transplant Proc. 2005;37(5):2272–4.
5. Gurunluoglu R, Rosen MJ. Recipient vessels for microsurgical flaps to the abdomen: a systematic review. Microsurgery. 2017;37(6):707–16.
6. Alleyne B, Ozturk CN, Rampazzo A, Johnson J, Gurunluoglu R. Combined submuscular tissue expansion and anterior component separation technique for abdominal wall reconstruction: long-term outcome analysis. J Plast Reconstr Aesthet Surg. 2017;70(6):752–8.
7. Wooten KE, Ozturk CN, Ozturk C, Laub P, Aronoff N, Gurunluoglu R. Role of tissue expansion in abdominal wall reconstruction: a systematic evidence-based review. J Plast Reconstr Aesthet Surg. 2017;70(6):741–51.
8. Aliotta RE, Gatherwright J, Krpata D, Rosenblatt S, Rosen M, Gurunluoglu R. Complex abdominal wall reconstruction, harness-

ing the power of a specialized multidisciplinary team to improve pain and quality of life. Hernia. 2019;23(2):205–15.
9. Oikawa K, Ohkohchi N, Kato H, Orii T, Shimaoka S, Kawagishi N, Asakura T, Takayama J, Satomi S. Graft weight/recipient body weight ratio (G/R ratio) in living-related liver transplantation for pediatric patients: abdominal wall closure in cases with a large G/R ratio. Transplant Proc. 1998;30(7):3209–10.
10. Kimata Y, Uchiyama K, Sekido M, Sakuraba M, Iida H, Nakatsuka T, Harii K. Anterolateral thigh flap for abdominal wall reconstruction. Plast Reconstr Surg. 1999;103(4):1191–7.
11. Ng RW, Chan JY, Mok V, Li GK. Clinical use of a pedicled anterolateral thigh flap. J Plast Reconstr Aesthet Surg. 2008;61(2):158–64.
12. Levi DM, Tzakis AG, Kato T, Madariaga J, Mittal NK, Nery J, Nishida S, Ruiz P. Transplantation of the abdominal wall. Lancet. 2003;361(9376):2173–6.
13. Broyles JM, Berli J, Tuffaha SH, Sarhane KA, Cooney DS, Eckhauser FE, Lee WP, Brandacher G, Singh DP, Sacks JM. Functional abdominal wall reconstruction using an innervated abdominal wall vascularized composite tissue allograft: a cadaveric study and review of the literature. J Reconstr Microsurg. 2015;31(1):39–44.
14. Molitor M, Oliverius M, Sukop A. Abdominal wall allotransplantation. Biomed Pap Med Fac Univ Palacky Olomouc Czech Repub. 2018;162(3):184–9.
15. Carlsen BT, Farmer DG, Busuttil RW, Miller TA, Rudkin GH. Incidence and management of abdominal wall defects after intestinal and multivisceral transplantation. Plast Reconstr Surg. 2007;119(4):1247–55; discussion 1256–8.
16. Fishbein TM, Bodian CA, Miller CM. National sharing of cadaveric isolated intestinal allografts for human transplantation: a feasibility study. Transplantation. 2000;69(5):859–63.
17. Cipriani R, Negosanti L, Pinto V, Sgarzani R, Gelati C, Contedini F. Abdominal wall transplantation and technique. In: Pinna AD, Ercolani G, editors. Abdominal solid organ transplantation: immunology, indications, techniques and early complications (cap 26). Cham: Springer International; 2015. p. 379–89.
18. Cipriani R, Contedini F, Santoli M, Gelati C, Sgarzani R, Cucchetti A, Lauro A, Pinna AD. Abdominal wall transplantation with microsurgical technique. Am J Transplant. 2007;7(5):1304–7.
19. Tzakis AG, Kato T, Nishida S, Levi D, Madariaga J, De Faria W, Nery J, Neff G, Kirk AD, Ruiz P. Campath-1H in intestinal and multivisceral transplantation: preliminary data. Transplant Proc. 2002;34(3):937.
20. Selvaggi G, Levi DM, Cipriani R, Sgarzani R, Pinna AD, Tzakis AG. Abdominal wall transplantation: surgical and immunologic aspects. Transplant Proc. 2009;41(2):521–2.
21. Park SH, Eun SC. Abdominal wall transplant surgery. Exp Clin Transplant. 2018;16(6):745–50.
22. Singh DP, Mavrophilipos VD, Zapora JA, Berli J, Broyles J, Chopra K, Sabino J, Matthews J, Buckingham EB, Maddox JS, Bluebond-Langner R, Silverman RP. Novel technique for innervated abdominal wall vascularized composite allotransplantation: a separation of components approach. Eplasty. 2014;14:e34.

Part VII

Uterus Transplantation

Deceased Donor Uterus Transplantation

29

Giuseppe D'Amico, Luca Del Prete, Elliott Richards, Stephanie Ricci, Cristiano Quintini, Andreas Tzakis, Anil Vaidya, and Tommaso Falcone

29.1 Introduction

The Cleveland Clinic trial on uterus transplantation (UT) (NCT02573415) is the first one in the USA that investigates outcomes after deceased donation (DD). Our group decided to deepen cadaveric donation to overcome donor comorbidity in a life-enhancing surgical procedure and not life-saving. Importantly, we strongly believe that this is a fundamental research area considering the outstanding results published in the first case series of UT from living donation (LD).

This feasibility study aims to enroll ten patients who will undergo UT at Cleveland Clinic. We estimated that, due to organ shortage, compatibility, and practical considerations (distance, cold ischemia time, blood type, viral serology status), 75 subjects will need to be enrolled to perform 10 uterine transplants within 3 years. We expected that at least 50% of the subjects screened will not qualify as transplant candidates. Consequently, we anticipated that approximately 75–100 candidates will need to be screened within our clinic. Calculating the donor availability of approximately one every other month, this would mean we needed to list 18 recipients initially. The recruiting started on October 2015 and study completion will be on October 2023. The first transplant was performed on February 2, 2016.

The aims of our study are:

1. To evaluate the feasibility and safety of UT from DD for women with absolute uterine factor infertility (AUFI).
2. To ascertain whether uterine transplantation from deceased donors can support 1–2 pregnancies and live births for the recipient using embryos resulting from pre-transplantation in vitro fertilization, specifically to report.
3. To assess whether pregnancies resulting through IVF and uterine transplantation have an increased risk of pregnancy complications.
4. To assess whether infants born from uterine transplantation have an increased risk of neonatal complications.

The primary outcome is the number of successful live births after UT and in vitro fertilization (IVF), whereas the secondary outcome is the rate of pregnancy complications after IVF and UT. In particular, we focused on the development of gestational hypertension, pre-eclampsia, intrauterine growth restriction, premature rupture of membranes, preterm delivery, and intrauterine fetal demise. Another secondary outcome considered is the rate of neonatal complications in the offspring, with high consideration of birth defects, perinatal infections, low birth weight, neonatal death, and neonatal intensive care unit admissions.

29.2 Cleveland Clinic Protocol

29.2.1 Recipient Selection

The most common indication in clinical trials of uterus transplantation is congenital absence of the uterus, such as mullerian agenesis, although there are many causes of absolute uterine factor infertility (UFI) [1]. Recent studies of interested candidates show a diverse group of interested patients including those with acquired UFI; e.g., those who underwent a hysterectomy for obstetric or gynecologic conditions [2]. Before uterus transplantation, the only option for patients with UFI to have a biologically related child was a gestational carrier. However, this option is not available to many people in the world. The ethical issues related to uterus transplantation have been extensively reviewed [3, 4]. The gen-

G. D'Amico (✉) · L. Del Prete · C. Quintini · A. Tzakis
A. Vaidya
Department of General Surgery, Transplantation Center, Digestive Disease and Surgery Institute, Cleveland Clinic, Cleveland, OH, USA
e-mail: damicog@ccf.org; delprel@ccf.org; quintic@ccf.org; tzakisa@ccf.org; vaidyaa2@ccf.org

E. Richards · S. Ricci · T. Falcone
Obstetrics and Gynecology and Women's Health Institute, Cleveland Clinic, Cleveland, OH, USA
e-mail: richare@ccf.org; riccis@ccf.org; falcont@ccf.org

© Springer Nature Switzerland AG 2023
R. Gurunian et al. (eds.), *Reconstructive Transplantation*, https://doi.org/10.1007/978-3-031-21520-9_29

eral principles of implementation of uterus transplantation have been outlined by American Society for Reproductive Medicine position statement on uterus transplantation [5]. The Cleveland Clinic exclusively uses deceased donors in their transplant program for reasons outlined in previous publications [6–8]. To summarize these documents: the technical procedure for procurement of a uterus in a living donor is associated with risk, both physical and psychologic, that we feel must be improved before implementing living donors in our program. In 2020, we reported the first birth from a deceased donor transplant program in the USA and the second in the world [9].

All recipients are pre-screened to confirm they meet study criteria such as age and menopausal status. The patient then is given a formal in-person assessment by members of our multidisciplinary team that includes transplant surgeons, gynecologic surgeons, reproductive endocrinologists, psychologists, bioethicists, social workers, and maternal-fetal medicine specialists. A physical exam is performed to assess vaginal length and need for dilation. The patient then progresses through several steps in order to be accepted as a transplant recipient (Fig. 29.1). It is important to exclude patients at risk for vascular disease or an underlying disease that may recur with anti-rejection drugs. A history of hypertension, diabetes, HIV, hepatitis B/C, mycobacteria, current tobacco use, high BMI, prior malignancy (except for early stage cervical cancer), prior uterus transplant, and low lying pelvic kidney also increases risk and therefore patients with these conditions are excluded. If the patient completes this screening phase, she moves to assisted reproductive technology in order to obtain sufficient embryos to achieve at least 1 pregnancy (our program currently has a requirement of six cryopreserved embryos).

29.2.2 Donor Selection

The donor selection for a deceased donor program is similar to living donor with some modification. In general, a history of infertility, recurrent pregnancy loss, and any chronic medical conditions that can affect vascular survival are excluded. The BMI upper limit is not as important for a deceased donor program and donors are accepted for uterus donation if they are a candidate for other intra-abdominal organ donation. In addition, premenopausal status is more important for deceased donor than living donor. In living donor programs, estrogen may be given to postmenopausal women in order to increase the diameter of the uterine arteries. This requires weeks of hormonal treatment to achieve the desired effect. As with living donors, infectious disease investigation including assessment of Zika virus risk is required. CMV status is preferred to match with the appropriate recipient. Only after extensive counseling and in the case of no other suitable candidates does our program allow uteri from CMV positive donors to be transplanted into CMV negative recipients. The donor uterus is assessed with imaging to rule clinically important uterine pathology. Imaging to assess vascular patency of vessels to the uterus is also required. As is typical of deceased donor programs, the protocol is similar to other organs (Fig. 29.2).

29.2.3 Post-Transplant Process for Pregnancy

The viability of the organ is monitored by ultrasound. Rejection is monitored with cervical biopsies. When it is deemed acceptable to proceed (typically after 6 months), an embryo transfer is performed. Embryo transfers may be

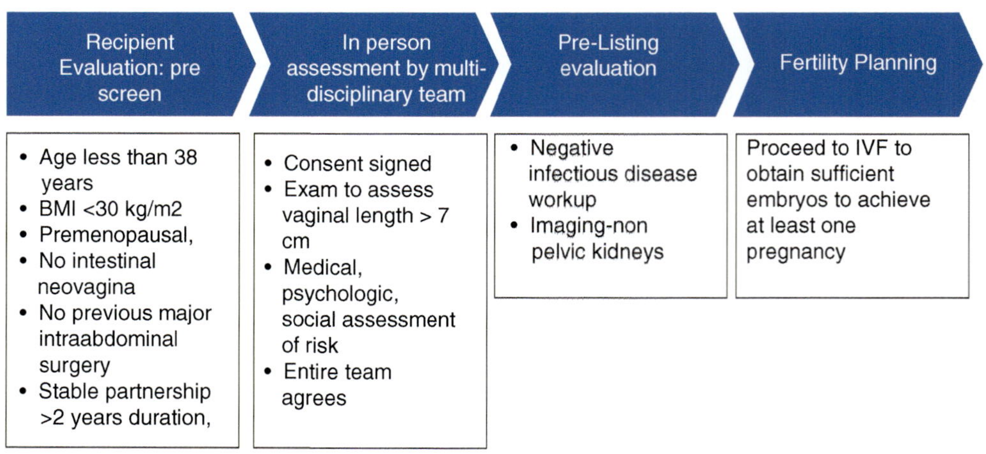

Fig. 29.1 Recipient assessment

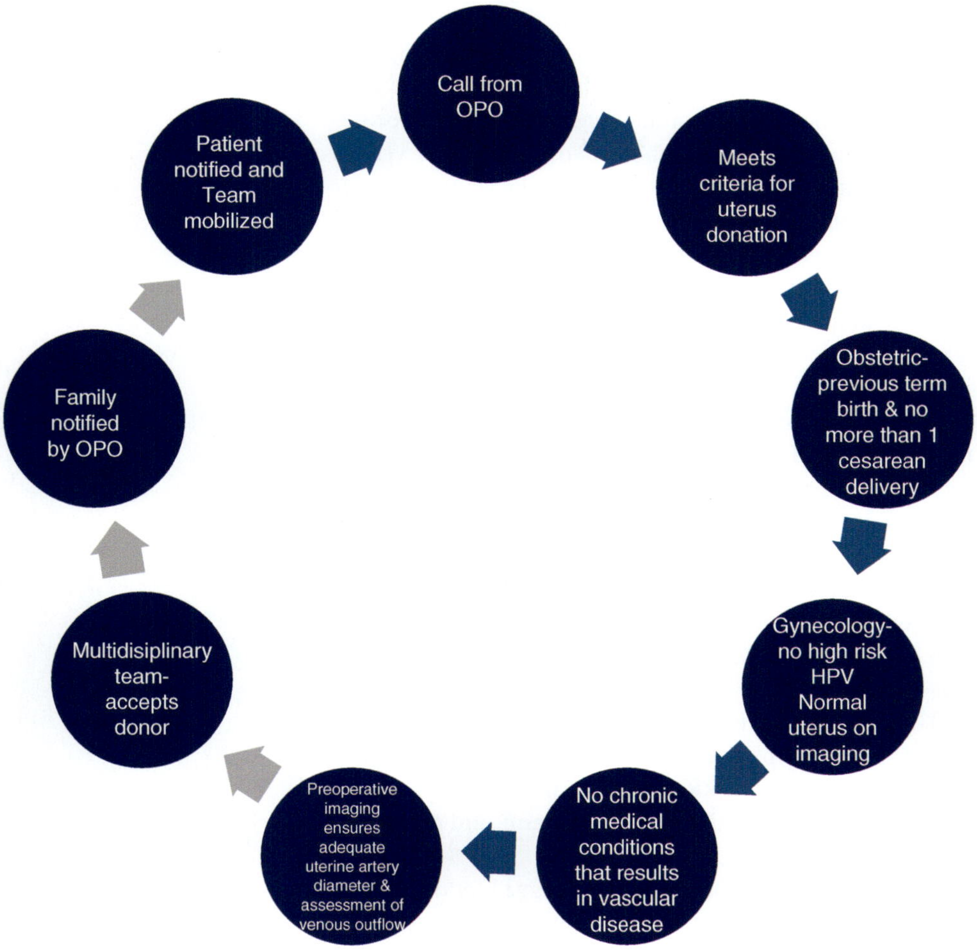
Call from OPO
Meets criteria for uterus donation
Obstetric-previous term birth & no more than 1 cesarean delivery
Gynecology-no high risk HPV Normal uterus on imaging
No chronic medical conditions that results in vascular disease
Preoperative imaging ensures adequate uterine artery diameter & assessment of venous outflow
Multidisiplinary team-accepts donor
Family notified by OPO
Patient notified and Team mobilized

Fig. 29.2 Deceased donor selection

challenging because of stenosis between the upper donor vagina and recipient. Vaginal anastomotic stenosis has been successively treated in our patients with use of vaginal dilators and/or surgical revision under anesthesia. Other programs have reported use of self-expanding vaginal stents to treat vaginal stenosis [10].

Perinatal outcomes resemble those seen with other solid organ transplantation, and anti-rejection drugs are managed similar to other transplant recipients who are pregnant. Our program uses tacrolimus, azathioprine, and prednisone during pregnancy. Renal function tests can become abnormal and therefore requires close (weekly) monitoring with adjustment of tacrolimus. Preterm birth and low birth weight are the most common perinatal complications. Neonatal outcomes have not revealed any unique features related to transplantation. Cesarean section is performed with all deliveries. The uterus is removed after 1–2 deliveries and usually performed at the time of Cesarean section, though interval hysterectomy is also considered acceptable.

29.2.4 Operative Management and Surgical Technique

29.2.4.1 Procurement

Once a donor is identified, a 200 mg miconazole intravaginal suppository or miconazole 2% vaginal cream will be placed into the posterior fornix of the vagina. The povidone-iodine solution vaginal disinfection will be performed in the operating room before and after the hysteroscopy which will be done at the outset of the case prior to performing an abdominal incision on the donor for multiorgan recovery. If the donor has had a normal transvaginal ultrasound within the past year or a preoperative ultrasound, then the donor hysteroscopy is not necessary. A second 200 mg miconazole intravaginal suppository will be inserted in the operating room. The donor will also receive Micafungin 100 mg IV on call to the operating room.

The uterus procurement technique has been conceptualized to preserve both uterus graft and life-saving organs, giving priority to the latter [11]. Furthermore, uterus is the last organ procured and vaginal section is made only after all the other organs and graft are already harvested to avoid contamination. The most important concept of uterus procurement is to not compromise the venous return. The venous return is optimally obtained from the uterine veins. However the utero-ovarian or ovarian veins are removed as a potential alternative source. The uterine veins originate from the internal iliac vein and move medially and have a variable course in its relationship to the ureter. Furthermore the uterine vein may be a single trunk such as deep uterine vein or tributaries. In a living donor this dissection is tedious and requires a lot of time in order not to damage the ureter. In a deceased donor the ureter is cut before it enters the parametrium and all tissues surrounding the uterus are taken en bloc so that the venous return is not compromised.

Uterus procurement takes place in 6 steps:

Step 1: Dissection of the ureters from the pelvic brim

Maximal exposure is obtained with a reverse arrow incision (Tzakis incision), a xiphoid-pubic with bilateral extension from the pubis to the 12th rib.

The purpose of this step is to avoid separating the distal ureters from the parametrium while preserving adequate length of ureters for the kidney transplants.

Step 2: Ligation of the round ligaments and dissection of the bladder

The round ligament on the uterus is tagged for orientation and utilized during transplantation to anchor the graft to the recipient round ligament. It is crucial that the parametrium with the uterine vessels is never opened but kept attached to the uterus.

Step 3: Dissection of the utero-ovarian and ovarian vessels

The ovaries are detached and separated from the utero-ovarian veins, which are carefully preserved in case they are needed for the outflow of the graft.

Step 4: Identification and ligation of the obliterated umbilical vessels

The lowermost identifiable structure of the specimen is the obliterated umbilical vessels. These are ligated distally at the level of the bladder. These vessels are important landmarks as they invariably lead to their respective uterine artery.

Step 5: Dissection of the internal iliac vessels

The internal iliac artery and vein are recovered 1–2 cm distal to the bifurcation. The gluteal, obturator, and superior rectal branches of the internal iliac artery are carefully ligated or oversewn. The parametrium is kept intact as the dissection proceeds in order to protect the network of minute veins.

Step 6: Dissection of the rectovaginal and vesicovaginal space

Dissection of the vesicovaginal and rectovaginal space takes place contemporaneously and facilitates the delineation of the uterine pedicles. An umbilical tape is placed around the vagina to facilitate its transection during the final removal of the graft.

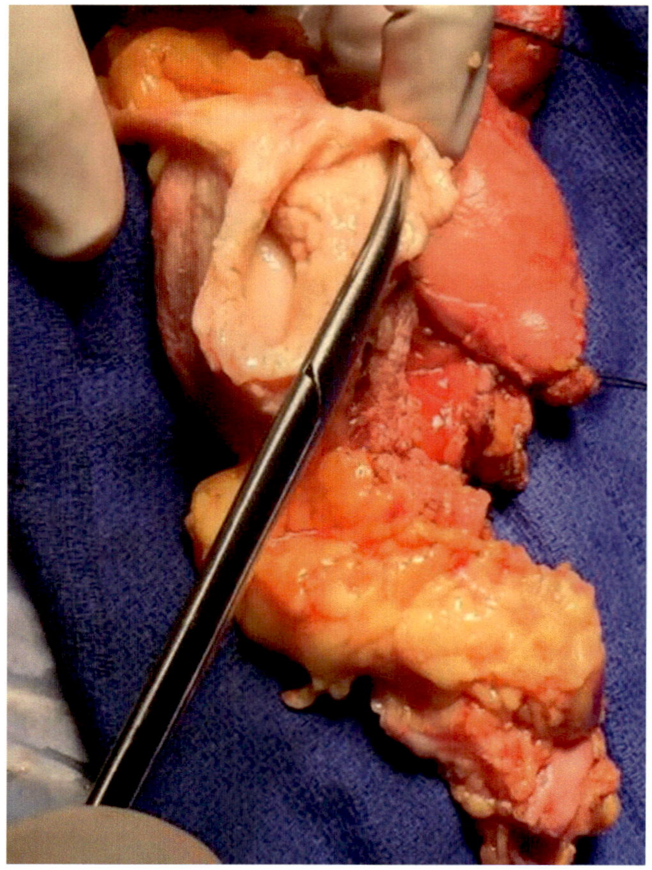

Fig. 29.3 Donor's vagina. Its section occurred as last part of the multiorgan procurement and it should be reopened at the time of vagina re-anastomosis in the recipient

The closure of the graft's vagina will take place after core cooling but before placement in preservation solution. It will only be reopened at the time of the vaginal re-anastomosis in the recipient. Graft's vagina is depicted in Fig. 29.3.

Importantly, the sacrifice of the ovaries and long vascular pedicles harvesting, including gonadal vessels and internal iliac vessel, do not represent a problem in the cadaveric uterus procurement.

Uterus procurement steps and uterus graft after DD procurement are depicted in Figs. 29.4 and 29.5, respectively. Typically procurement in a deceased donor takes less than 2 hours.

29.2.4.2 Transplant

On admission to the hospital the recipient's vulva and vagina will be prepped for 2 min using 10% povidone-iodine solution followed by insertion of 200 mg miconazole intravaginal suppository. This process will be repeated intraoperatively. Subjects with an iodine allergy will have the vulva and vagina prepped using baby shampoo.

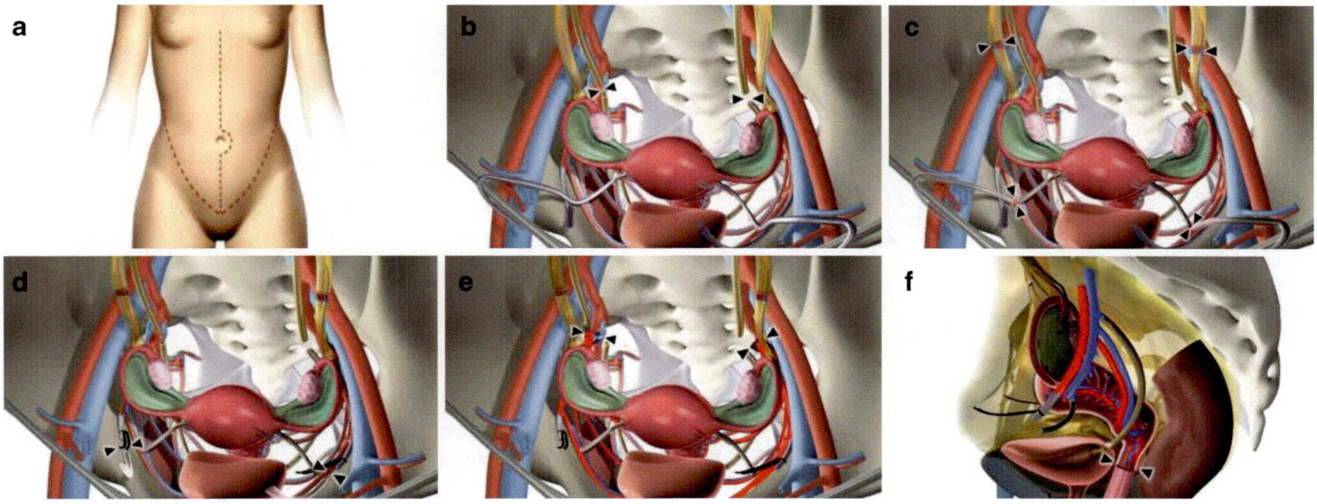

Fig. 29.4 (**a**) Reverse arrow Tzakis incision; (**b**) step 1, dissection of the ureters from the pelvic brim; (**c**) steps 2 and 3, ligation of the round ligaments, dissection of the bladder and of the utero-ovarian and ovarian vessels; (**d**) step 4, identification and ligation of the obliterated umbilical vessels; (**e**) step 5, dissection of the internal iliac vessels; (**f**) step 6, dissection of the rectovaginal and vesicovaginal space

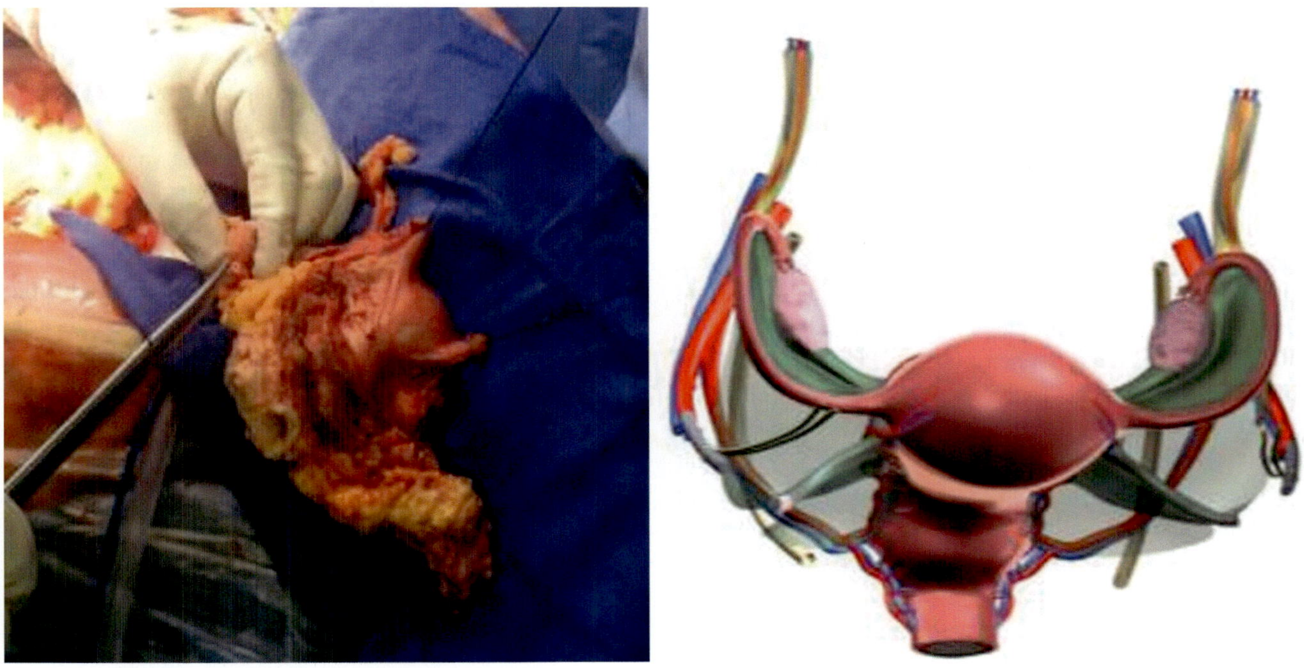

Fig. 29.5 Uterus graft after deceased donor procurement. Gonadal vessels and internal iliac vein can be procured without affecting life-saving organ procurement or donor morbidity. The ovaries are removed during backtable

The transplant will take place within 7 h of recovery of the uterus from the DD.

The iliac vessels will be exposed bilaterally as will the vagina/neovagina of the recipient. The uterine vessels of the donor will be anastomosed to the iliac vessels of the recipient bilaterally. The vault of the vagina of the donor will be anastomosed to the vagina of the recipient. This will allow for a functioning uterus with adequate blood supply which is connected to a functional vagina. The uterus will be perfused after unilateral artery and vein are anastomosed. Either the left or right arterial and venous anastomosis will be completed and the uterus will be re-perfused prior to contralateral vascular anastomosis. If the uterine vessels (arteries or veins) are inadequate for anastomosis, the utero-ovarian vessels may be used for anastomosis. When all anastomoses are completed, an ultrasound of the graft will be performed in the operating room. In addition, another ultrasound will be performed during postoperative day (POD) 0. Graft and recipient's vessels and vaginal cuff before anastomosis are depicted in Fig. 29.6.

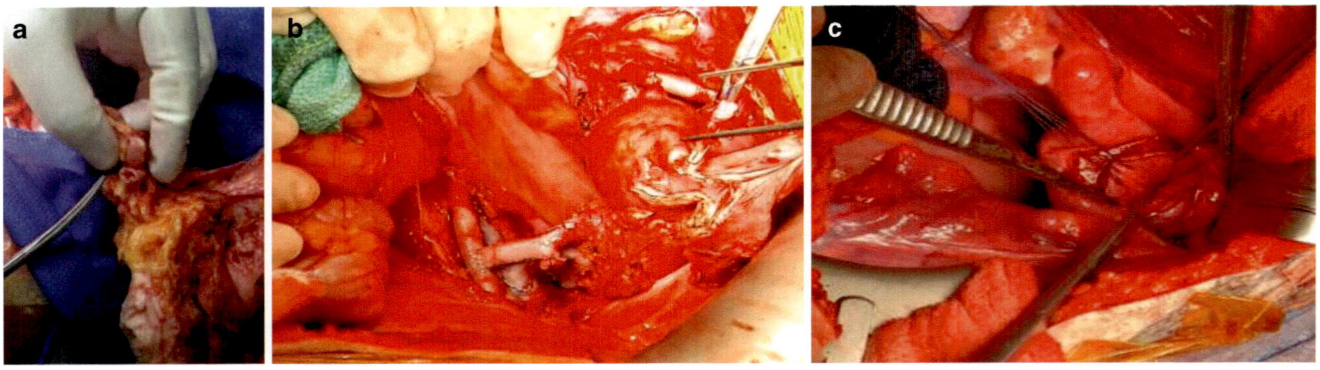

Fig. 29.6 (**a**) The internal iliac artery and vein are recovered 1–2 cm distal to the bifurcation. The parametrium is kept intact as the dissection proceeds in order to protect the network of minute veins. (**b**) Donor's internal iliac vessels are anastomosed with recipient's external iliac vessels. The wide caliber makes the vascular anastomosis easier and less prone to complication. (**c**) Vaginal cuff prepared for anastomosis

29.2.5 Immunosuppression

The immunosuppression treatment will begin with induction and then continue with maintenance treatment. Thymoglobulin 1.5 mg/kg intravenous (IV) will be started on POD 0. For the first thymoglobulin dose, the subject will be pre-medicated 30 min prior with hydrocortisone 200 mg IV, diphenhydramine 50 mg IV, and acetaminophen 500 mg per os (PO). Thymoglobulin will also be given on POD 2 and 4. On POD 2, the patient will be pre-medicated 30 min prior to receiving thymoglobulin with hydrocortisone 100 mg IV, diphenhydramine 50 mg IV, and acetaminophen 500 mg PO. On POD 4, the subject will be pre-medicated 30 min prior to receiving thymoglobulin with diphenhydramine 50 mg IV and acetaminophen 500 mg PO. Doses will be adjusted for thrombocytopenia, if the platelet count is <25,000 the dose will be cut in half; if the platelet count is <15,000 the dose will be held for 24 h and the platelet count will be reassessed. Platelet infusions can be considered but these subjects are young, with no coagulation problems or renal insufficiency, so the risk of intracranial bleeding from thrombocytopenia is minimal.

Tacrolimus will be administered orally with a starting dose of 1–2 mg twice a day. Levels will be followed closely and adjusted accordingly to achieve a 12 h trough level of 7–11 ng/mL.

Methylprednisolone will be administered IV from induction to POD 5 at the dose of 1000 mg, 50 mg, 40 mg, 30 mg, 20 mg, and 20 mg respectively. Prednisone 20 mg PO will be administered daily thereafter.

Mycophenolate mofetil (MMF) will be started orally post-operatively as 1000 mg every 12 h. As an option, calcineurin inhibitors can be replaced with mTOR inhibitors, if the calcineurin inhibitors are not tolerated: sirolimus will be started with a loading dose of 5 mg once daily and then maintenance dose of 1–2 mg daily, or everolimus will be started at 1–2 mg every 12 h. Medications will be adjusted to maintain trough levels of 7–10.

The cervix provides a simple and non-invasive method of evaluating the graft for rejection. Speculum examination will be performed 2 weeks after the transplant and then monthly until ready to begin embryo transfers for pregnancy. If there is a concern for graft viability or rejection, this exam and biopsy may be performed sooner or more frequently during follow-up than anticipated. During pregnancy, the cervix and vagina will be inspected and biopsied at least once per trimester. Following delivery, cervical and/or vaginal biopsy monitoring will decrease to every 3 months (+/− 1 month) until the decision is made on a second pregnancy or medical/surgical hysterectomy is performed.

Mild to moderate rejection will be treated with a steroid cycle and increased tacrolimus dose. For a severe rejection, thymoglobulin will be ordered. If the transplant team feels it is safe, a second course of thymoglobulin may be administered with the research team's unanimous approval. A third course of thymoglobulin will not be administered unless the entire clinical team is in agreement and the DSMB also approves. A clinical decision will be made to remove the graft if the rejection progresses, does not regress, or recurs despite treatment. Because the uterus is not a vital organ, the threshold of graft removal will be lower than in the case of the vital organs.

29.2.6 Follow-Up

If the subject opts to keep the uterus for a second pregnancy, from the time of the first childbirth, there will be a wait time of a minimum of 12 months prior to attempting a second pregnancy.

The visit schedule will be every 3 months. During the follow-up visits the subject will be examined by the transplant surgeon and gynecologist and have cervical and/or vaginal biopsies and follow-up testing including blood testing, ultrasounds, and if recommended, abdominal CT or MRI. If a hysterectomy was performed, no further biopsies will be needed.

In addition, during the 12-month follow-up visit post-transplant, a consult with psychiatry will be scheduled. Rating scales will be administered for quantitative assessment of anxiety, depression, personality disorder, and quality of life and spousal/partner support. In addition to being administered during phase I and 12 month follow-up time points, the additional administration of these rating scales can vary pending psychiatry's recommendation.

In conjunction with the subject's follow-up, the baby will be brought in for follow-up as well. A neonatologist will assess the baby 3 months (+/−1 month) after birth. After the initial follow-up, subsequent appointments will be determined by the neonatologist as needed.

Once immunosuppression is stopped, after 1–2 successful live births (or sooner if clinical circumstances favor removal) a hysterectomy procedure will be performed, the study will end and the patient will be followed as standard of care.

29.2.7 Ethical Problems in Cadaveric Uterus Donation

The choice between utilizing a cadaveric graft or a living donor represents one key decision point [12]. We have elected to pursue the deceased donor option and thereby avoid all of the risks to the donor associated with living donation. This is especially relevant given the instance of ureteral injury to a living donor recorded in many uterine transplant studies. We do recognize that other research groups have chosen the living donor route and understand the clinical and scientific merits of that approach. Our decision was based in part on the ethical premise of "first do no harm." A concept that applies to considerations for both the donor and recipient. We have developed a system of education and informed consent to discuss the risk–benefit analysis based on our current understanding of the potential complications that may arise with either a living or deceased donor.

A common challenging problem with other composite tissue donation is represented by the consent to organ donation [13].

Importantly, the substituted judgment of donor's family members is not well-accepted and commonly utilized as in other aspects of surrogate medical decisions in organ donation. Indeed, surrogate decision-making is seldom applied in other aspects of reproductive medicine. However, uterus transplantation is in its infancy. The public's attitude toward this new opportunity and women's opinions of uterus donation could quickly evolve, making the consent to uterus donation an overcame dilemma.

Closing Questions (Q) and Answers (A)

Q: How were the transplants funded?

A: Funding is internally to fund 10 transplants.

Q: How many patients have you screened?

A: More than 300 patients were screened before making the final list.

Q: How many patients were approved and how many are on the waiting list?

A: We listed a total of 16 patients. We have already transplanted 8 women, whereas 4 patients are in the waiting list and four withdrew.

Q: Is there any obstacle to the expansion of the program?

A: To date, the major problem to expand the program is represented by funding.

Q: How many actual patients did receive uterus transplant so far?

A: Eight patients have been transplanted with all grafts procured from deceased brain donor in a setting of multiorgan donation.

Q: Functional outcomes, live births?

A: 6/6 of the viable grafts have had a functional success developing a neo-menarche. Two grafts were removed before they could develop menstruation. Four patients became pregnant and delivered 4 healthy babies.

Q: Did you experience any unique problems or challenges encountered?

A: The first and fifth patients underwent hysterectomy because of fungal infection and graft vascular thrombosis, respectively.

Q: What are the strengths of your program?

A: We are a cohesive multidisciplinary team.

Q: What did you change over time?

A: The most important change was in the procurement. Originally, we did much more dissection before cold ischemia was induced. Now we wait until all organs are removed, then we remove the uterus. Furthermore, in our first case, reperfusion occurred after the vascular pedicles of both sides were anastomosed. However, starting from our second case, we decided to reperfuse the graft after the creation of arterial and venous anastomosis in one side, thus we reduce significantly the warm ischemia time.

Q: What will you not repeat in the future?

A: No change.

Q: How do you see the future of uterus transplant?

A: This will be a standard procedure.

References

1. Hur C, Rehmer J, Flyckt R, Falcone T. Uterine factor infertility: a clinical review. Clin Obstet Gynecol. 2019;62(2):257–70.
2. Arian SE, Flyckt RL, Farrell RM, Falcone T, Tzakis AG. Characterizing women with interest in uterine transplant clinical trials in the United States: who seeks information on this experimental treatment? Am J Obstet Gynecol. 2017;216(2):190–1.
3. Farrell RM, Johannesson L, Flyckt R, Richards EG, Testa G, Tzakis A, et al. Evolving ethical issues with advances in uterus transplantation. Am J Obstet Gynecol. 2020;222(6):584.e1–5.
4. Richards EG, Agatisa PK, Davis AC, Flyckt R, Mabel H, Falcone T, et al. Framing the diagnosis and treatment of absolute uterine factor infertility: insights from in-depth interviews with uterus transplant trial participants. AJOB Empir Bioeth. 2019;10(1):23–35.
5. Practice Committee of the American Society for Reproductive Medicine. Electronic address: asrm@asrm.org, Practice Committee of the American Society for Reproductive Medicine. American society for reproductive medicine position statement on uterus transplantation: a committee opinion. Fertil Steril. 2018;110(4):605–10.
6. Flyckt RL, Farrell RM, Perni UC, Tzakis AG, Falcone T. Deceased donor uterine transplantation: innovation and adaptation. Obstet Gynecol. 2016;128(4):837–42.
7. Flyckt R, Kotlyar A, Arian S, Eghtesad B, Falcone T, Tzakis A. Deceased donor uterine transplantation. Fertil Steril. 2017;107(3):e13.
8. Ricci S, Bennett C, Falcone T. Uterine transplantation: evolving data, success, and clinical importance. J Minim Invasive Gynecol. 2021;28(3):502–12.
9. Flyckt R, Falcone T, Quintini C, Perni U, Eghtesad B, Richards EG, et al. First birth from a deceased donor uterus in the United States: from severe graft rejection to successful cesarean delivery. Am J Obstet Gynecol. 2020;223(2):143–51.
10. Fronek J, Janousek L, Kristek J, Chlupac J, Pluta M, Novotny R, et al. Live birth following uterine transplantation from a nulliparous deceased donor. Transplantation. 2021;105(5):1077–81.
11. D'Amico G, Quintini C, Eghtesad B, Hashimoto K, Ricci S, Flyckt R, et al. Uterus recovery from deceased donor: simple technique securing safety of vital organs and uterus graft. J Am Coll Surg. 2021;232(3):e1–6.
12. Bruno B, Arora KS. Ethical implications of donor type for uterus transplantation: why we should remain wary of using living donors. Yale J Biol Med. 2020;93(4):587–92.
13. Bruno B, Arora KS. Uterus transplantation: the ethics of using deceased versus living donors. Am J Bioeth. 2018;18(7):6–15.

Uterus Transplant: The Dallas Experience

30

Pratik Mehta, Liza Johannesson, and Giuliano Testa

30.1 Introduction

Uterus transplant (UTx) was first conceived as a treatment for patients with absolute uterine factor infertility (AUFI). AUFI can either be congenital or acquired. Congenital AUI is most commonly the result of Mayer–Rokitansky–Kuster–Hauser syndrome and affects roughly 1/5000 women. Acquired AUI is the result of hysterectomy or uterus loss due to benign or obstetric complications. In the United States it is estimated that of the 62 million women of reproductive age, between 1 and 5% may have AUFI. Women who suffer from AUFI are unable to conceive and are forced into either surrogacy or adoption to acquire parenthood. Uterus transplant was devised as a novel treatment to help these women experience gestation and give birth. The basic outline of UTx is as follows.

Prior to UTx the potential recipients undergo in vitro fertilization to require embryos. These embryos are then cryopreserved in the lab. This step is done to make certain that there is reproductive potential present. During the transplantation process, the donor's uterus is removed and implanted into the recipient. The uterine graft may come from either a deceased donor or a living donor. The recipient is started on immunosuppressants to prevent rejection of the uterine graft. Following a monitoring protocol the recipient undergoes serial uterine graft biopsies to assess for acute cellular rejection. Once the first menstrual period is obtained and the recipient has fully recovered from the surgery, embryo transfer is performed. If the embryo transfer is successful and the recipient becomes pregnant, the mother and fetus are monitored as a high risk pregnancy with the goal of delivery by cesarean section. While a second pregnancy can be attempted, this decision requires consideration between the mother and medical team. The decisions regarding a second pregnancy and timing of graft hysterectomy are made jointly between the medical team and recipient, considering recipient/couple preference, immunosuppression-related concerns, maternal and antenatal concerns, and total recipient-graft time. The uterus graft is removed following completion of pregnancies to minimize the risk of infections and to discontinue the use of immunosuppressants.

The first attempt from a living donor was performed in Saudi Arabia in 2000 and the first attempt from a deceased donor was performed in Turkey in 2011 [1, 2]. These early studies helped to demonstrate that the transplanted uterus was capable of achieving menses, while attempts at pregnancy were mixed. These attempts paved the way for the first clinical trial for UTx, reported by the Swedish group [3]. The Swedish clinical trial resulted in the first live birth after UTx in 2014 and established the feasibility of uterine transplantation as a cure to absolute uterine factor infertility.

Given the pioneering work of the Swedish group there was interest in furthering the field with a US clinical trial. The Dallas Uterus Transplant Study (DUETS) was initiated in November 2015 with research approval through the Baylor University Medical Center Ethics Committee and Institutional Review Board. The Dallas Uterus Transplant Study at Baylor University Medical Center was announced on January 29th, 2015. IRB approval was obtained later the same year with enrollment being initiated in 2016. Philanthropic support was provided by Baylor Health Care System Foundation. The trial would cover investigations, surgery, hospital stay, medications, and follow-up visits but would not cover in vitro fertilization (IVF), travel, accommodation, or loss of income. The clinical trial was designed as a prospective study to treat AUFI through UTx resulting in live birth. Primary endpoints include graft survival, recipient survival, and number of live births. Secondary endpoints include number of clinical pregnancies, miscarriages, and rejection episodes. Members of the Swedish group provided significant insight and contributed to the launching of this study. There were five distinct clinical stages in the study: screening, transplant, pregnancy, delivery to explant, and

P. Mehta · L. Johannesson · G. Testa (✉)
Annette C. and Harold C. Simmons Transplant Institute, Baylor University Medical Center, Dallas, TX, USA
e-mail: Liza.johannesson@bswhealth.org; Giuliano.Testa@bswhealth.org

© Springer Nature Switzerland AG 2023
R. Gurunian et al. (eds.), *Reconstructive Transplantation*, https://doi.org/10.1007/978-3-031-21520-9_30

follow-up. Following the announcement of the clinical trial there was a tremendous amount of interest not only from potential recipients, but also from non-directed donors [4].

Since the inception of the Baylor program there have been over 2800 calls or emails requesting further information on being either a donor or recipient. The initial screening was performed by phone or through online survey. The study had two rounds of enrollment, with 10 recipients for each enrollment period. Recipients were offered both living donor and deceased donor options for uterine transplant. Between the two rounds 1050 recipients and 399 donors completed the initial screening. Ultimately, 18 recipients underwent a living donor uterus transplant and 2 underwent a deceased donor transplant. In November 2017 a live birth following UTx was achieved as a result of our study [5]. This milestone event marked the first birth to occur in the United States and the first one to replicate the success in Sweden. To date, 12 babies have been born through the Dallas Uterus Transplant Study. Early lessons learned helped create new surgical techniques and management strategies that ultimately helped improve uterus transplant outcomes.

30.1.1 Patients

30.1.1.1 Donor and Recipient Selection

A deliberate well-constructed screening and evaluation process needs to be implemented in any investigational study. The Dallas Uterus Transplant Study had two enrollment periods, each ultimately approving 10 recipients for transplants. Our screening process had five stages: subjective health screening, objective health screening, initial selection committee meeting, in vitro fertilization for potential recipients, and final selection committee meeting [4]. Given the experimental nature and paucity of previous results, careful diligence was paid adequately informing and consenting the subjects of the study during multiple stages of screening. The design, construction, and implementation of the study were grounded in the principles of medical ethics. Initial contact with potential recipients or donors was made through a nurse coordinator. This initial encounter introduced the participants to the structure and timeline of the study, highlighted the known risk/complications, informed them of previous international experience with uterus transplant, and finally provided a brief overview of the operation. Participants who completed this preliminary step were then moved into the first step of screening, the subjective health screening.

The subjective health screen consisted of a health history questionnaire and an informed consent form. Participants also submitted any related medical records. Inclusion and exclusion criteria for the study were used for screening (Table 30.1). Furthermore, each applicant was reviewed by the primary investigator to determine eligibility to continue onto stage 2.

Table 30.1 Selection criteria for recipients

Inclusion criteria	Exclusion criteria
Diagnosis of absolute uterine infertility (AUI) with at least one functioning ovary	Hx of diabetes mellitus type I and II by medical history or elevated hemoglobin A1c blood test
Women of childbearing age 20–40	Hypersensitivity to tacrolimus, thymoglobulin, or everolimus
No active human 142 papillomavirus (HPV) or active cervical dysplasia present	BMI >30
Negative for gonorrhea, chlamydia, and syphilis	Active infection
HSV-2 negative or have a history of HSV-2 with no current symptoms	Seropositive for HIV, HBV, or HCV
Subjects have received counseling regarding infertility alternatives to uterine transplant such as adoption or surrogate pregnancy	History of solid organ or bone marrow transplant
Willing to undergo in vitro fertilization	Unable to undergo in vitro fertilization
Evaluation by a fertility specialist and determined to have good ovarian reproductive potential	Unwilling or unable to comply with study requirements
Subject must have the ability to fund either through third party coverage or through their own personal financing, any expenses associated with assisted reproduction services provided to them	Subject with technical obstacles as per anatomical malformations, which pose a high surgical risk in the judgment of the investigator
Subject meets psychological recipient criteria	Alcohol or drug abuse within last 12 months, smoking within the last 3 months
Subject must be willing to complete questionnaires about their infant's growth and development and return them to the study team	Per investigator's discretion any pre-existing clinical or medical conditions that would pose the subject at an increased risk. For example, hypertension or cancer within past 5 years

Stage 2 consisted of a medical workup comprising of physical examinations, imaging studies, blood tests, immunological tests, infectious testing, drug screen, PAP screen, electrocardiogram, and urinalysis (Table 30.2). The participants were examined by the transplant surgeon, gynecological oncologist, and psychiatrist. The transplant surgeon and gynecologist separately performed another informed consent discussion at this time. Participants were explained the risks of the operation, previous complications reported in the literature, expected length of hospital stay, and expected recovery from the procedure. Again, participants were informed of the experimental nature of uterine transplant and the unknown outcome for both recipients and donors. Finally, during stage 2 the participants met with the psychologist to

Table 30.2 Medical workup for both potential donor and recipients

Stage 2 Medical workup	
Health care professional evaluation	Physical examination
	Pelvic examination
	Psychological evaluation (including an in-depth interview and standardized questionnaires)
Imaging	Chest X-ray
	Computed tomography, abdomen, and pelvis, MRI (added later)
	Vaginal ultrasound
	Doppler ultrasound
	Transabdominal ultrasound
Blood tests	Complete blood count with differential
	Comprehensive metabolic panel
	Gamma-glutamyl transferase
	Lipid panel
	Prothrombin time/international normalized ratio
	Partial thromboplastin time
	Hemoglobin A1C
Immunological testing	ABO blood groups Rh antigens
	Human leukocyte antigens
Viral, bacterial, and fungal testing	Syphilis
	Chlamydia and gonorrhea (neisseria gonorrhoeae culture)
	Herpes simplex virus 1 and 2
	Hepatitis C virus RNA by polymerase chain reaction
	Surface antigen of the hepatitis B virus
	Cytomegalovirus IgM and IgG
	Epstein–barr virus IgM and IgG
	HIV
	Fungal screening
	Urine culture
	Rubella
	Tuberculosis (T-SPOT)
Drug screen	Serum alcohol test
	Urine drug test
Other tests	Pap smear with co-testing for human papillomavirus
	Urinalysis
	Electrocardiogram

undergo an evaluation which included an in-depth interview and standardized psychological questionnaires.

In stage 3 initial selection committee met and suitable candidates were selected based on medical and psychological clearance. Recipient candidates were then referred for the reproductive endocrinologist to initiate the IVF process in stage 4. The goal of IVF was for the recipient to have at minimum two embryos of day 5–6 blastocytes of satisfactory quality as determined by biopsy and PGS testing. Finally, in stage 5, recipients were matched with either a directed living donor or an altruistic living donor. If no living donor was matched with a potential recipient, she was placed on a list for deceased donor matching. The final decision to proceed with uterine transplant was determined at the selection committee.

The previously published Dallas experience highlighted characteristics of the first enrollment period [4]. The paper highlighted the tremendous interest in uterine transplant among donor and recipients. This interest only increased after published reports of the first live birth in the United States following successful uterine transplant. The majority of applicants were screened out prior to stage 2 and thus avoided unnecessary and costly testing. Of the 20 recipients selected, 18 had congenital AUFI caused by MRKH. Two recipients had acquired AUI after undergoing hysterectomy for benign disease. Mean age of the selected recipients was 29.8 years and all were either married or in a committed relationship. Interestingly of the 18 selected living donors, 17 of them were non-directed donors and 1 was a directed donor (friend). Mean age of the living donors was 37.9 years. All living donors had at least one successful pregnancy and had completed their family planning. Two recipients received uteri from deceased donors (Table 30.3).

30.1.1.2 Donor Hysterectomy and Complications

Prior to the Dallas Uterus Transplant Study, only living donor uterine grafts had resulted in successful live births. The recent success by the group in Brazil has highlighted the potential debate between living and deceased donation [6]. The benefit of deceased donation is the elimination of risk to a healthy donor in a non-life saving or preserving transplant. Living donors must fully understand the surgical, mental, and financial risks associated with transplantation. The condition that a living donor must have completed her family planning generally makes the living donors slightly older. Deceased donation yields a pool of potential younger donors with less risk factors for atherosclerotic disease. However deceased donors cannot be scheduled ahead of time, thus making coordination and mobilization of the multiple teams required for uterine transplant more difficult.

In the Dallas Uterus Transplant Study all recipients were afforded the opportunity for either a living donor transplant or a deceased donor if an adequate immunological match could not be found. In total 18 living donor hysterectomies were performed; the first 13 utilized an open technique and the final 5 adopted a robot-assisted approach. In the 5 robotically assisted hysterectomies, the uteri were extracted through the vagina [7].

The living donor hysterectomy operation is a fusion of the lessons learned during other living donor transplants (liver/kidney) and of the widely practiced gynecology surgery, the radical hysterectomy. The procedure requires increased focus on meticulous dissection of the vascular pedicles completely to ensure adequate inflow and outflow of the graft.

Table 30.3 Donor characteristics and surgical outcomes

Donor	Age	Number of previous pregnancy	Donor type	Hysterectomy approach	LOS days	Inpatient readmission within 30 days? (Y/N)	Return to OR? (Y/N)
D01	42	2	NDLD	Open	5	N	N
D02	55	3	NDLD	Open	5	N	N
D03	45	3	NDLD	Open	5	Y	Y
D04	35	2	NDLD	Open	4	N	N
D05	36	4	NDLD	Open	6	Y	Y
D06	30	1	DD	Procurement	N/A		
D07	39	4	NDLD	Open	5	N	N
D08	44	2	DD	Procurement	N/A		
D09	35	7	NDLD	Open	4	N	N
D10	48	2	NDLD	Open	5	N	N
D11	32	5	NDLD	Open	4	N	N
D12	33	2	DLD	Open	7	N	N
D13	39	4	NDLD	Open	4	N	N
D14	32	1	NDLD	Open	3	N	N
D15	42	2	NDLD	Open	5	Y	Y
D16	30	1	NDLD	Robotic	3	Y	Y
D17	31	3	NDLD	Robotic	6	N	N
D18	38	2	NDLD	Robotic	3	N	N
D19	32	2	NDLD	Robotic	3	N	N
D20	38	2	NDLD	Robotic	3	N	N

NDLD non-directed living donor, *DD* deceased donor, *DLD* directed living donor

Obtaining length must be done carefully to avoid injury when the ureter is circumferentially dissected off the vascular pedicle. Arterial inflow for the graft relied on the uterine artery taken in conjunction with a patch of the internal iliac artery. Venous outflow can be obtained by using either the superior uterine vein (aka utero-ovarian vein) and/or the inferior uterine vein (aka uterine vein). Significant portion of the operative times is spent on dissection of the uterine veins while avoiding injury to the ureter. Once appropriate length on the vascular pedicles is obtained, the uterus is transected below the level of the cervix. Vascular clamps are placed on the vessels, the uterus graft is placed on ice, and it is transported to the recipient room. The uterus graft is then flushed with cold preservation solution through the uterine artery. The first 4 transplants were flushed with KPS (kidney perfusion solution), while the remaining were flushed with HTK (histidine–tryptophan–ketoglutarate) solution. Flow and blanching are carefully assessed to determine viability of the graft and if the recipient operation can proceed. Following hemostasis, the donor is then closed and taken to the ICU for recovery.

Donor complications between the open and robotic approach were carefully reviewed. The average donors' length of stay was 4.2 days with no difference appreciated with surgical approach. Median blood loss for open approach was 0.8 L and 0.1 L for robotic assisted. Only one patient, donor 9, required a blood transfusion for symptomatic anemia. The most common complication was UTI requiring outpatient antibiotic therapy (donors 2,3,4,5,10,13). A total of 4 donors in the study had a complication requiring readmission, 2 for each of the open and robotic approach [7, 8]. Donor 3 had a vagina cuff dehiscence >90 days after surgery that required transvaginal repair. Donor 5 developed fecal impaction that required manual decompression. The 2 readmissions following robotic donors were secondary to ureteral issues. Donor 15 had a ureteral clot, presumably from stent placement at time of surgery, and required placement of a ureteral stent. Donor 16 suffered a thermal injury at both ureters that caused a urine leak. Donor 16 underwent ureteral stent placement as well. While we had no ureteral complications from the open technique, at least one of the robotic cases can be attributed to ureter injury at the time of hysterectomy. While this is a rare event, ureter complications have been well documented during open hysterectomies in other studies [9, 10]. In our study while robotic donors had longer surgical times, the donors did have less blood loss, shorter hospital stay, and quicker return to work. The uterine graft outcomes were comparable, and the donors had a superior cosmetic result.

30.1.1.3 Recipient Uterine Transplant and Complications

The recipient operation begins with a lower midline laparotomy with the patient in lithotomy position. Exposure of the bilateral external iliac arteries and veins is performed. The uterine artery with a patch of donor internal iliac artery is anastomosed to the external iliac artery in an end-to-side fashion on each side. Originally the inferior uterine vein was used as the outflow but later the best outflow (either inferior or superior uterine vein) as determined by visual inspection

Table 30.4 Recipient UTx outcomes

Recipient	Date of UTx	Donor type	Donor operation	Vessels used for anastomosis	Live birth (number of children)	Graft survival (30 days/1 year)	Clinical pregnancy	Miscarriage
R1	Sep 2016	NDLD	Laparotomy	RSUV, LIUV	Graft loss	N/N	N/A	N/A
R2	Sep 2016	NDLD	Laparotomy	RIUV, LSUV	Graft loss	N/N	N/A	N/A
R3	Sep 2016	NDLD	Laparotomy	RSUV, LIUV	Graft loss	N/N	N/A	N/A
R4	Sep 2016	NDLD	Laparotomy	RSUV, LSUV	Yes (1)	Y/Y	1	0
R5	Dec 2016	NDLD	Laparotomy	RSUV, LSUV	Yes (2)	Y/Y	4	2
R6	Jun 2017	DD	Multi-organ retrieval	RSUV/RIUV, LIUV	Yes (1)	Y/Y	1	1
R7	Aug 2017	NDLD	Laparotomy	RIUV, LSUV	Yes (1)	Y/Y	1	0
R8	Nov 2017	DD	Multi-organ retrieval	RSUV/RIUV, LIUV	Graft loss	N/N	N/A	N/A
R9	May 2018	NDLD	Laparotomy	RIUV, LIUV	Yes (1)	Y/Y	1	0
R10	May 2018	NDLD	Laparotomy	RSUV, LSUV	Graft loss	N/N	N/A	N/A
R11	Oct 2018	NDLD	Laparotomy	RSUV, LIUV	Yes (1)	Y/Y	1	0
R12	Nov 2018	DLD	Laparotomy	RIUV, LIUV	Ongoing pregnancy	Y/Y	1	1
R13	Dec 2018	NDLD	Laparotomy	RSUV, LSUV	Yes (1)	Y/Y	1	0
R14	Dec 2018	NDLD	Laparotomy	RSUV, LSUV/LIUV	Graft loss	N/N	N/A	N/A
R15	Feb 2019	NDLD	Laparotomy	RSUV, LIUV	Yes (1)	Y/Y	1	0
R16	April 2019	NDLD	Robotic assisted	RSUV/RIUV, LSUV	Yes (1)	Y/Y	1	0
R17	May 2019	NDLD	Robotic assisted	RSUV, LSUV	Awaiting embryo transfer	Y/Y	2	2
R18	June 2019	NDLD	Robotic assisted	RSUV/RIUV, LSUV	Yes (1)	Y/Y	1	0
R19	Aug 2019	NDLD	Robotic assisted	RSUV/RIUV, LIUV	Ongoing pregnancy	Y/Y	1	0
R20	Aug 2019	NDLD	Robotic assisted	RSUV, LSUVx2	Ongoing pregnancy	Y/Y	1	0

NDLD non-directed living donor, *DD* deceased donor, *DLD* directed living donor, *RSUV* right superior uterine vein, *RIUV* right inferior uterine vein, *LSUV* left superior uterine vein, *LIUV* left inferior uterine vein

was used on either side. Table 30.4 highlights the venous anastomosis used with each recipient; 7 of the 13 recipients had more than one venous outflow on each side. Arterial anastomosis was performed with 7–0 prolene and the venous anastomosis was done with a running 8–0 prolene suture. Following reperfusion, the vaginal cuff of the uterus graft is attached to the recipient's vagina with 0 Vicryl suture. The uterus is then fixated to the round/sacrouterine ligament, paravaginal connective tissue, and the bladder peritoneum. A low dose heparin drip is initiated and continued during the admission. Finally, an implantable Doppler is placed on one of the uterine arteries to continually monitor arterial flow during the hospitalization.

Despite careful planning and the assistance of the Swedish team, initial outcomes were poor [11]. The first three uterus grafts were lost due to vascular compromise. The result of an in-depth analysis of each case was published and helped identify potential factors for graft loss: (a) Poor preoperative venous imaging, (b) atherosclerosis of uterine artery, and (c) venous outflow obstruction.

(a) In the early cases CT angiogram was used preoperatively and helped define the arterial inflow but was insufficient in defining the venous diameter and length. An MRI with venous phase helped better define the uterine veins preoperatively. (b) Arterial plaque was encountered at the origin of the uterine artery complicating the anastomosis in recipient 2. Using a segment of internal iliac artery proximal to the takeoff of the uterine artery would presumably allow for a larger lumen free of plaque. (c) Two of the early graft losses, recipients 1 and 3, were felt to be related to venous congestion due to poor outflow. Since the uterine and utero-ovarian veins can be thin walled, a finer suture was used for the anastomosis. Dissection of the donor veins also included taking a patch of the thicker internal iliac vein to perform the anastomosis upon. Also, the recipient venotomy was widened and moved from the superior aspect of the external iliac vein to a more medial site, preventing kinking of the vein when the uterus was pulled caudally and sewn in place.

After careful review of the first three cases, changes were made to help mitigate the presumed reason for vascular compromise. Ultimately, the fourth recipient had a functional uterine graft and would go on to have the first live birth from the study [5]. The outcomes improved for the remaining recipients, but challenges still arose.

In the remaining 16 uterine transplant recipients there were three further graft losses. Recipients 8 and 10 had uterine grafts with patent vasculature but failed to adequately reperfuse Both donor 8 and 10 were older females and donor 10 was additionally a deceased donor; graft failure from these donors was attributed to poor selection. Finally, recipient 14 had a well perfused uterus graft but developed postoperative bleeding from a branch off the uterine artery. She was taken back for control of bleeding, but the uterine graft suffered irreversible ischemic injury and was eventually explanted.

Of the 14 recipients who underwent a technically successful uterus transplant, other complications were also present. Intraoperative bladder injuries occurred in recipients 6 and 17 during dissection of the vagina vault. These were repaired immediately and had uneventful recovery. The most common complication encountered was strictures of the vaginal anastomosis that required surgical dilations in eight patients.

Table 30.5 Rejection episodes of UTx recipients

Recipient	Rejection POD	Steroid cycle length (days)	Resolved (Y/N)
R4	155	6	Y
R5	615/548	3/3	Y
R6	331	3	Y
R11	105	3	Y
R12	23	3	Y
R13	19	3	Y
R15	31	2	Y
R18	94	10	Y
R20	21/29	7/1	Y

POD postoperative day, *Y* yes, *N* no

30.1.1.4 Immunosuppression Protocol

Immunosuppression use in pregnancy has been studied in kidney transplant recipients since 1958 [12]. Immunosuppression regimens in uterus transplant recipients have mimicked those of kidney transplant with both induction and maintenance immunosuppression. Recipient immunosuppression involved induction with thymoglobulin (1.5 mg/kg intravenously every 2 days × 3) and corticosteroids. Both medications were started in the operating room following reperfusion of the uterine graft. Thymoglobulin is categorized as category C (risk not ruled out), with lack of information on the risk of fetal harm or reproduction. Therefore, recipients did not undergo embryo transfer within 3 months of thymoglobulin treatment.

Maintenance immunosuppression initially included tacrolimus (0.2 mg/kg orally daily, initial trough 7–12 ng/mL), mycophenolic acid (720 mg orally twice a day), and a steroid taper over 35 days. Mycophenolate was then converted over to azathioprine prior to delivery due to the teratogenic risk. Following conversion, it was advised to wait 3–6 months before attempting conception. Mycophenolate was eliminated from the maintenance regimen. Instead tacrolimus and azathioprine were used as maintenance immunosuppression with no difference in rejection episodes [13].

Rejection episodes were treated with high dose corticosteroids. We encountered 11 rejection episodes in nine recipients in our study. All rejection episodes resolved with high dose steroid cycle (Table 30.5). Given the use of tacrolimus, renal function was monitored in the recipients. Recipient 4 and 6 had evidence of acute kidney injury based on a higher than expected creatinine level. Tacrolimus goal was adjusted lower and may account for the delayed rejection episodes we saw in these patients. No other significant side effects of immunosuppression were appreciated in our study. Immunosuppression was stopped before graft hysterectomy.

30.1.1.5 Monitoring Protocol

Of the 14 technically successful urine transplants the median hospital length of stay was 6 days. These patients were followed under a protocol established at the onset of our study. In the immediate post-operative hospital setting patients underwent daily physical exams and blood draws for pertinent labs. The implantable Doppler placed at the time of surgery was continuously monitored during the hospitalization. On the first and fifth post-operative day the patient underwent a Doppler ultrasound of the graft, both transvaginal and transabdominal, to confirm adequate perfusion of the graft. Additionally, the first cervical biopsy was performed on fifth post-operative day and compared with the US results from the same day. After discharge, the patient was re-evaluated every 2 weeks for the first month and then every 4 weeks. Protocol US and cervical biopsies were performed every 2–4 weeks. When the patient was deemed ready embryo transfer was scheduled and the patient was closely followed by reproductive medicine (see below). Obstetrics performed prenatal visits every 2–3 weeks during pregnancy. Fetal growth, biophysical profiles, and umbilical artery Doppler were performed. During pregnancy cervical biopsy was performed during gestational week 12–14 and week 24–26. Delivery through cesarean section is targeted at a gestational age of 36–38 weeks.

30.1.1.6 Embryo Transfer

Once the recipient has achieved menses and that patient has recovered from the surgery, the uterine graft is technically ready for embryo transfer. Given the previous history of pregnancy with other transplants, the American Society of Transplant in 2005 recommended a 1-year waiting period between solid organ transplant and conception [12]. Earlier trials, such as a Swedish group, followed the 1 year waiting period as well. However, uterus transplant is a temporary graft that is judged on the birth of a healthy baby and not on long term graft function. Ideally, the time the uterine graft is in the recipient (recipient-graft time) should be minimized to reduce the potential adverse effects of immunosuppression medications. The Dallas Uterus Study sought to decrease the recipient-graft time by implementing earlier embryo transfer. In the Dallas study the time from Uterus transplant to embryo transfer was tailored to the individual patient based on post-operative recovery, stable graft function, immunosuppression regimen, infectious disease susceptibility, and minimization of recipient-graft time [14].

Recipients underwent in vitro fertilization prior to uterine transplant, and acceptable blastocytes were confirmed. The process of embryo transfer begins with endometrium preparation with oral estrogen therapy. Once adequate endometrial thickness was obtained (at least 7 mm), there was no dominant follicle or signs of ovulation, and progesterone levels were low, embryo transfer was scheduled. Natural progesterone was vaginally administered for 5 complete days before embryo transfer. Nine to twelve days following embryo transfer, blood tests were performed to detect the pregnancy hormone, HCG. The levels of the pregnancy hormone and the estrogen and progesterone levels were closely monitored. At 8 weeks gestation, the recipient underwent an ultrasound evaluation to see if there was viable pregnancy. If there are any remaining frozen embryos, they were used for a second pregnancy or for another attempt if the first embryo transfer was unsuccessful.

30.1.1.7 Live Births

To date, 12 children have been born from 11 recipients in the Dallas study. Median gestational age at birth was 36 weeks and 6 days with a 5 min APGAR score of 9. Birth weight remained appropriate for gestational age of all children. All children are currently healthy with ages between 1 week and 3 years. Maternal and obstetric complications are highlighted in Table 30.6. Of the 11 recipients who have given birth 8 have completed all desired pregnancies and have had the graft uterus explanted.

30.1.2 Lessons Learned

The Dallas Uterus Transplant Study helped to transform uterine transplant from an experimental procedure to a more established treatment option for women with AUFI [15]. The study was the first to verify the groundbreaking work performed by the Swedish group. The Dallas study also resulted in the first live birth following uterus transplant in the United States. Additionally, it has been the only study to date that resulted in live births from both deceased and living donors. This study now represents the largest UTx experience in the United States and the world. It has helped the field continue to grow, with results being replicated in many US and international centers. This type of endeavor requires a strong multidisciplinary team comprising of reproductive medicine,

Table 30.6 Pregnancy complications and infant outcomes

Case no	Maternal age at delivery (y)	Maternal complications	Obstetric complications	Infant gender	Gestational age (w.d)	Birthweight (g)	Apgar (1 min/5 min)	Time from Utx to delivery (days)
4	31	Proteinuria, vaginal bleeding	PTD	Male	33.1	1995	8/9	432
5	29	None	None	Female	36.6	2920	9/9	439
5	31	None	None	Female	38	3370	9&9	1171
6	39	GHTN	None	Female	38	3470	9&9	1059
7	28	GDM	None	Female	35.6	2860	8/8	761
9	25	None	CI, PTL, PTD	Female	30.6	1770	7/8	404
11	21	None	None	Male	37.2	3140	8/8	365
13	32	None	None	Male	37.0	2960	8/9	464
15	32	Preeclampsia	Previa	Female	36.6	2400	8&9	445
16	32	GHTN	Polyhydramnios	Male	37.0	3025	4&9	422
18	34	None	Previa, PTL, PTD	Male	32.4	2350	7&8	335

w.d weeks.days, *GHTN* gestational hypertension, *GDM* gestational diabetes, *Previa* placenta previa, *CI* cervical incompetence, *PTL* preterm labor, *PTD* preterm delivery, a delivery for a maternal medical, obstetrical, or fetal indication transplantation, gynecology, obstetrics, and medical ethics. The contributions of our nurse clinic managers and the rest of the nursing support cannot be understated as well. The Dallas study's true strength came from a desire from all parties to tirelessly work toward advancement of the field. The early challenges faced by the study required an in-depth analysis of each case. It was during this time that institutional support was paramount and ultimately lead to success of the study.

Throughout the study, refinements were made to improve outcomes. Review of our three initial cases helped to modify our technical aspects of the donor and recipient operation. Through increased experience we were able to modify the venous outflow to include the uterine vein and/or the utero-ovarian vein on each side. In our last five cases we converted the donor operation from an open approach to a robotic approach with similar outcomes. After making changes to our immunosuppression protocol, we were able to considerably shorten the amount of time to embryo transfer. Ultimately this allowed us to decrease the time between uterine transplant and uterine graft removal following successful pregnancies.

The changes made helped us to create procedural advancements that ultimately lead to the delivery of 12 live births after uterine transplant. Despite these tremendous results we faced challenges that were harder to overcome. Review of the 6 graft losses reveals 5 of them had donors over the age of 40. While three of the graft losses were from presumed technical challenges, the other two were felt to be poor grafts. The quality of the graft and its response to ischemia-reperfusion are not clearly understood. While there has been success with older donors, as seen in one of our patients as well, further studies may be needed for better utilization of such organs.

The future of uterine transplant appears to be quite strong. While uterine transplant is not a "lifesaving transplant" it is a "life-giving" transplant. In the United States millions of women suffer from acquired absolute uterine infertility (AUI). In our study 18 of the 20 recipients suffered from congenital AUI and only two from acquired AUI. The hope is uterine transplant can be offered to recipients for a wider range of indications. Keeping the safety and comfort of donors in mind, the use of robotic and minimally invasive techniques for the donor hysterectomy is likely to continue. As the donor operation has become more standardized, the hope is that its complications, especially ureteral complications, will also become a rare event.

Ultimately, increased utilization will depend significantly on acceptance of uterus transplant as a standard fertility treatment. The Dallas study has shown that uterus transplant should no longer be considered an experimental procedure. "Life-giving" uterus transplant should be considered a definitive treatment for absolute uterine factor infertility.

References

1. Ozkan O, Akar ME, Ozkan O, et al. Preliminary results of the first human uterus transplantation from a multiorgan donor. Fertil Steril. 2013;99:470–6.
2. Fageeh W, Raffa H, Jabbad H, et al. Transplantation of the human uterus. Int J Gynaecol Obstet. 2002;76:245–51.
3. Brannstrom M, Johannesson L, Bokstrom H, et al. Livebirth after uterus transplantation. Lancet. 2015;385:607–16.
4. Johannesson L, Wallis K, Koon EC, et al. Living uterus donation and transplantation: experience of interest and screening in a single center in the United States. Am J Obstet Gynecol. 2018;218:331e1–7.
5. Testa G, McKenna GJ, Gunby RT Jr, et al. First live birth after uterus transplantation in the United States. Am J Transplant. 2018;18:1270–4.
6. Ejzenberg D, Andraus W, Baratelli Carelli Mendes LR, et al. Livebirth after uterus transplantation from a deceased donor in a recipient with uterine infertility. Lancet. 2019;392(10165):2697–704.
7. Johannesson L, Koon EC, Bayer J, et al. DUETS (dallas uterus transplant study): early outcomes and complications of robot-assisted hysterectomy for living uterus donors [published online ahead of print, 2020 Mar 2]. Transplantation. 2020;105(1):225–30. https://doi.org/10.1097/TP.0000000000003211.
8. Ramani A, Testa G, Ghouri Y, et al. DUETS (dallas uterus transplant study): complete report of 6-month and initial 2-year outcomes following open donor hysterectomy. Clin Transpl. 2020;34(1):e13757.
9. Brännström M, Johannesson L, Dahm-Kähler P, et al. First clinical uterus transplantation trial: a six-month report. Fertil Steril. 2014;101:1228–36.
10. Brucker SY, Brännström M, Taran FA, et al. Selecting living donors for uterus transplantation: lessons learned from two transplantations resulting in menstrual functionality and another attempt, aborted after organ retrieval. Arch Gynecol Obstet. 2018;297:675–84.
11. Testa G, Koon EC, Johannesson L, et al. Living donor uterus transplantation: a single center's observations and lessons learned from early setbacks to technical success. Am J Transplant. 2017;17:2901–10.
12. McKay DB, Josephson MA, Armenti VT, August P, Coscia LA, Davis CL, et al. Reproduction and transplantation: report on the AST consensus conference on reproductive issues and transplantation. Am J Transplant. 2005;5:1592–9.
13. Mölne J, Broecker V, Ekberg J, Nilsson O, Dahm-Kähler P, Brännström M. Monitoring of human uterus transplantation with cervical biopsies: a provisional scoring system for rejection. Am J Transplant. 2017;17:1628–36.
14. Johannesson L, Wall A, Putman JM, et al. Rethinking the time interval to embryo transfer after uterus transplantation—DUETS (dallas uterus transplant study). BJOG. 2019;126:1305–9.
15. Testa G, McKenna G, Johannesson L, et al. The evolution of transplantation from saving lives to fertility treatment. Ann Surg. 2020;272(3):411–7. https://doi.org/10.1097/SLA.0000000000004199.

Live Birth from the World's First-Ever Successful Uterus Transplant and the Following Second Case from Turkey: Technical Aspects, Surgical and Obstetric Outcomes

31

Ömer Özkan, Özlenen Özkan, and Nasuh Utku Dogan

31.1 Introduction

Infertility related to absence of uterus affects 3–5% of all young women of reproductive age and until recently no treatment for this condition has been available [1]. Surrogacy and adoption are alternative methods, although surrogacy is not legal in many countries, and adoption does not establish a genetic link between mother and child. After the first successful uterus transplantation in Turkey on September 2011, studies in this field accelerated significantly, and successful transplantations and consequently live births were reported from different parts of the world [2–4]. Most uterus transplants involve live donors, although several advantages make deceased donor transplantation a reasonable option, mainly by eliminating surgical risks to the live donor.

In this chapter we described in detail the surgical procedures, previous failed pregnancies, methods for overcoming pregnancy failure, and, most importantly, the birth of a healthy infant in the first-ever uterus transplantation from a deceased donor and also summarized briefly the second case performed in our unit.

When did the program start?

The idea of uterus transplantation was first conceived while dealing with significant number of patients with Mayer–Rokitansky–Küster–Hauser (MRKH) syndrome. Since 2005 our team has been performing genital reconstruction in women with vaginal agenesis. Over 100 women with vaginal agenesis have received bowel and intestinal neovaginal reconstruction. Thus, a special patient registry had already been created for women with congenital mullerian agenesis. The uterus allotransplantation program first started in 2009. The official permissions were obtained from Akdeniz University Ethical Committee and Turkish Ministry of Health for three patients. Patients eligible for the uterus transplantation project were selected from this registry, and pre-transplantation work-up was carried out for each candidate, as previously reported [2, 5]. During a 6-month period, discussions were held with the candidates about the experimental nature of this trial. The patients and their families were informed about the details, risks, and complications related to the transplantation surgery and immunosuppression treatment. They were also informed regarding pregnancy complications under immunosuppression, the potential inability to achieve pregnancy, and the potential need for subsequent hysterectomy. The couples also were informed about the available treatment choices.

How were the transplants funded?

There is no established, official uterus transplantation program and no legislation particularly for uterus transplantation. Two uterus transplantations were all funded by Turkish Ministry of Health with further support from Akdeniz University, Faculty of Medicine.

Is the program still active?

Our program is still active. We are recruiting women with vaginal agenesis and other etiologies (mostly women undergoing hysterectomy for obstetric hemorrhage).

How many patients have you screened?

Up to now, over 200 patients have been screened and 153 have been included in the registry.

How many patients were approved and how many are on the waiting list?

So far, 45 patients have been approved and are on the waiting list.

Is there any obstacle to the expansion of the program?

Because of the potential risks and complications in a live donor, we performed the two uterus transplant procedures from cadaveric donors. However, there are a limited number of available cadaveric uterus donors. Moreover, there is no

Ö. Özkan (✉) · Ö. Özkan
Department of Plastic, Reconstructive, and Aesthetic Surgery, Akdeniz University School of Medicine, Antalya, Turkey

N. U. Dogan
Department of Gynecology, Faculty of Medicine, Akdeniz University, Antalya, Turkey

© Springer Nature Switzerland AG 2023

R. Gurunian et al. (eds.), *Reconstructive Transplantation*, https://doi.org/10.1007/978-3-031-21520-9_31

established legislation particularly for uterus transplantation and one should obtain special permission to perform this kind of transplantation in Turkey.

31.2 Patients

So far, we have performed two uterus transplantations and we are actively recruiting new candidates in our program. We have been collaborating and cooperating with Turkish Ministry of Health to launch uterus transplant legislation. In 2011 September our team performed the first successful uterus transplantation in Turkey which was followed by further successful transplantations and consequently live births from different parts of the world [2–4]. Most of the uterus transplants involve live donors but several advantages make deceased donor transplantation a reasonable option, particularly by eliminating surgical risks to the live donor.

Case 1

The uterus transplantation from a deceased donor performed in Turkey in September 2011 was the first such procedure in the world, and only the second trial after the failed attempt in Saudi Arabia, as previously reported [2, 6]. The first recipient was a 21-year-old female with MRKH syndrome without any previous illnesses. Two years before the transplantation she had undergone vaginal reconstruction with jejunal segment. Preoperatively she had normal blood tests (including normal renal function, normal FSH, E2, AMH levels). The renal function and anatomy were normal before the transplantation procedure. Basic fertility work-up for the patient and her spouse was all within normal limits. The result of her karyotype analysis was 46, XX. She was a nonsmoker with a BMI of 21 kg/m^2. Her screening tests were negative for infection with human immunodeficiency virus (HIV), hepatitis B and C virus, toxoplasma, rubella, and cytomegalovirus. She passed a thorough psychiatric examination and was found to be stable by the counselor. She was selected to be first among the three candidates because of the match with the donor's blood group and HLA. The donor was a 22-year-old nulliparous brain-dead woman who sustained cerebral trauma in a traffic accident. She was pretested for blood group type, human leukocyte antigen (HLA) matching, and screening for toxoplasma, rubella, cytomegalovirus (CMV), human immunodeficiency virus (HIV), and hepatitis B and C. She revealed no signs of latent or acute infection. The donor's and recipient's blood groups were the same, and they shared three HLAs (donor: HLA-A*03, HLA-A*11; HLA-B*08, HLA-B*51; HLA-DRB1*03, HLA-DRB1*15; recipient: HLA-A*03, HLAA* 32; HLA-B*08, HLA-B*18; HLA-DRB1*03, HLA-DRB1*11). Anti-HLA reactive antibodies and retrospective crossmatching were negative. Transabdominal ultrasound performed in the intensive care unit revealed the uterus had no structural abnormalities such as myoma uteri or uterine anomaly. A cervical smear was inspected for the presence of cervical lesions and human papillomavirus (HPV) types 16, 18, 31, 33, and 45 using the nucliSENS Easy Q HPV v1 assay (BioMerieux) to get a reliable and prompt result.

31.3 Surgical Technique

The uterine procurement was performed as the first procedure from the donor including long vascular pedicles of common iliac artery and veins. The harvest took 120 min. Transfer time of the allograft was 30 min. A median abdominal incision was performed in the recipient. The external iliac artery and vein were dissected. After back-table preparation of the uterine allograft, it was placed in the orthotopic position. Vaginal part of the graft was sutured to the apex of previously created jejunal neovagina. Sacrouterine ligaments were secured to sacrum to create three-dimensional stable neo-uterus. After positioning and securing the ligaments, vascular anastomosis was performed between the recipient's external iliac vessels and the donor's hypogastric vessel pedicle, in an end-to-side manner. During the back-table preparation and positioning of the uterine graft, the length of the hypogastric artery pedicle (including uterine vessel pedicle) was adjusted and a smooth curve (3 cm length longer than the straight distance) was created to avoid tension at the anastomosis and also a loose vessel graft. After vascular anastomosis, round ligaments were sutured to inguinal ligament of the recipient. A wide anterior bladder peritoneal flap retrieved generously from donor was sutured to parietal peritoneum of the recipient. Bilateral salpingectomy was also performed to prevent any possible ectopic pregnancy. The fixation of the anterior bladder pillar is an important step of the procedure to tailor and to position the uterine graft properly in a three-dimensional manner. We described and published this part of the surgery previously and our technique was also adopted by the Swedish team who visited our clinic after our successful uterus transplantation procedure [2, 7]. Right after the de-clamping of the arterial bulldogs, the perfusion of the uterus was observed both clinically with the change of the color from pale yellow to red and also confirmed by intraoperative color-Doppler ultrasonography scan (Fig. 31.1). We also retrieved a rectangular sentinel skin graft from the donor and transplanted this onto the anterior thigh of the recipient in order to monitor any possible rejection externally.

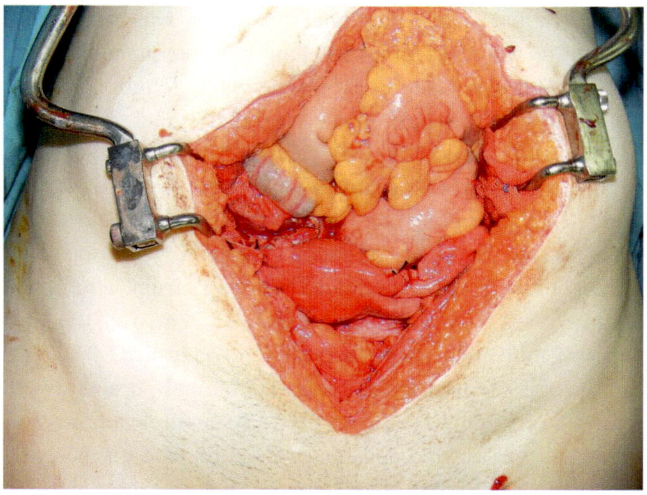

Fig. 31.1 Intraoperative view of the transplanted uterus

31.4 Immunosuppression Protocol

Immunosuppression induction with a 2.0 mg/dL daily dose of thymoglobulin was administered intraoperatively, adjusted based on the CD3 levels, and stopped on day 10. An initial intraoperative dose of 1000 mg of prednisolone was administered and then reduced to 20 mg 1 week after surgery. Tacrolimus (0.2 mg/kg) was not started simultaneously but rather on day 7 to decrease the rate of complications related to immunosuppressive therapy. For the first postoperative 10 days, fluconazole (200 mg/100 mL IV infusion), piperacillin/tazobactam (4.5 g IV every 8 h), cotrimoxazole (10 mg/kg per day IV), oral nystatin drops, and oral valacyclovir tablets were administered for prophylaxis. Maintenance immunosuppression therapy consisted of tacrolimus (0.2 mg/kg with plasma levels 15–20 ng/mL), mycophenolate mofetil (2 g/day), and prednisolone (20 mg/day). Cotrimoxazole (2.5 mg/kg per day orally) was administered for the first 6 months. Subcutaneous heparin was administered for antithrombotic prophylaxis.

31.5 Monitoring Protocol

Follow-up observation included routine tests, uterine artery Doppler ultrasound, biopsies, and speculum examination of the cervix. For acute rejection monitoring, biopsy was taken from the transplanted vagina every 2 weeks for the first 3 months. No endometrial biopsies were taken during the first 3 months to decrease the risk of infection due to relatively higher immunosuppressive doses. Thereafter, patient was evaluated with endometrial biopsy every 3 months. The mucosa of the transplanted vagina at month 6 demonstrated a few lymphocytes around the capillaries, but there was no fibrinoid necrosis. The endometrial biopsy at 6 months revealed vacuolization of the glandular epithelium and edematous stroma. The patient was also checked weekly for any signs, symptoms, and findings of infection with regular urine and throat cultures, during follow-up evaluations. The patient acquired the first menstrual cycle 20 days after the procedure. Her menstruation was irregular for the next two menstrual cycles after the first menstrual cycle.

The first embryo transfer (ET) attempt, performed 18 months after the transplantation, yielded an increase in human chorionic gonadotropin (hCG) up to 35 IU/L with no ultrasonographic sign of pregnancy. Following failed attempts and five pregnancies (miscarriages at 7–8 weeks), the ET attempts were suspended and the underlying etiology was investigated. Interestingly, the growth of the gestational sac always lagged behind the normal fetal pole, and all five pregnancies resulted in miscarriages at nearly 8 weeks gestation, all of which suggested a possible placentation problem and/or blood outflow obstruction. Static magnetic resonance imaging of the uterus revealed normal anatomic findings. Perfusion computed tomography (256-slice helical SOMATOM Definition Flash CT, Siemens Medical Solutions, Erlangen, Germany) revealed an obstructed blood outflow, particularly in the left anterolateral part of the uterus. In order to overcome this blood flow obstruction, a new venous outflow from the uterus to the central venous pool was planned. Following receipt of informed consent and a detailed discussion with the patient, the plan for vascular augmentation surgery was reported to both Turkish Ministry health authorities and Akdeniz University Ethical Commitee and IRB approval was obtained. On November 2018 an exploratory laparotomy was performed, followed by dissection of a vein originating from the left utero-ovarian pedicle. A saphenous vein graft (4 mm in diameter and 13 cm in length) was harvested and used as an interpositional vein graft between one of the branches of the utero-ovarian veins (end-to-end) and the left ovarian vein (end-to-side). After the anastomosis of the saphenous vein graft to the utero-ovarian vein, the left ovarian was clamped and end-to-side anastomosis was performed. Total clamping time and anastomosis to left ovarian vein were 15 min. After the anastomosis, the patency of the vessels on both sides (both vein and artery) was confirmed with intraoperative Doppler ultrasonography. During the operation, apart from relative enlargement, the position/location and blood flow of the uterus were normal. The anastomosis worked well, both intraoperatively and postoperatively which were all confirmed with Doppler ultrasonography. Follow-up perfusion computed tomography performed 3 months after the operation demonstrated the resolution of venous congestion on the fundal side and a significant decrease in uterine volume (154 cm^3) compared to the pre-operative period (280 cm^3). On December single euploid embryo transfer attempt was performed under ultrasonographic guidance. Blood β-hCG level was 923 IU/L 13 days after the embryo transfer. Clinical pregnancy and fetal cardiac activity were confirmed 28 days after the last embryo transfer. The patient received prednisolone (5 mg/day), azathioprine (50 mg/day followed by 100 mg/day in the second trimester), and tacrolimus (2 mg/day, target serum dose 5–7 ng/mL) treatments throughout the pregnancy. The patient's kidney functions also remained stable and were within normal limits all throughout non-gravid phase and during pregnancy. We regularly checked renal functions during the index pregnancy. We also checked regularly for symptoms of rejection (a watery, foul smelling discharge). The sentinel skin graft from the donor implanted on the recipient's anterior thigh during the time of uterus transplantation served as a means for observing a possible rejection episode. To note, no clinical rejection episode occurred in the period from uterus transplantation to hysterectomy. In the first trimester, gross examination of the cervix was considered to be adequate for the follow-up of rejection, and cervical biopsy was planned for the second trimester. However, this could not be performed because of the preterm premature rupture of membranes and potential risk of infection. Serial speculum examination of the cervix was normal, and complete blood counts, particularly eosinophil counts, were within normal limits. The dosage of tacrolimus was adjusted according to the blood levels. As we could not monitor rejection with serial cervical biopsies, we did not decrease the doses of immunosuppressive drugs in the second trimester. Due to the intrauterine growth restriction, deteriorated Doppler ultrasonography findings, and suspected preeclampsia, cesarean section was planned at 28 weeks gestation. After a detailed discussion with the patient, hysterectomy was planned, and informed consent was obtained. On June 4, 2020, surgery began with a midline incision after the onset of regional anesthesia. Adhesions were lysed. The bladder peritoneum was close to the lower uterine segment, and the planned uterine incision site was vascularized. Therefore, a classical vertical fundal incision was made. A 760 g male fetus with Apgar score of 7–8-8 was delivered. After delivery, the umbilical cord was sutured, the fundal incision was closed, and we proceeded with hysterectomy. The patient's position was changed to low-lithotomy from supine. Adhesions were lysed, and normal anatomy was restored. Round ligaments were divided, the retroperitoneum was entered, and ureteral traces were visualized. The bladder peritoneum was dissected off, while the ovaries were left in situ. Salpingectomy had been performed previously in the first uterus transplant surgery. The uterine arteries were ligated close to the entrance to the uterus. The venous anastomosis between left ovarian vein and utero-ovarian vein was subsequently ligated. The sacrouterine ligaments were ligated and cut. A sponge was introduced from the neovagina. The previous line of the vaginal-neovagina lining was identified, and a circumferential colpotomy was carried out. The uterus was then removed along with recipient's vagina. Every effort was made to excise the whole length of recipient's vagina. The cuff of neovagina (jejunal graft) was sutured and closed. Topical hemostatic agents (Surgicel) were applied, and two drains were left in place after hemostasis. Total operative time was 130 min, and total blood loss was 400 mL. Two units of packed red cells were transfused intraoperatively. Postoperative broad-spectrum antibiotics (ceftriaxone 2 g i.v. and metronidazole 1500 mg i.v.) together with low molecular weight heparin (enoxaparin 4000 IU s.c./day) were administered. Intra-abdominal drains were removed on the third postoperative day. Immunosuppression treatment was tapered and finally discontinued on the postoperative seventh day. After delivery, the neonate was transferred to the NICU. The infant was successfully discharged from the NICU 79 days after delivery in good condition, weighing 2475 g. Sentinel skin graft from the donor was gradually rejected after delivery and cessation of the immunosuppressants. It has been 18 months since the birth of baby. Both mother and baby have been in good condition (Fig. 31.2). The renal functions of the mother were normal (creatinine 0.69 mg/dL, BUN 15 mg/dL, and creatinine clearance 117 mL/min) in the last follow-up.

Case 2

In July 2021, the second uterus transplant was performed in our unit. The donor was a 37-year-old multiparous brain-dead woman (four previous live births) because of ruptured intracranial aneurysm. She was pretested for blood group type, human leukocyte antigen (HLA) matching, and screening for toxoplasma, rubella, cytomegalovirus (CMV), human immunodeficiency virus (HIV), and hepatitis B and C. She revealed no signs of latent or acute infection. The same surgical technique was followed except anastomosis of two ovarian veins (right and left) to both external iliac veins. She

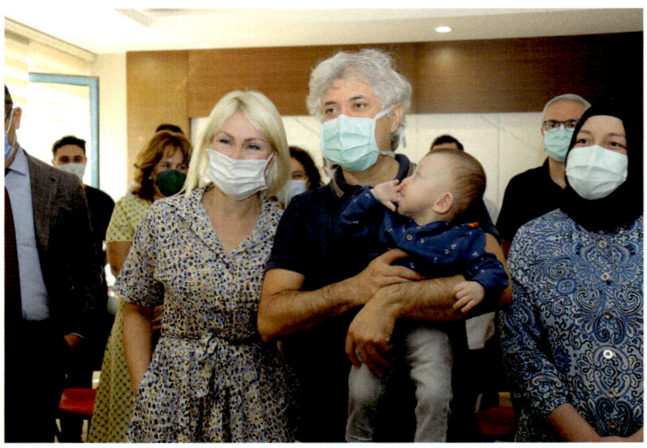

Fig. 31.2 The baby, mother, Prof Dr. Omer Ozkan, and Prof Dr. Ozlenen Ozkan 1 year after the birth of the baby

had a vaginal length of 6 cm established previously by frank dilatation. Her postoperative course has been uneventful with a viable uterine allograft 4 months after the surgery. She had two menstrual bleeding. We are expecting to perform ETs 6 months following the surgery.

31.6 Remarks

This chapter describes the course of the first successful uterus transplantation from a deceased donor. The first case described possesses a number of important and unique features, including the use of a deceased donor and live birth after failed attempts handled with the use of vein graft in order to restore venous outflow. This was also the first case of uterus transplantation with a live birth after jejunal vagina construction, representing a pioneer case. Following our success, experience in uterus transplantation has increased exponentially, and this approach has now become a viable option rather than merely an experimental concept. So far, around 80 such transplantations have been reported and more than 30 infants have been successfully delivered, four from cadaveric donors [8]. The importance of deceased donor uterus transplantation lies in the fact that it poses no harm to the donor and allows harvest of long vascular pedicles, thus improving the chance of successful patent vascular anastomosis.

The first donor surgeries in Sweden lasted more than 10 h, and the donors were transferred to ICU units after the procedures [9]. Recently, minimally invasive surgery has been adapted to uterine retrieval surgery, although operative times are still long. In a report by a team from Sweden, part of the donor surgery commenced with robotic surgery lasting 360 min [10]. For safety reasons, due to the extended time spent in the Trendelenburg position (360 min), the surgery was converted and completed with laparotomy. The total duration of donor surgery was 12 h, with 400 cc blood loss. The same group recently published their experience with eight more robotic donor surgeries. However, the median duration of surgery was still 10.5 h, the final parts still being completed with median laparotomy [11].

In addition, a number of complications such as ureteric injuries, ureterovesical fistula formation, and vaginal cuff dehiscence have been reported from live donor surgeries [9, 12]. In order to retrieve longer vascular pedicles, donor surgeries included the removal of the ovaries, thus putting young donor women into a menopausal state requiring prolonged exogenous estrogen use and involving a possible increased future cardiovascular risk and mortality [13, 14]. In the light of all these drawbacks of live donor uterus transplantation, deceased donor transplantation can avoid potential harm to the donor and increase the chance of successful vascular anastomosis with the help of longer vascular grafts.

In our first case, after five failed pregnancies, investigation of the etiology revealed an area of venous congestion in the fundal region of the transplanted uterus. The first static radiological studies including magnetic resonance imaging showed no anatomical problem. However, subsequently perfusion computed tomography demonstrated venous congestion and an area of venous pooling in the fundal area of the uterus. A vascular venous graft was used in order to overcome the venous congestion. The resolution of the previously congested area and a relative decrease in the size of the uterus at follow-up perfusion computed tomography were all indicative of a real venous insufficiency. The underlying condition could be a mechanical obstruction due to a kinking or a thrombotic event but during the revision surgery the gross venous outflow and arterial vasculature were all checked with intraoperative Doppler ultrasonography and the uterine venous and arterial vasculature were normal. The importance of this case is the presence of regional venous congestion area that was treated with vascular augmentation and presentation of a new exit strategy to establish a healthy pregnancy before removing uterine graft after failed pregnancy attempts. In this way an important cause of infertility was eliminated by improving vascularity in a small regional area of the uterus with the help of vascular augmentation.

Achieving pregnancy is an important step in uterus transplantation trials but the real success and proof of an established treatment of uterine-related infertility is the birth of a healthy baby. Previous reports have described a number of patients with pregnancy attempts resulting in recurrent miscarriages, without successful delivery of a baby [15–17]. To the best of our knowledge, this is the first uterus transplantation case involving a successful birth after vascular revision of uterine venous outflow following recurrent miscarriages.

In case of recurrent pregnancy failures in uterine-related infertility, in addition to routine evaluation of recurrent pregnancy losses, the presence of a venous outflow obstruction should be checked before removing the graft. Perfusion computed tomography may serve as a good tool for evaluating blood inflow and outflow characteristics of the transplanted uterus. Vascular revision in these patients may increase the possibility of ongoing pregnancies.

The drawbacks of the deceased uterus transplant are a relatively low number of multiorgan donors, a shorter time for pre-operative evaluation of the donor, logistic problems concerning organ transfer, and that less experience has been achieved with this procedure [18]. Adapting the organ retrieval order without impairing vital organ outcomes will shorten the cold ischemia duration of the uterus [19]. As the number of live births from deceased uterus transplants increases, the opportunities to compare both live and deceased donor transplants will also increase.

One possible criticism of the first case may involve the follow-up of the recipient for 9 years without removal of the uterus. There is an increased risk of infections in the course of treatment, malignancy even after discontinuing immunosuppression, and a potential risk for nephrotoxicity. However, post-transplant malignancy rates in renal transplant recipients are comparable to those of the non-transplanted population, particularly for recipients aged 20–30 years and receiving immunosuppression for less than 10 years [20, 21]. Removal of the uterus was discussed with the patient after failed attempts during the course of follow-up. All the risks were explained in detail, but the patient opted to keep the uterine graft. Interestingly, the patient stated that she felt positive about herself due to experiencing menstrual cycles despite previous unsuccessful embryo transfer attempts.

31.7 Lessons Learned

31.7.1 What Are the Strengths of Your Program?

The most important strengths of our program are our previous experiences with respect to composite tissue transplant. We had the opportunity to follow different kinds of tissue in every possible scenario. Moreover, we have a significant number of women with vaginal agenesis in our registry which gave us opportunity to choose the most appropriate candidate in these two uterus transplant patients.

31.7.2 What Did You Change Over Time?

In our first case, nulliparous status of the donor was not the ideal choice and likely contributed to the long waiting period till the birth of the baby. In the second uterus transplant, instead, uterus from multiparous donor was retrieved in order to increase the chances of live birth. Moreover, finding of a possible venous outflow obstruction in our first case led us to perform ovarian venous anastomosis as a second venous drainage.

31.7.3 What Will You Not Repeat in the Future?

Because of all these drawbacks, multiparous donor was chosen in our second uterus transplant.

31.7.4 How Do You See the Future of VCA?

The most important limiting factor of deceased donor uterus transplant is the low number of cadaveric donors. Moreover, use of immunosuppressants poses a significant risk of nephrotoxicity and tumor formation. There are ongoing studies of artificial uterus and tissues which will exclude the use of immunosuppressants and problematic dissections in live donor.

31.8 Conclusion

Deceased donor uterus transplantation is a reasonable approach for treating uterine factor-related infertility, and the two cases are presented here, one with the delivery of a healthy infant, which will take its place as the first-ever successful uterus transplant in the literature. Even in the absence of blood flow disorder under normal physiological conditions, in case of recurrent miscarriages, regional vascular augmentation by arterial or venous supercharging may be required in order to overcome regional mis-perfused regions determined by imaging studies.

References

1. Saravelos SH, Cocksedge KA, Li TC. Prevalence and diagnosis of congenital uterine anomalies in women with reproductive failure: a critical appraisal. Hum Reprod Update. 2008;14(5):415–29.
2. Ozkan O, Akar ME, Ozkan O, Erdogan O, Hadimioglu N, Yilmaz M, et al. Preliminary results of the first human uterus transplantation from a multiorgan donor. Fertil Steril. 2013;99(2):470–6.
3. Brannstrom M, Johannesson L, Bokstrom H, Kvarnstrom N, Molne J, Dahm-Kahler P, et al. Livebirth after uterus transplantation. Lancet. 2015;385(9968):607–16.
4. Ejzenberg D, Andraus W, Baratelli Carelli Mendes LR, Ducatti L, Song A, Tanigawa R, et al. Livebirth after uterus transplantation from a deceased donor in a recipient with uterine infertility. Lancet. 2019;392(10165):2697–704.
5. Erman Akar M, Ozkan O, Aydinuraz B, Dirican K, Cincik M, Mendilcioglu I, et al. Clinical pregnancy after uterus transplantation. Fertil Steril. 2013;100(5):1358–63.
6. Fageeh W, Raffa H, Jabbad H, Marzouki A. Transplantation of the human uterus. Int J Gynaecol Obstet. 2002;76(3):245–51.
7. Ozkan O, Dogan NU, Ozkan O, Mendilcioglu I, Dogan S, Aydinuraz B, et al. Uterus transplantation: from animal models through the first heart beating pregnancy to the first human live birth. Womens Health (Lond). 2016;12(4):442–9.
8. Malasevskaia I, Al-Awadhi AA. A new approach for treatment of woman with absolute uterine factor infertility: a traditional review of safety and efficacy outcomes in the first 65 recipients of uterus transplantation. Cureus. 2021;13(1):e12772.
9. Brannstrom M, Johannesson L, Dahm-Kahler P, Enskog A, Molne J, Kvarnstrom N, et al. First clinical uterus transplantation trial: a six-month report. Fertil Steril. 2014;101(5):1228–36.
10. Brannstrom M, Dahm-Kahler P, Kvarnstrom N, Akouri R, Rova K, Olausson M, et al. Live birth after robotic-assisted live donor uterus transplantation. Acta Obstet Gynecol Scand. 2020;99(9):1222–9.
11. Brannstrom M, Kvarnstrom N, Groth K, Akouri R, Wiman L, Enskog A, et al. Evolution of surgical steps in robotics-assisted donor surgery for uterus transplantation: results of the eight cases in the Swedish trial. Fertil Steril. 2020;114(5):1097–107.
12. Chmel R, Novackova M, Janousek L, Matecha J, Pastor Z, Maluskova J, et al. Revaluation and lessons learned from the first 9 cases of a Czech uterus transplantation trial: four deceased donor and 5 living donor uterus transplantations. Am J Transplant. 2019;19(3):855–64.

13. Puntambekar S, Puntambekar S, Telang M, Kulkarni P, Date S, Panse M, et al. Novel anastomotic technique for uterine transplant using utero-ovarian veins for venous drainage and internal iliac arteries for perfusion in two laparoscopically harvested uteri. J Minim Invasive Gynecol. 2019;26(4):628–35.
14. Wei L, Xue T, Tao KS, Zhang G, Zhao GY, Yu SQ, et al. Modified human uterus transplantation using ovarian veins for venous drainage: the first report of surgically successful robotic-assisted uterus procurement and follow-up for 12 months. Fertil Steril. 2017;108(2):346–56 e1.
15. Favre-Inhofer A, Rafii A, Carbonnel M, Revaux A, Ayoubi JM. Uterine transplantation: review in human research. J Gynecol Obstet Hum Reprod. 2018;47(6):213–21.
16. Daolio J, Palomba S, Paganelli S, Falbo A, Aguzzoli L. Uterine transplantation and IVF for congenital or acquired uterine factor infertility: a systematic review of safety and efficacy outcomes in the first 52 recipients. PLoS One. 2020;15(4):e0232323.
17. Chmel R, Cekal M, Pastor Z, Chmel R Jr, Paulasova P, Havlovicova M, et al. Assisted reproductive techniques and pregnancy results in women with Mayer-rokitansky-kuster-hauser syndrome undergoing uterus transplantation: the Czech experience. J Pediatr Adolesc Gynecol. 2020;33(4):410–4.
18. Jones BP, Saso S, Quiroga I, Yazbek J, Smith JR. Limited availability of deceased uterus donors: a UK perspective. Transplantation. 2020;104(8):e250–e1.
19. Testa G, Anthony T, McKenna GJ, Koon EC, Wallis K, Klintmalm GB, et al. Deceased donor uterus retrieval: a novel technique and workflow. Am J Transplant. 2018;18(3):679–83.
20. Agraharkar ML, Cinclair RD, Kuo YF, Daller JA, Shahinian VB. Risk of malignancy with long-term immunosuppression in renal transplant recipients. Kidney Int. 2004;66(1):383–9.
21. Engels EA, Pfeiffer RM, Fraumeni JF Jr, Kasiske BL, Israni AK, Snyder JJ, et al. Spectrum of cancer risk among US solid organ transplant recipients. JAMA. 2011;306(17):1891–901.

Part VIII

Penis Transplantation

Conventional Surgical Techniques and Emerging Transplantation in Complex Penile Reconstruction

32

Nima Khavanin and Richard J. Redett

32.1 Introduction

32.1.1 Conventional Surgical Techniques

The Russian surgeon Nikolaj Bogoraz reported the first attempted total penile reconstruction in 1936 [1]. He used a bipedicle flap of abdominal tissue with a rib cartilage graft to provide stiffness for sexual intercourse. An important first step in penile reconstruction, this attempt fell short of attempting urethral reconstruction or taking measures to restore protective and/or erogenous sensation. Since then several breakthroughs including the "tube within a tube" design for creation of the neourethra [2] and novel microsurgical techniques have vastly expanded our toolkit in complex genitourinary reconstruction, enabling substantial improvements in functional and esthetic outcomes.

As the collective experience increased, it was no longer enough to simply measure success as flap survival. The emphasis shifted instead toward the functional and esthetic outcomes of the reconstruction. In their 1987 article, Gilbert and colleagues [3] described five criteria for the ideal phallic reconstruction that have since then become widely adopted:

1. A reproducible, single-stage procedure.
2. Creation of a neourethra that allows for voiding while standing.
3. A neo-phallus with erogenous and tactile sensibility.
4. The ability to partake in penetrative sexual intercourse.
5. A satisfactory esthetic result.

Free tissue transfer using the radial forearm free flap, anterolateral thigh flap, fibular osteocutaneous flap, and latissimus dorsi myocutaneous flap has become workhorses in penile reconstruction. These procedures allow for the transfer of a large amount of tissue with relatively minimal donor site morbidity [4, 5]. At least at the surface, each of the conventional techniques for phalloplasty has the potential to achieve the above listed goals set forth by Gilbert. The reality however is an unreliable outcome that often fails to meet one or more of our reconstructive goals.

These procedures can technically be performed in as few as one stage; however, many surgeons prefer staging them in 3 or more procedures in an attempt to minimize complications. These typically include: initial flap transfer, tissue debulking, corona/glans-"plasty," urethral lengthening/anastomosis, and/or the insertion of a penile prosthesis. Even in the most skilled of hands, complication rates exceed 40%, with urethral fistulas (≥30%), urethral strictures (~10%), and complications related to the penile prosthesis (≥40%) accounting for the majority of the morbidity [4, 6].

With these limitations of conventional penile reconstruction in mind, the need for a better solution becomes clear. We continue to fall short on delivering a successful, single-stage procedure particularly with regard to the successful urinary transport and the ability to achieve an erection. To that end, penile reconstruction represents the first true solution to the reconstructive challenge set forth by Gilbert over 30 years ago. In this chapter, we aim to review our experience in still burgeoning field of penile transplantation. We will review our experience performing the most extensive penis, scrotum, and partial abdominal wall transplantation to date and provide insight into our methods for patient selection, technical considerations for the procedure, and out post-operative protocols.

32.1.2 History of Penis Transplantation

The earliest animal models for penile transplantation were developed in 2000s. The feasibility of allogeneic penile transplantation through nonvascular anastomosis and subsequently arterial anastomosis to the distal corpus spongiosum were first demonstrated in a rodent model [7, 8]. Autotransplantation rat models were also developed to assess the

N. Khavanin · R. J. Redett (✉)
Department of Plastic and Reconstructive Surgery, Johns Hopkins University School of Medicine, Baltimore, MD, USA
e-mail: rjr@jhmi.edu

© Springer Nature Switzerland AG 2023
R. Gurunian et al. (eds.), *Reconstructive Transplantation*, https://doi.org/10.1007/978-3-031-21520-9_32

viability and functionality of re-planted phalluses [9]. Since then, the development of a canine model [10], deceased donor anatomic studies [10], and an ex vivo model to assess graft rejection [11] has helped to bridge the gap between bench and bedside in preparation for the first few cases of penis transplantation.

The first in human procedure was attempted in 2006 in China. A 44-year-old man who had lost his penis following a traumatic injury underwent a technically successful procedure. Nonetheless, the graft was explanted just 2 weeks after the surgery due to psychological rejection [12]. In 2015, the second penis transplant was performed in South Africa on a 21-year-old man with a penile injury sustained during cultural circumcision [13]. Two years following this procedure, the recipient reported the ability to urinate and to achieve erections, orgasms, and ejaculation [14]. In 2017, the same group in South Africa performed its second (world third) penis transplantation [15]. In the United States, a partial penis transplant to a 64-year-old man who had underwent oncologic penectomy was performed in 2016 [16]. Six months following the operation that patient had recovered sensation, was voiding successfully, and reported partial erectile function.

The penis transplantation program at the Johns Hopkins University School of Medicine was started in 2013 to meet the needs of wounded military personnel who were returning to the United States with large and complex genitourinary and abdominal wall defects from IEDs. To date we have screened many patients including one patient who underwent the world's most extensive penis transplantation including the entire penis, scrotum, and parts of the abdominal wall in 2018 (Fig. 32.1).

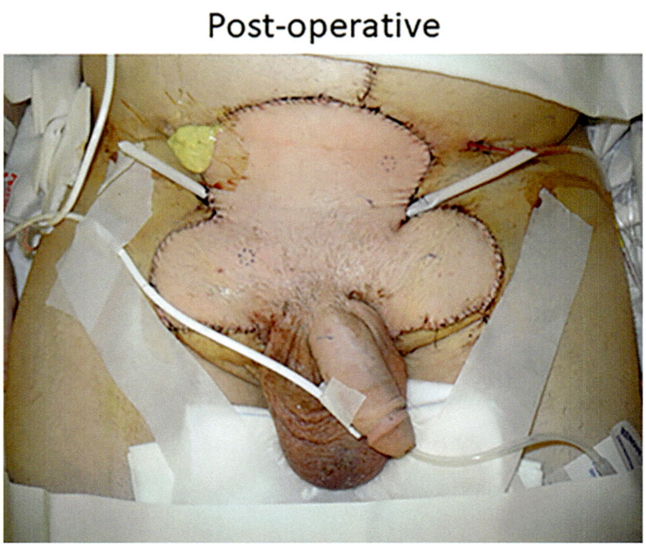

Fig. 32.1 Immediate post-operative result of the world's first penis, scrotum, and lower abdominal wall transplantation. Continuous near-infrared spectroscopy monitored tissue oxygen saturation in the distributions of the dorsal penile and external pudendal vessels independently. The donor and recipient urethras were anastomosed over a 16-French Foley catheter

32.2 Technical Considerations

32.2.1 Indications

Most discussions on the indications for penis transplantation have focused on traumatic etiologies. In this cohort, extremity amputation or other injuries may have compromised conventional donor sites for phalloplasty, leaving patients with few or no alternatives.

Oncologic extirpation remains another important avenue for potential transplantation. We have recently expanded our own eligibility criteria to include patients who are in remission 5-years following oncologic penectomy. The largest study to date on recurrence in penile cancer found that all recurrences tend to occur within 5 years of the initial resection [17]. Given that all remaining native penile skin can be resected before transplantation, the risk of locoregional recurrence should be negligible, even in the setting of systemic immunosuppression.

We have also expanded our indications to include men with congenitally ambiguous genitalia or true micropenis. As we discussed earlier, even the most sophisticated techniques for conventional penile reconstruction are fraught with urinary complications and issues related to penile prostheses [4, 18]. Although there are greater risks with penis transplantation, this may be outweighed by the improved function and esthetics of a transplanted phallus. At this time, further deliberation on the use of penile transplantation in transgender men is warranted. The lack of proximal corpora nearly guarantees that a transgender man will not be able to achieve an erection after transplantation.

Traditionally vascularized composite allotransplantation has been considered a last resort after several failed conventional procedures [19]. This thought process has been questioned recently, as there are considerable downsides to undergoing multiple failed reconstructive attempts before transplantation, including more extensive scarring of the native soft tissues and potential injuries to the donor vessels and nerves [20]. Furthermore, we believe that surgeons should preserve conventional reconstructive options as a contingency plan in the event of allograft failure. Without long-term data on graft longevity we should also make sure to preserve several "back-up" options in the event of immunologic rejection.

32.2.2 Patient Selection and Pre-Operative Evaluation

Our protocol for human penile allotransplantation has been approved by the Johns Hopkins Institutional Review Board. Potential candidates are identified through review of existing patients in the Johns Hopkins medical system in addition to referrals from the United States military and other outside providers. Once identified, potential patients undergo a rigorous screening process including evaluation by a multidisciplinary penile transplant team that includes plastic surgery, urology, transplant surgery, transplant medicine, mental health, and infectious disease. History and physical exams are carried out by both plastic surgery and urology, and the patient undergoes comprehensive infectious testing. Once a candidate is deemed appropriate, additional pre-operative evaluation includes cardiology workup with echocardiogram and electrocardiogram, pulmonary function testing and chest X-ray, HLA typing and panel-reactive antibody testing, and imaging including CTA of the abdomen and pelvis, lumbosacral plexus MRI, and MR neurography of the pelvis.

For several ethical and/or practical reasons [21, 22], candidates for penis transplantation are currently limited to adults aged 18 or older. The cumulative risks of a transplant are greater in children than adults due to the extended exposure to immunosuppression over their lifetime, and it is not clear when a child can provide adequate consent to such a life altering procedure. Additionally, pediatric penile transplant is complicated by issues related to donor matching. It would be inappropriate to transplant an adult phallus onto a child, but the use of an age-congruent phallus risks issues related to an age-incongruent phallus in adulthood. Finally, we do not yet know what the lifespan of a penis transplant is, and childhood recipients are likely to require at least one additional transplant in adulthood.

In addition to a full medical evaluation, potential patients are also screened by psychology, sexual psychology, and social work as a part of their multidisciplinary evaluation. Safer sex counseling is an essential part of recipient care because certain sexually transmitted infections may be particularly devastating to an immunocompromised host. Given the intimate nature of penile transplants, sexual partners and others close to the patient should be involved in care if the recipient so wishes. Relationship counseling can similarly be an essential component of pre- and post-transplant care. This also provides an opportunity to ensure the recipient has a stable and strong support network to aid with emotional adjustment post-operatively.

32.2.3 Donor Considerations

Limited donor availability represents a major hurdle for any type of transplantation. Several factors in addition to the traditional HLA matching further complicate the issue when specifically dealing with the topic of penis transplantation. The donor phallus must be healthy without vascular disease, sexually transmitted infection, and/or complications of diabetes. Additionally, attention should be paid to recipient's esthetic preferences. The appearance of donor phallus must be congruent with the recipient's desired appearance and discussed frankly before listing in order to limit psychological stresses.

32.2.4 Surgical Technique

Given its anatomical complexity, penile transplantation presents unique challenges such as how proximal the graft will need to be performed. Anastomosing a distal portion of the penis requires fewer structural anastomoses than that of the entire penis with portions of the pelvic floor. The indication for transplantation also plays a role in the surgical decision-making. Larger grafts may be required to address wartime injuries with extensive damage to the perineum and abdominal wall, and in congenital anomalies, there may be extensive scarring from multiple prior surgeries and insufficient tissue development to provide adequate proximal corpora anastomosis. There is not a single solution in penile transplantation for every patient, and the details of graft design should be tailored to the individual patient at hand.

The penis has three main vascular perfusion territories which have been previously described in detail [23]. The first includes the shaft and scrotal skin which is vascularized by the external pudendal arteries—branches of the femoral arteries bilaterally. The glans and corpus spongiosum are supplied by the dorsal arteries, and the corpora cavernosa are supplied by the cavernous arteries. These latter two both originate from the pudendal arteries; however, each may require its own vascular anastomosis depending on the proximal extent of the graft. Venous outflow similarly depends upon the extent of the transplant. In a mid-shaft transplantation, outflow could be limited to as little as the deep and superficial dorsal veins, whereas in the most extensive penis, scrotum, and abdominal wall transplantation performed to date the dorsal veins were anastomosed in addition to the bilateral saphenous veins [24]. Similar to penile replantation, the donor dorsal penile nerves can be coapted with the recipient dorsal penile nerves. The donor urethra can be anastomosed with the recipient urethra in a spatulated fashion consistent with primary anastomotic urethroplasty. The tunica albuginea, Buck's fascia, dartos fascia, and skin are also anastomosed between donor and recipient tissues.

In our first patient (Fig. 32.1), the graft was procured by transecting the corporal bodies and urethra well behind the pubic bone, dissecting the scrotal skin off the donor testes, and incorporating a portion of the lower abdominal wall from just below the umbilicus down to the genitalia. Once the allograft was procured, the recipient team prepared the surgical site and exposed the required vessels and nerves. The first step of the transplantation was to perform the urethroplasty. The donor and recipient urethra were spatulated and interrupted anastomosed over a 16-French Foley catheter. The corporal anastomosis was performed next with a suture repair of the tunica albuginea. Our first vascular anastomoses included anastomosis of both donor dorsal arteries and veins to the recipient's deep inferior epigastric arteries and veins. The deep inferior epigastric system was used as his native dorsal vessels were destroyed by the blast injury.

Next, the dorsal nerves of the graft were coapted to the recipient's dorsal nerves. At this stage, indocyanine green angiography was used to evaluate perfusion of the graft. Our assessment demonstrated perfusion of the glans and most of the shaft but inadequate perfusion of the groin, abdomen, and scrotal tissues. As such, the left donor external pudendal artery was taken with a segment of femoral artery and revascularized by end-to-side anastomosis to the recipient femoral artery. Repeat angiography confirmed perfusion of the entire graft, and the final skin closure was performed.

Post-operatively graft perfusion was monitored through hourly assessments including appearance, temperature, color, capillary refill, and assessment of Doppler signals in the dorsal penile and external pudendal vessels. Continuous near-infrared tissue spectroscopy using the ViOptix T.Ox (ViOptix, Inc., Newark, CA) was used to monitor tissue oxygenation saturations within the distributions of the dorsal penile and external pudendal vessels.

32.2.5 Antimicrobial Therapy

Pre-operatively patients undergo a chlorhexidine gluconate bath and receive a dose intravenous cefazolin that is repeated every 4 h during the operation. If either the donor or recipient screen positive for MRSA colonization, antibiotic prophylaxis is exchanged to intravenous vancomycin and ciprofloxacin. Prophylaxis is continued with the above regimen for 71 h post-operatively. Recipients who test positive for any staphylococcal aureus strain in their nares receive mupirocin twice daily to the nares for 5 days.

Antiviral prophylaxis includes valacyclovir 500 mg twice daily for 12 months. Testing is performed for herpes simplex virus I/II, varicella zoster virus, Epstein–Barr virus, and cytomegalovirus, and prophylaxis can be adjusted as needed based on these results. Seropositive patients receive intravenous ganciclovir for 2 weeks followed by valganciclovir for 6 months before transitioning to valacyclovir for the final 6 months. Pneumocystis prophylaxis is with daily trimethoprim–sulfamethoxazole 400 mg/80 mg for a total of 12 months. Alternative regimens include dapsone 100 mg daily or atovaquone 1500 mg daily if patients are unable to tolerate first-line therapy. Anti-candida prophylaxis is with fluconazole 800 mg loading dose followed by 400 mg daily for 1 month.

32.2.6 Immunosuppression Protocol

At our center, recipients are treated with an immunomodulatory regimen consisting of monoclonal antibody induction, calcineurin inhibitor (tacrolimus) monotherapy maintenance, and a donor bone marrow cell infusion 2 weeks after the transplant. Specifically, our patient underwent induction therapy with a single dose of alemtuzumab (Campath-1H™, Millennium Pharma, Cambridge, MA) 30 mg over 2 h for lymphocyte depletion given immediately before transplantation in the operative room. Additionally, 1000 mg of intravenous methylprednisolone was administered before graft reperfusion. He was started on tacrolimus maintenance therapy on the day of transplantation with a target trough between 10 and 15 mg/mL.

Skin biopsies were performed at weeks 1, 2, 3, 4, 6, 12, 24 to monitor for acute cell mediated rejection of the graft. Episodes of erythema and rash post-operatively were treated with topical clobetasol +/− topical tacrolimus, at no point the patient requires an increase in systemic tacrolimus or additional steroid bolus.

32.2.7 Donor Bone Marrow Transfusion and Chimerism Analysis

At the time of graft procurement, donor vertebral bodies from T8 to L4 were also resected for processing and bone marrow cell isolation. The vertebrae were stored between 2° and 8 °C for a total of 26 h before processing. The protocol for progenitor cell isolation from the donor vertebrae has been previously described in detail [25]. After processing, the product contained 4.2×10^{10} nucleated cells, including: 1.23% CD34+ and 10.23% CD3+ cells with 3 mL of RBCs.

On post-operative day 14, bone marrow was infused intravenously at a dose of 5.7×10^{6} CD34 + cells/kg without any adverse events.

Blood testing for peripheral chimerism was performed post-operatively on weeks 1 and 2 (prior to bone marrow infusion) as well as on weeks 3, 4, 6, and 7 and months 3 and 6. The details of this chimerism analysis have been previously described at length [24]. Evaluations at weeks 1, 2, and 3 yielded a small percentage of donor DNA (<5%), which is below the linear quantification range of the assay. At week 4, CD3+ separated T cell analysis showed 8% mixed chimerism, but none was detected by week 6 with subsequent test remaining without evidence of donor DNA.

32.3 Lessons Learned

The field of penis transplantation is still in its infancy, and each new patient continues to teach us a great deal about its potential as well as its current limitations. Many questions remain regarding the long-term longevity of these grafts and the potential need for re-transplantation or other salvage procedures. Nonetheless, short term outcomes have been reassuring thus far.

32.3.1 Clinical Outcomes

Apart from the first penis transplantation that was removed due to psychological rejection, at the time of writing this article, all other instances of penis transplantation have been reportedly successful. Urinary transport is generally achieved without complication in penile transplantation, as is the case in penile replantation and primary anastomotic urethroplasties where two healthy urethral segments are approximated. This is unlike phalloplasty, which uses tubularized skin for urethral reconstruction and involves high complication rates as previously mentioned. Case series demonstrated that natural erections are attainable after penile replantation for traumatic amputations [26], as has been the case with the limited series of penile transplantations [24].

At our center, it has now been more than 2 years since our first patient underwent transplantation (Fig. 32.2). He experiences near-normal erections and is able to achieve orgasm, with substantial improvements in self-reported pleasure scores [24]. He has normal sensation to the shaft and tip of the penis and can successfully localize touch sensation. Neurosensory testing reveals that the glans has near-normal sensibility to one-point moving touch and somewhat lower results with one-point static touch. Sensation in the shaft has recovered to higher thresholds than in the glans. The patient is able to urinate while standing, without straining, frequency, or urgency and with a strong stream.

32.3.2 Building a Successful Program

The cornerstone of the success of our penis transplantation program is the support of our hospital and school of medicine. Our first in human transplantation was the culmination of over 5 years of work in cadaver and animal models and the organization of many dozens of physicians, nurses, therapists, researchers, and administrators. Our multidisciplinary vascularized composite allotransplantation team has over 10 years of experience in the management of upper extremity transplantation. Our clinical transplantation program is bolstered by a strong basic and translational research laboratory that has developed large and small animal models for penis, face, limb, and abdominal wall transplantation. The development of robust animal models has enabled research aimed at monitoring tissue rejection and decreasing the burden of immunosuppression as we optimize chimerism protocols.

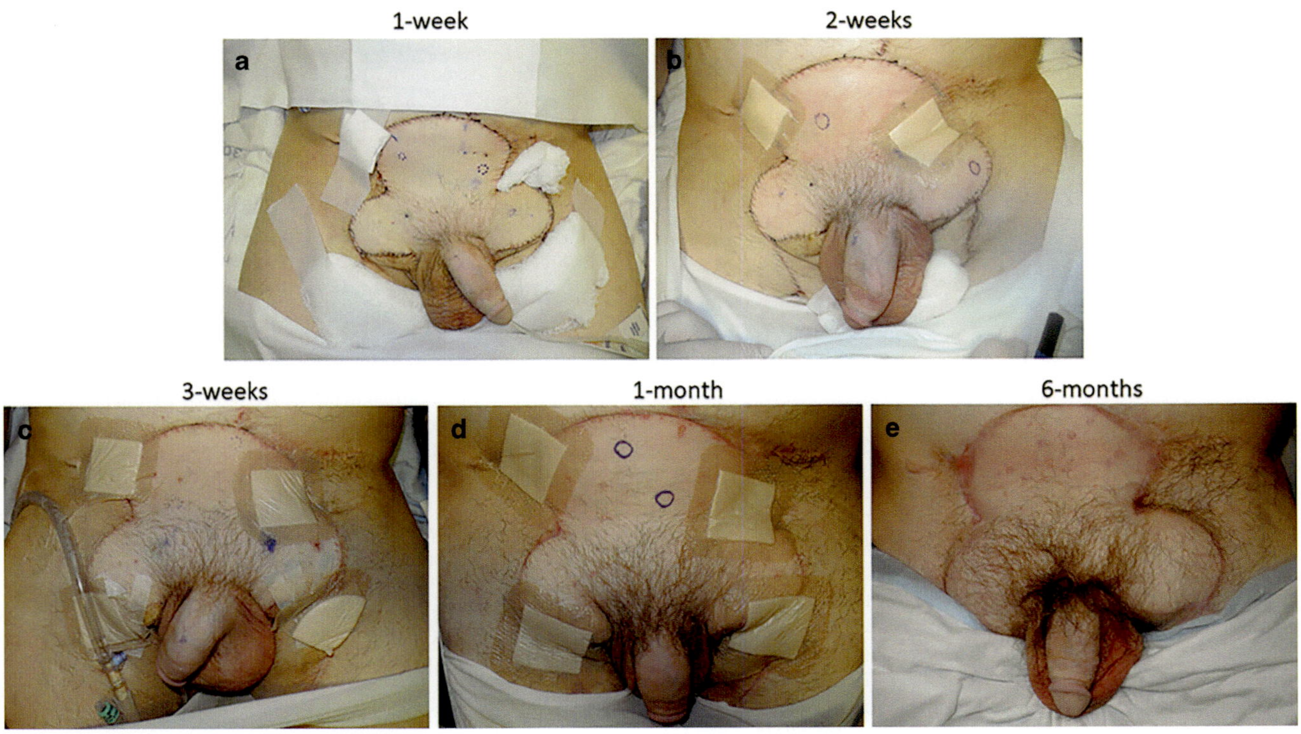

Fig. 32.2 Post-operative follow-up at 1 week (**a**), 2 weeks (**b**), 3 weeks (**c**), 1 month (**d**), and 6 months (**e**). The graft has healed uneventfully without any evidence of immunologic rejection. He is now over 2-years post-operative and reports near-normal erections as well as intact protective and erogenous sensation with the ability to achieve orgasm. He is able to urinate while standing without any evidence of complications

32.3.3 Conclusion

Nearly 90 years after the first attempted penile reconstruction, and 30 since Gilbert and colleagues outlined the five criteria to achieve ideal phallic reconstruction, it would appear that the surgical community has finally realized its goal of the ideal penis reconstruction. Penile transplantation represents a single-stage procedure that allows the recipient to void while standing, provides protective and erogenous sensation as well as the ability to achieve and erection, and results in an unmatched esthetic outcome. Although still a young field with many unanswered questions, its early success represents a new opportunity for many patients to finally "feel whole" [27] again after facing incredible hardships.

References

1. Bogoraz N. On complete plastic reconstruction of a penis sufficient for coitus. Sov Surg. 1936;8:303–9.
2. Gillies H. Congenital absence of the penis. Br J Plast Surg. 1948;1(1):8–28.
3. Gilbert DA, Horton CE, Terzis JK, Devine CJ Jr, Winslow BH, Devine PC. New concepts in phallic reconstruction. Ann Plast Surg. 1987;18(2):128–36. https://doi.org/10.1097/00000637-198702000-00006.
4. Yao A, Ingargiola MJ, Lopez CD, Sanati-Mehrizy P, Burish NM, Jablonka EM, et al. Total penile reconstruction: a systematic review. J Plast Reconstr Aesthet Surg. 2018;71(6):788–806. http://www.ncbi.nlm.nih.gov/pubmed/29622476.
5. Kropp B, Cohn JE, Wang W, Sokoya M, Ducic Y. Free tissue transfer penile reconstruction. Semin Plast Surg. 2019;33(1):24–9. http://www.ncbi.nlm.nih.gov/pubmed/30863209.
6. Monstrey S, Hoebeke P, Selvaggi G, Ceulemans P, Van Landuyt K, Blondeel P, et al. Penile reconstruction: is the radial forearm flap really the standard technique? Plast Reconstr Surg. 2009;124(2):510–8. http://www.ncbi.nlm.nih.gov/pubmed/19644267.
7. Sonmez E, Nasir S, Siemionow M. Penis allotransplantation model in the rat. Ann Plast Surg. 2009;62(3):304–10. http://www.ncbi.nlm.nih.gov/pubmed/19240530.
8. Koga H, Yamataka A, Wang K, Kato Y, Lane GJ, Kobayashi H, et al. Experimental allogenic penile transplantation. J Pediatr Surg. 2003;38(12):1802–5. http://www.ncbi.nlm.nih.gov/pubmed/14666472.
9. Akyurek M, Ozkan O, Safak T, Ozgentas HE, Dunn RM. The penile flap in the rat: description and autotransplantation. Ann Plast Surg. 2005;55(1):94–100; discussion 101. http://www.ncbi.nlm.nih.gov/pubmed/15985799.
10. Zhao Y, Hu W, Zhang L, Guo F, Wang W, Wang B, et al. Penis allotransplantation in beagle dog. Biomed Res Int. 2016;2016:1489204. http://www.ncbi.nlm.nih.gov/pubmed/26977412.
11. Sopko NA, Matsui H, Lough DM, Miller D, Harris K, Kates M, et al. Ex vivo model of human penile transplantation and rejection: implications for erectile tissue physiology. Eur Urol. 2017;71(4):584–93. http://www.ncbi.nlm.nih.gov/pubmed/27432525.
12. Hu W, Lu J, Zhang L, Wu W, Nie H, Zhu Y, et al. A preliminary report of penile transplantation: part 2. Eur Urol. 2006;50(5):1115–6; discussion 1116. http://www.ncbi.nlm.nih.gov/pubmed/17106949.
13. Bateman C. World's first successful penis transplant at Tygerberg hospital. S Afr Med J. 2015;105(4):251–2. http://www.ncbi.nlm.nih.gov/pubmed/26294859.
14. van der Merwe A, Graewe F, Zühlke A, Barsdorf NW, Zarrabi AD, Viljoen JT, et al. Penile allotransplantation for penis amputation following ritual circumcision: a case report with 24 months of follow-up. Lancet (London, England). 2017;390(10099):1038–47. http://www.ncbi.nlm.nih.gov/pubmed/28823494.
15. Ngaage LM, Elegbede A, Sugarman J, Nam AJ, Cooney CM, Cooney DS, et al. The Baltimore criteria for an ethical approach to penile transplantation: a clinical guideline. Transpl Int. 2019;33(5):471–82. http://www.ncbi.nlm.nih.gov/pubmed/31646681.
16. Cetrulo CL, Li K, Salinas HM, Treiser MD, Schol I, Barrisford GW, et al. Penis transplantation: first US experience. Ann Surg. 2018;267(5):983–8. http://www.ncbi.nlm.nih.gov/pubmed/28509699.
17. Leijte JAP, Kirrander P, Antonini N, Windahl T, Horenblas S. Recurrence patterns of squamous cell carcinoma of the penis: recommendations for follow-up based on a two-Centre analysis of 700 patients. Eur Urol. 2008;54(1):161–8. http://www.ncbi.nlm.nih.gov/pubmed/18440124.
18. Bluebond-Langner R, Redett RJ. Phalloplasty in complete aphallia and ambiguous genitalia. Semin Plast Surg. 2011;25(3):196–205. http://www.ncbi.nlm.nih.gov/pubmed/22851911.
19. Tuffaha SH, Cooney DS, Sopko NA, Bivalacqua TJ, Lough DM, Cooney CM, et al. Penile transplantation: an emerging option for genitourinary reconstruction. Transpl Int. 2017;30(5):441–50. http://www.ncbi.nlm.nih.gov/pubmed/28130926.
20. Diaz-Siso JR, Borab ZM, Plana NM, Parent B, Stranix JT, Rodriguez ED. Vascularized composite allotransplantation: alternatives and catch-22s. Plast Reconstr Surg. 2018;142(5):1320–6. http://www.ncbi.nlm.nih.gov/pubmed/30511987.
21. Marchac A, Kuschner T, Paris J, Picard A, Vazquez MP, Lantieri L. Ethical issues in pediatric face transplantation: should we perform face transplantation in children? Plast Reconstr Surg. 2016;138(2):449–54. http://www.ncbi.nlm.nih.gov/pubmed/27465167.
22. Amaral S, Levin LS. Pediatric and congenital hand transplantation. Curr Opin Organ Transplant. 2017;22(5):477–83. http://www.ncbi.nlm.nih.gov/pubmed/28719391.
23. Tuffaha SH, Sacks JM, Shores JT, Brandacher G, Lee WPA, Cooney DS, et al. Using the dorsal, cavernosal, and external pudendal arteries for penile transplantation: technical considerations and perfusion territories. Plast Reconstr Surg. 2014;134(1):111e–9e. http://www.ncbi.nlm.nih.gov/pubmed/24622570.
24. Redett RJ, Etra JW, Brandacher G, Burnett AL, Tuffaha SH, Sacks JM, et al. Total penis, scrotum, and lower abdominal wall transplantation. N Engl J Med. 2019;381(19):1876–8. http://www.ncbi.nlm.nih.gov/pubmed/31693813.
25. Gorantla VS, Schneeberger S, Moore LR, Donnenberg VS, Zimmerlin L, Lee WPA, et al. Development and validation of a procedure to isolate viable bone marrow cells from the vertebrae of cadaveric organ donors for composite organ grafting. Cytotherapy. 2012;14(1):104–13. http://www.ncbi.nlm.nih.gov/pubmed/21905958.
26. Sopko NA, Tuffaha SH, Lough D, Brandacher G, Lee WPA, Bivalacqua TJ, et al. Penile allotransplantation for complex genitourinary reconstruction. J Urol. 2017;198(2):274–80. http://www.ncbi.nlm.nih.gov/pubmed/28286074.
27. The Associated Press. US veteran 'feeling whole' year after penis transplant. Newyork, NY: The Associated Press; 2019; https://apnews.com/780c0fb67f5245e0acd4213b0780997c.

Part IX

Miscellaneous Special

33 Future Directions of Vascularized Composite Allotransplantation

Andrea Sisti

33.1 Introduction

Organ reconstruction is very challenging for patients suffering from severe and extensive injuries. For these patients, it is necessary to use non-autogenous sources as reconstructive material because autologous tissues are not usually sufficient. Recent advances in microsurgery and transplant immunology provided the opportunity to offer the patient different reconstructive options. Vascularized composite allotransplantation (VCA) is a reconstructive option that allows the replacement of similar composite tissues, which is one of the basic and essential principles in plastic surgery [1, 2]. VCA aims to recreate esthetics and function in the recipient site [3]. VCA is the process of the transplantation of various tissues as a functional unit from a deceased brain dead donor to a recipient [4]. It should be noticed the differences between VCA and solid organ transplantation (SOT), such as liver or renal transplantation [5]. Early and subsequent developments in SOT and VCA were as the results of plastic surgeons' contribution. One of the early kidney transplantations between identical twins was performed by a US plastic surgeon, Joseph E. Murray, in 1995 [6]. On September 23, 1998, the first successful hand transplantation was performed by Dr. Jean-Michel Dubernard in Lyon, France [7–9]. Four months later, on January 24, 1999, a hand transplantation was performed at the Jewish Hospital of Louisville, USA [10]. In 2005, Dr. Bernard Devauchelle and Dubernard performed a partial face transplant and in 2010, a Spanish team led by Dr. Juan Barret performed the first full-face transplant [5, 11]. Since then, more than 145 upper extremities, 45 partial/total facial transplantations, and several other types including hand, larynx, abdominal wall, lower extremities, partial eye (non-vascularized), uterus, and penis with scrotum transplantations have been performed worldwide [3, 7, 12–19]. The main challenges for patients undergoing VCA are: the prevalence of acute rejection, which is more than 80% in hand and face transplantation during the first year, and the requirement of lifelong immunosuppression (IS) and long-term chronic rejection, which has been reported in several patients [17, 20, 21]. VCA offers the highest level of reconstruction, decreased number of revisions compared to traditional methods, and presents new opportunities for the treatment of complex tissue and functional defects [3, 22–26]. Therefore, unique opportunities provided by VCA support further development in this area.

Since the first historical attempts, a lot of progress has been made in VCA research including using animal models, translational research, and clinical outcome studies [27, 28]. In order to find the best outcome, it is vital to investigate the main challenges related to VCA.

33.2 Rejection

The allogeneic tissue is recognized by the recipient's immune system and the alloimmune response is activated. These immune responses are initiated by ABO (blood group) antigens and the human leucocyte antigens (HLA) [29]. VCAs have specific structural, molecular, and cellular attributes that lead to a distinct rejection response pattern [22, 30]. Jacoby et al. [27] recently suggested a precise diagnosis of rejection through measurement of donor-specific antibodies, complement protein deposition in allograft tissue, donor-derived cell-free DNA, and hair chimerism assays.

Unlike in other solid organ transplantation, VCAs are composed of multiple tissues with different immunogenic and functional properties, including skin, muscles, bones, nerves, blood vessels, bone marrow, lymph nodes, and tendons [25, 31].

One unique characteristic of transplantation is the usage of skin/mucosa as a monitoring tool to detect rejection (observing for rash, edema, or erythema) [32–34]. *The skin* is proven to be extremely immunogenic [32, 35]. Langerhans cells, dermal dendritic cells, macrophages, innate cells (mast

A. Sisti (✉)
Department of Surgery, University of Texas Medical Branch (UTMB), Galveston, TX, USA

© Springer Nature Switzerland AG 2023
R. Gurunian et al. (eds.), *Reconstructive Transplantation*, https://doi.org/10.1007/978-3-031-21520-9_33

cells, NK cells, NKT cells, γδ-T cells), and memory T cells comprise the skin-resident immune system [36].

It was demonstrated that T cells residing in the recipient site play a key role in skin allograft rejection. The number of T cells belonging to the skin is much higher than in the peripheral circulation and they can result in allograft rejection, led by the immune response [37].

In a recent study, Etra et al. [37] explained the basic mechanisms of rejection in VCA. They demonstrated that acute and chronic rejection are possible immunologic consequences of VCA.

Acute rejection was reported in most of VCA's recipients (75–88%) while a small percentage of patients (7.3%) receiving renal transplant (SOT) was diagnosed by acute rejection in the first year after the transplant [23, 37, 38]. Combination of tissue biopsy and clinical assessment is used for acute rejection diagnosis in VCA recipients [23]. Changes in the skin including maculopapular variably erythematous rash with edema is typically used for clinically diagnosis of acute rejection [37].

Several classification systems are used to classify histological rejection samples [39–43]. In particular, the Banff classification grades the histopathological features of acute rejection on a scale from 0 (no features of rejection) to 4 (frank necrosis of epidermis) [29, 40].

In addition to examination of the recipient's skin changes, biomarkers are also used to monitor the recipient patient under immunosuppression. These biomarkers are common to all transplants and include:

1. markers of the morbidity of immunosuppression (hypertension, hyperlipidemia, renal biochemistry, glucose function tests, white cell count),
2. markers of immunosuppressive compliance and dosing (medication levels of tacrolimus, for instance),
3. immunological system markers (donor-specific antibodies and peripheral blood chimerism), and,
4. diagnostic markers of rejection (histological assessment by biopsy).

The mechanisms of *chronic rejection* of VCA are not completely understood. Chronic rejection targets preferentially the skin (dermal sclerosis, adnexal atrophy, necrosis) and vessels (graft vasculopathy) and may cause graft dysfunction, often resulting in ischemic graft loss [44]. Cutaneous findings include scaly plaques, bruise-like or purpuric skin lesions, necrotic ulcerations, sclerodermoid and dyschromic lesions reminiscent of graft-versus-host disease, finger thinning, and nail loss [44].

Graft vasculopathy (GV) is one of the most consistent pathological outcomes that result in irreversible allograft dysfunction and eventual loss [45, 46]. It was demonstrated that GV is a multifactorial entity shared between acute and chronic rejection [46].

GV involves C4d deposition and donor-specific antibody (DSA) formation. From a recent literature review by Ng ZY [45], 6% (13 of 205) of all VCA patients reported to have developed GV at a mean of 6 years post-transplantation and 46% of these patients have either lost or had their VCAs removed. They also reported that neither C4d nor DSA alone was predictive of GV development. GV progress is not reversible by the current IS therapy and its progress cannot be stopped after diagnosis, which often leads to allotransplantation loss.

33.3 Immunosuppression

Originally, for SOT, azathioprine and prednisone were used, but then the discovery of cyclosporine in 1976 dramatically changed the available resources spectrum and opened to a new IS era [29]. At the beginning, the same IS therapies used for SOT were used for VCA; however, they were then modified specifically for VCA. For a comprehensive review of all the IS drugs used in VCA, please refer to the work developed by Mathes et al. [6].

In order to protect the transplant from the cytokine excess observed after surgery, IS in recipients is performed through lymphocyte-depleting induction therapy, during the peri-transplantation period.

The maximum immune load is at the highest level immediately after the transplantation. Therefore, drugs are administrated immediately to decrease the T-cell and B-cell population and the antibody response. Normally, T-cell depletion through antibody-mediated induction therapy using antithymocyte globulin and Campath-1H is used. Other reagents such as basiliximab (interleukin-2 receptor blocker) or alemtuzumab (anti-CD52 monoclonal antibody) were recently used. After the induction, the maintenance phase is to prevent acute and chronic rejections throughout the lifespan of the transplant. The IS maintenance is performed through triple-drug therapy (tacrolimus, mycophenolate mofetil, and prednisone) [37].

Lifelong immunosuppression (IS) risks are usually susceptible to patients undergoing VCA [24]. The use of IS drugs inhibits the immune system and therefore protects the allograft but decreases the body's overall ability to fight infection and tumors [6]. The *common complications* of IS are opportunistic infections and systemic complications [29, 47]. Infections include cytomegalovirus, clostridium difficile enteritis, herpes simplex, cutaneous mycosis, and osteomyelitis. The metabolic complications include hyperglycemia, diabetes, hyperlipidemia, hyperparathyroidism, Cushing syndrome, osteonecrosis, and impaired renal function. In a study performed by Benedict and Magill, they found out that 90% of upper extremity transplantation patients had some post-transplant metabolic complication [48]. Moreover, they found out that 75% of patients receiving tacrolimus experience anorexia, nausea, vomiting, diarrhea, and abdominal discomfort [48], and the risk of developing nonmelanoma skin cancer or chronic kidney disease is higher in VCA patients compared to the general population.

33.4 Ischemia-Reperfusion Injury (IRI)

VCA is particularly susceptible to *ischemia-reperfusion injury (IRI)* since it involves the transplantation of highly metabolically active tissues [49]. It was reported that IRI is one of the primary determinants of tissue survival in VCA because it triggers an inflammatory cascade which eventually results in tissue dysfunction, poor graft function, and survival.

IRI is driven by the innate immune response and is a major concern in VCA [50]. The initial lack of oxygen supply and ATP, followed by the secondary cellular insult after reperfusion, results in the release of heat shock proteins, radical oxygen species, and damage-associated molecular patterns. The activation of pattern recognition receptors, such as Toll-like receptors (TLRs), on macrophages, neutrophils, and natural killer cells, enhances proinflammatory cytokine, chemokine, and adhesion molecule programs which leads to further leukocyte recruitment. TLRs regulate the activation of antigen-presenting cells (APCs), which increase antigen-specific T-cell frequency, often in concert with the complement cascade. A key factor of the complement-promoting IRI disease is the activation of the membrane attack complex. This phenomenon stimulates cell death, the release of chemotactic agents and anaphylatoxins as well as neutrophil recruitment and mast cell degradation. Depending on the tissue type, VCAs display disparate susceptibility against cold ischemia with the muscle component being the least tolerant.

It is well-known that there is no effective treatment for IRI [49]. Currently, the main strategies to combat IRI are the prevention and minimization by reducing ischemia time and the metabolic activity of tissue during storage. As an example, static cold storage (SCS) and limiting ischemia time could mitigate the risk of IRI.

33.5 Strategies Proposed to Improve VCA Outcomes

Several techniques were recommended to reduce the prevalence of rejection and to improve the VCA outcomes, as summarized in Table 33.1 [49].

Table 33.1 Strategies proposed to improve VCA outcomes

Strategy	References
Machine perfusion	[49, 51, 52]
Cryopreservation	[49, 51]
Local immunosuppression (local IS)	[30, 53]
Targeted immunosuppression	[54]
Costimulation blockade (CoB)	[30]
Hematopoietic cell transplantation (HCT)	[30]
Cell therapy [including adipose-derived stem cells (ADSCs) and stromal vascular fraction (SVF), regulatory T cells, bone marrow-derived mesenchymal stem cells (BM-MSCs), dendritic cells (DCs), bone marrow transplantation, donor recipient chimeric cell (DRCC) therapy]	[30, 55, 56]
Transfer of donor lymph node (LN)	[57]
Decellularization/recellularization	[4]
Nerve regeneration [through nerve guidance conduits, fibrin glues, stem-cell therapy, electrical stimulation, tacrolimus (FK506), and hormonal therapy]	[58]

33.6 Machine Perfusion Technique and Cryopreservation

The *machine perfusion technique* aims to preserve organ viability through the provision of oxygen and nutrients and the removal of metabolic by-products. Organs are mechanically perfused using a perfusion solution, providing nutrients, and washing out potential toxins, before transplantation [51]. The perfusion can be hypothermic (0–12 °C), midthermic (13–24 °C), subnormothermic (25–34 °C), or normothermic (35–38 °C) [51]. The goal of *cryopreservation* is to slow down the deterioration of graft tissue by reducing the rate of metabolism by freezing the graft to temperatures below 0 °C. Cryopreservation uses very low temperatures (≤ -80 °C) to reduce the metabolic activity and therefore slowing down the biologic functions while maintaining the structures of cells and tissues. However, cryopreservation can damage cells and anatomical structures due to extracellular and intracellular ice [51]. Other preservation techniques have been described by Burlage et al. [51] An ideal preservation solution could lower the occurrence of IRI in VCA by protecting the microvasculature and reducing ROS generation [49]. Several chemical materials including Dextran 40, deferoxamine, LK-614, allopurinol, and glutathione have been used to lower the ROS (reactive oxygen species) production and protect the endothelial cells following reperfusion.

33.7 Modulating Immunosuppression

Local IS and targeted IS therapies are significant innovations. Considering the easy accessibility through the skin, VCAs are ideal candidates for *local IS* [30, 53]. Local IS strategies, such as topical application of IS or the use of a local drug delivery system, can minimize systemic exposure to IS while maintaining sufficient levels at the graft site to prevent rejection. Tacrolimus-laden hydrogel, topical formulations of CyA and tacrolimus, hydrogen sulfide, and steroid creams have been used for this purpose. It should be noted that while local IS reduces the need for systemic IS, they are not capable of inhibiting the occurrence of chronic vascular rejection.

Targeted immunosuppression uses innovative drug delivery systems (DDS) to overcome the systemic toxicity of the IS drugs [54]. Site-specific DDS are proved to reduce systemic toxicity and promote VCA survival. These findings suggest that targeted delivery could increase patient compliance and potentially decrease toxicity in VCA recipients.

Targeted immunosuppression in VCA represents a promising approach for improving patient compliance and graft survival while reducing systemic toxicity and the risk of rejection.

33.8 Innovative Strategies to Regulate the Immune System to a Mitigate VCA Rejection

Novel approaches to minimize rejections in VCA using the modulation of the cell population have been proposed in recent years [17]. Parallel transplant of the donor marrow with VCA is one of the major strategies to minimize VCA rejection. This strategy stimulates the development of bone marrow chimerism and promotes the recipient's tolerance to donor tissues [3]. This in turn helps to reduce the incidence of rejection in the VCA host.

In 2021, Matar et al. [30] proposed new immune strategies to improve VCA outcomes using *hematopoietic cell transplantation (HCT), costimulation blockade (CoB), and cell therapy*.

Hematopoietic cell transplantation [30] or HCT (infused bone marrow, cytokine "mobilized" cells, or vascularized bone marrow) induces a state of mixed chimerism, in which donor and host-derived cells coexist in a state of tolerance without a host versus graft allo-response (rejection) or graft-versus-host disease (GVHD) [55, 56]. Following the induction of mixed chimerism and immune tolerance, transplantation of a subsequent donor allograft is accepted without additional IS [30].

Jundziłł et al. [56] used the vascularized skin allograft model to compare the tolerogenic effects of allogeneic bone marrow transplantation into immunoprivileged compartments (intracapsular, intragonadal, intrathecal). The authors observed that transplantation of donor bone marrow cells into immunoprivileged compartments delayed rejection of vascularized skin allograft and inducted donor-specific chimerism [56].

Donor recipient chimeric cell (DRCC) therapy is a novel therapeutic approach for the maintenance of chimerism and extension of VCA survival. This technique was studied by Cwykiel et al. [55], which evaluated the efficacy of DRCC therapy created by fusion of donor and recipient derived bone marrow cells in chimerism and tolerance induction in a rat VCA model.

Rats were randomly divided into 4 groups. Group 4 got DRCC therapy with 7-day anti-αβTCR monoclonal antibody and cyclosporine A protocol, whereas the animals in the other groups got other IS therapies or were left untreated. Group 4 presented the longest average VCA survival (79.3 ± 30.9 days). The authors concluded that a single dose of DRCC therapy induced long-term multilineage chimerism and extended VCA survival [55].

Costimulation blockade [30] (CoB) has recently been proposed as an alternative method to standard calcineurin inhibitor (CNI) therapy. Belatacept, a CTLA4-Ig fusion protein was recently shown to confer improved graft and patient survival compared to CNI in renal transplant patients. CoB-based therapy blocking either the CD28-CD80/86 or CD40-CD154 pathways has shown promising results in animal VCA models.

Adipose-derived stem cells (ADSCs), stromal vascular fraction (SVF), regulatory T cells, bone marrow-derived mesenchymal stem cells (BM-MSCs), and dendritic cells (DCs) are among different regulatory cell populations that have been studied in VCA models [30]. Chen et al. [59] researched the prevention of allograft rejection using *ADSCs and SVF* to modulate the immune system to prevent allograft rejection in a VCA model. Allograft pre-treatment with SVF enhances allograft survival through suppression of T lymphocyte proliferation and infiltration and augmented immunomodulatory cytokine secretion as well as induction of Treg expression and CD31 and VEGF-A expressions. This treatment modality may be a key adjunct in the introduction and maintenance of immunotolerance in VCA [59]. They demonstrated that ex-vivo treatment of allografts with SVF or ADSC prolonged allograft survival in contrast to medium control cohorts. They observed increased levels of immunomodulatory cytokines and enhanced VEGF-A and CD31 expression as well as reduced infiltration and proliferation of T lymphocytes along with raised Treg expressions.

In their recent study, Hu et al. [60] reported the use of *ADSCs* to improve the survival of allogeneic skin grafts. However, there is currently no consensus on the administration route of ADSCs. The authors studied the effectiveness of local injection and intravenous (IV) administration of ADSCs in improving the survival of allogeneic skin grafts in mice. They found out that ADSCs increased the survival of allogeneic skin grafts in mice regardless of the route of administration. This effect might be due to the anti-inflammatory and angiogenic effects of ADSCs.

After irradiation therapy, injections of donor-derived allogeneic *mesenchymal stromal cells* causing a state of chimerism in recipients have been shown to improve allograft survival of a pig hindlimb [32]. Furthermore, prolonged allograft survival upon repetitive high-dose application of bone marrow-derived mesenchymal stem cells (MSCs) in a pig hemifacial model has been reported [32].

Soares et al. [61] used an established rat hindlimb model for allotransplantation. In the absence of long-term pharmacologic immunosuppression, they found out significant prolonged rejection-free allograft survival with a single perioperative ex-vivo infusion of bone marrow-derived mesenchymal stem cells through the allograft vasculature. *DCs* have been used for tolerance induction to alleviate the requirement for chronic immunosuppression in VCA [62]. While injection of mature DCs rapidly increases T-cell activity in humans and promotes transplant rejection, the injection of immature DCs acts as an immunosuppressant and inhibits T-cell activity. In addition to immature DCs, mesenchymal stem cells were also found to have a positive effect on allotransplantation of solid organs and bone marrow via cytokine expression which decreases the alloreactive effector lymphocytes and increases CD4+/CD25+/FoxP3 Tregs. Despite the promising findings, the efficacy of cell-based therapies varies greatly across studies, partly due to different methods of cell isolation and purification techniques, source, route, timing of administration, and combining immunosuppressive therapy.

In a recent study, Olariu et al. [57] hypothesized that the *transfer of donor lymph node (LN)* might be used to promote lymphangiogenesis and influence rejection in vascularized composite allotransplantation (VCA). Their experiments on rats showed that graft rejection started significantly later in D:LN+ transplanted rats as compared to the D:LN- group. The D:LN+ group showed a higher level of VEGF-C and better lymphangiogenesis compared to the D:LN- group. Furthermore, the donor LN+ group showed increased levels of circulating and skin-resident donor T regulatory cells [57]. This study suggests that VCA LNs may be potential targets for future research aimed to decrease the allotransplants' rejection rate.

Decellularization/recellularization constitutes another attractive strategy to avoid lifelong immunosuppressive medications and is one of the most promising topics in VCA research [4]. The objective of decellularization/recellularization methodology is to develop immunogenic-free biological substitutes that will restore, maintain, or improve tissue and organ function. Sodium dodecyl sulfate (1%) is typically used for the decellularization process. Mechanical agitation lyses cells and destroys cell–matrix adhesive proteins and therefore it is used to facilitate decellularization. The first indicator of the effective removal of cells from the VCA is the progressive change of its color to a white or even transparent color during decellularization [4]. Fat can be removed by treating the VCA with a polar solvent, 2- propanol, initially described for isolated adipose tissue decellularization.

The immunological response of the decellularized scaffolds remains poorly understood. There have been few successful attempts to recellularization and transplantation of these scaffolds. Generally, successful transplantation needs prior recellularization. A good recellularization technique requires the removal of all cellular materials, while the extracellular matrix composition and architecture are preserved to the maximum extent possible. Vascular integrity and mechanical properties/strength need to be preserved as well.

Recellularization would require repopulation with multiple cell types in different compartments to form a complex cellular architecture; therefore, adult tissue stem cells, such as the adipose-derived stem cells and mesenchymal stem cells, are considered to hold great potential in repopulating the engineered VCA due to their potential to generate the different cell types. In addition, these stem cells not only directly participate in mesenchymal tissue regeneration but also modulate the host immune response to the engineered constructs. Although decellularization/recellularization was tested only by a few groups on human VCA models, its potential is very promising for the future.

33.9 Nerve Regeneration

Nerves appear to be less immunogenic than grafted skin, tendon, muscle, and bone [63]. One of the limitations of VCAs is the limited nerve regrowth across long distances which results in poor regeneration and functional recovery [64]. As an example, Arun et al. [58] found out that in VCAs, reperfusion of tissues is not sufficient to restore their function. The re-gaining of function rather depends on the *nerve regeneration*, which in turn allows motor function and skin sensation [58]. Although nerve damage is usual during the transplant, there are potential strategies to improve the regenerative process after the surgical coaptation (tension-free repair) of the donor and recipient nerves in an end-to-end fashion. Several techniques such as nerve guidance conduits, fibrin glues, stem-cell therapy, electrical stimulation, tacrolimus (FK506), and hormonal therapy have been used to promote nerve regeneration [58, 64].

FK-506 is a calcineurin phosphatase inhibitor and an IS drug that inhibits the activation of T-cell proliferation through binding and inhibition of calcineurin. Interestingly enough, FK506 has an effect on nerve regeneration in a dose-dependent, calcineurin-independent mechanism, through systemic and local administrations [58]. The precise mechanism mediating the neuroregenerative effect of FK506 is still unclear [65]. FK506 has neuroprotective and neurotrophic actions that can accelerate nerve regeneration and enhance nerve regeneration following nerve allotransplantation. Treatment with tacrolimus significantly improved motor and sensory neuronal regeneration, as well as histomorphometric indices including myelinated axon number [66, 67].

Nephrotoxicity, hyperglycemia, and central nervous system toxicity are potential side effects of tacrolimus.

33.10 Eye Transplantation

There is no treatment available for blindness due to optic nerve atrophy or retinal ganglion cell loss, caused by end-stage glaucoma, traumatic optic atrophy, or by other diseases [19]. Numerous studies have been published on face and hand transplant, but only a few on eye transplantation [7, 19, 68–74]. Human whole eye transplantation (WET, Fig. 33.1) is one of the last frontiers of VCA [71]. To date, WET is still a highly experimental procedure, so the possible outcomes and the occurrence of rejection or infections remain uncertain [69]. Rare WET attempts in humans as xenotransplants and one partial eye non-vascularized allotransplant have been reported [19]. Some research groups have conducted significant experiments on WET [7, 19, 70, 72, 73], such as the works developed by Davidson et al. [72] and Siemionow et al. [73] on the feasibility of WET on human cadavers. Animal experiments on WET have been performed on cold-blooded invertebrate eye transplantation animal models (salamander, toad, frog) and mammalian eye transplantation animal models (rabbit, rat, canine, sheep, swine) [19]. In 2019, Zor et al. [70] used a rodent model to demonstrate the technical feasibility and viability of whole eye transplantation. They also [7] investigated the immunological behavior of ocular tissues in WET. The authors found out that potential risks of this procedure could be an immune rejection and graft failure, or graft survival in the absence of optic nerve regeneration [7]. Although there are several vital challenges for WET in humans [69], the goal of providing vision to blind recipients is worth the effort of future research on this topic.

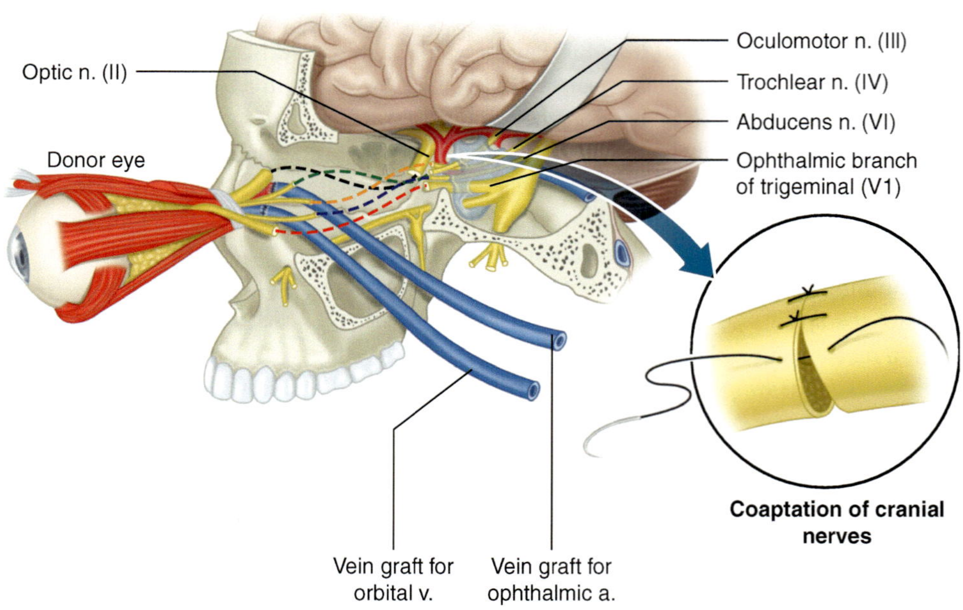

Fig. 33.1 Whole eye transplantation (WET)

33.11 Limitations

Unlike solid organ transplants (e.g., liver and heart transplants), VCAs are considered life-enhancing, rather than life-saving procedures; therefore, they are exposed to potential ethical issues, considering all the risks of lifelong immunosuppression [28, 32]. The near certainty of the development of serious side effects, including malignancy, a shortened life expectancy, and the eventual loss of the graft to rejection complicate the calculation of the risk vs. benefit ratio [48]. For upper extremity VCA, research has shown that the quality of life typically goes down for the first 3 months following the transplant and that patients routinely underestimate the challenges. In some cases, low quality of life post-transplantation brought patients to ask for transplant removal. Benedict and Magill [48] have described the ethical issues related to the upper extremity and craniofacial VCA.

The concerns include questions around the procurement of grafts, patient selection, proper consent, data sharing, patient experiences and quality of life, and pediatric VCA.

Long-term immunosuppression and years of physiotherapy are necessary for upper limb transplant patients. It also requires intense, long-term patient participation and commitment. Therefore, this information should be shared with patients when informed consent is required. The consent should be for a dynamic continuous cooperation between the team and the patient, rather than for the surgical procedure stand-alone.

Another main limitation of VCA research is the need to study outcomes from disparate groups and the small number of patients [31]. Furthermore, the complications criteria are not validated [31].

Similar to other solid organ transplants, VCA requires a multi-disciplinary team and a major institutional commitment, which is not available in many research centers.

33.12 Conclusions

VCA is a reconstructive option for patients suffering from severe and extensive injuries, aiming to recreate esthetics and function in the recipient site. Despite many advancements in the field of VCA, acute rejection occurs in over 80% of all upper extremity and face transplants within the first-year post-transplantation. As time passes and more long-term outcomes are available, high incidence of chronic rejection is observed in VCA patients. Promising strategies have been proposed to improve the outcomes in order to better understand the rejection mechanism and therefore prevent the allotransplant loss, but additional research on the mechanisms of immunologic tolerance is required. These life-enhancing transplantations require more diverse studies to get to the definitive and final application in humans.

References

1. Cetrulo CL Jr, Ng ZY, Winograd JM, Eberlin KR. The advent of vascularized composite allotransplantation. Clin Plast Surg. 2017;44:425–9.
2. Gorantla VS, Plock JA, Davis MR. Reconstructive transplantation: evolution, experience, ethics, and emerging concepts. In: Subramaniam K, Sakai T, editors. Anesthesia and perioperative care for organ transplantation. New York, NY: Springer; 2017. p. 539–52.
3. Grajek M, Bula D, Zeman M, Maciejewski A. Limitations and limits and of vascularized composite allotransplantations: can we reach the holy grail? Curr Opin Organ Transplant. 2020;25:609–14.
4. Lupon E, Lellouch AG, Acun A, et al. Engineering vascularized composite allografts using natural scaffolds: a systematic review. Tissue Eng Part B Rev. 2021;28:677. Epub ahead of print. PMID: 34238047. https://doi.org/10.1089/ten.TEB.2021.0102.
5. Nordham KD, Ninokawa S. The history of organ transplantation. Proc (Bayl Univ Med Cent). 2022;35:124–8.
6. Mathes DW, Butler PEM, Lee AWP. Transplantation in plastic surgery. In: Gurtner G, Neligan PC, editors. Plastic surgery: principles, vol. 1. 4th ed. Amsterdam: Elsevier Health Sciences; 2017.
7. Zor F, Karagoz H, Kapucu H, Kulahci Y, Janjic JM, Gorantla VS. Immunological considerations and concerns as pertinent to whole eye transplantation. Curr Opin Organ Transplant. 2019;24:726–32.
8. Siemionow M. The past the present and the future of face transplantation. Curr Opin Organ Transplant. 2020;25:568–75.
9. Dubernard JM, Owen E, Herzberg G, et al. Human hand allograft: report on first 6 months. Lancet. 1999;353:1315–20.
10. Jones JW, Gruber SA, Barker JH, Breidenbach WC. Successful hand transplantation. One-year follow-up. Louisville hand transplant team. N Engl J Med. 2000;343:468–73.
11. Barret JP, Gavaldà J, Bueno J, et al. Full face transplant: the first case report. Ann Surg. 2011;254:252–6.
12. Govshievich A, Saleh E, Boghossian E, et al. Face transplant: current update and first Canadian experience. Plast Reconstr Surg. 2021;147:1177–88.
13. Horen SR, Lopez J, Dorafshar AH. Facial transplantation. Facial Plast Surg. 2021;37:528–35.
14. Fullerton ZH, Tsangaris E, DeVries CEE, et al. Patient-reported outcomes measures used in facial vascularized composite allotransplantation: a systematic literature review. J Plast Reconstr Aesthet Surg. 2021;75(1):33–44. https://doi.org/10.1016/j.bjps.2021.09.002. Epub ahead of print. PMID: 34753682.
15. Woo SH, Kim YW, Cheon HJ, et al. Process of obtaining social consensus and 3-year functional outcomes of the first hand allotransplantation in Korea. J Korean Med Sci. 2021;36:e6.
16. Alberti B, Hoyle V. Face transplants: an international history. J Hist Med Allied Sci. 2021;76:319.
17. Kueckelhaus M, Fischer S, Seyda M, et al. Vascularized composite allotransplantation: current standards and novel approaches to prevent acute rejection and chronic allograft deterioration. Transpl Int. 2016;29:655–62.
18. Girard AO, Lake IV, Lopez CD, et al. Vascularized composite allotransplantation of the penis: current status and future perspectives. Int J Impot Res. 2021;34:383. https://doi.org/10.1038/s41443-021-00481-0. Epub ahead of print. PMID: 34711953.
19. Bourne D, Li Y, Komatsu C, et al. Whole-eye transplantation: a look into the past and vision for the future. Eye (Lond). 2017;31:179–84.
20. Shokri T, Saadi R, Wang W, Reddy L, Ducic Y. Facial transplantation: complications, outcomes, and long-term management strategies. Semin Plast Surg. 2020;34:245–53.

21. Tchiloemba B, Kauke M, Haug V, et al. Long-term outcomes after facial allotransplantation: systematic review of the literature. Transplantation. 2021;105:1869–80.
22. Issa F. Vascularized composite allograft-specific characteristics of immune responses. Transpl Int. 2016;29:672–81.
23. Honeyman C, Stark H, Wang HC, Hester J, Issa F, Giele H. Biomarker and surrogate development in vascularised composite allograft transplantation: current progress and future challenges. J Plast Reconstr Aesthet Surg. 2021;74:711–7.
24. Chim H, Amer H, Mardini S, Moran SL. Vascularized composite allotransplant in the realm of regenerative plastic surgery. Mayo Clin Proc. 2014;89:1009–20.
25. Siemionow MZ, Kulahci Y, Bozkurt M. Composite tissue allotransplantation. Plast Reconstr Surg. 2009;124:e327–e39.
26. Kaufman CL, Bhutiani N, Ramirez A, et al. Current status of vascularized composite Allotransplantation. Am Surg. 2019;85:631–7.
27. Jacoby A, Cohen O, Gelb BE, Ceradini DJ, Rodriguez ED. Vascularized composite allotransplantation and immunobiology: the next frontier. Plast Reconstr Surg. 2021;147:1092e–3e.
28. Kuo Y-R. Future directions in vascularized composite allotransplantation field. In: Cheng M-H, Chang K-P, Kao H-K, editors. Resection and reconstruction of head & neck cancers. Singapore: Springer; 2019. p. 165–77.
29. Iyer S. Vascularised composite allotransplants: transplant of upper extremities and face. Indian J Plast Surg. 2015;48:111–8.
30. Matar AJ, Crepeau RL, Mundinger GS, Cetrulo CL Jr, Torabi R. Large animal models of vascularized composite allotransplantation: a review of immune strategies to improve allograft outcomes. Front Immunol. 2021;12:664577.
31. https://www.myast.org/public-policy/vascularized-composite-allotransplantation-vca-research.
32. Iske J, Nian Y, Maenosono R, Maurer M, Sauer IM, Tullius SG. Composite tissue allotransplantation: opportunities and challenges. Cell Mol Immunol. 2019;16:343–9.
33. Kauke M, Safi AF, Zhegibe A, et al. Mucosa and rejection in facial vascularized composite allotransplantation: a systematic review. Transplantation. 2020;104:2616–24.
34. Kauke-Navarro M, Tchiloemba B, Haug V, et al. Pathologies of oral and sinonasal mucosa following facial vascularized composite allotransplantation. J Plast Reconstr Aesthet Surg. 2021;74:1562–71.
35. Yang JH, Eun SC. Therapeutic application of T regulatory cells in composite tissue allotransplantation. J Transl Med. 2017;15:218.
36. Richmond JM, Harris JE. Immunology and skin in health and disease. Cold Spring Harb Perspect Med. 2014;4:a015339.
37. Etra JW, Raimondi G, Brandacher G. Mechanisms of rejection in vascular composite allotransplantation. Curr Opin Organ Transplant. 2018;23:28–33.
38. Fischer S, Lian CG, Kueckelhaus M, et al. Acute rejection in vascularized composite allotransplantation. Curr Opin Organ Transplant. 2014;19:531–44.
39. Bejarano PA, Levi D, Nassiri M, et al. The pathology of full-thickness cadaver skin transplant for large abdominal defects: a proposed grading system for skin allograft acute rejection. Am J Surg Pathol. 2004;28:670–5.
40. Cendales LC, Kanitakis J, Schneeberger S, et al. The Banff 2007 working classification of skin-containing composite tissue allograft pathology. Am J Transplant. 2008;8:1396–400.
41. Cendales LC, Kirk AD, Moresi JM, Ruiz P, Kleiner DE. Composite tissue allotransplantation: classification of clinical acute skin rejection. Transplantation. 2006;81:418–22.
42. Kanitakis J, Petruzzo P, Jullien D, et al. Pathological score for the evaluation of allograft rejection in human hand (composite tissue) allotransplantation. Eur J Dermatol. 2005;15:235–8.
43. Schneeberger S, Kreczy A, Brandacher G, Steurer W, Margreiter R. Steroid- and ATG-resistant rejection after double forearm transplantation responds to Campath-1H. Am J Transplant. 2004;4:1372–4.
44. Morelon E, Petruzzo P, Kanitakis J. Chronic rejection in vascularized composite allotransplantation. Curr Opin Organ Transplant. 2018;23:582–91.
45. Ng ZY, Lellouch AG, Rosales IA, et al. Graft vasculopathy of vascularized composite allografts in humans: a literature review and retrospective study. Transpl Int. 2019;32:831–8.
46. Kollar B, Kamat P, Klein HJ, Waldner M, Schweizer R, Plock JA. The significance of vascular alterations in acute and chronic rejection for vascularized composite allotransplantation. J Vasc Res. 2019;56:163–80.
47. Broyles JM, Alrakan M, Ensor CR, et al. Characterization, prophylaxis, and treatment of infectious complications in craniomaxillofacial and upper extremity allotransplantation: a multicenter perspective. Plast Reconstr Surg. 2014;133:543e–51e.
48. Benedict J, Magill G. Upper extremity and craniofacial vascularized composite allotransplantation: ethics and immunosuppression. Emerg Top Life Sci. 2019;3:681–6.
49. Datta S, Fitzpatrick AM, Haykal S. Preservation solutions for attenuation of ischemia-reperfusion injury in vascularized composite allotransplantation. SAGE Open Med. 2021;9:1–13.
50. Kadono K, Gruszynski M, Azari K, Kupiec-Weglinski JW. Vascularized composite allotransplantation versus solid organ transplantation: innate-adaptive immune interphase. Curr Opin Organ Transplant. 2019;24:714–20.
51. Burlage LC, Tessier SN, Etra JW, Uygun K, Brandacher G. Advances in machine perfusion, organ preservation, and cryobiology: potential impact on vascularized composite allotransplantation. Curr Opin Organ Transplant. 2018;23:561–7.
52. Rezaei M, Figueroa B, Orfahli L, et al. Composite vascularized allograft machine preservation: state of the art. Curr Transplant Rep. 2019;6:265–76.
53. Safi AF, Kauke M, Nelms L, et al. Local immunosuppression in vascularized composite allotransplantation (VCA): a systematic review. J Plast Reconstr Aesthet Surg. 2021;74:327–35.
54. Taddeo A, Tsai C, Vögelin E, Rieben R. Novel targeted drug delivery systems to minimize systemic immunosuppression in vascularized composite allotransplantation. Curr Opin Organ Transplant. 2018;23:568–76.
55. Cwykiel J, Jundzill A, Klimczak A, Madajka-Niemeyer M, Siemionow M. Donor recipient chimeric cells induce chimerism and extend survival of vascularized composite allografts. Arch Immunol Ther Exp (Warsz). 2021;69:13.
56. Jundziłł A, Klimczak A, Sonmez E, Brzezicki G, Siemionow M. The positive impact of donor bone marrow cells transplantation into immunoprivileged compartments on the survival of vascularized skin allografts. Arch Immunol Ther Exp (Warsz). 2021;69:28.
57. Olariu R, Tsai C, Abd El Hafez M, et al. Presence of donor lymph nodes within vascularized composite allotransplantation ameliorates VEGF-C-mediated lymphangiogenesis and delays the onset of acute rejection. Transplantation. 2021;105:1747–59.
58. Arun A, Abt NB, Tuffaha S, Brandacher G, Barone AAL. Nerve regeneration in vascularized composite allotransplantation: current strategies and future directions. Plast Aesthet Res. 2015;2:226–35.
59. Chen J, Wang Y, Hu H, Xiong Y, Wang S, Yang J. Adipose-derived cellular therapies prolong graft survival in an allogenic hind limb transplantation model. Stem Cell Res Ther. 2021;12:94.
60. Hu JL, Kwon ST, Kim SW, Nam HJ, Kim BJ. Effects of administration route of adipose-derived stem cells on the survival of allogeneic skin grafts in mice. Transplant Proc. 2021;53(7):2397–406.
61. Soares MA, Massie JP, Rifkin WJ, et al. Ex vivo allotransplantation engineering: delivery of mesenchymal stem cells prolongs rejection-free allograft survival. Am J Transplant. 2018;18:1657–67.

62. Vyas KS, Mohan AT, Morrison SD, Tran DC, Mardini S. Cell-based therapies in vascularized composite allotransplantation. J Reconstr Microsurg. 2018;34:642–50.
63. Yan Y, Wood MD, Moore AM, et al. Robust axonal regeneration in a mouse vascularized composite allotransplant model undergoing delayed tissue rejection. Hand (N Y). 2016;11:456–63.
64. Tung TH, Mackinnon SE. Stem cell-based approaches to enhance nerve regeneration and improve functional outcomes in vascularized composite allotransplantation. Curr Opin Organ Transplant. 2018;23:577–81.
65. Rau CS, Kuo PJ, Wu SC, et al. Enhanced nerve regeneration by exosomes secreted by adipose-derived stem cells with or without FK506 stimulation. Int J Mol Sci. 2021;22(16):8545.
66. Zuo KJ, Shafa G, Chan K, et al. Local FK506 drug delivery enhances nerve regeneration through fresh, unprocessed peripheral nerve allografts. Exp Neurol. 2021;341:113680.
67. Glaus SW, Johnson PJ, Mackinnon SE. Clinical strategies to enhance nerve regeneration in composite tissue allotransplantation. Hand Clin. 2011;27(4):495–509, ix.
68. Bravo MG, Granoff MD, Johnson AR, Lee BT. Development of a new large-animal model for composite face and whole-eye transplantation: a novel application for anatomical mapping using indocyanine green and liquid latex. Plast Reconstr Surg. 2020;145:67e–75e.
69. Sivak WN, Davidson EH, Komatsu C, et al. Ethical considerations of whole-eye transplantation. J Clin Ethics. 2016;27:64–7.
70. Zor F, Polat M, Kulahci Y, et al. Demonstration of technical feasibility and viability of whole eye transplantation in a rodent model. J Plast Reconstr Aesthet Surg. 2019;72:1640–50.
71. Canavero S. Total eye transplantation for the blind: a challenge for the future. Med Hypotheses. 1992;39:201–11.
72. Davidson EH, Wang EW, Yu JY, et al. Total human eye allotransplantation: developing surgical protocols for donor and recipient procedures. Plast Reconstr Surg. 2016;138:1297–308.
73. Siemionow M, Bozkurt M, Zor F, et al. A new composite eyeball-periorbital transplantation model in humans: an anatomical study in preparation for eyeball transplantation. Plast Reconstr Surg. 2018;141:1011–8.
74. Davidson EH, Wang EW, Yu JY, et al. Clinical considerations for vascularized composite allotransplantation of the eye. J Craniofac Surg. 2016;27:1622–8.

34 Ethical Considerations of Living Donation in Vascularized Composite Allotransplantation

Maureen Beederman, Chad M. Teven, and Lawrence J. Gottlieb

34.1 Introduction

In 1972, Mark Siegler introduced a new field of clinical medical ethics to help clinicians navigate the clinical–ethical challenges that often arise during patient care [1]. Since then, several ethical frameworks have been developed specifically aimed at improving ethical decision-making. The widely recognized framework expressed by Beauchamp and Childress (1979) underlines four principles to aid in managing ethical challenges: respect for autonomy, beneficence, nonmaleficence, and justice [2]. While this model has been broadly applied to address wide-ranging ethical challenges, its practical effectiveness in clinical medicine remains limited by strict adherence to moral principlism rather than accounting for clinical variables [3].

In an effort to mediate ethical analysis in a clinical-informed manner, Jonsen et al. proposed a novel framework the so-called four-quadrant approach [4]. In this model, each of the four quadrants represents a clinically relevant topic (i.e., medical indications, patient preferences, quality of life, contextual features), and each topic has its own set of questions to be considered (Table 34.1) [5]. The objective is for clinicians to link specific details of the clinical picture to underlying core ethical principles, facilitating exploration of patient values and wishes. Ideally, this results in medically and ethically sound decisions with which all parties (e.g., clinician, care team, patient/family) are in agreement. The "four-quadrant" approach is advantageous in that it can be practically applied to a wide range of clinical scenarios [6]. Here, we employ the "four-quadrant" approach to facilitate ethical analysis of live donation in vascularized composite allotransplantation (VCA). VCA denotes the transplantation of multiple tissue types, often a combination of the follow-

Table 34.1 The four quadrant approach to ethical case analysis [4]

Medical indications	Patient preferences
Principles addressed: beneficence and nonmaleficence Considerations: • Medical diagnosis/problem • Time course of medical problem (emergent vs. acute vs. chronic) • Goals of treatment and potential treatment options • Prognosis with and without different treatments • Balance between medical interventions helping vs. harming patient	*Principles addressed: respect for patient autonomy* Considerations: • Patient knowledge about medical diagnosis/problem, including risks/benefits/ alternatives for treatment • Informed consent obtained • Patient competence and ability to make decisions regarding care • Patient preferences regarding treatment options vs. no treatment • Patient past preferences (especially important if patient without capacity) • Assigned surrogate for patient without capacity
Quality of life	Contextual features
Principles addressed: beneficence, nonmaleficence, and respect for patient autonomy Considerations: • Subjective nature of quality of life • Return "normalcy" of life differs for each patient—Must consider physical, mental, social deficits • Treatment options vs. no treatment and impact on quality of life • Judgment about quality of life for a patient unable to make decisions—Provider might have biases • Spectrum of comfort-care and pain relief to medically assisted dying when poor outlook for patient quality of life	*Principles addressed: justice and fairness* Considerations: • Conflicts of interest (personal, professional) • Role of family members (non-surrogates) in medical decision-making • Financial factors and allocation of scarce resources as part of medical treatment options • Other factors that can influence decision-making: Religion, research, legal, medical education, publicity

M. Beederman (✉) · L. J. Gottlieb
Section of Plastic and Reconstructive Surgery, The University of Chicago Medicine, Chicago, IL, USA
e-mail: mbeederman@bsd.uchicago.edu; lgottlie@surgery.bsd.uchicago.edu

C. M. Teven
Northwestern University Feinberg School of Medicine, Chicago, IL, USA
e-mail: chad.teven@northwestern.edu

© Springer Nature Switzerland AG 2023
R. Gurunian et al. (eds.), *Reconstructive Transplantation*, https://doi.org/10.1007/978-3-031-21520-9_34

ing: skin, bone, cartilage, tendon, ligament, muscle, and/or neurovascular structures. Unlike deceased donor VCA, living donor VCA also requires consideration of the donor as a patient, requiring utilization of the four-quadrant approach for both donor and recipient (Table 34.2) [7].

Living donation in solid organ transplantation has become a widely accepted practice in the USA and around the world. Benefits to the organ recipient are well established and include increased organ availability, reduced wait times on the transplant list, and superior short-term and long-term outcomes compared to deceased donor transplantation [8]. Live donation also results in shorter ischemia times, improved human leukocyte antigen (HLA) matching, and the potential to achieve immune tolerance [9, 10]. Unlike deceased donor organ transplantation, living donation not only affects the recipient but also affects an otherwise healthy individual—the donor. Therefore, the medical and ethical interests of the donor must be carefully considered to minimize donor morbidity and ensure the benefits to both parties outweigh risks inherent to live donation [11]. Recognizing the unusual ethical circumstances surrounding live donation, the Transplantation Society offered guidelines regarding living organ donation in two documents. The first, developed during the 2004 Amsterdam Forum, highlighted care for live kidney donors [12]. At the 2005 Vancouver Forum, a second document was produced to address living donation of other solid organs (i.e., lung, intestine, liver, and pancreas) [13].

Table 34.2 Four-quadrant ethical analysis for donor/recipient patients in living donor VCA

Donor	*Medical indications*	*Patient preferences*
	• None—unless patient was already planning to undergo cosmetic procedure for removal of donated tissue	• Potential esthetic/functional improvement from removal of donated tissue • Similar risk profile, long-term morbidity as conventional free flap harvest • Protect donor autonomy while ensuring no coercion and appropriate understanding
	Quality of life	*Contextual features*
	• Donor site morbidity • Psychological benefits (e.g., altruism, volunteerism)	• Media/publicity surrounding VCA
Recipient	*Medical indications*	*Patient preferences*
	• Potential improved HLA matching • Shorter wait time/higher organ supply • Improved surgical scheduling/reduced ischemia time • No donor site morbidity • Ability to "replace like with like," improved appearance/functional results	• Reduced number of surgeries and subsequent surgical risks to achieve acceptable reconstruction • Psychological (e.g., altruism, volunteerism, personal autonomy, ability to enhance quality of life) • Potential esthetic/functional improvement from removal of donated tissue
	Quality of life	*Contextual features*
	• Lifelong immunosuppression and resultant infectious, neoplastic, and metabolic complications • Potential for future immune tolerance and decreased need for immunosuppression	• Media/publicity surrounding VCA

Recent advances in the field of transplant medicine have facilitated safe transplantation of human tissue beyond solid organs. The most frequent vascular composite allografts to date have been applied in the context of face and hand transplantation, usually for devastating trauma and resultant deformity. Unlike solid organ transplantation, the idea of living donor VCA has historically been considered implausible as it would result in unacceptably high donor morbidity (i.e., disfigurement and functional loss) [14]. More recently, however, with increased success in hand and face transplantation as demonstrated in the face and upper extremity transplantation sections (Sects. 34.2.1 and 34.2.4), VCA has been performed using a variety of tissues across the body for novel indications. It is these types of living donor VCA with more acceptable donor morbidity that are the focus of this chapter. Examples include abdominal wall tissue (for breast reconstruction) [15], omentum (scalp repair) [16], uterus [17], and fasciocutaneous radial forearm tissue (hemifacial reconstruction) [18]. Despite successful outcomes, these cases have raised legal and ethical concerns with respect to living donation in VCA. Particularly, compared to solid organ transplantation, the benefits of live donor VCA are less clear. Unlike solid organ transplantation, which may be life-saving for the recipient, VCA generally improves quality of life (QOL) of the recipient. This may be considered less rewarding than life preservation. Nevertheless, donors may benefit from feelings of altruism, volunteerism, and protection of personal autonomy [8]. Whether these benefits outweigh risks to the donor, however, is questionable. Despite an elusive risk/benefit calculus for live donor VCA, in 2013 the U.S. Department of Health and Human Services declared that vascular composite allografts are akin to solid organs from a transplantation perspective, effectively lifting formal legal prohibition on living donation in VCA [19].

Due to the recent successes in VCA and reduced legal barriers to live donation, the number of living donation VCA operations is expected to rise going forward. It will be important to ensure continued safety of all parties (i.e., donor and recipient). First, ongoing examination of the medical feasibility of live donor VCA and the risks and benefits to both donor and recipient are key [8]. Next, adherence to established transplantation protocols and guidelines for living donation is recommended to optimize safety and outcomes [8]. Additionally, reconstructive surgeons performing live donor VCA must be able to identify and navigate the complex ethical issues that arise regarding both recipients and donors. This chapter aims to highlight the ethical considerations of live donor VCA by employing the "four-quadrant" ethical framework approach to facilitate ethical analysis in a clinically informed manner.

34.2 Analysis of Vascularized Composite Allotransplantation Using Four-Quadrant Approach to Ethical Decision-Making

34.2.1 Medical Indications

The first quadrant, medical indications, refers to the medical information related to the case and patient. This includes a patient's diagnosis and prognosis, other (non-VCA) options for treatment, and predicted outcomes. In the context of living donor VCA, there are two patients to consider: donor and recipient. Therefore, it is crucial to include both patients in the discussion of the principles of beneficence and nonmaleficence.

As has been previously described, patients who are candidates for VCA traditionally suffer from severe disfigurement and have often exhausted other reconstruction options [20]. For some patients, including those who have undergone multiple attempts at autologous reconstruction, patients who have sustained extensive burn injuries, or pediatric patients, there is a paucity of autologous tissue available with which to perform reconstruction [21]. The option of VCA in these cases allows surgeons to follow one of the core principles of plastic surgery: to replace like with like. Living donor VCA can also prevent additional donor site morbidity in the already injured recipient, providing tissue that the recipient might not have (or that has already been used) for reconstruction. In addition, the paucity of deceased donors available for VCA transplantation, as well as the importance of esthetic matching to provide optimal results, makes the option of living donor VCA attractive. Many of the other benefits of living donation for solid organ transplantation, including improved HLA matching, reduced ischemia time, and the potential for immune tolerance, also relate to living donor VCA.

The concept of living donation is often at odds with the principles of beneficence and nonmaleficence as they relate to the living donor. This has been described in living kidney donors. The donor is taking on the risks of anesthesia and surgery, often without a direct physical benefit. Some of these risks could be ameliorated using a concept described by Testa et al. in their paper "Elective Surgical Patients as Living Organ Donors: A Clinical and Ethical Innovation" [22]. Here they describe the idea of performing donor nephrectomies on patients undergoing anesthesia and surgical risk for another, nonrelated reason (cholecystectomy). One can foresee a similar situation with living donor VCA, where a patient undergoing an abdominoplasty donates their abdominal tissue to another patient who desires autologous breast reconstruction but does not have enough native tissue. Currently, this has only been performed between identical twins to avoid the risks of lifelong immunosuppression [15].

34.2.2 Patient Preferences

This quadrant relates specifically to patient autonomy and the importance of informed decision-making. With living donor VCA it is again important to consider the patient preferences of both donor and recipient.

Patient autonomy allows recipients to decide whether they want to incur the risks of surgery and risks of immunosuppression that accompany VCA. It has been shown that potential recipients are likely to assume more risk for certain deceased donor transplants (face, bilateral hands) than others (unilateral hand, foot) [23]. This is likely to be the case with living donor VCA as well. Additionally, living donor VCA may provide acceptable cosmetic and functional reconstructive results when no autologous reconstructive options are available or could only be performed in multiple surgical procedures. For example, if a burn patient had significant contractures and soft tissue deficits, reconstruction using a free flap from the patient's relative (deep inferior epigastric artery perforator flap, anterolateral thigh flap) would allow for avoidance of staged procedures and/or use of tissue expanders. Patients therefore may prefer to reduce the risks associated with multiple surgeries and anesthesia, rather than the risks associated with immunosuppression.

The morbidity associated with certain types of VCA (full face, partial face, hand) is too great for these to be considered appropriate for living donation. However, donors may be willing to assume more risk when the benefits to the recipient are greater. Interestingly, the donor risks associated with certain types of currently allowed living solid organ donation (lung, liver, intestines, pancreas) are likely greater than those associated with living donor VCA. From the vast experience that plastic surgeons have with autologous free flap reconstruction, we have the knowledge to provide donors with information about the expected morbidity and long-term outcomes of living VCA. For example, if a patient wanted to donate a fibula for long bone or mandibular reconstruction, the risks of fibula harvest are well known and allow the donor to make an informed decision and exercise their autonomy.

Similar to solid organ transplantation donor guidelines [11], potential VCA donors should undergo a vigorous screening process, including psychosocial evaluation, to ensure that they are appropriately exercising their autonomy. Donors need to be free of coercion and have a thorough understanding of risks and benefits. The importance of protecting donor rights and decision-making is highlighted by Bruno and Arora, who outline the ethical considerations of both deceased and living donor uterine transplantation [24]. Conversely, several publications highlight the dichotomy between treatment of living organ donors and cosmetic surgery patients, both of whom are commonly otherwise healthy individuals opting to assume the risks associated with surgery in order to attain personal fulfillment and psychological benefit [25, 26].

34.2.3 Quality of Life

It is important to recognize that living donor VCA—and VCA more generally—is not a life-saving procedure. Rather, these surgeries aim to correct physical or functional disabilities, improve symptoms, and improve the quality of the recipient's life. The argument that VCA is not life-saving, but rather "life-enhancing" has been made by critics, who believe that the risks accompanying lifelong immunosuppression outweigh the benefits provided to the recipient. The risks associated with VCA, and whether these could be justified by subjective improvements in the recipient's quality of life, were frequently debated in the early days of VCA [27]. The balance between risk and improvement in quality of life for the recipient is likely no different when it comes to living donor VCA.

At the present time, the most common type of living donor VCA performed is uterine transplantation in patients with uterine factor infertility [28]. Recipients of uterine transplants are in the relatively unique circumstances of not being expected to be on lifelong immunosuppressive drugs. After delivery of a baby, a hysterectomy is performed, and immunosuppressive medication is stopped. For these patients, the risks inherent in the procedure and the temporary immunosuppression are outweighed by the benefits and improved quality of life of a gestational pregnancy despite the fact that other options for childbearing exist (surrogacy, adoption).

Since the first successful hand transplantation in 1998, the transplant and medical ethics communities have worked to establish guidelines for VCA, where the risk–benefit calculus for lifelong immunosuppression is based upon the improvement in patient function and quality of life [29]. Given the current limitations of immunosuppression and its associated risks, we believe it is helpful to group patients who may require living donor VCA into two categories: (1) patients who have previously undergone solid organ transplantation and thus, are already experiencing the risks of lifelong immunosuppression and (2) those patients who are not. For patients in the former group, no additional risk from immunosuppression is incurred with living donor VCA. In these patients, the risk of living donor VCA is analogous to prior VCAs performed between identical twins, where there is a reduced risk from immunosuppression. For patients in the latter group (those not on immunosuppression), we believe the risks from immunosuppression must be offset by the benefits gained by living donor VCA reconstruction. The risks of immunosuppression, as well as chronic rejection, will also depend on other factors such as the age of the recipient patient, as the lifelong risk is greater for younger recipients. Most patients with malignancies would not be candidates for VCA transplants, living or not. Those with a remote history of malignancy would need to be counseled on the potential increased risk of recurrence with immunosuppression.

With continued progress in immunosuppression and tolerance, it is plausible that the future risks of lifelong immunosuppression could be minimized or ultimately entirely disappear [30, 31]. One study surveying hand surgeons found that hand allotransplantation was more widely accepted if it were to be performed without standard immunosuppression or in patients who had previously undergone solid organ transplantation [32]. It is possible that acceptance of living donor VCA would follow similar trends. Without the risks of immunosuppression, the benefits to the recipient ought to be directly weighed against the risks and potential morbidity to the donor. Moving forward, a discussion regarding prognosis and expected outcomes may be preferentially focused on living donor morbidities, rather than recipient morbidities from immunosuppression.

For living VCA donors, quality of life improvements is primarily psychological in nature and is likely similar to those of solid organ living donors. These include the notions of altruism, volunteerism, and enhancing another individual's quality of life. Of note, improvements in donor quality of life may also be considered in the "patient preferences" box of the four-quadrant model. Additionally, for some potential VCA donor sites (abdominal free flap), there are certain cosmetic benefits, which may improve the quality of life for the donor as well.

34.2.4 Contextual Features

Living donor VCA would likely be accompanied by considerable media attention and publicity, similar to deceased donor VCA. This may result in a breach of patient confidentiality (for both recipient and donor). Media attention also potentially creates a conflict of interest for the hospital and the surgical team planning to perform the procedure. It is essential that the best interests of the recipient, as well as the donor, are prioritized for all decisions related to living donor VCA. Furthermore, as the concept of living donor VCA becomes more mainstream, it may be accompanied by media commentary like that which occurred in the early days of facial transplantation.

Furthermore, one of the notable barriers to deceased donor hand and face transplantation has been the cost-effectiveness of the procedure [32]. Because living donor VCA would entail the harvest of free tissue from one patient in preparation for transfer to another—procedures commonly performed by plastic surgeons and managed in hospital facilities—the costs associated with surgery and post-operative care of these patients could be expected to be lower.

34.3 Conclusions

Living donor VCA will likely continue to become a more common topic of discussion, given the successes of deceased donor VCA over the past 10–15 years. We believe that it is no longer a matter of "if" living donation VCA becomes a viable option, but rather "when." Further, we believe that living donor VCA is ethically permissible in certain situations. It is imperative, however, to remember that both recipient and donor are patients to whom the four-quadrant framework should be applied. Both patients must have a thorough and complete understanding of the risks and benefits associated with the procedures, as well as attendant post-operative morbidity and complications. For the recipient, the major risk of lifelong immunosuppression would have to be discussed in detail. An argument against living donor VCA is that these procedures are life-enhancing versus life-saving, and that the risks associated with immunosuppression thus do not outweigh the benefits gained by the patient. However, we believe this same argument may be made for patients who are on dialysis and undergo renal transplantation. Patient preferences and quality of life are key considerations in the four-quadrant approach to ethical decision-making, and for some patients, the long-term risks associated with immunosuppression are tolerated to "feel whole" and improve esthetic and functional outcomes.

For donor patients, the risks of VCA flaps (e.g., abdominal-based flaps, fibula flaps, radial forearm flaps) are well known, and donors can be provided with detailed information regarding surgical technique, post-operative recovery, potential complications, and long-term morbidity. Moreover, given plastic surgeons' vast experience with free tissue transfer, VCA flaps can be harvested with relatively low donor morbidity, particularly compared to some solid organ transplantations. However, special attention must still be paid to the type of tissue being transplanted, which is an integral component of the decision-making process. This is key as certain VCA flaps are likely to be potentially more harmful to a donor than others, or result in additional morbidity. For example, the transfer of forearm tissue (i.e., radial forearm free flap) is fundamentally different from the transfer of a uterus. More specifically, removal of the uterus in a woman of childbearing age renders the donor unable to bear children, whereas transfer of forearm tissue results in no such deficit. Another example is the transfer of abdominal tissue for breast reconstruction in a separate individual. The risks of abdominal tissue transfer are not insignificant (e.g., hernia, bulge, weakness). Additionally, the donation of abdominal tissue may limit a donor's own reconstructive options in the future, should one be diagnosed with breast cancer. As living donor VCA becomes more of a reality, additional issues are likely to arise in the context of specific types of tissue transfer. As with all types of living donor transplantation, the risks to the donor must be carefully considered relative to the potential benefits to be gained by the recipient.

Perhaps the first actual expedition into this field—outside of twin-based living donor VCA—will be in patients who have previously undergone solid organ transplantation (i.e., and are therefore already immunosuppressed). In our view, this may be particularly useful in pediatric patients who obtain an organ from a parent or relative. If such patients require additional tissue (e.g., for abdominal closure after liver transplantation), an additional VCA from the liver donor may be harvested. The potential clinical scenarios for living donor VCA are vast, and as each donor–recipient pair is unique, it is important to tailor the discussion of medical indications, patient preferences, quality of life, and contextual features accordingly.

Currently, the notion of living donor VCA remains largely theoretical. Other than living donor uterus transplantation, which only requires transient immunosuppression, there have only been a few case reports detailing living donor VCA—the majority of which have been between siblings that are identical twins. In the coming years, we posit that living donor VCA will increase in frequency, a point highlighted by the recent modification of the Organ Procurement and Transplantation Network protocols that specifically includes living VCA donors [33]. However, because other types of living donor VCA have not yet been performed widely, an inherent and important limitation to this paper lies in a paucity of specific examples to detail and to which to apply the four-quadrant approach. Rather, our aim is to provide a broad framework to help clinicians with ethical decision-making related to this topic as it arises. In the future, as theory becomes reality, and more living donor VCA is performed, we hope to have the opportunity to discuss this ethical framework in the context of actual clinical cases, which we believe would facilitate a more targeted and specific discussion of the issues surrounding the utilization of various types of VCA tissue.

References

1. Siegler M. Clinical medical ethics: its history and contributions to American Medicine. J Clin Ethics. 2019;30(1):17–26.
2. Beauchamp T, Childress J. Principles of biomedical ethics. 7th ed. New York: Oxford Press; 2010.
3. Page K. The four principles: can they be measured and do they predict ethical decision making? BMC Med Ethics. 2012;13:10. Published 2012 May 20.
4. Jonsen A, Siegler M, Winslade W. Clinical ethics: a practical approach to ethical decisions in clinical medicine. 6th ed. New York: McGraw-Hill; 2006.
5. Jonsen AR, Siegler M, Winslade W. Clinical ethics. 8th ed. New York: McGraw-Hill; 2015.
6. Teven CM, Gottlieb LJ. The four-quadrant approach to ethical issues in burn care. AMA J Ethics. 2018;20(1):595–601. Published 2018 Jun 1.
7. Beederman M, Teven CM, Gottlieb LJ. Four-quadrant approach squared: ethical analysis of living donation in vascularized composite allotransplantation. Plast Reconstr Surg. 2022;149(6):1244e–50e.
8. Pomahac B, Alhefzi M, Bueno EM, McDiarmid SV, Levin LS. Living donation of vascularized composite allografts. Plast Reconstr Surg. 2018;142(3):405e–11e.
9. Kawai T, Sachs DH, Sykes M, Cosimi AB, Immune Tolerance Network. HLA-mismatched renal transplantation without maintenance immunosuppression. N Engl J Med. 2013;368(19):1850–2.
10. Cecka JM. The OPTN/UNOS renal transplant registry. Clin Transpl. 2005:1–16.
11. Abecassis M, Adams M, Adams P, et al. Consensus statement on the live organ donor. JAMA. 2000;284(22):2919–26. https://doi.org/10.1001/jama.284.22.2919.
12. Ethics Committee of the Transplantation Society. The consensus statement of the amsterdam forum on the care of the live kidney donor. Transplantation. 2004;78(4):491–2.
13. Pruett TL, Tibell A, Alabdulkareem A, et al. The ethics statement of the vancouver forum on the live lung, liver, pancreas, and intestine donor. Transplantation. 2006;81(10):1386–7.
14. Organ Procurement and Transplantation Network. https://optn.transplant.hrsa.gov/resources/by-organ/vascular-composite-allograft/vcas-from-living-donors/. Accessed 25 Jun 2020.
15. Allen RJ Jr, LoTempio MM, Craigie JE, Allen RJ Sr. Transplantation in identical twins: another option for breast reconstruction. Plast Reconstr Surg. 2008;122(4):1019–23.
16. Buncke HJ, Hoffman WY, Alpert BS, Gordon L, Stefani AE. Microvascular transplant of two free scalp flaps between identical twins. Plast Reconstr Surg. 1982;70(5):605–9.
17. Testa G, Koon EC, Johannesson L, et al. Living donor uterus transplantation: a single center's observations and lessons learned from early setbacks to technical success. Am J Transplant. 2017;17(11):2901–10.
18. Amin A, Bassiouny M, Sallam K, Ghally G, El-Karaksy H, El-Haddad A. Living related hemi-face skin transplant using radial forearm free flap for a xeroderma pigmentosa patient: early outcome. Head Neck Oncol. 2010;2:18. Published 2010 Jul 13.
19. Final Rule. https://optn.transplant.hrsa.gov/governance/about-the-optn/final-rule/. Accessed 25 Jun 2020.
20. Gottlieb L, Agarwal S. Autologous alternatives to facial transplantation. J Reconstr Microsurg. 2012;28(1):49–61.
21. Siemionow M, Unal S, Agaoglu G, Sari A. A cadaver study in preparation for facial allograft transplantation in humans: part I. what are alternative sources for total facial defect coverage? Plast Reconstr Surg. 2006;117(3):864–75.
22. Testa G, Angelos P, Crowley-Matoka M, Siegler M. Elective surgical patients as living organ donors: a clinical and ethical innovation. Am J Transplant. 2009;9(10):2400–5.
23. Brouha P, Naidu D, Cunningham M, Furr A, Majzoub R, Grossi FV, Francois CG, Maldonado C, Banis JC, Martinez S, Perez-Abadia G, Wiggins O, Kon M, Barker JH. Risk acceptance in composite-tissue allotransplantation reconstructive procedures. Microsurgery. 2006;26(3):144–9; discussion 149–50.
24. Bruno B, Arora KS. Ethical implications of donor type for uterus transplantation: why we should remain wary of using living donors. Yale J Biol Med. 2020;93(4):587–92.
25. Testa G, Carlisle E, Simmerling M, Angelos P. Living donation and cosmetic surgery: a double standard in medical ethics? J Clin Ethics. 2012;23(2):110–7.
26. Ross LF, Glannon W, Gottlieb LJ, Thistlethwaite JR Jr. Different standards are not double standards: all elective surgical patients are not alike. J Clin Ethics. 2012;23(2):118–28.
27. Agich GJ, Siemionow M. Until they have faces: the ethics of facial allograft transplantation. J Med Ethics. 2005;31(12):707–9. https://doi.org/10.1136/jme.2005.011841.
28. Lewis HC, Cendales LC. Vascularized composite allotransplantation in the United States: a retrospective analysis of the organ procurement and transplantation network data after 5 years of the final rule. Am J Transplant. 2020;21(1):291–6.
29. The United States position. Position paper of the American society for reconstructive microsurgery on facial transplantation. South Med J. 2006;99(4):430.
30. Cetrulo CL Jr, Drijkoningen T, Sachs DH. Tolerance induction via mixed chimerism in vascularized composite allotransplantation: is it time for clinical application? Curr Opin Organ Transplant. 2015;20(6):602–7.
31. Leonard DA, Kurtz JM, Cetrulo CL Jr. Achieving immune tolerance in hand and face transplantation: a realistic prospect? Immunotherapy. 2014;6(5):499–502.
32. Bertrand AA, Sen S, Otake LR, Lee GK. Changing attitudes toward hand allotransplantation among north American hand surgeons. Ann Plast Surg. 2014;72(Suppl 1):S56–60.
33. Organ Procurement and Transplantation Network. Briefing to the OPTN Board of Directors on modify living donor policy to include living VCA donors. 2000. https://optn.transplant.hrsa.gov/media/4199/bp_202012_modify-living-donor-policy-to-include-living-vca-donors.pdf. Accessed 6 Mar 2021.

Correction to: Face Transplantation: Cleveland Clinic Experience

Nicholas R. Sinclair, Raffi Gurunian, Antonio Rampazzo,
Bahar Bassiri Gharb, Brian Gastman, Risal Djohan,
Frank Papay, and Maria Z. Siemionow

Correction to:
Chapter 3 in: R. Gurunian et al. (eds.), *Reconstructive Transplantation*, https://doi.org/10.1007/978-3-031-21520-9_3

The author's name Maria Z. Siemionow was unfortunately excluded from the author group in Chapter 3. The initially published version has now been corrected.

The updated original version for this chapter can be found at
https://doi.org/10.1007/978-3-031-21520-9_3

© Springer Nature Switzerland AG 2023
R. Gurunian et al. (eds.), *Reconstructive Transplantation*, https://doi.org/10.1007/978-3-031-21520-9_35

Index

© Springer Nature Switzerland AG 2023
R. Gurunian et al. (eds.), *Reconstructive Transplantation*, https://doi.org/10.1007/978-3-031-21520-9

GPSR Compliance

The European Union's (EU) General Product Safety Regulation (GPSR) is a set of rules that requires consumer products to be safe and our obligations to ensure this.

If you have any concerns about our products, you can contact us on ProductSafety@springernature.com

In case Publisher is established outside the EU, the EU authorized representative is:

Springer Nature Customer Service Center GmbH
Europaplatz 3
69115 Heidelberg, Germany

Batch number: 10756390

Printed by Printforce, the Netherlands